PRINCIPLES OF
SURGICAL
ONCOLOGY

PRINCIPLES OF SURGICAL ONCOLOGY

Edited by

Ronald W. Raven, O.B.E., T.D.

Former Member of Council, Royal College of Surgeons of England
Consulting Surgeon, Royal Marsden Hospital and Institute
of Cancer Research
Consulting Surgeon, Westminster Hospital
London, England

PLENUM MEDICAL BOOK COMPANY
New York and London

Library of Congress Cataloging in Publication Data

Main entry under title:

Principles of surgical oncology.

Includes bibliographies and index.
1. Oncology. 2. Cancer–Surgery. I. Raven, Ronald William. [DNLM: 1. Neoplasms–Surgery. QZ268 R253p]

RC254.P64	616.9'92	77-1804
ISBN-13: 978-1-4684-2303-7	e-ISBN-13: 978-1-4684-2301-3	
DOI: 10.1007/978-1-4684-2301-3		

CONTRIBUTORS

Y. S. BAKHLE, Department of Pharmacology, Institute of Basic Medical Sciences, Royal College of Surgeons of England, London, England

R. W. BALDWIN, Professor of Tumor Biology, Cancer Research Campaign Laboratories, The University of Nottingham, Nottingham, England

BARRY BARBER, Chief Management Scientist, North East Thames Regional Health Authority, London, England

ENZO BONMASSAR, Immunochemotherapy Section, Laboratory of Experimental Chemotherapy, Drug Research and Development Division of Cancer Treatment, National Cancer, Institute, Bethesda, Maryland

R. D. BULBROOK, Department of Endocrinology, Imperial Cancer Research Fund Laboratories, London, England

DENIS BURKITT, Geographical Pathology Unit, Department of Morbid Anatomy, St. Thomas' Hospital Medical School, London, England

E. J. DAVISON, Department of Electrical Engineering, University of Toronto, Toronto, Canada

THOMAS J. DEELEY, Director, South Wales Radiotherapy and Oncology Service, Velindre Hospital, Cardiff; South Glamorgan Health Authority; Lecturer, Welsh National School of Medicine, Wales

HAROLD ELLIS, Professor of Surgery, University of London, Westminster Medical School, London, England

I. W. F. HANHAM, Consultant in Oncology and Radiotherapy, Westminster Hospital, London, England

DAVID P. HOUCHENS, Immunochemotherapy Section, Laboratory of Experimental Chemotherapy, Drug Research and Development Division of Cancer Treatment, National Cancer Institute, Bethesda, Maryland

O. A. N. HUSAIN, Consultant Pathologist, Regional Cytology Centre, St. Stephen's Hospital, London, England

MICHAEL HUTT, Geographical Pathology Unit, Department of Morbid Anatomy, St. Thomas' Hospital Medical School, London, England

CRAWFORD JAMIESON, Consultant Surgeon St. Thomas and Hammersmith Hospitals, Senior Lecturer in Surgery, Royal Postgraduate Medical School, London, England

ADALBERT KOESTNER, Department of Veterinary Pathobiology, Ohio State University, Columbus, Ohio

ARNOLD LEVENE, Consultant Pathologist, The Royal Marsden Hospital, London, England

DENNIS V. PARKE, Department of Biochemistry, University of Surrey, Guildford, Surrey, England

RONALD W. RAVEN, Member of Council, Royal College of Surgeons of England; Consulting Surgeon, Royal Marsden Hospital and Institute of Cancer Research; Consulting Surgeon, Westminster Hospital, London, England

P. R. SALMON, Senior Lecturer in the Department of Medicine, University of Bristol, Bristol Royal Infirmary, Bristol, England

ERIC SAMUEL, Forbes Professor of Medical Radiology, University of Edinburgh and the Royal Infirmary, Edinburgh, Scotland

A. A. SHIVAS, University of Edinburgh Medical School, Edinburgh, Scotland

D. Y. WANG, Department of Endocrinology, Imperial Cancer Research Fund Laboratories, London, England

G. P. WARWICK, Institute of Cancer Research (Royal Cancer Hospital), Chester Beatty Research Institute, London, England

WOLFGANG WECHSLER, Max-Planck Institut für Hirnforschung, Abteilung für Allgemeine Neurologie, Köln, West Germany

D. C. WILLIAMS, Head of Research Department, The Marie Curie Memorial Foundation, Oxted, Surrey, England

PREFACE

The synthesis during the present decade of different arts and sciences to form oncology as a multidisciplinary subject is of profound importance for coordinating the clinical and research efforts to control a number of diseases that cause high mortality and morbidity in the human race and to elucidate their causation. These diseases traditionally have been grouped together under the general term of *cancer,* without any scientific reason and irrespective of many differences existing between them. The word *cancer,* because it is synonymous with diseases that cause suffering and death, naturally generates fear in people throughout the world. Cancer fortunately has a changing face caused by the realization that these diseases are different diseases with variable etiology and prognosis; they need different kinds of treatment, and even prevention is a practical proposition. The time has therefore come to delete the term *cancer* from our terminology as unscientific and unhelpful and to substitute *oncological diseases* governed by the system of knowledge designated oncology. This conforms also with the designations used for other groups of diseases.

In the divisions of oncology an important place is held by surgical oncology because many oncological diseases require surgical treatment alone, or in combination with radiotherapy and chemotherapy. Combination therapy is being used effectively for an increasing number of these diseases, and this trend will become more pronounced as chemotherapy develops. The results achieved with available chemicals and present dosage schedules are impressive. Serious side effects, however, do occur, so we need new chemicals with tumor specificity without damaging normal tissues. More information is required also about their administration and dosage. The surgical oncologist as a leading member of the oncological team must keep abreast of this rapidly expanding therapeutic knowledge and practice.

The contributions from different sciences to oncology are considerable and of tremendous importance for the surgical oncologist in his work. For instance, he must be familiar with carcinogens and carcinogenesis in the same way as knowledge of infections and inflammation is essential. The biochemistry of human oncological diseases is a rapidly growing subject with far-reaching effects upon investigations, diagnosis, and treatment. This and other sciences are unfolding the mysterious biological nature of the diseases we are treating daily. We must learn to discern the practical implications of scientific advances and apply them without delay to our work in the clinic. Our scientific knowledge requires a wide base for this understanding, in addition to enabling original contributions to be made to oncology. Participants in the clinic and laboratory are integral parts of a feedback system composed of clinicians and researchers. Education and training in surgical oncology is emerging as a definite discipline to conform with these new circumstances. Graduates in greater numbers desire teaching programs embodying theory and practice. They have different objectives, for while some surgeons will embrace this speciality for full-time work, others will seek this knowledge to help them as general and specialist surgeons having the responsibility of treating many patients with these diseases as part of their overall interests. It seems that more academic appointments in surgical oncology are required in addition to those already established in departments of surgery and oncology.

The contents of this book demonstrate the building up of this well-defined system of knowledge and the principles forming the foundation of surgical oncology. It is hoped the book will prove to be a valuable companion for graduates in their oncological training and contribute in this way to the maintenance of a high standard of care for patients with oncological diseases.

The editor expresses his warmest thanks to the authors of the various chapters for their valuable work, to the publisher for the excellent production, and to Miss Joan Gough-Thomas, M.A., his secretary, for her unfailing help.

RONALD W. RAVEN

London, England

CONTENTS

Chapter 1

ONCOLOGY— A GENERAL SURVEY

RONALD W. RAVEN

Oncology is a multidisciplinary subject where different arts and sciences are synthesized for the study of neoplastic diseases. This is the vehicle for all the scientific knowledge concerning the etiology, development, and behavior of these diseases which has accrued throughout many centuries. This knowledge is interpreted for, and related to, the care of patients including diagnosis, treatment, and prognosis. The identification of etiological factors by research enables preventive action to be taken against these diseases.

The emergence of this new subject is changing traditional attitudes towards cancer. Indeed, cancer has acquired a new look and this terminology no longer has any scientific value. Oncology encompasses many different diseases of diverse etiology, manifestation, and prognosis which require various forms of treatment. The term "oncological diseases" should now be substituted for "cancer," which has lost any meaning it may have possessed, in addition to causing considerable fear, and even despair.

The constant acquisition of new knowledge about these diseases and the practical application to the care of patients and its relevance to the community require different disciplines and practical skills. Consequently, oncology is divided into divisions and subdivisions (Table 1).

Ronald W. Raven • Member of Council, Royal College of Surgeons of England; Consulting Surgeon, Royal Marsden Hospital and Institute of Cancer Research; Consulting Surgeon, Westminster Hospital, London, SW1, England.

TABLE 1. Divisions of Oncology

Research oncology
  Laboratory
  Clinical
  Epidemiology
Clinical oncology
  Medical oncology
  Radiological oncology
  Surgical oncology
Social oncology
  Education and training
  Rehabilitation
  Prevention

Research Oncology

The present position of oncology must be viewed in the perspective of history which extends throughout two millenia and was built up by the slow accumulation of scientific data. While we move towards the solution of the most complex biological problems, patient, painstaking research is essential, without looking necessarily for a spectacular breakthrough. In certain areas at present we may not possess the scientific knowledge and methodology to make further advances but must await the discovery of new clues. A relevant example is an understanding of the mechanism of hormonal control systems in carcinoma of the breast, prostate, and other viscera, which is essential for meaningful treatment.

Advances in scientific knowledge should be assessed by centuries, rather than decades, when the growth of oncology is studied. Hippocrates and his school (470–375 B.C.) attempted a classification of tumors; and Celsus (53 B.C.–A.D. 7) distinguished benign from malignant tumors. Little further knowledge was gained for many succeeding centuries because of the lack of scientific instruments and methodology. Discoveries depended upon clinical observation and description, which enabled Percivall Pott (1775) to associate scrotal skin cancer with soot from chimneys. This is the basic contribution to chemical carcinogenesis.

In the nineteenth century the discovery of the microscope initiated another advance when Johannes Müller (1838) classified tumors according to their cellular structure. Speculative thought was also directed to etiological factors by Rudolph Virchow (1847), who propounded the theory of local irritation, and Julius Cohnheim (1877–80), who expounded the theory of embryonal rests.

In the twentieth century there was a massive expansion of scientific work producing spectacular discoveries about tumors. Chemical carcinogenesis is probably the outstanding discovery, for we know that not only do chemicals cause tumors, but they can also cure them. The initial observation of Percivall Pott was emphasized by Yamagiwa and Ichikawa (1916) who produced an epithelioma in the skin of rabbit's ear by applying coal tar. This sequence culminated in the isolation and synthesis of the pentacyclic hydrocarbon 3:4 benzpyrene by Kennaway *et al.* (1932) who correlated chemical structure with carcinogenicity. Many more chemical carcinogens, natural and synthetic, are now known.

Tumor virology has attracted considerable research interest based upon the discovery of a transmissible avian tumor by Rous (1910) and the later work on viruses by Gye (1925). There is no proof yet that a malignant human tumor is caused by a virus.

Several sciences, in addition to clinical observation, have built up this basic knowledge in oncology, and these include physiology, pathology, virology, and chemistry. During recent years important discoveries have been made by epidemiological research regarding environmental carcinogens; it is considered that about 70% of human oncological diseases are caused by them and thus are preventable. Endocrinology is of outstanding importance in the etiology and treatment of breast and prostate carcinoma, in addition to others where more information is required. The earlier observations were made by surgeons on this relationship. John Hunter (1786) stated that the initial secondary sexual structure of the male genital tract is dependent in some way upon the presence of the functional testis. Berthold (1849) suggested that a substance was produced by testicular tissue which affected the prostate through the blood stream, thus indicating hormonal action. White (1895) performed orchidectomy to influence the growth rate of the human prostate; and Huggins and Clarke (1940) demonstrated that prostate tumors in animals were androgen dependent and controlled by estrogens.

Endocrine surgery and the administration of synthetic hormones have brought considerable relief to many females with breast carcinoma. Nearly a century has elapsed since Nunn (1882) reported the case of a female age 30 years with an advanced ulcerating breast carcinoma and multiple skin nodules which underwent "general shrinking" following a severe emotional upset caused by the sudden death of her husband, and she also had a very early menopause. The linkage with endocrine organs is obvious here. Schinzinger (1889) suggested oophorectomy for breast carcinoma and Beatson (1869, 1902) wrote, "We must look in females to the ovaries as the seat of the exciting cause of carcinoma, certainly of the mamma." He reported marked regression of breast carcinoma following oophorectomy. In subsequent years spectacular regression in disseminated breast carcinoma has followed oophorectomy, adrenalectomy, and hypophysectomy. It is of profound significance that manipulating the hormonal control systems in these ways can reverse carcinoma to apparently normal tissue and stability is maintained for many years, but not permanently. These systems are retained by about 40% of breast carcinomas, since their receptor sites for the hormones can be demonstrated in the cell membrane and cytoplasm, and their presence is a good indication that the carcinoma will respond to endocrine ablation and therapy.

Hormonal control systems are being sought for other tumors, including pulmonary and renal, for they may prove to be susceptible to endocrine therapy. For example, an oat–cell carcinoma of the lung produces adreno-cortico-trophic hormones (ACTH) and vasopressin (ADH) and other hormones which cause recognizable and treatable clinical syndromes.

Immunology attracts increasing attention by researchers and clinicians, who now carry out with new techniques intricate investigations at the cellular level. Antigenic substances can be identified in neoplastic cells which are absent in normal cells but are usually too weak to be used by the host to control the tumor. Therefore, methods are now being sought to enhance this action, but we cannot speak yet of immunotherapy. There is considerable interest, nevertheless, in immunodiagnosis with the identification of tumor-specific antigens. For example, the presence of α-fetoprotein is considered to be specific for primary liver cell carcinoma.

Other scientific disciplines are contributing to oncological knowledge at the present time. These include developmental and molecular biology, enzymology, and clinical investigation where there must be a continuous feedback to the laboratory. This interdisciplinary approach on the scale indicated here is essential for the solution of the remaining perplexing problems in oncology. Teamwork is the key, where clinicians and laboratory and field workers are together to share their knowledge and use their skills.

Clinical Oncology

This subject has greatly expanded and is therefore divided into three divisions, characterized by the chief treatment modalities of surgery, medicine, and radiology. There must be, however, complete collaboration and teamwork between them, especially with the increasing indications for combined treatment.

Medical Oncology

Chemotherapy is the central method of treatment, which is rapidly expanding because of the impressive results in a variety of diseases, including solid tumors, when used alone or in combination with surgery and radiotherapy. It is also concerned with general supportive treatment for many patients, in addition to investigations, diagnosis, and other aspects of management. Research and teaching activities are pursued also, and several academic departments have been established for all this work.

Radiological Oncology

Radiotherapy is the central method of treatment, which is used alone or combined with surgery and chemotherapy in many oncological diseases. It is also concerned with investigations, diagnosis, teaching, and radiobiological research. Academic departments have been in existence for many years.

Surgical Oncology

Surgical treatment is the central method of treatment practiced by both general and specialist surgeons. The majority of oncological diseases require surgical treatment alone, or combined with radiotherapy and chemotherapy. In addition to this work, investigations, diagnosis, teaching, and research are an integral part. The subject is a synthesis of scientific and clinical knowledge required by the surgical oncologist, in addition to the technical skills necessary in operative treatment; it is discussed in greater detail later in this chapter.

Social Oncology

This subject brings together oncological work which is connected chiefly with the community and has expanded considerably with the realization of its importance.

Professional Education

The extent and importance of oncological knowledge requires a special place in the medical curriculum for medical undergraduates and in the nursing curriculum. There are many teaching and training facilities available for the requirements of different groups of graduates. Courses of training are arranged in branches of oncology in hospitals having special facilities for this work. In addition to clinical work including the various treatment disciplines, facilities are necessary for clinical, laboratory, and epidemiological research for those graduates wishing to undertake this. There are numerous well-designed short courses in oncology, symposia dealing with special subjects, and congresses, national and international, which provide ample opportunities for communication and discussion. All members of the caring professions take part in these meetings, which provide an interdisciplinary approach to the problem.

An important development is the institution of education and training in nursing oncology, for the full collaboration of nurses is essential in the teamwork for patient care in the hospital and the community.

Public Education

Over recent decades an increasing awareness has developed for this particular form of education, and considerable effort is now expended on numerous educational programs for lay people. It is essential for people to understand more clearly the ways in which oncological diseases affect them and recognize warning symptoms and signs. They must know also how to act under various conditions so that early advice is received. For the prevention of these diseases full collaboration of the public is necessary; they must know how to keep healthy and avoid the well-known carcinogenic substances.

Rehabilitation

The object of therapy of all oncological diseases is the restoration of patients to lives of good quality and longevity. Rehabilitation begins when the diagnosis is first established. This subject is dealt with in chapter 17.

Prevention

During recent years emphasis is placed on the importance and practicality of preventing oncological diseases, as about 70% are caused by environmental carcinogens. This subject is considered in chapter 8, and is of obvious interest to the surgical oncologist.

The Theory of Oncology

A system of knowledge has been built up, with derivations from multiple scientific disciplines, where laws are emerging for guidance and doctrine for teaching. In this system there is considerable certainty based upon scientific data, but adequate room remains for speculative ideas. New ideas are needed and we must never close our minds to those which seem unusual, or even novel.

Oncology theory must be related with practice so that patients are helped by any new developments without delay; a constant feedback from laboratory to clinic is essential, and more patient-orientated research is necessary. A study of various subjects in this book reveals the extent of the scientific contributions to oncology. Carcinogenesis is a key subject of great academic interest and practical importance. The emergence of trans-placental carcinogenesis, where various chemicals cross the placental barrier to interact with fetal cells and produce tumors in children and young adults, is of profound significance. Epidemiology is closely associated, for it is used to identify carcinogens in our environment, followed by migrant studies to separate these agents from racial and genetic factors. The outstanding value of population studies is exemplified by the lung–tobacco cancer investigations in Great Britain.

Reference has been made to the important contributions of immunology, endocrinology, and other scientific disciplines to oncological theory and practice.

The Practice of Oncology

This comprises the three chief treatment disciplines of surgery, radio-therapy, and chemotherapy, which are used singly, but more frequently in combination.

The Surgical Oncologist

The majority of oncological diseases require surgical treatment, either alone or in combination, so that the role of the surgical oncologist is important and extensive. These diseases are of great complexity and may be lethal, requiring the display of theoretical knowledge allied to technical skills in diagnosis and treatment. This extends far beyond the mere excision of a tumor into regions of endocrinology, immunology, biochemistry, and others.

The Art of Surgery

The development of present-day operations for various oncological diseases is a major part of the brilliant history of surgery which extends over a period of less than a century, as shown in Table 2.

These radical operations, designed on knowledge of the basic medical sciences, anatomy, physiology, and pathology, replaced the local operations for tumors which produced poor results from recurrent disease. This is clearly illustrated by carcinoma of the breast treated by local mastectomy

TABLE 2. Oncological Operations in History

Surgeon	Year	Operation
Billroth	1881	Subtotal gastrectomy
Halsted	1890	Radical mastectomy
Schlatter	1897	Total gastrectomy
Von Mickulicz	1898	Esophago-gastrectomy
Wertheim	1900	Radical hysterectomy
Miles	1908	Abdomino-perineal excision of rectum
Torek	1913	Esophagectomy
Trotter	1913	Partial pharyngectomy
Graham & Singer	1933	Pneumonectomy

at the end of the last century, where a high percentage of recurrences occurred in the chest wall and stimulated Halsted to develop radical mastectomy. The work of Miles on the pathology of carcinoma of the rectum with his detailed studies of the lymphatic spread of the disease led him to design and perform his abdomino-perineal excision operation, which remains as the standard operation for this disease with a high survival rate in the earlier stages.

These radical operations were performed without the tremendous benefits of modern anesthesia, antibiotic therapy, and blood, electrolyte, and fluid-replacement therapy enjoyed in surgical work today. The value of postoperative recovery wards and intensive care units is also stressed, for their remarkable contribution to surgical practice. Teamwork is the keynote for successful surgery where surgeons, anesthetists, nurses, and technicians take vital responsibilities.

Since these radical operations were introduced, advances in surgical technique have occurred for their development and improvement. For example, thoracic surgery led to new approaches for esophagectomy procedures. The partial pharyngectomy operations have been extended so that laryngo-pharyngectomy and laryngo-esophago-pharyngectomy operations are performed today where plastic and reconstructive surgical techniques are used to restore deglutition. Considerable work has been expended on organ transposition and transplantation. The best replacement for the whole esophagus is the stomach, which is transposed to the neck where a pharyngo-gastric anastomosis is performed. An alternative procedure is the transposition of part of the colon. Liver transplantation can be performed for a hepatoma which is operable, and kidney transplantation for bilateral tumors of the kidney.

A Present Challenge

It is a salutary exercise to challenge the end results of the surgical treatment of tumors and to change methods when this is indicated. The place of radical operations in the surgery of oncological diseases is being challenged today, where there is a tendency to adopt local operations for carcinoma in sites which include the breast and rectum. The answer is being sought to the question of whether lymph node block dissection should be performed. Before this question can be answered more information is required concerning the function of the lympho-reticular system in relation to oncological diseases. There are no scientific data yet available to support immunotherapy for oncological diseases, and this must not be used as an argument in favor of local as opposed to radical operations. In the present state of knowledge it is very unwise to return to the local operations for malignant tumors which proved so unsatisfactory at the turn of the century. When metastatic lymph nodes can be excised, this should be carried out, and the value of radical operations is reemphasized here.

Staging Systems of Diseases

Surgical staging is essential for planning treatment, assessment of prognosis, and clinical trials. Furthermore, it has been demonstrated that when accurate staging has been introduced for various affected sites, this usually leads to better end results. An outstanding example of this is carcinoma of the cervix uteri. The TNM classification system has been adopted internationally, but more emphasis is now being placed on surgical staging combined with histological tumor grading, for this usually gives a more accurate assessment and guidance for treatment. Hodgkins' disease is staged by laparotomy, where the involved lymph node groups are identified, liver biopsy is done, and splenectomy is carried out; at the same time the ovaries are transposed from the pelvis in females where pelvic radiation is necessary. The same procedure is done for patients with lymphosarcoma where there is splenomegaly.

Accurate surgical staging should be done in breast carcinoma, where clinical trials are carried out and prognosis is assessed. When accurate measurements of the hormonal and immunological status of the patient are available, these should be incorporated in the system of staging.

Laparotomy staging of carcinoma of the stomach, colon, and rectum should be done to provide an accurate assessment of the intraperitoneal spread of the disease by direct extension to other organs and tissues, metastatic lymph node involvement, and metastases in other organs. When the disease in adjacent tissues and regional lymph nodes cannot be excised with the primary tumor, metal markers are placed in these situations so that accurate postoperative radiotherapy and chemotherapy can be given. It is important to establish systems of surgical staging for both national and international adoption, so that methods of treatment can be compared and modified when this is indicated.

Combined Therapy

An increasing number of patients with various oncological diseases require combined treatment for optimum results. The surgical oncologist cannot work in isolation, for teamwork is essential with medical and radiological oncologists. He requires, therefore, basic knowledge of radiotherapy and chemotherapy including the indications for their use and the end results of this treatment.

Impressive advances in knowledge are being made by radiobiological research which considerably influence clinical radiotherapy used alone or in combination with other treatments. Fast neutron therapy is being developed as a method of obtaining better tumor control in certain sites (Morgan, 1973). Methods are being sought to increase the sensitivity of tumors to irradiation. There are indications that adjuvant chemotherapy, with adriamycin and bleomycin for example, may have this effect. The most effective sensitizer at present, however, is hyperbaric oxygen, although its use is more complex and time consuming than conventional methods (Henk, 1973).

For the treatment of malignant tumors in the head and neck teamwork is essential; this region is an excellent example where surgery, radiotherapy, and chemotherapy all have an important place. Treatment decisions are made by joint consultation when the diagnosis is established and, according to the stage of the disease, this is directed to cure or palliate, so that the contribution of each method of therapy has to be assessed. The method of radiotherapy must also be considered; many lesions are treated by external irradiation, but this may have to be supplemented by interstitial irradiation. Combined surgery and radiotherapy is indicated for many tumors, especially for those that are more advanced in the mouth, larynx, and hypopharynx. Increasing emphasis is placed on the value of preoperative radiotherapy with a tumor dose of 4,000 rads, which does not interfere with satisfactory healing after operation. Many carcinomas in the mouth, especially when they do not extend beyond the mucosa, heal with radiotherapy; when the regional lymph nodes are enlarged a block dissection is necessary. In general, preoperative is preferable to postoperative radiotherapy, but when a dose of 6,000 rads has been given, there are problems to solve when surgery is done. These include necrosis of skin flaps, pharyngeal fistula, and rupture of the carotid arteries. The risk of the last complication is lessened by muscle cover performed at the operation.

It is now realized that preoperative radiotherapy may improve the prognosis in carcinoma of the rectum, especially in the more advanced lesions. On the other hand, the value of radiotherapy in the management of breast carcinoma is being strongly debated. There is some promise of better results when preoperative radiotherapy is given in urological tumors, including the kidney, bladder, and prostate. More data are required from controlled clinical trials to solve these problems.

Chemotherapy is the most spectacular development in oncology during recent decades and profoundly affects the work of the surgical oncologist because of its proved value in many oncological diseases, including solid tumors, and its important part in combined treatment. Surgical infusion and perfusion techniques have been developed to treat tumors of the head and neck and the extremities with chemicals; sometimes the results are spectacular.

Large carcinomas in the thoracic esophagus are a good example of the value of combined treatment. A gastrostomy is instituted first under local anesthesia, so that the patient's nutritional state is maintained throughout radiotherapy and chemotherapy. This is allowed to close following tumor regression and the restitution of normal deglutition. Gastric carcinoma regresses with chemical treatment and radiotherapy, which are helpful in treating patients with inoperable tumors and residual disease following gastrectomy. Chemotherapy with 5-fluorouracil or combination therapy is used routinely for residual, recurrent, and metastatic colonic carcinoma.

Chemotherapy gives considerable relief to patients with disseminated breast carcinoma. Local and metastatic tumors regress and bone pain is relieved; complete remissions occur in many patients. A notable recent development is the introduction of adjuvant chemotherapy in the management of breast carcinoma in stage 2, but further observations are now necessary to determine whether any untoward side effects are produced. If these are proved negative, adjuvant chemotherapy can be introduced into the treatment program of many patients with stage 1 carcinoma with possible benefit to those who have unsuspected systemic disease. It is certain that combined treatment will continue to develop, especially when new and safer chemicals, easy to administer over long periods, become available. The surgical oncologist will be aware of these advances, so that new treatment can be introduced quickly into clinical practice.

Additional Interests

The surgical oncologist is concerned with many other oncological subjects which are mentioned briefly here.

Investigations and Diagnosis

An extensive range of investigations is available for the diagnosis of oncological diseases in all stages of development. Emphasis is rightly placed on the importance of diagnosing subclinical diseases by various screening procedures including cytology and radiology. Good examples are cytology of the uterus and mammography for breast carcinoma. Increasing use is being made of indirect methods of diagnosis such as serological tests for carcinofetal proteins found in primary carcinoma of the liver, bronchus, stomach, pancreas, and gallbladder.

Conventional methods of radiology, endoscopy, cytology, and biopsy give accurate diagnostic results in patients with local diseases. The EMI-Scanning System is of great value in the localization of primary and metastatic brain tumors and is likely to become important for other regions of the body.

The diagnosis of systemic disease is highly important for treatment planning, so that occult metastases are detected in the skeleton, liver, lungs, and elsewhere using scintiscans, ultrasonography, and measurements of tumor-indexing substances such as circulating polypeptides and urinary hydroxyproline. Bone marrow cytology is proving to be increasingly important in lymphomas and in carcinomas of the lung, breast, stomach, and elsewhere.

The recognition of various clinical syndromes caused by tumors, even when occult, is now possible, and the causative polypeptide hormones can be measured.

Immunology

There is considerable interest in the relationship of immunology to oncological diseases. It is premature to speak of immunotherapy for these diseases, but assay systems are now available for the detection of tumor marker substances, thus initiating immunodiagnosis (see chapter 12).

References

Beatson, G. T. (1896). *Lancet* **2**:104.
Beatson, G. T. (1902). *Br. Med. J.* **2**:1300.
Berthold, A. A. (1849). *Arch. f. Anat. Physiol. U., Wissensch. Med., Berlin* **42**:672.
Celsus, A. A. C. (25 B.C.–A.D. 50). *De Medicina* W. G. Spencer, trans. (1935–38). Heinemann (Loebs Classical Library), London.
Cohnheim, J. F. (1877–80). *Vorlesungen über allgemeine Pathologie*. A. Hirschwald, Berlin.
Cook, J. W., Hieger, I., Kennaway, E. L., and Mayneord, W. V. (1932). *Proc. Royal Soc., London,* **Series B 3**:111; 455.
Gye, W. R. (1925). *Lancet* **2**:109.
Henk, J. M. (1973). Tumour oxygenation and radiotherapy. In *Modern Trends in Oncology* (R. W. Raven, ed.), Vol. 1, part 2, chap. 10. Butterworth, London.
Hippocrates (470–375B.C.). (a) Littre, E. (1939–61) *Oeuvres Complètes d'Hippocrate. Traduction Nouvelle avec le Texte Grec en Regard. . . .* J. B. Bailliere, Paris. (b) Works with English translation (1923–31) (W. H. S. Jones and E. T. Withington, eds.). Heinemann (Loebs Classical Library), London.

Huggins. C. B., and Clarke. P. J. (1940). *J. Exp. Med.* **72**:747.

Hunter J. (1786). *Observations on Certain Parts of the Animal Oeconomy,* 1st Ed., p. 38. London.

Morgan, R. L. (1973). Fast neutron therapy. In *Modern Trends in Oncology* (R. W. Raven, ed.), Vol. 1, part 2, chap. 11. Butterworth, London.

Müller, J. (1838). *Uber den feinern Bau und die Formen der Krankhaften Geschwälste,* Lief 1. G. Reimer, Berlin.

Nunn, T. W. (1882). *On Cancer of the Breast,* p. 103 (Case 44). Churchill, London.

Pott, P. (1775). *Chirurgical Observations.* Carnegy, London.

Rous, F. P. (1910). *J. Exp. Med.* **12**:696.

Schinzinger (1889). *Verh. Dtsch. Ges. Chir.* **18**:28.

Virchow, R. L. K. (1847). *Virchows Arch. Pathol. Anat.* **1**:94.

White, J. W. (1895). *Trans. Amer. Surg. Assoc.* **13**:103.

Yamagiwa, K., and Ichikawa, K. (1916). *Verh. Jap. Pathol. Ges.* **6**:169.

Chapter 2

ANATOMICAL ASPECTS

HAROLD ELLIS

Introduction

It goes without saying that a detailed knowledge of the anatomy of the part is a vital prerequisite for a surgeon before he undertakes an operation in a particular region. One of the most unpleasant experiences is to watch a so-called surgeon working in the depths of the abdomen or the neck without knowing where he is or where vital structures are located; it is in this situation that terrible disasters may occur. Yet it is a strange symptom of modern medical education that anatomy is denigrated and that time spent in its study is constantly reduced. Even in surgical training programs there is an undoubted move towards curtailment of anatomical teaching. While not denying that a surgeon requires a wide basic education in the course of his training, I would personally feel happier having a surgeon operating upon me who knew the detailed anatomy of the area concerned than one with less anatomical knowledge, but with a profound comprehension of my molecular biology.

In this chapter it is obviously impossible and undesirable to enumerate the detailed anatomy of every viscus which may require excisional procedures for cancer; a surgeon has his own reference sources before carrying out a major ablation in an area in which he does not have daily familiarity. Rather, a number of features of topographical anatomy which are of importance to the oncologist in general will be highlighted.

Harold Ellis • Professor of Surgery in the University of London at the Westminster Medical School, London, SW1, England.

The Lymphatic System

Because of its importance in the spread of malignant disease, it is obvious that the oncologist requires an intimate knowledge of the lymphatic pathways.

The lymphatic system is made up of lymph vessels, lymph nodes, and lymphoid collections which lie along the length of the alimentary canal.

Lymph capillaries are found in most tissues of the body, the only exceptions being those structures which do not possess a blood supply (the epidermis, and its appendages of hair and nails, the cornea, articular cartilage), together with the pulp of the spleen, the bone marrow, and the central nervous system. The capillaries commence as blind-ending ducts within the tissue spaces with a diameter rather larger than that of blood capillaries. These fine-walled tubes, made up of a single layer of endothelial cells, are capable of absorbing colloid material as well as solid particles such as bacteria. Usually the lymph contained within these capillaries is a colorless, clear fluid, but that within the lymphatics of the small bowel has a milky appearance due to the presence of fat; this fluid is named chyle and the lymph vessels are called lacteals. The lymphatic capillaries link up to form lymphatic trunks which nearly always drain through one or more sets of lymph nodes before entering the venous blood stream; the exceptions are some of the lymphatic drainage pathways of the thyroid gland and of the esophagus.

The large collecting lymphatics have three coats, similar to those found in veins. The intima comprises a flattened endothelium, with a thin surrounding of fibrous tissue. The media contains smooth muscle cells and there is an adventitia of fibrous tissue. These larger vessels have their own blood supply and nerve network; the blood supply accounts for the inflammatory changes of lymphangitis. The lymph vessels contain numerous semilunar paired valves.

The lymph vessels drain into two major channels, the thoracic duct, and the right lymphatic duct, which empty into the left and right brachiocephalic veins, respectively, at their origin from the junction of the internal jugular and subclavian veins.

The thoracic duct (Figure 1) is the left principal collecting vessel of the lymphatic system and is larger by far than the right lymphatic duct. It commences as an elongated sac, the cisterna chyli, into which drain the right and left lumbar lymphatic trunks. The cisterna has a length of about 5 cm and overlies the bodies of the first and second lumbar vertebrae immediately to the right of the abdominal aorta and it is overlapped anteriorly by the medial edge of the right crus of the diaphragm. From the cisterna the thoracic duct runs proximally through the aortic hiatus. It ascends through the posterior mediastinum, having the azygos vein on its

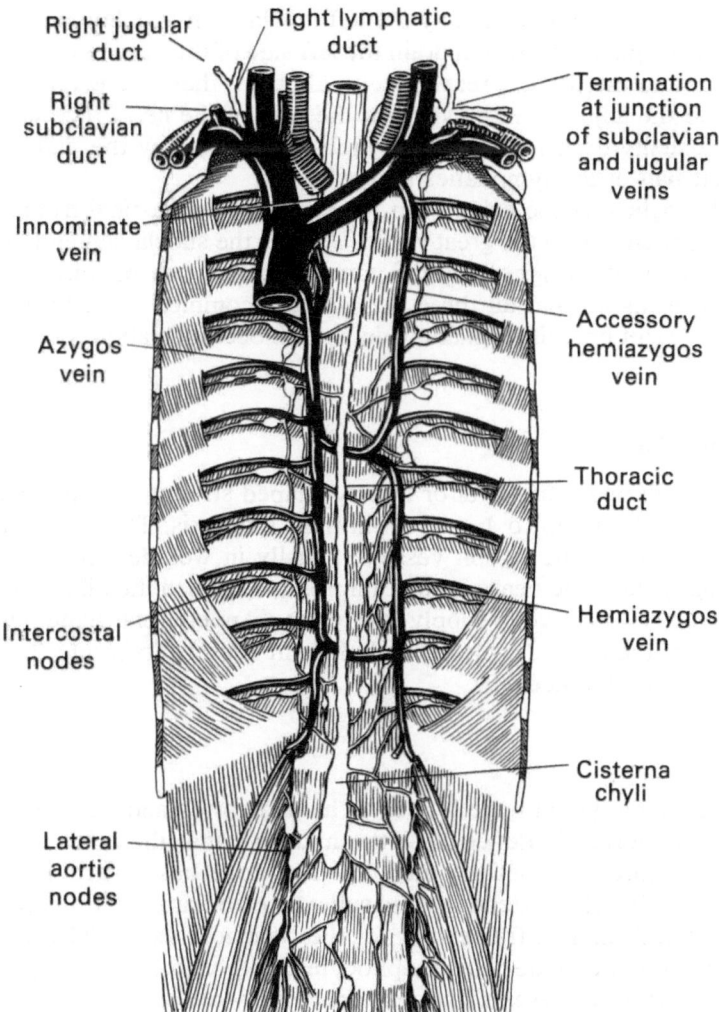

Right jugular duct

Right lymphatic duct

Right subclavian duct

Termination at junction of subclavian and jugular veins

Innominate vein

Azygos vein

Accessory hemiazygos vein

Thoracic duct

Intercostal nodes

Hemiazygos vein

Cisterna chyli

Lateral aortic nodes

Figure 1. The thoracic duct.

right side and the descending aorta on its left, with the vertebral column immediately posterior. In front lie the diaphragm and esophagus. At the level of the fifth thoracic vertebra, the duct slopes to the left and ascends along the left side of the esophagus into the neck. The duct then passes laterally behind the carotid sheath, descends over the subclavian artery, and empties into the junction of the left subclavian and internal jugular veins. The duct has several valves with a constant one at its entry into the venous system which prevents reflux of blood into the thoracic duct.

The thoracic duct is joined by the left jugular, left subclavian, and left mediastinal lymph trunks which drain the left side of the head and neck, the upper limb, and the thorax, respectively, although these trunks may open directly into the adjacent large veins at the root of the neck. The thoracic duct thus usually drains the whole lymphatic field below the diaphragm, and the left half of the lymphatics above it.

On the right side the subclavian, jugular, and mediastinal trunks may open independently into the great veins. Usually the subclavian and jugular trunks first join into a right lymphatic duct, and this may be joined by the mediastinal trunk so that all three then have a common opening into the origin of the right brachio-cephalic vein, which occurs in about one-fifth of the population.

The Lymph Nodes

The lymph nodes are oval or kidney-shaped structures which vary in size from 1 or 2 mm up to 1 or 2 cm in their long axis. They are situated along the course of the lymph vessels, usually in well-defined congregations. Usually the node bears a slight impression termed the hilum through which an artery and vein supply the node. An efferent lymph vessel emerges from the hilum, while several afferent vessels drain into the node around its circumference.

Structure

On section a lymph node is seen to have a cortex and a rather darker medulla. The cortex is deficient at the hilum so that the efferent lymph vessel drains directly from the medulla. The node has a fibrous capsule from which trabeculae extend into its substance and are continuous with a fine reticulum forming a framework for the lymphoid tissue. The majority of cells within the node are lymphocytes, although macrophages and plasma cells are also present. The cells are densely packed in the cortex and here form lymphatic follicles. The center of each follicle contains larger, more lightly staining cells which divide rapidly; these are termed the germinal centers. In conditions of antigenic stimulation, the node increases in size and becomes more vascular, and there is a proliferation in the number of germinal centers.

Lymphatic Drainage of the Skin

The lymphatic drainage of the skin and subcutaneous tissues forms a definite pattern made up of a number of zones (Figure 2). The midline of the body, front and back, demarcates lymph drainage laterally into the right

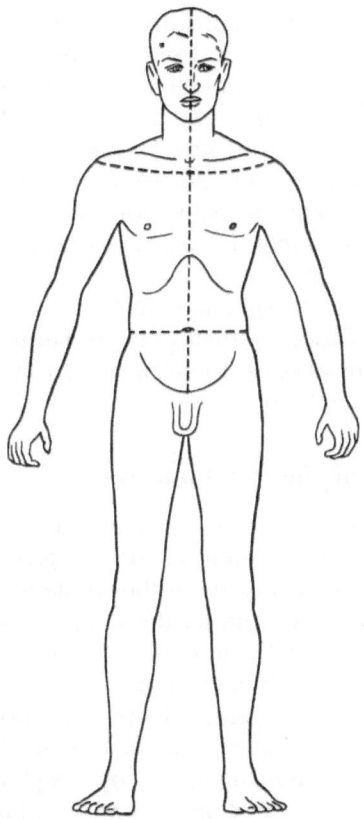

Figure 2. Zones of cutaneous lymph drainage.

and left sides. Each side can then be further divided by the line of the clavicles, continued on to the dorsum of the upper thorax, and by an imaginary line down around the body of the level of the umbilicus. The area above the clavicular line drains into the deep cervical lymph nodes which connect via the jugular lymphatic trunk into the thoracic duct on the left side and into the right lymphatic duct on the right. The area between the clavicular line and the umbilical line, including the upper limb and the skin of the breast, drains into the axillary lymph nodes and thence to the subclavian lymphatic trunk which enters the thoracic duct on the left and the right lymphatic duct on the right. The skin below the umbilical line, including the perineum and genitalia, drains into the inguinal lymph nodes on the same side. These drain into the iliac nodes and thence into the lumbar lymphatic trunk.

It is obvious, therefore, that the whole of the skin and subcutaneous tissues of the body drain into three groups of lymph nodes only; the deep cervical, the axillary, and the inguinal. Most areas drain into only one group, but midline structures, for example the perineum, drain to the corresponding nodes on the right and left side. Certain areas may, indeed, drain into four groups of nodes; a cutaneous malignant tumor at the umbilicus, or the area corresponding posteriorly in the midline of the lumbar region, may drain to both axillary and both inguinal node groups; similarly, a lesion in the suprasternal region, or the corresponding midline point posteriorly, may drain into the axillary or deep cervical nodes on both sides.

Of course, blockage of lymphatic vessels or nodes by malignant deposits, or as a result of irradiation, or their previous surgical removal may force lymph to find other pathways of drainage so that atypical involvement of more distant nodes may take place.

Lymphatic Drainage of the Head and Neck

The lymph nodes of the head and neck comprise the terminal deep cervical group of nodes and a number of outlying groups. The deep cervical nodes are the final drainage pathway for the whole region. They empty into the jugular lymph trunk and drain all the lymph vessels of the head and neck, either directly or indirectly, after passing through one of a number of outlying groups associated with the venous trunks of the head and neck.

The deep cervical lymph nodes (Figure 3) lie along the carotid sheath in close relationship to the internal jugular vein. These nodes may be divided into a superior group, mostly lying deep to the sterno-mastoid muscle, with some nodes extending beyond its anterior border, and an inferior group. The former includes the large jugulo-digastric node which is located at the junction of the common facial vein with the internal jugular vein. It is the main pathway for lymphatic drainage from the pharyngeal tonsil and is concerned also with lymph drainage of the tongue. Efferents from the upper deep cervical lymph nodes pass either to the lower deep cervical group or directly to the jugular trunk. The inferior group of nodes lies deep to the lower part of the sterno-mastoid muscle but also extends into the subclavian triangle and is therefore related to the brachial plexus and the subclavian vessels. One node in this group is situated in the region of the intermediate tendon of the omohyoid (the jugulo-omohyoid node) and is particularly concerned with lymph drainage of the tongue.

The lower group of deep cervical lymph nodes may be involved in metastatic disease of the lung, mediastinum, esophagus, stomach, and other abdominal viscera. These nodes are not the normal pathway of drainage for these structures but become implicated secondarily when there is a blockage of normal lymph drainage and probably represent retrograde spread. Although the lower deep cervical group of nodes and the apical

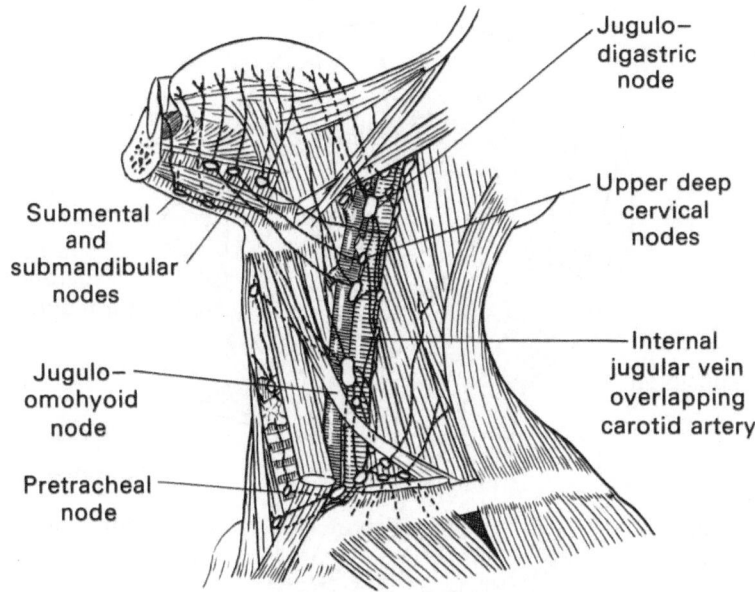

Figure 3. The deep cervical lymphatic chain.

group of axillary nodes are closely related, they represent different zones of lymph drainage; when one group is involved by drainage from the other area, this indicates lymphatic blockage of the normal pathways.

In addition to this main deep cervical group, there exists a horizontal group of nodes which encircle the junction of the head and neck and which are named, according to their position, the submental, submandibular, superficial parotid (or preauricular), mastoid (or retroauricular), and suboccipital nodes (Figure 4). These nodes drain the superficial tissues of the head, and their efferents then pass to the deep cervical nodes (although some lymph vessels, as already noted, pass directly to the deep cervical nodes and bypass the horizontal groups).

In addition, there are series of vertically placed nodes which drain the deep structures of the head and neck; these are the superficial cervical nodes, lying along the external jugular vein, which serve the parotid and the lower part of the ear and drain into the deep cervical group. Along the front of the neck lies another group of vertically disposed nodes, which includes the infrahyoid (on the thyro-hyoid membrane), the prelaryngeal, and the pre- and paratracheal nodes. These drain the thyroid, larynx, trachea, and part of the pharynx and empty into the deep cervical group. The retropharyngeal nodes lie vertically behind the pharynx and drain the back of the nose, the pharynx, and the eustachian tube.

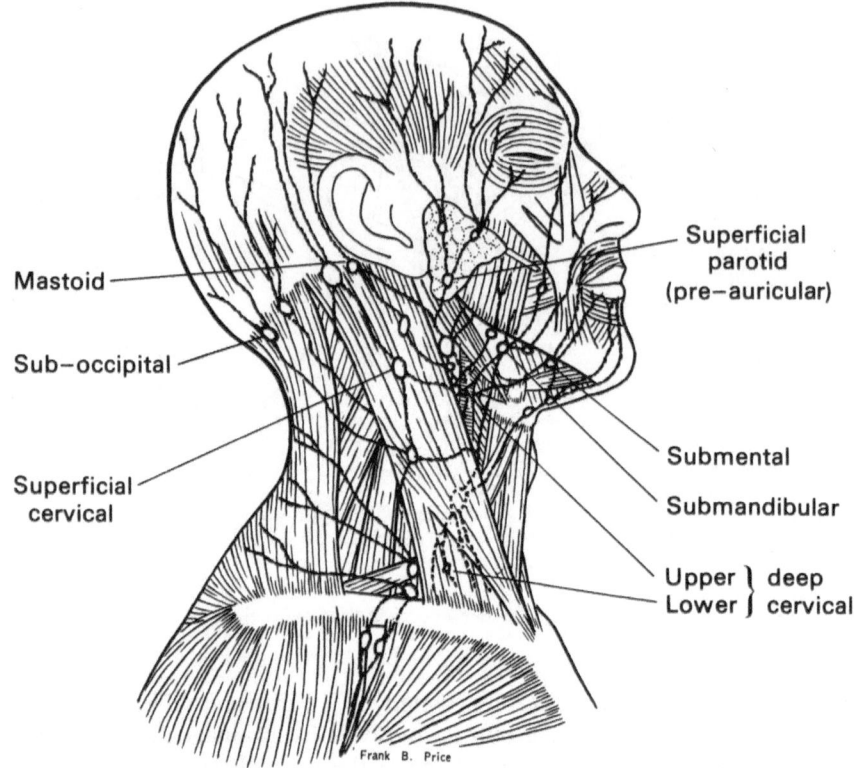

Figure 4. The superficial cervical lymph nodes.

The efferents of all these vertically disposed chains drain into the deep cervical lymph nodes.

The drainage of some areas of particular importance now requires mention in more detail.

The Lips

The upper lip and the lateral part of the lower lip drain into the submandibular nodes. The central part of the lower lip (together with the floor of the mouth and the tip of the tongue) drains into the submental group of nodes, which receive afferents from both sides of the median plane; these drain to the submandibular and jugulo-omohyoid nodes.

The Tonsil

The tonsillar lymph nodes pierce the bucco-pharangeal fascia and drain to the upper deep cervical lymph nodes, in particular the jugulo-digastric node at the angle of the mandible. Since this node is affected in tonsillitis it is the most common lymph node in the body to undergo pathological enlargement.

The Tongue

The drainage zones of the tongue can be grouped into three areas: (1) The tip drains to the submental nodes; (2) the anterior two-thirds of the tongue in front of the vallate papillae drains to the submental and submandibular nodes, and thence to the lower nodes of the deep cervical chain, particularly the jugulo-omohyoid node; and (3) the posterior one-third of the tongue drains to the upper nodes of the deep cervical chain.

There is rich anastomosis across the midline between the lymphatics of the posterior one-third of the tongue so that a tumor on one side readily metastasizes to the contralateral nodes. In contrast, there is little cross-communication in the anterior two-thirds of the tongue, where tumors situated more than 1.5 cm from the midline do not metastasize to the opposite side of the neck until late in the disease.

The Larynx

The lymphatics of the larynx are separated into an upper and lower group by the vocal cords. The supraglottic area is drained by vessels which accompany this superior laryngeal vein and empty into the upper deep cervical lymph nodes. The infraglottic zone similarly drains in company with the inferior vein into the lower part of the deep cervical chain. Lymphatics from the anterior part of the lower larynx also empty into small prelaryngeal and pretracheal nodes, which drain in turn into the deep cervical group. The vocal cords themselves are firmly bound down to the underlying vocal membranes, and lymph channels are therefore absent in this region. This accounts for the clearly defined watershed between the upper and lower zones of lymph drainage.

The Parotid Salivary Gland

The lymph drainage of the parotid salivary gland ends in the superficial and deep cervical lymph nodes, but these vessels may be interrupted in their course by two or three nodes which lie on the surface and within the substance of the parotid salivary gland.

The Thyroid Gland

The lymph vessels of the thyroid gland pass to the prelaryngeal nodes just above the thyroid isthmus and to the pretracheal and paratracheal nodes. Some drainage may occur into the brachio-cephalic nodes related to the thymus in the superior mediastinum. Laterally, the thyroid gland drains by vessels accompanying the superior thyroid vein to the deep cervical nodes. Some vessels may pass directly into the thoracic and right lymphatic duct.

Lymphatic Drainage of the Breast

The importance of the lymphatic drainage of the breast in the spread of carcinoma in this organ can hardly be overstressed, yet it is still the subject of confusion in many standard surgical and anatomical texts. This is the result of descriptions which were based on postmortem dissection studies or on the autopsy investigation of patients with widely disseminated carcinoma. Modern investigations, based on intravital techniques with dyes and radioactive gold, have destroyed much of the mystique surrounding this subject and have shown that lymph drainage of the breast, like that of any other organ, passes along lymphatics which accompany its blood supply. There is no clinical significance, for example, to the subareolar plexus described by Sappey (as the result of mercury injection into the lactating breast) which he believed drained the breast parenchyma. Many authors described lymph drainage from the breast passing centripetally to this plexus and thence to the axilla. This subcutaneous network communicates with lymphatics around the lactiferous ducts, which are important as a secretion-absorbing mechanism particularly during pregnancy, but there is no evidence of any essential confluent point in the lymphatic drainage of resting breast tissue to the areolar region. Similarly, there is no evidence of lymphatic drainage passing from the breast to lymphatics of the fascia over pectoralis major. Minute lymphatics do occur in this region which probably represent lymphatic drainage of the fascia itself. Large lymphatics leave the posterior aspect of the breast along the larger perforating blood vessels, but there is no suggestion of any plexus formation.

The following description is based largely on the excellent account given by Turner-Warwick (1959):

> The breast receives its blood supply from three principal sources; the axillary vessels, the internal mammary vessels and a small contribution from the lateral perforating branches of the intercostal vessels. The lymphatic drainage takes place in these three directions and is roughly proportional to the blood supply from each of the three sources. Most lymphatic drainage passes to the axillary nodes, next important is the drainage to the parasternal nodes and there is also a small and inconstant drainage to the posterior intercostal nodes.

The Axillary Lymph Nodes

The nodes in the axilla provide terminal drainage for the whole of the upper limb as well as the breast. They number between 20 and 30 and are divided, in a rather arbitrary manner, into five groups (Figure 5): *(1) The lateral group.* These are four to six in number and are grouped medially and posterior to the axillary vein. They drain to the central and apical groups; *(2) the pectoral (or anterior) group.* Again four to six in number, they lie along the lower border of pectoralis minor in relation to the lateral thoracic vessels; this group drains to the central and apical groups; *(3) the subscapular (or posterior) group.* This collection of six or seven nodes accompanies the subscapular vessels along the posterior wall of the axilla and drains to the apical and central nodes; *(4) the central group.* These are three or four nodes lying in the axilla. This group receives drainage from the other three clumps of nodes, and in turn its efferents empty into the apical group; *(5) the apical group.* This group consists of up to twelve nodes that lie along the medial side of the axillary vein behind and above the pectoralis minor.

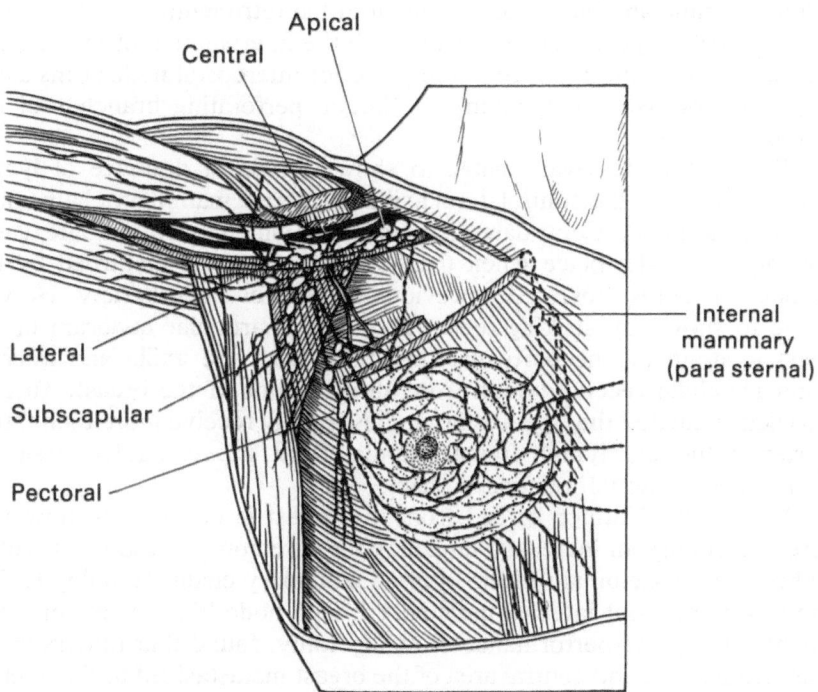

Figure 5. The axillary nodes and lymph drainage of the breast.

It receives the efferents of the other axillary lymph node groups and also directs drainage from the breast. Its efferents form the subclavian trunk.

The lymphatics of the main axillary pathway arise in the lobules of the breast and pass to the pectoral group; some lymph may pass directly to the subscapular nodes. A few lymph vessels pass directly from the upper part of the breast to the apical nodes.

The Parasternal (Internal Mammary) Lymph Nodes

These nodes lie along the internal mammary vessels from the fifth space upwards. They are usually situated between the costal cartilages but may lie behind them. These nodes receive lymph from lymphatic vessels which accompany the anterior perforating vessels and also from those which run with the lateral perforating branches of the upper intercostal vessels. Below the fifth intercostal space the internal mammary chain is poorly developed. The upper three or four spaces have small posterior intercostal lymph nodes which lie between the necks of the ribs close to the vertebrae.

Perforating lymph vessels leave the posterior aspect of the breast without forming any plexus arrangement in the retromammary plane; they pass through the pectoralis major to reach the internal mammary chain. A small and inconstant drainage to the posterior intercostal nodes runs along lymphatic vessels accompanying the lateral perforating branches of the intercostal vessels.

Turner-Warwick was unable to show significant drainage of lymph from one breast to the contralateral axilla or internal mammary chain under normal conditions. Contralateral metastases which occur in late cases probably only take place when the normal drainage is disturbed by the presence of metastases, or by previous surgery or radiotherapy. He was unable to show any striking tendency for any particular quadrant of the breast to drain in one particular direction. Both the axilla and internal mammary chain receive lymph from all quadrants of the breast. Turner-Warwick estimated that the axillary nodes usually receive more than three-quarters of the total lymph drainage of the breast, the remainder passing to the ipsilateral internal mammary chain.

When actual tumor spread from the breast is considered, however, there is certainly an increased tendency for carcinoma of the inner half of the breast to disseminate to the internal mammary chain. Handley (1972), who has carried out internal mammary lymph node biopsies in some 900 patients during the performance of mastectomy, found that tumors in the inner hemisphere and central area of the breast metastasized to the internal mammary nodes more than twice as often as do primary tumors in the outer hemisphere—the figures are 29% for the upper inner quadrant, 35%, for the lower inner quadrant, 15% for the upper outer quadrant, 13% for the lower outer quadrant, and 32% for the central region. In those patients with axillary lymph node metastases, there is again an obvious predominance of spread to the internal mammary chain from the medial half of the breast. In the 495 patients in this category there were positive internal mammary node biopsies; in 48% of upper inner quadrant, 71% of lower inner quadrant, 22% of upper outer quadrant, 20% of lower outer quadrant, and 45% of central tumors.

Lymphatic Drainage of the Lower Limb

The whole of the lower limb drains into the inguinal lymph nodes which also drain lymph from the lower anterior and latero-abdominal wall from the level of the umbilicus downwards, from the gluteal region, the penis, the scrotum, the vulva, the perineum, and the lower part of the anal canal. Drainage from the central areas may pass to both groins and there is a rich anastomosis across the midline. The inguinal lymph nodes may be divided into a superficial and deep group. The superficial nodes lie in the superficial fascia of the thigh grouped around the termination of the saphenous vein and its tributaries. The nodes vary in number from 2–25. They drain by means of efferent lymphatics, principally into the external iliac group of nodes which run along the course of the external iliac vein. Some drainage passes into the deep inguinal nodes which lie beneath the deep fascia on the femoral triangle. These deep nodes are small and lie along the course of the femoral vein. The largest and most constant member of this chain is the gland of Cloquet which lies in the femoral canal immediately medial to the femoral vein.

Lymphatic Drainage of the Alimentary Canal and Its Adnexae

The lymph vessels within the abdomen accompany the major arterial trunks, and the lymphatic drainage of the abdominal viscera bears a correspondingly close relationship to the arterial supply. The lymph nodes are arranged in numerous intermediary groups, situated along the corresponding arteries, with terminal lymph nodes which lie in relation to the abdominal aorta. The lateral aortic group of lumbar lymph nodes receive efferents from the outlying groups in relation to the iliac arteries as well as the drainage from the viscera supplied by the lateral branches of the aorta; they therefore drain the urogenital organs and posterior abdominal wall. The paraaortic lymph nodes drain the viscera supplied by the anterior branches of the aorta and are grouped in relation to the coeliac, superior mesenteric, and inferior mesenteric arteries at their origins. Their function is to drain the abdominal part of the alimentary canal and its adnexae.

The Stomach

The lymph vessels of the stomach form a rich plexus in the submucosa from which drainage takes place to lymph nodes situated mainly along the greater and lesser curvatures. These nodes may be divided into three main groups. The first lies as a ring around the cardia (the "cardiac necklace") together with nodes of the upper end of the lesser curvature along the left gastric vessels. The second group includes the subpyloric and hepatic nodes. The subpyloric nodes are four or five in number and lie in the angle between the first and second parts of the duodenum in relation to the gastro-duodenal artery. The hepatic nodes are situated in the lesser omentum along the course of the hepatic artery. Nodes of the third group lie along the greater curvature of the stomach and are congregated particularly along the pyloric end of the greater curvature and in the gastrosplenic omentum in relation to the hilum of the spleen. The subpyloric nodes and those situated along the lesser curvature are most often implicated in gastric carcinoma.

Although there is a continuous connection between the lymphatics of the whole of the stomach, lymph tends to flow from the right part of the stomach towards the lesser curvature and from the left towards the greater curvature. The stomach is divided into three drainage zones (Figure 6): The first area comprises the superior two-thirds of the stomach which drains along the left and right gastric vessels to the paraaortic nodes, the pyloric region also communicating with the hepatic nodes; the second area comprises the right two-thirds of the inferior one-third of the stomach, which drains along the right gastro-epiploic vessels to the subpyloric nodes and then to the aortic group; the third area comprises the left one-third of the inferior one-third of the stomach, which drains along the short gastric and splenic vessels and then via the suprapancreatic nodes to the aortic group.

This extensive lymphatic drainage and the technical impossibility of its complete removal is one of the serious problems in dealing with gastric carcinoma. Involvement of the nodes along the splenic vessels can be dealt with by removal of the spleen, the gastrosplenic and lieno-renal ligaments, and the body and tail of the pancreas. Lymph nodes along the gastro-epiploic vessels are removed by excising the greater omentum. However, involvement of the nodes around the aorta, the head of the pancreas, and the porta hepatis may render the carcinoma incurable.

The Intestine

The arrangement of lymph nodes is relatively uniform in the small and large intestines. Numerous small nodes lie near, or even on, the wall of the

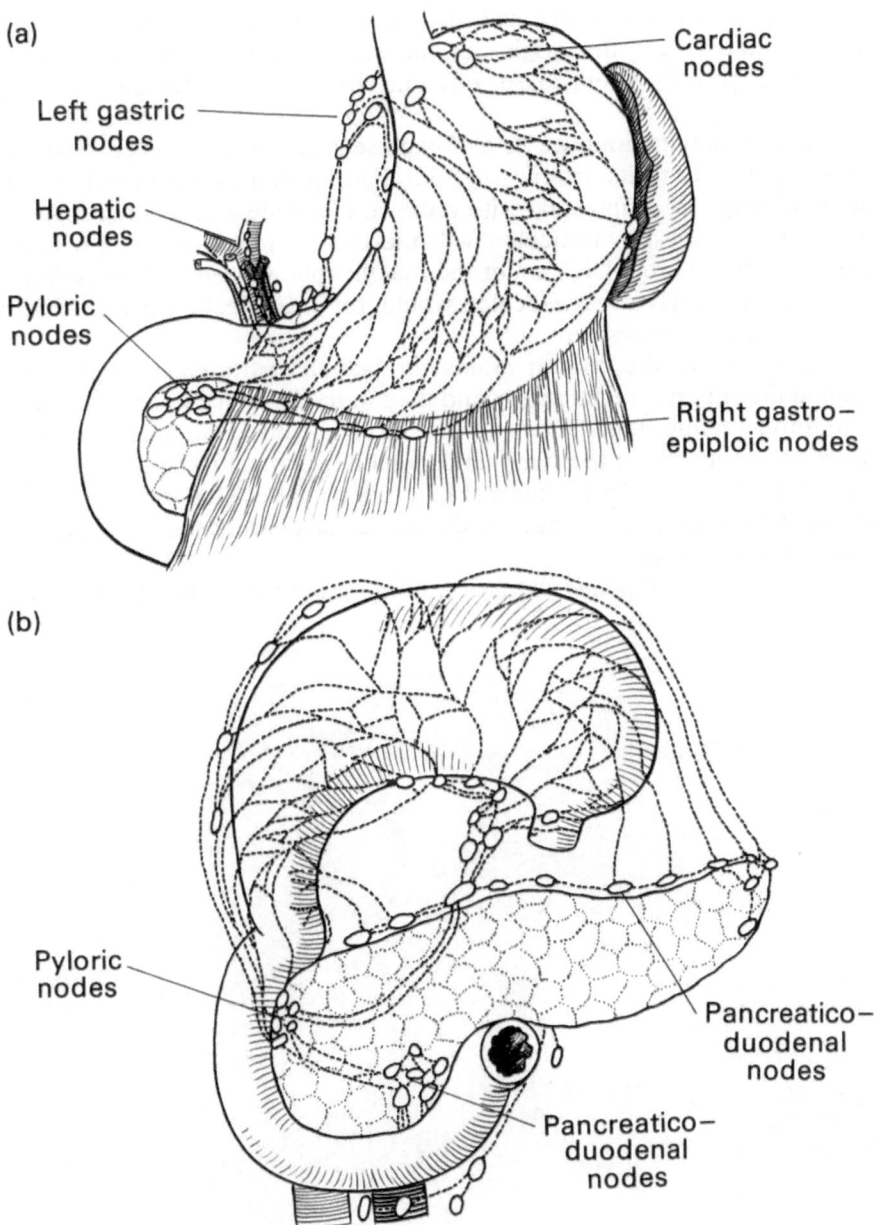

Figure 6. Lymphatic drainage of the stomach.

intestine which drains to intermediary placed and rather larger nodes along the vessels of the mesentery and mesocolon and then to clumps of lymph nodes situated near the origins of the superior and inferior mesenteric arteries (Figure 7). From these, efferent vessels link up to drain into the cisterna chyli.

The lymphatic drainage field of each segment of intestine corresponds fairly accurately to its arterial supply. High ligation of the vessels to the involved segment of intestine with removal of a wide surrounding segment of the mesentery or mesocolon will therefore remove the lymph nodes which drain the area. Division of the middle colic vessels and resection of the wedge of transverse mesocolon would, for example, be performed for a tumor of the transverse colon.

The bulk of the rectum drains through the pararectal lymph nodes around the superior rectal artery and then to the inferior mesenteric nodes. The lower rectum, together with the anal canal above the mucocutaneous junction, drains along the lymphatics which accompany the middle rectal vessels to nodes along the internal iliac artery. Below the mucocutaneous junction the lymphatic drainage of the anal canal descends to the superficial inguinal lymph nodes.

Retrograde lymphatic extension to the groin nodes may take place in

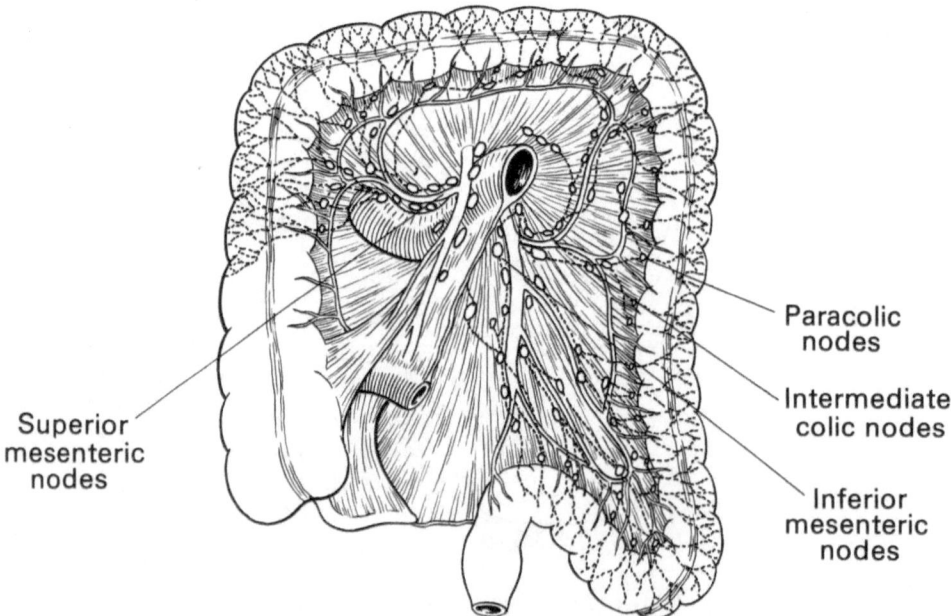

Superior
mesenteric
nodes

Paracolic
nodes

Intermediate
colic nodes

Inferior
mesenteric
nodes

Figure 7. Lymph drainage of the large bowel.

advanced cases of carcinoma of the rectum, when the upward lymphatic flow is blocked by extensive metastases in the pararectal and inferior mesenteric nodes.

The Liver

The collecting lymphatic vessels of the liver are divided into superficial lymph vessels, which run in the subserous connective tissue over the surface of the organ, and deep lymph vessels in the accompanying tributaries of the portal vein and branches of the hepatic artery. The subfascial lymph vessels drain to nodes around the termination of the inferior vena cava and to the hepatic nodes at the porta hepatis. There are also connections to the coeliac nodes and, in addition, lymph vessels on the diaphragmatic aspect of the liver may enter the thoracic duct directly. The deep lymph vessels accompany the hepatic veins to end in nodes around the termination of the inferior vena cava, while other lymphatics descend to terminate in the hepatic lymph nodes.

The Gallbladder and Bile Duct

These drain to the hepatic nodes, especially to the prominent cystic lymph node which can usually be discovered at operation in relation to the cystic duct.

The Pancreas

The pancreas has a particularly rich lymphatic drainage which passes through the pancreaticosplenic nodes situated in the hilum of the spleen and into the pancreaticoduodenal nodes placed between the head of the pancreas and the C-loop of the duodenum. Other vessels drain into the superior mesenteric group of paraaortic lymph nodes.

The Urinary Tract

The Kidney

The lymphatics of the kidney are divided into a superficial system, draining the perirenal fat, a second system beneath the fibrous capsule, and a third in the renal substance itself. The vessels drain to lymph nodes behind the renal pelvis at the hilum and thence to the nodes lying along the aorta and inferior vena cava at the level of the renal vessels. The lymph from the upper part of the ureter joins the renal drainage; other vessels pass directly to the lateral aortic nodes. More distally, the ureteric lymph drains to the common iliac nodes and its pelvic portion drains to the external and internal iliac lymph nodes.

The Bladder

The lymph vessels of the bladder form plexuses which lie in the mucus, intramuscular, and the extramuscular planes. Drainage passes principally to the external iliac nodes, although some might pass directly into the internal or common iliac groups.

The Prostatic Lymphatics

These lymphatics terminate principally in the internal iliac and sacral nodes, although some drainage passes with the lymphatics of the bladder to the external iliac nodes.

Lymphatic Drainage of the Genitalia

The Male Reproductive Organs

Testis. The testis arises from the germinal ridge of mesoderm in the posterior wall of the abdomen, medial to the developing kidney. As the testis enlarges, it also undergoes a caudal migration and descends into the scrotum in the ninth month of fetal life. During this migration it drags with it its arterial supply, which arises from the aorta just caudal to the origin of the renal arteries. The corresponding testicular vein drains into the inferior vena cava on the right and into the left renal vein on the left side. The lymphatic drainage of the testis obeys the usual rule and follows the vascular pedicle of the organ; the testicular lymphatics therefore pass to the paraaortic lymph nodes at the level of the renal vessels. Free communication occurs between the lymphatics on either side and there is also a plentiful anastomosis with the paraaortic intrathoracic nodes and, in turn, with the deep cervical nodes, so that spread of malignant disease from the testis to the root of the neck is not rare. It should be noted that a unilateral block dissection of the paraaortic nodes in the treatment of testicular tumors has no basis in anatomy because of this rich lymphatic communication across the midline; modern therapy of the regional nodes in such cases comprises irradiation of both the ipsi- and contralateral lymph node areas.

The vas deferens and the epididymis are supplied by the artery to the vas which arises from the inferior vesical branch of the internal iliac artery. This vessel anastomoses with the testicular artery and this cross-connection means that ligation of the testicular artery is not necessarily followed by testicular atrophy. The lymphatic drainage of the epididymis, the vas, and the tunica vaginalis passes to the internal iliac nodes, then via the common iliac nodes to the paraaortic chain. Note that there is no communication whatsoever with the inguinal lymph nodes.

Scrotum and Penis. The skin of this area drains by lymphatics which accompany those of the perineal skin along the course of the external pudendal arteries to the superficial inguinal nodes. The lymphatics of the glans penis drain to the deep inguinal and external iliac chain.

The Female Reproductive Organs

The Ovary. This organ drains in a similar manner to the testis; its lymphatics pass along the ovarian artery to the paraaortic chain.

The Uterus (Figure 8). This organ contains two sets of lymphatic vessels, comprising a superficial network lying beneath the peritoneum and

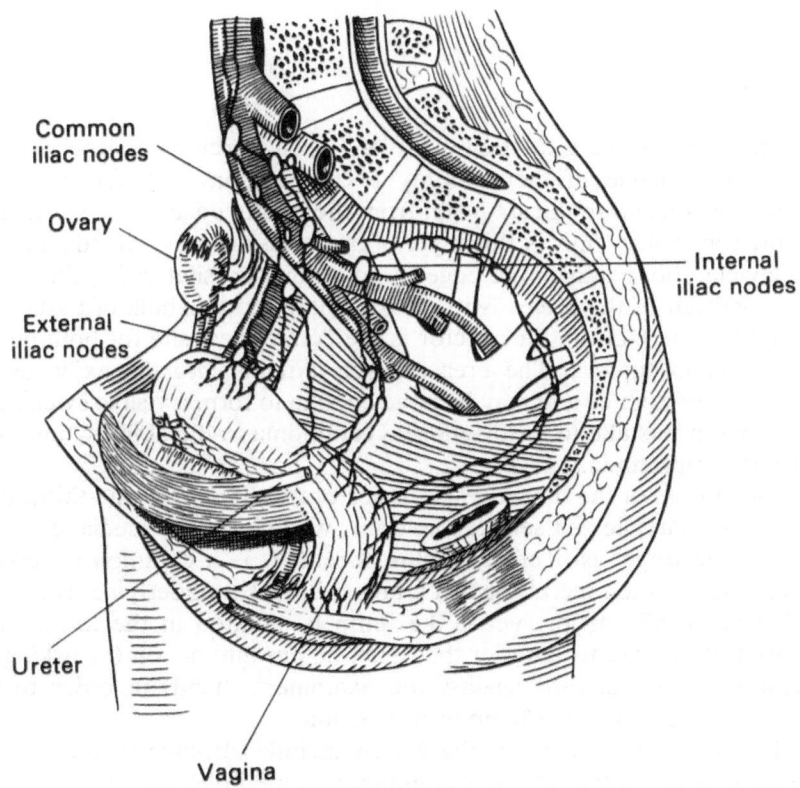

Figure 8. Lymph drainage of the female pelvis.

a deep plexus in the substance of the uterine muscles. The fundus, together with the Fallopian tube, has similar drainage to the ovary, but in addition the region of the fundus at the site of its attachment to the tube is drained by lymphatics which pass along the round ligament to reach the superficial inguinal nodes. It is thus always essential to examine the inguinal nodes in a suspected carcinoma of the corpus uteri.

The body of the uterus drains via lymphatics in the broad ligament to nodes which lie alongside the external iliac vessels.

The lymphatics draining the cervix uteri pass in three directions; laterally in the broad ligament to the external iliac nodes, postero-laterally along the uterine vessels to the internal iliac nodes and posteriorly along the recto-uterine folds to the sacral nodes.

The Vagina. This may be divided into three lymphatic zones; the upper third drains to the external and internal iliac nodes, the middle third to the internal iliac nodes (along the vaginal artery), and the lower third, together with the lymphatics of the vulva and skin of the perineum, to the superficial inguinal nodes. It should be noted that these drainage areas are not sharply demarcated one from the other.

The Breast

Much of the surgical treatment of breast carcinoma depends on a detailed knowledge of the anatomy of this region. The female breast overlies the second to the sixth rib, from the lateral edge of the sternum to the anterior axillary line. A thin layer of breast tissue may extend almost to the clavicle above and to the edge of latissimus dorsilaterally. The upper outer quadrant of the breast is its thickest part and this bulk of tissue may account for the fact that this sector is the commonest site for both benign and malignant tumors. The breast tissue extends into the axilla as the axillary tail of Spence and may be large enough to form a visible swelling. It is a common mistake to misdiagnose a carcinoma in the axillary tail for an enlarged lymph node.

Two-thirds of the breast rests on pectoralis major and one-third, in its lower outer part, lies on serratus anterior, while its lower medial edge just overlaps the upper part of the rectus sheath. It is a common mistake in clinical examination merely to test a breast lump for underlying fixation by tensing pectoralis major, yet if the lump is situated in the lower outer quadrant, it is serratus anterior that must be put into action (by asking the patient to press forward against the examiner's hand) in order to test underlying fixation of the lump in this region.

Congenital anomalies of the breast include absence of one or both sides, and asymmetry, which is common in a mild degree, although rarely one breast may be twice the size of the other. Accessory nipples along the nipple line are commonly seen, although accessory breasts are much more unusual. Accessory breast tissue is about twice as common in females as in males and the anomaly may be familial.

Many accessory breasts comprise a small nipple and areola only; in other instances there is a glandular epithelium which may connect through a nipple via a duct system. In such cases lactation may occur and infants may be suckled from them. Where there is glandular parenchyma benign and malignant tumors of the accessory breast may occur.

Structure

The breast is made up of 15 to 20 lobes, each of which drains by a lactiferous duct onto the nipple, which is surrounded by the pigmented areola. The bulk of the nipple is made up of smooth muscle fibers which, on contraction, produce erection of the nipple and help to empty the milk sinuses. The skin of the areola contains large sebaceous glands which become prominent during pregnancy and lactation and not infrequently become infected (the glands of Montgomery).

The lobes of the breast are supported in a connective tissue so intimately blended that there is no plane of dissection in the breast itself.

The deep aspect of the breast is separated from the fascial covering of pectoralis major and serratus anterior by a layer of loose areolar tissue which accounts for the mobility of the breasts on the chest wall. Once in this plane the surgeon can readily separate the breast tissue from the underlying muscle.

Blood Supply (Figure 9)

The arterial supply of the breast is derived from three sources; branches of the axillary, internal mammary, and intercostal arteries. The axillary artery provides a small superior thoracic branch from its first part, a pectoral branch of its acromiothoracic artery from its second part, and a lateral thoracic branch, which passes down the lateral border of the pectoralis minor, from its third part. The subscapular artery, which is the largest branch of the axillary artery, runs down the lateral border of the scapula and is accompanied in the lower part of its course by the nerve to latissimus dorsi. Although this artery has no part to play in the blood supply of the breast, it is associated with the posterior group of axillary lymph nodes and it, together with its accompanying vein, may give rise to troublesome bleeding during the course of axillary clearance in a radical or extended simple mastectomy.

The internal mammary artery gives off perforating branches to supply

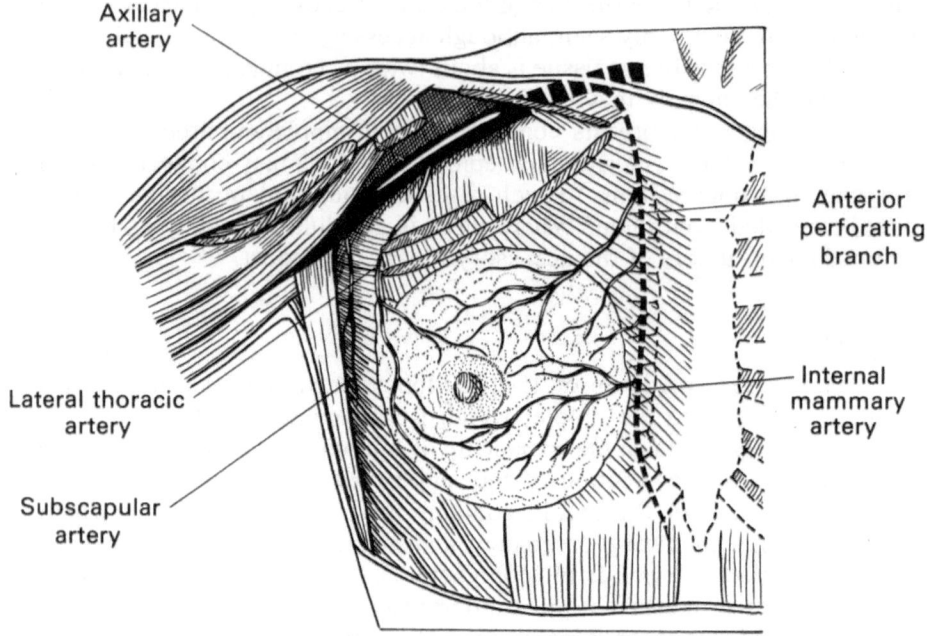

Figure 9. Blood supply of the breast.

the breast via the first, second, third, and fourth intercostal spaces. These branches traverse pectoralis major to reach the breast along its medial edge. The first and second perforators are the largest of these branches. Secondary perforators are usually found in the upper interspaces about 2.5 cm (1 in.) lateral to the main perforators.

Small mammary branches arise from the intercostal arteries via their lateral perforating branches in the second, third, and fourth intercostal spaces.

The venous drainage corresponds to the arterial supply. (Lymphatic drainage of the breast is considered above on p. 24.)

The Liver

To the oncologist, the liver represents one of the commonest sites of blood-borne metastases; to the oncological surgeon malignant disease of the liver presents an important surgical challenge. It is with these practical considerations in mind that the following section has been prepared. After a brief account of the conventional anatomy of the liver, consideration will be given to its segmental anatomy, which is of importance in major hepatic resections, and to the details of its blood supply.

The liver is the largest solid organ in the body. From the anterior aspect it is somewhat triangular in shape and lies principally in the upper right quadrant of the abdomen. It is related by its domed upper surface to the diaphragm, which separates it from the pleura, lungs, pericardium, and heart. Its postero-inferior (or visceral) surface abuts against the abdominal esophagus, the stomach, duodenum, hepatic flexure of the colon and the right kidney and suprarenal, as well as carrying the gallbladder. Tumors of all these structures not infrequently invade the adjacent visceral aspect of the liver.

The surface markings of the normal liver comprise a line which runs from the tip of the right tenth rib to just below the left nipple, which defines its lower border; the upper border follows a line which passes just below the nipple on each side.

The liver is divided into a larger right and smaller left lobe separated superiorly by the falciform ligament, and postero-inferiorly by an H-shaped arrangement of fossae (Figure 10). To the right and anteriorly lies the fossa for the gallbladder. To the right and posteriorly is the groove in which lies embedded the inferior vena cava. To the left and anteriorly lies the fissure

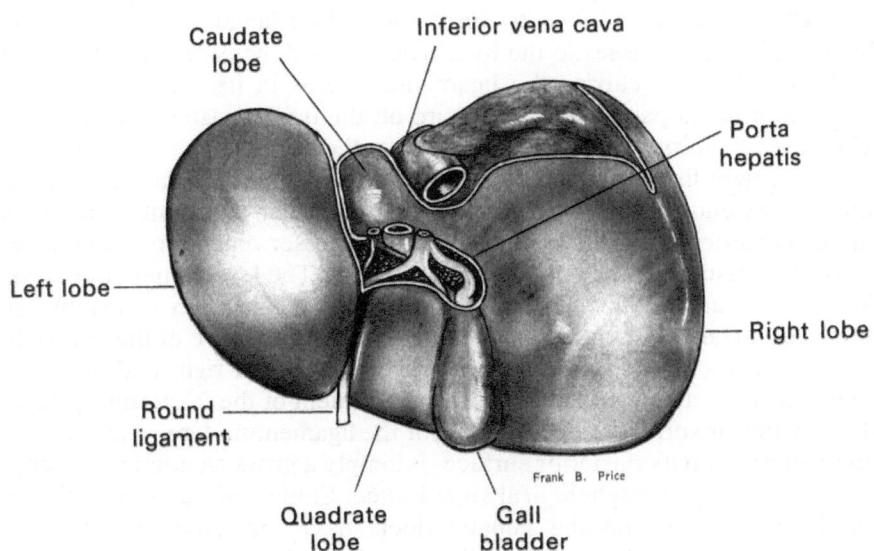

Figure 10. The inferior aspect of the liver.

which contains the ligamentum teres. To the left and posteriorly is the fissure for the ligamentum venosum. The crossbar of the H is the porta hepatis and the limbs of this H mark out two subsidiary lobes on the visceral aspect of the liver. These are the quadrate lobe anteriorly and the caudate lobe posteriorly.

The ligamentum teres represents the obliterated remnants of the left umbilical vein, whose function is to bring blood from the placenta back to the fetus. The ligamentum venosum is the fibrous remnant of the ductus venosus which functions in fetal life to shunt blood from this left umbilical vein to the inferior vena cava, thus short-circuiting the liver. The grooves for the ligamentum teres, ligamentum venosum, and inferior vena cava thus represent the pathway of the fetal venous trunk and are therefore continu-, ous in the adult.

Lying in the porta hepatis are three main structures; anteriorly lies the common hepatic duct, posteriorly the portal vein, and, sandwiched between, the hepatic artery. In addition there are autonomic nerve fibers, lymphatic vessels, and lymph nodes.

Peritoneal Attachments (Figure 11)

The liver is encased in peritoneum except for a small posterior bare area, which represents the zone where peritoneum from the diaphragm is reflected on it as the upper and lower layers of the coronary ligament. To the right, these layers fuse to form the right triangular ligament. The falciform ligament passes to the liver from the umbilicus rather to the right of the midline and carries the ligamentum teres in its free border. The ligamentum teres passes into its fissure on the inferior aspect of the liver, while the falciform ligament proceeds over the dome of the liver and then splits. Its right limb joins the upper layer of the coronary ligament, and its left limb extends as the long, narrow, left triangular ligament which then passes posteriorly and to the right to join the lesser omentum in the upper end of the fissure for the ligamentum venosum. The lesser omentum arises from the fissures of the porta hepatis and the ligamentum venosum and passes as a sheet to be attached along the lesser curvature of the stomach.

The gross anatomical division of the liver into a right and left lobe, demarcated by a line passing from the attachment of the falciform ligament on the anterior surface to the fissures for the ligamentum teres and ligamentum venosum on its posterior surface, is simply a gross anatomical descriptive term with no morphological significance. Studies of the distribution of the blood vessels and the hepatic ducts have indicated that the true morphological and physiological division of the liver is into right and left lobes demarcated by a plane which passes through the fossa of the gallblad-

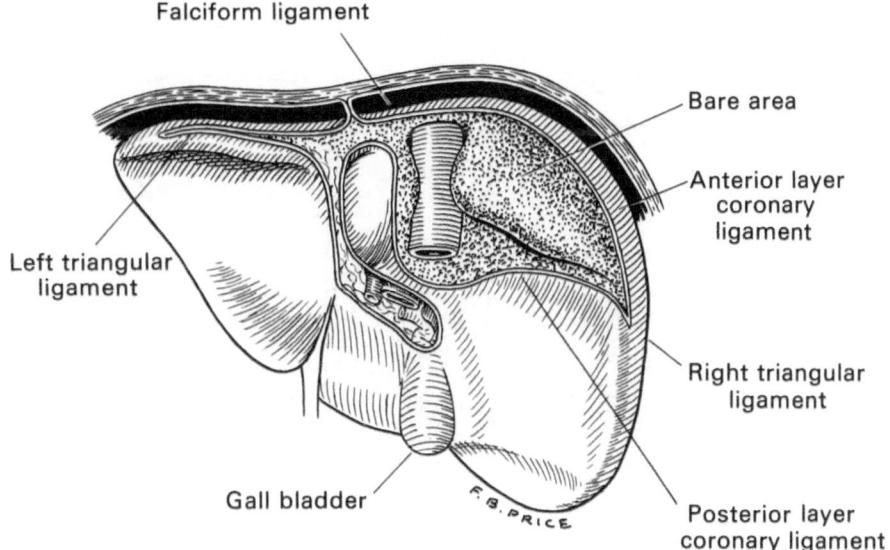

Figure 11. Peritoneal attachments of the liver.

der and the fossa of the inferior vena cava. Although these two lobes are not differentiated by any visible line on the dome of the liver, each has its own arterial and venous blood supply and separate biliary drainage. This morphological division lies to the right of the gross anatomical plane and in this the quadrate lobe comes to be part of the left morphological lobe of the liver while the caudate lobe divides partly to the left and partly to the right lobe (Figure 12).

Segmental Anatomy of the Liver

It is now proposed to discuss the morphological divisions of the liver in more detail. Four sets of vessels traverse the liver substance. The portal veins, hepatic arteries, and bile duct system form one pattern, whereas the hepatic veins have a rather different plan.

At the hilum of the liver, the hepatic artery, portal vein, and bile duct divide into right and left branches, and there is little or no anastomosis between the divisions on the two sides. From the region of the porta hepatis, the branches pass laterally and spread upwards and downwards throughout the liver substance, defining the two morphological lobes already described (Figures 13a and b).

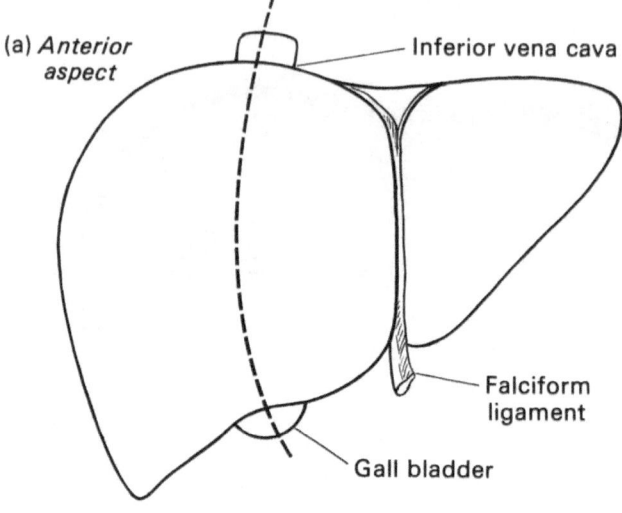

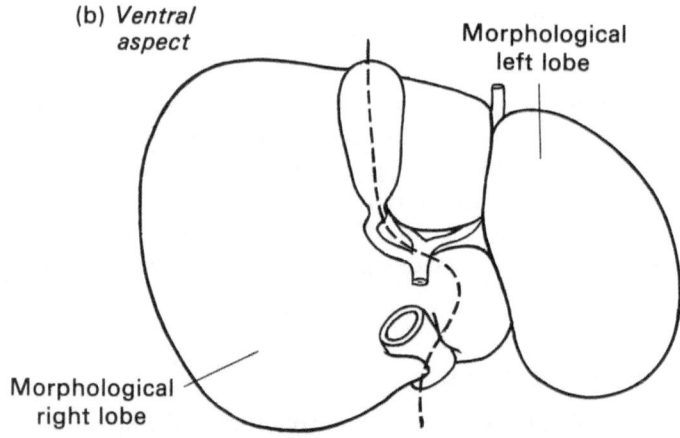

Figure 12. Morphological divisions of the liver. Note that the quadrate lobe is morphologically a part of the left lobe while the caudate lobe belongs to both right and left lobes.

Although further subdivisions of the liver can be described (for example, two segments, anterior and posterior, can be distinguished in the right true lobe of the liver) with still further subdivisions into further segments, these are of little practical importance in operative surgery and will not be dealt with more fully.

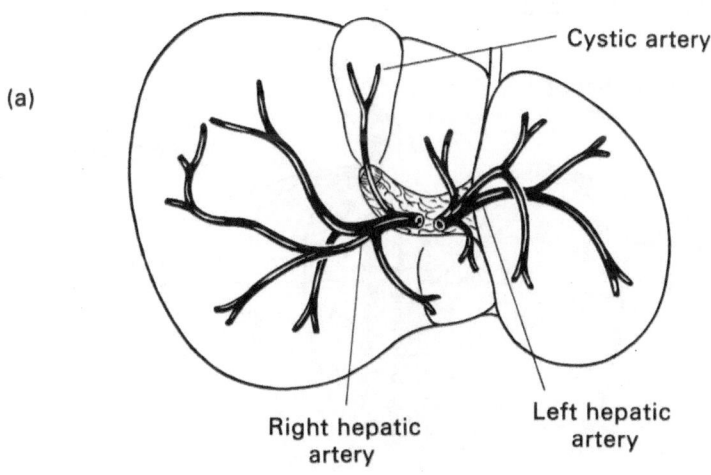

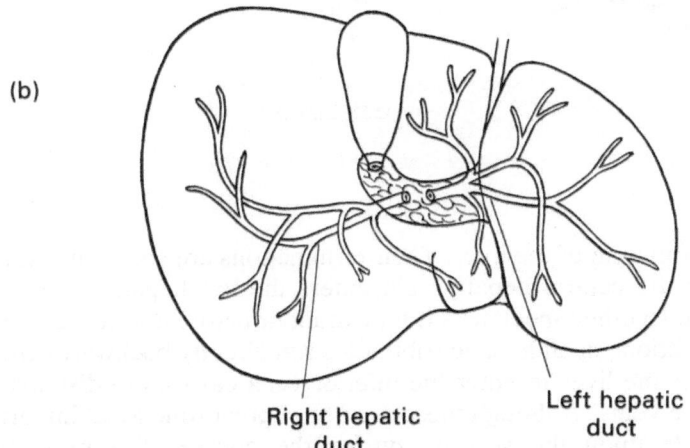

Figure 13. (a) Distribution of hepatic arteries. (b) Distribution of hepatic ducts. Note that the quadrate lobe is supplied exclusively by the left hepatic artery and drained by the left hepatic duct. The caudate lobe is supplied by each.

The Hepatic Venous System (Figure 14)

The hepatic veins are massive and their distribution is somewhat different from that of the portal hepatic arterial and bile duct system already described. There are three major hepatic veins, right, central, and left. These pass upwards and backwards to drain into the inferior vena cava at

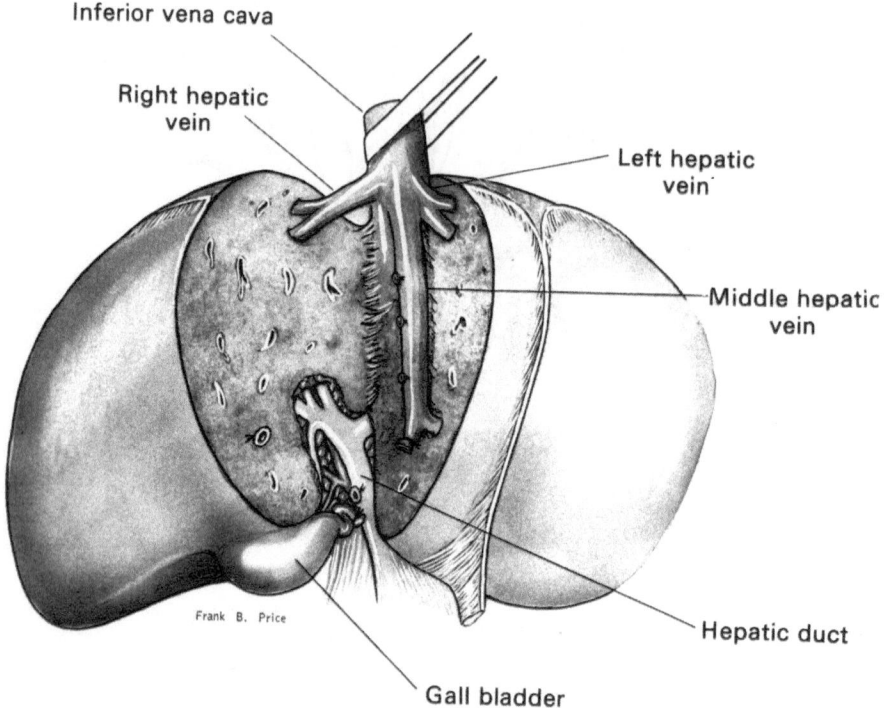

Figure 14. The hepatic venous system. Based on Edwards *et al.* (1975).

the superior margin of the liver. Their terminations are somewhat variable, but usually the central hepatic vein enters the left hepatic vein near its termination. In other specimens it may drain directly into the inferior vena cava. In addition, small hepatic tributaries run directly backwards from the substance of the liver to enter the inferior vena cava more distally to the main hepatic veins. Although these are not of great functional importance, they obtrude upon the surgeon during the course of a right hepatic lobectomy.

The three principal hepatic veins have three zones of drainage corresponding roughly to the right, middle, and left thirds of the liver. The plane defined by the falciform ligament corresponds to the boundary of the zones drained by the left and middle hepatic veins. Unfortunately for the surgeon, the middle hepatic vein lies just at the line of the principal plane of the liver between its right and left morphological lobes, and it is this fact which complicates the operation of right hepatic resection.

In carrying out resection of the left lobe of the liver, the left hepatic vein should be ligated and divided to the left of the falciform ligament, in this way damage to the central hepatic vein, which often drains directly into the left vein, can be avoided. In carrying out a right hemihepatectomy, section is performed roughly along the principal plane of the liver but the central vein must again be preserved to make certain that the half of the central segment of the liver, which is to be preserved, will maintain its hepatic venous drainage. It is therefore necessary to perform the operation somewhat to the right of the principal plane.

Anatomical Details of Right Hemihepatectomy

The main anatomical points in this procedure are as follows:

A right thoraco-abdominal incision is necessary, with division of the diaphragm as far as the opening of the inferior vena cava posteriorly.

The porta hepatis is dissected and the cystic duct and artery are ligated and divided followed by isolation, ligation, and division of the right hepatic duct and right hepatic artery.

The right division of the portal vein is then ligated and divided. At this stage a visible line of color change will be seen on the hepatic surface which helps to indicate the plane of hepatic division. It is important to appreciate that anatomical variations are common in the porta hepatis; for example, some 15% of patients have a right hepatic artery which arises from the superior mesenteric artery which enters the right lobe at the posterior aspect of the porta hepatis. Variations in the pattern of the gallbladder and bile ducts are also extremely common. The right triangular ligament and the layers of the coronary ligament are divided to liberate the right lobe from its diaphragmatic attachments. The right lobe of the liver is now displaced to the left to expose the inferior vena cava and the short hepatic veins running into it. These are divided. The termination of the right hepatic vein into the inferior vena cava is now dissected, and this is usually covered by a tongue of liver tissue which requires careful dissection. The right hepatic vein is ligated and divided, preserving the central hepatic vein. The hepatic substance is then divided, aiming the line of resection to the right lateral border of the inferior vena cava in order to leave a rim of hepatic substance covering the middle hepatic vein.

The Blood Supply of Liver Tumors

The source of blood supply to hepatic tumors is of importance and interest to oncologists from the point of view of surgical treatment, angiographic diagnosis, and the possibility of regional cytotoxic perfusion.

Hepatic arteriography can be performed via a Seldinger catheter threaded through the femoral artery into the coeliac axis. Superior mesenteric artery angiography is usually performed at the same time. Michels (1960), in a study of such angiograms, noted that 55% showed a normal "textbook" coeliac axis and major branches. In 25% of subjects some hepatic blood supply was derived from the left gastric artery, which either replaced the left hepatic artery or gave an additional supply by means of an accessory hepatic branch. Abnormalities of the right hepatic arterial supply occurred in 18% of subjects, the right hepatic artery being either derived from the superior mesenteric artery (11%) or there being an accessory right hepatic branch from this source (7%). There were other variants in the remaining 2% of subjects.

The arteriographic appearances of hepatic tumors were well described by Bosniak and Phanthumachinda (1966). Hemangioma gives the appearance of a large vascular tumor with an orderly circular arterial pattern; a localized hepatoma shows abnormal vascularity, pooling of contrast, and stretching and displacement of vessels; multicentric hepatomas can be difficult to differentiate from metastases, but they tend to be more vascular than metastases which, although sometimes quite vascular, often appear either as poorly vascularized or even as avascular filling defects.

There is still debate about the major source of arterial supply to hepatic tumors for very few studies have been carried out on human material. Arteriographic studies are limited by the fact that small tumors cannot be visualized *in vivo* and, for obvious reasons, injection studies on postmortem material are usually confined to extensive deposits. Healey (1965), in a study of 45 human livers with metastatic tumors, found that the specimens with generalized subcapsular infiltration or nodular infiltration had a decreased vascularity, whereas other specimens appeared to have a normal arterial supply. Portal venous channels were found to be completely excluded in the tumor area. Most experimental studies with transplanted tumors conclude that the hepatic artery is the major, if not the exclusive, source of supply (Assa, 1970). However, a recent important contribution was made by Ackerman (1974), who investigated the vascular supply of experimental, implanted Walker rat tumors of increasing size. He found that those less than 1 mm in diameter appear to exist without any blood supply, probably depending on diffusion from surrounding vessels for nourishment. As the tumors grow, angiogenesis occurs with a blood supply consisting of vessels developed from surrounding arterial or portal components and, in some instances, both these sources coexist and connect with each other. As the tumors become larger, the arterial supply becomes predominant and the portal vessels are generally displaced and obliterated. However, in occasional tumors, there may be a small portal component and portal vessels may play a role in supplying a growing edge of the tumor as it penetrates into the liver substance. As the tumor becomes massive, the well-organized pattern breaks down with the development of irregular arterial or portal channels, and a mixed supply may occur in these tumors. He concludes that there is a variability in the vascularity of metastatic tumors in the liver, depending to some extent on their size and rate of growth.

Umbilical Vein Cannulation

In fetal life, the umbilical vein carries blood from the placenta into the portal circulation. Immediately after birth the vein is still patent and can be employed for exchange transfusion, but soon after this it closes down and has always been regarded as being obliteratd in the adult. It can be demonstrated, however, that this cord can be entered and dilated by means of a probe as it lies in the free edge of the falciform ligament. The umbilical vein enters the left branch of the portal vein about 2.5 cm from its bifurcation in the hilum of the liver, and this entrance is sealed by a fibrous membrane which yields to gentle pressure on the dilator.

This relatively simple method of entering the portal venous system has been employed clinically in a number of different ways. Portal venous pressure can be measured and, indeed, in cases of portal hypertension, decompression of the portal venous system has been carried out as an emergency measure by shunting the vein, either into the upturned long saphenous vein, or into the jugular vein by means of a polythene tube. Repeated specimens of portal blood and thus radiological studies of the portal vascular tree can be obtained; repeated hepatograms may be performed to assess progress of treatment during cytotoxic therapy. The umbilical vein has also been employed for infusion of cytotoxic drugs (Bevan, 1973), although, as described above, it is likely that the hepatic artery is the main source of nutrition of the liver metastases, and the regression noted in these cases may be accounted for in the systemic effects of the cytotoxic agent.

References

Ackerman, N. B. (1974). The blood supply of experimental liver metastases. *Surgery* **75**:589.

Assa, J. (1970). Differential patterns of vasculature to liver tumours. *Br. J. Cancer* **24**:360.

Bevan, P. G. (1973). Cytotoxic perfusion of the liver via the umbilical vein for liver metastases in carcinoma of the colon. *Br. J. Surg.* **60**:369.

Bosniak, M. A., and Phanthumachinda, P. (1966). Value of arteriography in the study of hepatic disease. *Am. J. Surg.* **112**:348.

Edwards, E. A.. Malone, P. D., and MacArthur, J. D. (1975). *Operative Anatomy of the Abdomen and Pelvis.* Lea & Febiger, Philadelphia.

Handley, R. S. (1972). Observations and thoughts of cancer of the breast. *Proc. Royal Soc. Med.* **65**:437–444.

Healey, J. E. (1965). Vascular pattern in human metastastatic liver tumours. *Surg. Gynecol. and Obstet.* **120**:1187.

Michels, N. A. (1960). Newer anatomy of the liver: Variant blood supply and collateral circulation. *JAMA* **172**:125.

Sappey, M. P. C. (1874). *Anatomie, physiologie et pathologie des vaisseaux lymphatiques considérés chez l'homme et les vertébrés.* Paris.

Turner-Warwick, R. T. (1959). The lymphatics of the breast. *Br. J. Surg.* **46**:574–582.

Chapter 3

PHARMACOKINETICS —A PHYSIOLOGICAL FUNCTION OF LUNG

Y. S. BAKHLE

Boyle recognized the "genuine use of Respiration as the Ventilation of the Blood in its passage thorow the Lungs; in which passage it is disburthened of Excrementitious Steams" (Boyle, 1660) and Lower a few years later came to the additional conclusion that "the blood takes in air in its course through the lungs and owes its bright colour entirely to the admixture of air" (Lower, 1669). Ever since then investigations into the function of lung have concentrated on respiratory gas exchange. Only comparatively recently have some nonrespiratory functions of lung, for instance, its ability to act as a reservoir of blood and its ability to filter cellular debris from blood, been recognized and lucidly summarized by Heinemann and Fishman (1969). The newest function of lung to be studied is its ability to alter the biological activity of substances entering the lung either through the airways or, more importantly, through the pulmonary circulation. This ability has been called, for want of a better phrase, the pharmacokinetic function of lung (Bakhle and Vane, 1974), and it is this function that is discussed here.

The first relevant results were provided over 50 years ago by Starling and Verney (1925) as an epiphenomenon during their investigations into

Y. S. Bakhle • Department of Pharmacology, Institute of Basic Medical Sciences, Royal College of Surgeons of England, Lincoln's Inn Fields, London, WC2A 3PN, England.

secretion of urine by the cat isolated kidney. They could not maintain adequate perfusion of the isolated kidney with the cat's own blood unless they included the lungs in their pumped circuit and they postulated the detoxification of a blood vasoconstrictor substance by the lungs as the reason for this necessity. Almost 30 years later, when the blood vasoconstrictor substance had been identified as 5-hydroxytryptamine (5-HT), Gaddum et al. (1953) showed that the biological activity of 5-HT was indeed severely attenuated on passage through isolated lungs perfused with blood. The inactivation of 5-HT in the pulmonary circulation in vivo was later confirmed by Davis and Wang (1965) and Thomas and Vane (1967).

By that time Vane and his colleagues had already demonstrated the ability of the pulmonary circulation in vivo to inactivate hormones as different as noradrenaline, bradykinin, and prostaglandins and to activate angiotensin I by conversion to angiotensin II (for references see Bakhle and Vane, 1974). These experiments were the beginning of a detailed and systematic study of the metabolism of vasoactive hormones in lung. Work with isolated lungs and with subcellular fractions of lung homogenates soon established that the pharmacokinetic properties of the pulmonary circulation in vivo were due to the properties of the lung tissue itself. More recent experiments have demonstrated most elegantly that for noradrenaline (Hughes et al., 1969; Nicholas et al., 1974) and 5-HT (Strum and Junod, 1972; Cross et al., 1974) and for bradykinin and angiotensin I (Ryan et al., 1975) the cells responsible for the metabolic transformations are the endothelial cells of the pulmonary capillaries. These cells, which until now had been considered just as inert linings to the capillaries, have become the locus of highly active enzymic and uptake systems. Furthermore, the large surface area of the pulmonary capillaries which optimizes conditions for gas exchange also optimizes conditions for metabolism of blood-borne substrates by the endothelial cells. However, not all the metabolic functions have been identified with the endothelial cells, and with 40 different cell types in lung, there are still plenty of candidates for the sites of the other reactions.

Table 1 summarizes what is known at present about the types of substrate and their fate in the pulmonary circulation. This is not the place to expound the details of the mechanisms involved in the fate of each substrate; there are now several reviews in which this has been done most adequately (Bakhle and Vane, 1974; Fishman and Pietra, 1974; Junod, 1975). Instead, a few general points about the results summarized in the table are made, before discussing their clinical implications.

On the basis of their fate in the pulmonary circulation, Vane (1969) has classified vasoactive hormones into "local hormones," i.e., those that are essentially excluded from the arterial circulation by inactivation in the pulmonary circulation, such as bradykinin and 5-HT, and "circulating

TABLE 1. Effect of Passage through the Pulmonary Circulation on Biological Activity

Substrate	Activation	Inactivation	No change in activity
Peptides	Angiotensin I	Bradykinin	Angiotensin II Eledoisin: physalemin Oxytocin: vasopressin L Gastrin L Cholecystokinin
Amines		5-Hydroxytryptamine Tryptamine Noradrenaline Phenylethylamine Acetylcholine	α-Methyl-5-hydroxytryptamine Adrenaline: isoprenaline
Prostaglandins	Arachidonic acid Other PG precursors	Prostaglandins of E and F type	Histamine Prostaglandins of A type
Nucleotides		Adenosine monophosphate (AMP) Adenosine triphosphate (ATP)	
Steroids	Cortisone	Testosterone Estrogen Cortisol	
Basic drugs		By absorption Imipramine Chlorcyclizine Amphetamine By metabolism Methadone	

hormones,'' such as adrenaline and angiotensin II which pass freely through the pulmonary circulation and enter the systemic arterial circulation. This distinction is also apparent within classes of substrate. Thus, although noradrenaline is inactivated, adrenaline and isoprenaline pass through the pulmonary circulation without inactivation; angiotensin I is hydrolyzed to angiotensin II, but the product of this reaction, angiotensin II itself, is not hydrolyzed; prostaglandins of the E and F types are metabolized, but prostaglandins of the A type are unchanged. In each case only a small chemical difference ensures a considerable difference in pharmacokinetics.

Together with this specificity there is, as Table 1 shows, a wide range of enzymes present in the lung—peptidases, nucleotidases, monoamine oxidases, and drug and steroid oxidases. However, it has been made very clear that not every enzymic activity exhibited by homogenates of lung will be exhibited by the whole lung toward substrates in the pulmonary circulation. For instance, there are histamine-inactivating enzymes (Bennett, 1965) and angiotensin-II-inactivating enzymes (Bakhle, 1968) to be found in chopped or homogenized lung, but both these substrates pass unchanged through the lung (Hodge *et al.*, 1967; Biron *et al.*, 1969; Boileau *et al.*, 1970; Ferreira *et al.*, 1973). There is clearly an overriding factor, the transport of substrate to enzyme, that controls the fate of any given hormone in the pulmonary circulation and the analysis of this control is providing some of the most fascinating work in progress. This discrepancy between the presence of an enzyme in homogenates and its apparent absence in the whole tissue may be due to an "anatomical" separation of the enzyme from the substrate. For instance, if the histamine-inactivating enzymes are heavily concentrated in cells close to the mast cells where histamine is stored, or near bronchial smooth muscle where histamine acts, then since these are areas predominantly perfused through the bronchial circulation, histamine in the pulmonary circulation will be a relatively long way from the inactivating enzymes. This possibility, it is hoped, will be investigated by histochemical methods which are being devised for the localization of these enzymes in sections of lung. The alternative explanation is that there is a very specific transport mechanism which readily carries one substrate but not another to an intracellular enzyme. This seems to be the explanation for the difference between the fates of adrenaline and noradrenaline, the latter readily metabolized in endothelial cells, as already observed, and the former excluded from the cell because, presumably, the transport system which carries noradrenaline will not accept adrenaline.

Sometimes the pharmacokinetic activity of the lung considered in isolation is considerably less than that of other organs, for instance of the liver. This is particularly true for the metabolism of steroids and drugs.

However, in terms of the overall effect of each organ on the systemic blood level of a substrate, it must be remembered that the liver receives about 20% of the cardiac output whereas 100% of the cardiac output goes through the pulmonary circulation. The lung can therefore compensate for a lower intrinsic level of activity by the greater exposure of that activity to the substrate.

It is emphasized that this pharmacokinetic function is effective at physiological concentrations of substrates and has reserve capacity to deal with sudden increases of substrate; and it is effective, as the early experiments showed, *in vivo* and in all the species investigated, including man. It is not a pharmacological curiosity, but a physiologically significant control mechanism whose importance is still being realized.

There are at least three fascinating aspects of lung pharmacokinetics which can at best reflect a nonphysiological, but a nonetheless real, state; the release of active substances from lung, the binding of drugs to lung, and the whole question of the metabolism of exogenous chemicals entering through the airways. The best known example of release of active substances is the release of histamine, SRS-A, and prostaglandins from the lung during anaphylaxis (Bartosch *et al.*, 1933; Kellaway and Trethewie, 1940; Piper and Vane, 1969). Several other chemical and physical stimuli are known which cause the release of prostaglandin and prostaglandin-like substances from the lung into the systemic arterial circulation. Some of these are discussed later, but it is relevant here to note there is discussion as to whether the release of active substances into the systemic arterial circulation represents the overflow of substances intended only for intrapulmonary effect, or a true endocrine function of lung in which the substances released are designed for an effect on distant structures, e.g., the arterial smooth muscle of the systemic circulation. Tumors in lung seem to be particularly able to secrete hormones (ectopic endocrine syndrome), usually polypeptides; ADH, parathyroid hormone, ACTH, etc. Most of the hormones so secreted are not substrates for pulmonary metabolism and should not concern us here. However, the prevalence of such ectopic endocrine cells in lung tumors does suggest a latent endocrine potential in the lung (Said, 1974).

Drug metabolizing enzymes are present in lung tissue (Bend *et al.*, 1972), and some drugs are indeed metabolized after uptake by the perfused lung (Orton *et al.*, 1973). However, many others are neither metabolized nor taken up into cells, but are avidly removed from the perfusing blood by a process of binding to a readily accessible, but as yet unidentified, component of lung. This process is rapid and dependent on the chemical structure of the drug in so far as strongly basic amines are bound most avidly, and, most important from a therapeutic point of view, the binding is reversible. This property means that, for instance, imipramine already bound to lung can be displaced by chlorpromazine, another basic drug (Junod, 1972). Displacement could also be brought about by a suitably basic drug metabolite produced by the liver. Examples of drugs bound in this way to lung include the tricyclic antidepressants, propranolol and amphetamine (Hayes and Cooper, 1971; Orton *et al.*, 1973).

Although most of the work discussed here deals with the fate of exogenous and endogenous chemicals entering the lung through the pulmonary circulation, some drugs are given by inhalation, usually for their direct effect on bronchial smooth muscle, and many exogenous chemicals are inhaled in the average city air. The fate of an inhaled substrate may be entirely different from its fate in the pulmonary circulation. In one important instance, isoprenaline, which as already noted passes unchanged through the pulmonary circulation (Table 1), is metabolized to at least 30% when it is administered through the airway (Briant *et al.*, 1973). Thus, isoprenaline entering through the airways encounters a different set of cells, transport systems, and enzymes, and this is reflected in its metabolism. It also means that less isoprenaline is available to enter the circulation and cause unwanted side effects on the heart. More recently, steroids have been used in aerosol form to treat asthmatics with less systemic side effects than would result from oral administration. A particularly effective steroid is beclamethasone dipropionate (for references see Martin *et al.*, 1974) and, when administered intratracheally to rat isolated lungs, it is metabolized so rapidly that at 2 min after dosing only 50% is present unchanged and at 5 min only 30% is unchanged (Hartiala *et al.* 1976). Here too, then, entry through the airways seems to expose the substrate to a readily accessible set of enzymes and also perhaps, the lack of systemic side effects is due to the greater metabolism of the steroid *in situ* before it enters the circulation.

The practical implications for various human conditions of some of the reactions shown in the Table 1 are discussed below.

Peptides

One of the recent significant advances in the understanding of the renin–angiotensin system was the discovery of an active angiotensin-I-converting enzyme activity in the pulmonary circulation (Ng and Vane, 1967, 1968). This enzyme, as its name implies, converts inactive decapeptide, angiotensin I, to the highly active pressor octapeptide, angiotensin II, the biological effector of the renin–angiotensin system. This conversion is, therefore, a crucial step in the biological response to the release of renin. Since 1967 there has been a great deal of fundamental research on the properties of pulmonary converting enzyme (see Soffer, 1976), and one of the most important practical results has been the discovery of a potent inhibitor of converting enzyme in the venom of *Bothrops jararaca*, a

Brazilian snake (Ferreira *et al.*, 1970). The effect of such an inhibitor is to prevent the formation of angiotensin II and thus to prevent the biological response to renin release *in vivo*. For instance, in dogs with experimental renal artery constriction, the renin levels in blood rise rapidly, producing a rapid rise in systemic arterial blood pressure. However, treatment with the inhibitor of converting enzyme prevents the rise of blood pressure in spite of high blood levels of renin (Miller *et al.*, 1975). The inhibitor, however, does not affect the response to catecholamines or to other pressor agents.

Renal artery stenosis in man is also associated with high renin levels and hypertension. The converting enzyme inhibitor has been used success-fully as a diagnostic test for high renin hypertension (Gavras *et al.*, 1974). Essentially the inhibitor, now synthesized in the laboratory (Ondetti *et al.*, 1971), is injected intravenously and those patients whose hypertension was due to high levels of renin respond with a fall in blood pressure, whereas those hypertensives with normal renin levels do not respond. This proce-dure is much simpler than measuring renal vein renin and is as reliable in detecting high renin hypertensives. A further possible extension of this inhibition of converting enzyme would be to synthesize an analogue of the inhibitor with a greater duration of action—the present inhibitor has a half-life of about 3.5 h in man (Collier *et al.*, 1973)—and then the hypertension due to renal stenosis could be controlled until the stenosis was corrected surgically.

Another development which has great therapeutic potential is the use of the converting enzyme inhibitor in irreversible hemorrhagic shock (Errington and Rocha e Silva, 1974). Long-lasting hemorrhagic hypotension in dogs led to irreversible hemorrhagic shock, despite retransfusion of the lost blood, and all the untreated dogs died within 24 h of the retransfusion. Pretreatment with the converting enzyme inhibitor gave 100% survival for at least 3 days, i.e., no dog developed irreversible hemorrhagic shock and, more significantly from a therapeutic point of view, administration of the converting enzyme inhibitor at different times *after* hypotension had been established led to survival of at least 50% of the animals. The authors interpreted their results in terms of inhibition of the effects of renin which is known to be released during hemorrhage. Whatever the mechanism, the results are so striking that their significance for the treatment of hemor-rhagic shock in man, a not uncommon occurrence, is clear. More work must urgently be done on this aspect of converting enzyme inhibition.

Amines

The pulmonary inactivation of an amine, 5-HT, was the first example of pulmonary pharmacokinetics to be discovered in experimental animals, and the results obtained with this amine and with noradrenaline in animals are reproduced in man. Gillis and his colleagues (Gillis *et al.*, 1972) have demonstrated that both 5-HT and noradrenaline are removed from the pulmonary circulation in man and that immediately following heart–lung bypass more of each amine is removed. The increase in removal was correlated to the time spent on bypass but the researchers were not able, for technical and ethical reasons, to determine how long increased removal persisted after normal circulation had been restored. These results are some support for the author's long-held belief that much of the postperfusion syndrome is due to the exclusion of the metabolically active lung cells from the circulation and a consequent build-up of toxic substances in blood. A silicone membrane functions more than adequately as a gas-exchange interface, but it has no enzymic properties. However, the techniques of attaching enzymes to solid supports is advancing so rapidly that it should not be long before we are able to include in the bypass circuit a column of the relevant enzymes coupled to resin particles through which the blood could be pumped. The addition of a metabolic capability to the gas-exchange capability would certainly provide a better representation of the lung.

Two other factors shown to influence pulmonary inactivation of amines *in vivo* are pulmonary hypertension and gaseous anesthetics. In patients with pulmonary hypertension amine removal in the pulmonary circulation was higher than in patients with normal pulmonary pressure. Furthermore, when the cause of the pulmonary hypertension was corrected surgically and the pressure returned to normal limits, so did the removal of amine (Gillis *et al.*, 1974). The mechanism of this effect is, as yet, unknown.

The investigations into the basic mechanisms of amine removal and inactivation in lung have shown that the pulmonary endothelial cell membrane has a transport process for noradrenaline and 5-HT. Gaseous anesthetics are thought to have their effect by disrupting the structure of nerve cell membranes so that the ion-transport processes essential for the function of the nerve are hindered or prevented. Since gaseous anesthetics are nonspecific drugs, it was proposed that gaseous anesthetics might interfere with amine transport in the pulmonary endothelial cells (Bakhle and Vane, 1974). This suggestion has been supported by result obtained *in vitro* and *in vivo* (dogs) showing that halothane and nitrous oxide–oxygen mixtures inhibited the pulmonary inactivation of noradrenaline (Naito and Gillis, 1973; Bakhle and Block, 1976). The inactivation of prostaglandin E_2 was, however, not inhibited by halothane, showing that not all the membrane transport processes were affected. The practical significance of this effect of gaseous anesthetics has yet to be fully assessed, but certainly in the case of halothane any increase in the arterial levels of noradrenaline can only add to the factors predisposing to cardiac dysrhythmias.

Prostaglandins

Prostaglandins have been invoked in almost every physiological process but their therapeutic use is confined to their action on the pregnant uterus. The efficacy of prostaglandins given as intravenous infusions to induce labor or abortion has always presented a problem. The doses commonly used, 5–50 μg/ml, would give a concentration of 1–10 ng/ml entering the pulmonary artery (assuming a venous return of 5 liters/min); in man, as in other animals, the inactivation of prostaglandins in the lung is 80% or greater (Jose et al., 1976) which would suggest that no more than 0.2–2.0 ng/ml would reach the arterial circulation and the uterine smooth muscle. This is near or below the threshold of prostaglandin action on nonpregnant uteri. So, theoretically it is unlikely that prostaglandins in the doses administered should have any effect on uterine activity, but practically they are clearly effective. There seem at present to be two parts to an answer to this problem. The first is that the pregnant uterus may be more sensitive to prostaglandins than a nonpregnant uterus. The other part may lie in the biological activity of the metabolites of prostaglandin produced by the lung. These are much less active than the precursor prostaglandin on many smooth muscles, especially vascular smooth muscle, but on uterine smooth muscle at lease one metabolite, 13,14-dihydro-prostaglandin $F_{2\alpha}$, is as active as the parent prostaglandin (Bygdeman et al., 1974). So an action that would seem to inactivate the parent prostaglandins toward several tissues may, in fact, be producing a metabolite with biological activity directed towards a specific tissue. By a combination of these factors then, a greater sensitivity of the pregnant uterus and a more uterus-specific metabolite produced on transit through the pulmonary circulation, we may be able to explain why a mixture of very little prostaglandin and much more metabolite is so effective in stimulating the muscles of the pregnant uterus.

The idea that the pulmonary metabolism of prostaglandins may not merely be the removal of unwanted hormones but a purposeful change in the spectrum of their biological activity receives some support from the investigations into the effects of pregnancy on the pulmonary metabolism of prostaglandins. In rabbits, the vasodepressor responses to intravenous prostaglandin E_2 decreased during pregnancy (Bedwani and Marley, 1975), although the response to intraarterial prostaglandin was unaffected, suggesting an increased metabolism of prostaglandin E_2 in the lung. In homogenates of lungs from pregnant rabbits, the levels of prostaglandin-metabolizing enzymes increased as pregnancy progressed and, near term, the level of prostaglandin dehydrogenase was 20 times the level in nonpregnant animals (Sun and Armour, 1974). Furthermore, the levels of this enzyme in other tissues, liver and spleen, did not increase (Egerton-Vernon and Bedwani, 1975). In all cases the authors have interpreted this increase in the metabolizing capacity of the lung as a protective mechanism to shield the pregnant uterus from prostaglandin, particularly at or near term. It might equally be interpreted as a mechanism designed to produce, at or near term, a larger amount of a specifically oxytocic prostaglandin metabolite. Nevertheless, the change in the pulmonary metabolism is undisputed and so dramatic that it would seem to have some purpose. The question now arises as to whether or not analogous changes occur in human pregnancy and if inadvertent or deliberate interference in this metabolism can change the course of pregnancy or of labor. As an extension of this effect we must ask whether the pseudopregnant state caused by oral contraceptives causes similar changes in prostaglandin metabolism.

Let us consider the less physiological aspects of lung pharmacokinetics, in particular the release from lung of prostaglandin and prostaglandin-like substances induced by a variety of chemical and physical stimuli. Apart from anaphylaxis, the relevance of the other chemical stimuli of release even to pathological states in man is still speculative. What the animal experiments do, however, show is that lung tissue generally is capable of release, and the possibility of such release occurring in man cannot be discounted. For instance, the infusion of high concentrations of 5-HT (0.25–2 μg/ml) through isolated lung of rat and dog induced the release of prostaglandins and other unidentified spasmogens (Alabaster and Bakhle, 1970, 1976). Although such high concentrations of 5-HT are not normal, they are found in patients with carcinoid (Goble et al., 1955). The agents responsible for the carcinoid flush have always presented a problem; 5-HT itself did not seem appropriate and later both bradykinin (Oates and Butler, 1967) and prostaglandin (Sandler et al., 1968) were proposed as the causative agent. However, all three candidates are extensively (>90%) inactivated in the pulmonary circulation, and the flush must be due to an agent in the *arterial* circulation. If, as in the rat and the dog, high concentrations of 5-HT could cause the release of prostaglandin and other spasmogens in man, then even though the amine is itself inactivated, other active substances could be generated and appear in the pulmonary venous blood for distribution throughout the arterial circulation to act, perhaps, as skin vasodilators and produce the flush. The situation could be complicated by the presence of metastases in the lung which might drain directly into the pulmonary circulation and thus produce locally very high concentrations of 5-HT to induce release.

Another possible pathological role for spasmogen release arose from the same set of experiments on 5-HT-induced release. The release was prevented by known 5-HT antagonists like methysergide and, later, by ergotamine (Bakhle and Smith, 1972). The parallel between these results and the postulated involvement of 5-HT in migraine and the antimigraine properties of 5-HT antagonists led Sandler (1972) to propose that an analogous release might occur in migrainous subjects and that the released spasmogens would be the causative agents of the vascular changes in the migraine attack. This hypothesis has had its successes; for instance, tyramine and phenylethylamine, other amines implicated in dietary migraine, could also induce release and other antimigraine drugs will prevent release (Bakhle and Smith, 1972). However, clonidine, effective in some types of migraine, does not prevent release and the concentrations of amines required to produce release are high (0.25–50 μg/ml). Nevertheless, amine-induced release of spasmogen from lung may provide a useful model for antimigraine drugs of a certain type. The existence of a similar capability in human lung can only be determined by experiments on human tissue and has been delayed for that reason.

The physical stimuli inducing prostaglandin release from lung include embolization of the pulmonary circulation, hyperventilation, and hypoxia. Embolization of isolated lungs induces the release of prostaglandins into the lung effluent (Lindsey and Wyllie, 1970; Piper and Vane, 1971) and the release of prostaglandins *in vivo* has been deduced from the effects of aspirin and other similar anti-inflammatory agents which inhibit the synthesis of prostaglandins. The pulmonary vasoconstriction following embolization with platelet aggregates (Rådegran, 1972) or with barium sulfate (Nakano and McCloy, 1973) was abolished after treatment of the animal with aspirin, although physical blockage of the pulmonary capillaries could still be seen. Systemic hypotension often occurs in patients having steel hip-joint replacement when the steel pin is driven into the acrylic cement in the femur (Anonymous, 1974). One explanation of this is that fat cells and marrow fragments are dislodged at this time, enter the venous blood, and embolize the pulmonary circulation producing pulmonary vasoconstriction and systemic hypotension. Support for this hypothesis comes from the observation that the magnitude of the hypotension is reduced in those patients who had been treated with aspirin-like anti-inflammatory drugs before the operation (Modig *et al.*, 1973, 1974). This would certainly be compatible with the results obtained experimentally. If, *in vivo,* as in the isolated lung, prostaglandins of the E type appear in pulmonary venous blood, then they will produce systemic hypotension by their direct action on the peripheral vasculature. The contribution of the direct action of the released prostaglandins to the total fall in blood pressure is difficult to estimate.

Attempts, however, have been made to estimate it in the hypotensive response to hyperventilation in dogs (Said, 1974). In these experiments prostaglandin-like substances were detected in arterial blood during hyperventilation and after the P_{CO_2} in the arterial blood had been corrected to normal levels, about half of the fall in blood pressure remained. This could be abolished by treatment of the animal with aspirin. Similarly, aspirin treatment without adjustment of the CO_2 levels of the blood led to a reduction of about half in the hypotensive response to hyperventilation. From these results it would seem that a considerable portion of the systemic response is due to prostaglandins liberated from lung and it is, therefore, evidence for a definite endocrine function of lung. However, there is still active discussion as to the interpretation of these results and any conclusions that may be drawn from them.

Hypoxic pulmonary vasoconstriction is also accompanied by the release of prostaglandin-like substances, and the pulmonary vasoconstriction and bronchoconstriction *in vivo* in response to hypoxia are attenuated after treatment with aspirin (Said *et al.*, 1974). Whatever the final verdict may be on the endocrine aspects of the prostaglandin release, it is widely agreed that pulmonary responses to these stimuli are due to a great extent to prostaglandins formed in the lung. This statement, however, is not an adequate reflection of the complexity of the situation as the pulmonary responses are mostly due to contraction of smooth muscle, airway or vascular, whereas the prostaglandins appearing in pulmonary venous blood are mostly of the E type which would relax smooth muscle in lung as they do peripherally. Recently this complex situation was further complicated by the identification of a short-lived, highly active intermediate in prostaglandin synthesis which seems to be formed particularly when the lung prostaglandin-synthesizing enzymes are activated (Hamberg *et al.*, 1975). It might be, therefore, that many of the pulmonary responses are due to the short-lived intermediate and the systemic responses due to prostaglandins which are liberated into the arterial circulation.

What is most clearly demonstrated is that the lung is an organ capable of synthesizing and inactivating prostaglandins with apparently equal ease, removing or adding prostaglandins to the blood in the pulmonary circulation in response to stimuli arriving either in the pulmonary blood or through the airways.

Steroids and Basic Drugs

Many of the enzymes that metabolize drugs have as their natural substrates steroid hormones. The existence of steroid receptors in fetal lung (Giannopoulos, 1973; Giannopoulos *et al.*, 1973) and the importance of steroids in lung maturation (Liggins and Howie, 1972) have established the fetal lung as an important target organ for glucocorticoids. Recently, isolated lungs from adult rats were shown to take up the relatively inactive cortisone from the perfusate in the pulmonary circulation and reduce it to the more active cortisol which then reappeared in the lung perfusate (Nicholas and Kim, 1975). Most of the earlier work on steroid metabolism in the perfused lung had disclosed catabolic reactions (Pulkkinen, 1966; Miyabo *et al.*, 1975), but if this recent result can be supported it could be postulated that the lung can activate steroids and "export" them for an effect on peripheral target tissues. This would constitute an activation function of the pulmonary circulation analogous to the activation of angiotensin I by conversion to angiotensin II.

Drugs passing through the pulmonary circulation can be affected in the two ways already mentioned, by uptake and subsequent metabolism and by binding. As far as the drug-metabolizing enzymes in lung are concerned, they seem to be much like the better-described metabolizing enzymes in liver in their cofactor requirements (Bend *et al.*, 1972) and in their development with age (Fouts and Devereux, 1972). They seem, however, to be less readily induced than the liver enzymes (Bernardi *et al.*, 1972). Drug binding in the pulmonary circulation seems to have more obvious relevance to drug pharmacokinetics. The avidity and the reversibility of the binding will serve, firstly, to reduce the peak concentration of such drugs administered intravenously, secondly, to provide a store from which drugs will leak out slowly and, thirdly, to provide a possibility of drug interactions comparable with those already well documented for drugs avidly bound to plasma proteins.

As a general principle the problem of pulmonary inactivation of potential drugs must be kept in mind during drug evaluation procedures (Vane, 1970). Thus, compounds potent *in vitro* can be ineffective *in vivo* because they are largely inactivated, or removed, by the pulmonary circulation, and conversely, resistance to pulmonary inactivation can enhance the *in vivo* potency of a drug if its congeners are susceptible to inactivation. This principle has been clearly demonstrated in the work of Ondetti and Engel (1975) who synthesized an analogue of bradykinin, less potent than bradykinin *in vitro* but more potent *in vivo*. This paradox was resolved by discovering that the analog was less inactivated than bradykinin in the pulmonary circulation (Bakhle, 1976) and the consequently greater concentration of the analogue in the arterial blood more than compensated for its intrinsic lack of potency. Another way of turning pulmonary inactivation to therapeutic advantage would be in the design of bronchodilator drugs given by inhalation. The unacceptable cardiac side effects of isoprenaline led to the search for amines more specifically bronchodilator. An alternative aim would be to find compounds with bronchodilator activity but specifically inactivated in the pulmonary circulation. Such a drug, given by aerosol, would have its action on the bronchial smooth muscle and would then enter the bronchial venous blood and, with the rest of the venous return, pass through the pulmonary circulation before entering the coronary, or any other systemic arterial bed. Thus, even though this amine might have strong cardiac effects, it would be "automatically" inactivated before it arrived at the cardiac receptors. This "automatic" inactivation would also, of course, apply to amine absorption in the gut (90% of an aerosol dose of isoprenaline is swallowed; Blackwell *et al.*, 1974) as that would also pass through the pulmonary circulation, as well as the liver, before entering the arterial circulation.

Conclusion

The above is an overall view of those metabolic reactions of the lung which are capable of affecting the activity of many blood-borne hormones and drugs. This was not intended as an exhaustive review, but as an introduction to some aspects of lung pharmacokinetics which seem at present to have clinical relevance. Interest in lung pharmacokinetics has grown remarkably in the last few years, and the increased interest has been reflected in the growing research output (Junod and de Haller, 1975; Bakhle and Hartiala, 1976). No doubt, next year some of the hypotheses proposed here will be discredited and other aspects brought into a state where they have obvious clinical relevance.

For oncologists, at least three aspects would seem to have special interest—ectopic endocrine secretion by tumors in the lung, metabolism of drugs used in cancer chemotherapy, and the role of lung enzymes in the induction of lung cancer by inhaled carcinogens. The first aspect is relevant to the detection of malignant tissue in lung; an inappropriate level of a peptide hormone, for instance ACTH or ADH, may be the first sign of a tumor at a stage when it can still be treated surgically. Reductions in this level could be used to assess the amount of tumor remaining after treatment and thus the efficacy of the treatment, as is already done in choriocarcinoma. Metabolism of cancer chemotherapeutic agents by the lung has not yet been studied, but if such drugs are metabolized or inactivated by binding, then inhibition of these processes could lead to an increased therapeutic effect. For lung tumors in particular, the reasoning behind the use of inhaled steroids in asthmatic patients which has already been discussed could be applied to the administration of chemotherapeutic agents by inhalation. An increased local effect might be accompanied by diminished systemic side effects, a very real advantage with the potent cytotoxic agents.

The third aspect of lung metabolism relates to carcinogenesis and thus, by extension, to prevention rather than cure of lung tumors. It is now widely accepted that the polycyclic hydrocarbon carcinogens, in tobacco smoke for instance, need to be metabolically altered to the actual carcinogenic molecule. The enzymes needed for this transformation are present and are active in the lung, so that the connection between the inhaled carcinogen and lung cancer might seem to be clearly demonstrated. However, the lung also contains enzymes which convert the active carcinogenic molecules to inactive noncarcinogenic forms. Both these types of enzymes can be induced by the hydrocarbon itself or other enzyme inducers. There are, therefore, two opposing forces, one tending to carcinogenesis and the other protecting against it. Clearly the balance between these forces may be more important than the magnitude of either in isolation and much more information is needed on those factors, external or internal, which may affect this balance.

These remarks are admittedly speculative but they serve to emphasize again the widespread influence of lung pharmacokinetics and to illustrate the ways in which results of basic research could be applied to clinical problems. Now that something is known of the metabolic activities of normal lung, one can start to assess the effects of pathological states on these activities and eventually correlate disturbances in lung pharmacokinetics with the systemic effects of the disease. For the present, it is hoped that some of the author's enthusiasm is conveyed for the lung not as a simple, inert support for gas exchange between two surfaces, but as the locus of a wide range of enzymic and transport processes exerting an essential physiological control over the hormonal content of arterial blood. Perhaps the time has come to suggest that the pharmacokinetic function of the lung should no longer be described as a nonrespiratory function, but rather that gas exchange should be referred to as a nonpharmacokinetic function.

References

Alabaster, V. A., and Bakhle, Y. S. (1970). The release of biologically active substances from isolated lungs by 5-hydroxytryptamine and tryptamine. *Br. J. Pharmacol.* **40**:582–583P.

Alabaster, V. A., and Bakhle, Y. S. (1976). Release of smooth muscle contracting substances from isolated perfused lungs. *Eur. J. Pharmacol.* **35**:349–360.

Anonymous (1974). Acrylic cement and the cardiovascular system. Summary of report of working party on acrylic cement in orthopaedic surgery. *Lancet* **II**:1002–1004.

Bakhle, Y. S. (1968). Conversion of angiotensin I to angiotensin II by cell-free extracts of dog lung. *Nature (London)* **220**:919–921.

Bakhle, Y. S. (1976). The nature of the bradykinin inactivating system in isolated lungs. *Br. J. Pharmacol.* **56**:349–350P.

Bakhle, Y. S., and Block, A. J. (1976). Effects of halothane on pulmonary inactivation of noradrenaline and prostaglandin E_2 in anaesthetized dogs. *Clin. Sci. Mol. Med.* **50**:87–90.

Bakhle, Y. S., and Hartiala, J. (1976). The pharmacokinetic function of lung. *Proceedings of International Symposium at Turku, 1975. Agents and Actions.* **6**:493–559.

Bakhle, Y. S., and Smith, T. W. (1972). Release of spasmogenic substances induced by vasoactive amines from rat lungs. *Br. J. Pharmacol.* **46**:543–544P.

Bakhle, Y. S., and Vane, J. R. (1974). Pharmacokinetic function of the pulmonary circulation. *Physiol. Rev.* **54**:1007–1045.

Bartosch, R., Feldberg, W., and Nagel, E. (1933). Weitere Versuche über das Freiwerden eines histaminähnlichen Stoffes aus der durchströmten Lunge sensibilisieter Meerschweinchen beim Anlösen einer anaphylaktischen Lungenstarre. *Arch. für Physiol.* **231**:616–629.

Bedwani, J. R., and Marley, P. B. (1975). Enhanced inactivation of prostaglandin E_2 by the rabbit lung during pregnancy or progesterone treatment. *Br. J. Pharmacol.* **53**:547–554.

Bend, J. R., Hook, G. E. R., Easterling, R. E., Gram, T. E., and Fouts, J. R. (1972). A comparative study of the hepatic and pulmonary microsomal mixed-function oxidase systems in the rabbit. *J. Pharmacol. Exp. Ther.* **183**:206–217.

Bennett, A. (1965). The metabolism of histamine by guinea-pig and rat lung *in vitro*. *Brit. J. Pharmacol.* **24**:147–155.

Bernardi, M. de, Ferrara, A., and Manzo, L. (1972). Aspetti del farmacometabolismo polmonare nel coniglio adulto. *Boll. Soc. Ital. Biol. Sper.* **48**:102–105.

Biron, P., Campeau, L., and David, P. (1969). Fate of angiotensin I and II in the human pulmonary circulation. *Am. J. Cardiol.* **24**:544–547.

Blackwell, E. W., Briant, R. H., Connolly, M. E., Davies, D. S., and Dollery, C. T. (1974). Metabolism of isoprenaline after aerosol and direct intrabronchial administration in man and dog. *Br. J. Pharmacol.* **50**:587–591.

Boileau, J.-C., Campeau, L., and Biron, P. (1970). Pulmonary fate of histamine, isoproterenol, physalaemin and substance P. *Can. J. Physiol. Pharmacol.* **48**:681–684.

Boyle, R. (1660). New experiments physico-mechanicall, touching the spring of the air and its effects (made for the most part in a new pneumatical engine), pp. 350–352. H. Hall, Oxford.

Briant, R. H., Blackwell, E. W., Williams, F. M., Davies, D. S., and Dollery, C. T. (1973). The metabolism of sympathomimetic bronchodilator drugs by the isolated perfused dog lung. *Xenobiotica* **3**:787–799.

Bygdeman, M., Green, K., Toppozada, M., Wiqvist, N., and Bergström, S. (1974). The in fluence of prostaglandin metabolites on the uterine response to $PGF_{2\alpha}$. A clinical and pharmacokinetic study. *Life Sci.* **14**:521–531.

Collier, J. G., Robinson, B. F., and Vane, J. R. (1973). Reduction of the pressor effects of angiotensin I in man by synthetic nonapeptide (BPP_{9a} or SQ 20881) which inhibits converting enzyme. *Lancet* **I**:72–74.

Cross, S. A. M., Alabaster, V. A., Bakhle, Y. S., and Vane, J. R. (1974). Sites of uptake of ^{3}H-5-hydroxytryptamine in rat isolated lung. *Histochemistry* **39**:83–91.

Davis, R. B., and Wang, Y. (1965). Rapid pulmonary removal of 5-hydroxytryptamine in the intact dog. *Proc. Soc. Exp. Biol. Med.* **118**:799–800.

Egerton-Vernon, J. M., and Bedwani, J. R. (1975). Prostaglandin 15-hydroxydehydrogenase activity during pregnancy in rabbits and rats. *Eur. J. Pharmacol.* **33**:405–408.

Errington, M. L., and Rocha e Silva, M., Jr. (1974). On the role of vasopressin and angiotensin in the development of irreversible haemorrhagic shock. *J. Physiol.* **242**:119–141.

Ferreira, S. H., Greene, L. J., Alabaster, V. A., Bakhle, Y. S., and Vane, J. R. (1970). Activity of various fractions of Bradykinin Potentiating Factor against angiotensin I converting enzyme. *Nature (London)* **225**:379–380.

Ferreira, S. H., Ng, K. K. F., and Vane, J. R. (1973). The continuous bioassay of the release and disappearance of histamine in the circulation. *Br. J. Pharmacol.* **49**:543–553.

Fishman, A. P., and Pietra, G. G. (1974). Handling of bioactive materials by the lung. *N. Engl. J. Med.* **291**:884–890, 953–959.

Fouts, J. R., and Devereux, T. R. (1972). Developmental aspects of hepatic and extrahepatic drug metabolizing enzyme systems, microsomal enzymes and components in rabbit liver and lung during the first month of life. *J. Pharmacol. Exp. Ther.* **183**:458–468.

Gaddum, J. H., Hebb, C. O., Silver, A., and Swan, A. A. B. (1953). 5-Hydroxytryptamine. Pharmacological action and destruction in perfused lungs. *Q. J. Exp. Physiol.* **38**:255–262.

Gavras, H., Brunner, H. R., Laragh, J. H., Sealey, J. E., Gavras, I., and Vukovich, R. A. (1974). An angiotensin converting enzyme inhibitor to identify and treat vasoconstrictor and volume factors in hypertensive patients. *N. Engl. J. Med.* **291**:817–821.

Giannopoulos, G. (1973). Glucocorticoid receptors in lung. I. Specific binding of glucocorticoids to cytoplasmic components of rabbit fetal lung. *J. Biol. Chem.* **248**:3876–3883.

Giannopoulos, G., Mulay, S., and Solomon, S. (1973). Glucocorticoid receptors in lung. II. Specific binding of glucocorticoids to nuclear components of rabbit lung. *J. Biol. Chem.* **248**:5016–5023.

Gillis, C. N., Cronau, L. H., Greene, N. M., and Hammond, G. L. (1974). Removal of 5-hydroxytryptamine and norepinephrine from the pulmonary vascular space of man: Influence of cardiopulmonary bypass and pulmonary arterial pressure on these processes. *Surgery* **76**:608–616.

Gillis, C. N., Greene, N. M., Cronau, L. H., and Hammond, G. L. (1972). Pulmonary extraction of 5-hydroxytryptamine and norepinephrine before and after cardiopulmonary bypass in man. *Circ. Res.* **30**:666–674.

Goble, A. J., Hay, D. R., and Sandler, M. (1955). 5-Hydroxytryptamine metabolism in acquired heart disease associated with argentaffin carcinoma. *Lancet* **ii**:1016–1017.

Hamberg, M., Svensson, J., and Samuelsson, B. (1975). Thromboxanes, a new group of biologically active compounds derived from prostaglandin endoperoxides. *Proc. Nat. Acad. Sci. USA* **72**:2994–2998.

Hartiala, J., and Nienstedt, W. (1976). Metabolism of testosterone by human lung *in vitro*. *Int. J. Biochem.* **7**:317–319.

Hartiala, J., Uotila, P., and Nienstedt, W. (1976). Absorption and metabolism of steroids administered intratracheally to rat isolated lungs. *Br. J. Pharmacol.* **57**:442 P.

Hayes, A., and Cooper, R. G. (1971). Studies on the absorption, distribution and excretion of propranolol in rat, dog and monkey. *J. Pharmacol. Exp. Ther.* **176**:302–311.

Heinemann, H. O., and Fishman, A. P. (1969). Nonrespiratory functions of mammalian lung. *Physiol. Rev.* **49**:1–47.

Hodge, R. L., Ng, K. K. F., and Vane, J. R. (1967). Disappearance of angiotensin from the circulation of the dog. *Nature (London)* **215**:138–141.

Hughes, J., Gillis, C. N., and Bloom, F. E. (1969). The uptake and disposition of *dl*-noradrenaline in perfused rat lung. *J. Pharmacol. Exp. Ther.* **169**:237–248.

Jose, P., Niederhauser, U., Piper, P. J., Robinson, C., and Smith, A. P. (1976). Inactivation of prostaglandin $F_{2\alpha}$ in the human pulmonary circulation. *Br. J. Clin. Pharmacol.* **3**:342–343 P.

Junod, A. F. (1972). Accumulation of ^{14}C-imipramine in isolated perfused rat lung. *J. Pharmacol. Exp. Ther.* **183**:182–187.

Junod, A. F. (1975). Metabolism production and release of hormones and mediators in the lung. *Am. Rev. Respir. Dis.* **112**:93–108.

Junod, A. F., and de Haller, R. (1975). Lung metabolism *(Proceedings of the V International Symposium at Davos, 1974)*. Academic Press, New York/London.

Kellaway, C. H., and Trethewie, E. R. (1940). The liberation of a slow reacting smooth muscle stimulating substance in anaphylaxis. *Q. J. Exp. Physiol.* **30**:121–145.

Liggins, G. C., and Howie, R. N. (1972). A controlled trial of antepartum glucocorticoid treatment for prevention of the respiratory distress syndrome in premature infants. *Pediatrics* **50**:515–525.

Lindsey, H. E., and Wyllie, J. H. (1970). Release of prostaglandins from embolized lungs. *Br. J. Surg.* **57**:738–741.

Lower, R. (1669). *Tractatus de Corde Item de Motu & Colore Sanguinis et Chyli in Eum Transitu*, Vol. XVI, p. 220. J. Allestry, London.

Martin, L. E., Tanner, R. J. N., Clarke, T. J. H., and Cochrane, G. M. (1974). Absorption and metabolism of orally administered beclomethasone dipropionate. *Clin. Pharmacol. Ther.* **15**:267–275.

Miller, E. D., Jr., Samuels, A. I., Haber, E., and Barger, A. C. (1975). Inhibition of angiotensin-conversion and prevention of renal hypertension. *Am. J. Physiol.* **228**:448–453.

Miyabo, S., Kishida, S., and Hisada, T. (1975). Metabolism and conjugation of 20β-dihydrocortisol by various dog tissues *in vitro*. *J. Steroid Biochem.* **6**:143–146.

Modig, J., Busch, C., Olerud, S., and Saldeen, T. (1974). Pulmonary microembolism during orthopaedic trauma. *Acta Anaesthesiol. Scand.* **18**:133–143.

Modig. J., Olerud, S., and Malmberg, P. (1973). Sudden pulmonary dysfunction in prosthetic hip replacement surgery. *Acta Anaesthesiol. Scand.* **17**:276–282.

Naito, H., and Gillis, C. N. (1973). Effects of halothane and nitrous oxide on removal of noradrenaline from the pulmonary circulation. *Anesthesiology* **39**:575–580.

Nakano, J., and McCloy, R. B., Jr. (1973). Effects of indomethacin on the pulmonary vascular and airway resistance responses to pulmonary microembolization. *Proc. Soc. Exp. Biol. Med.* **143**:218–221.

Ng, K. K. F., and Vane, J. R. (1967). The conversion of angiotensin I to angiotensin II. *Nature (London)* **216**:762–766.

Ng, K. K. F., and Vane, J. R. (1968). Fate of angiotensin I in the circulation. *Nature (London)* **218**:144–150.

Nicholas, T. E., and Kim, P. A. (1975). The metabolism of ^{3}H-cortisone and ^{3}H-cortisol by the isolated perfused rat and guinea pig lungs. *Steroids* **25**:387–402.

Nicholas, T. E., Strum, J. M., Angelo, L. S., and Junod, A. F. (1974). Site and mechanism of uptake of ^{3}H-1-norepinephrine by isolated perfused rat lungs. *Circ. Res.* **35**:670–680.

Oates, J. A., and Butler, T. C. (1967). Pharmacologic and endocrine aspects of carcinoid syndrome. *Adv. Pharmacol.* **5**:109–128.

Ondetti, M. A., and Engel, S. L. (1975). Bradykinin analogs containing β-homo-amino acids. *J. Med. Chem.* **18**:761–763.

Ondetti, M. A., Williams, N. J., Sabo, E. F., Plušcec, J., Weaver, E. R., and Kocy, O. (1971). Angiotensin converting enzyme inhibitors from the venom of *Bothrops jararaca*. Isolation, elucidation of structure and synthesis. *Biochemistry* **10**:4033–4039.

Orton, T. C., Anderson, M. W., Pickett, R. D., Eling, T. E., and Fouts, J. R. (1973). Xenobiotic accumulation and metabolism by isolated perfused rabbit lungs. *J. Pharmacol. Exp. Ther.* **186**:482–497.

Piper, P. J., and Vane, J. R. (1969). Release of additional factors in anaphylaxis and its antagonism by anti-inflammatory drugs. *Nature (London)* **223**:29–35.

Piper, P. J., and Vane, J. R. (1971). The release of prostaglandins from lung and other tissues. *Ann. N. Y. Acad. Sci.* **180**:363–385.

Pulkkinen, M. O. (1966). Sulphate conjugation during pregnancy and under the influence of cortisone. *Acta Physiol. Scand.* **66**:120–122.

Rådegran, K. (1972). The effect of acetylsalicylic acid on the peripheral and pulmonary vascular responses to thrombin. *Acta Anaesthesiol. Scand.* **16**:140–146.

Ryan, J. W., Ryan, U. S., Schultz, D. R., Whitaker, C., Chung, A., and Dorer, F. E. (1975). Subcellular localization of pulmonary angiotensin-converting enzyme (kininase II). *Biochem. J.* **146**:497–499.

Said, S. I. (1974). Endocrine role of lung in disease. *Am. J. Med.* **57**:453–465.

Said, S. I., Yoshida, T., Kitamura, S., and Vreim, C. (1974). Pulmonary alveolar hypoxia: Release of prostaglandins and other humoral mediators. *Science* **185**:1181–1182.

Sandler, M. (1972). Migraine—a pulmonary disease? *Lancet* I:618–619.

Sandler, M., Karim, S. M. M., and Williams, E. D. (1968). Prostaglandins in amine-peptide-secreting tumors. *Lancet* II:1053–1054.

Soffer, R. L. (1976) Angiotensin converting enzyme. *Am. Rev. Biochem.* 73–94.

Starling, E. H., and Verney, E. B. (1925). The secretion of urine as studied on the isolated kidney. *Proc. Royal Soc., London* **Series B 97**:321–363.

Strum, J. M., and Junod, A. F. (1972). Radioautographic demonstration of 5-hydroxytryptamine-^{3}H uptake by pulmonary endothelial cells. *J. Cell Biol.* **54**:456–467.

Sun, F. F., and Armour, S. B. (1974). Prostaglandin 15-hydroxy dehydrogenase and Δ^{13}-reductase levels in the lungs of maternal, fetal and neonatal rabbits. *Prostaglandins* 7:327–338.

Thomas, D. P., and Vane, J. R. (1967). 5-Hydroxytryptamine in the circulation of the dog. *Nature (London)* **216**:335–338.

Vane, J. R. (1969). The release and fate of vasoactive hormones in the circulation. *Br. J. Pharmacol.* **35**:209–242.

Vane, J. R. (1970). The alteration or removal of vasoactive substances by the pulmonary circulation. In *Importance of fundamental principles in drug evaluation*. D. H. Tedeschi and R. E. Tedeschi, eds., pp. 217–236. Raven Press, New York.

PATHOLOGICAL ASPECTS
CONCEPTS IN TUMOR PATHOLOGY FOR THE SURGEON

A. A. SHIVAS

The surgeon of today is quickly coming to regard malignant diseases, and the role of surgery in treatment, very differently from his predecessor of even a decade ago. He no longer sees his work as the operative removal of every tumor cell, thereby producing a surgical cure of the disease. This reorientated approach has resulted not so much from the acquisition of new knowledge about cancer and its biology as from the reiteration of information which has long been available, but to varying degrees ignored, possibly because the implications were unpalatable. The cherished idea, as old as tumor surgery itself, that "early" excision of a malignant tumor, or sufficiently radical procedures in more advanced lesions, can in themselves offer cure to the patient, dies hard. With it there went an overreadiness to ascribe to surgical extirpation any long-term, symptom-free survival, further accorded the status of a "cure" at an interval as short as 5 years. It is many years since the tiny, elusive, or occasionally even undemonstrable bronchial carcinoma, with gross and widespread metastases, pointed clearly to the fact that hematogenous dissemination can occur when a primary neoplasm is very small, whether or not such dimension implies an "early" lesion in the biological or chronological sense. More recently it has become evident that this dissemination is not merely possible, but usual,

A. A. Shivas • University of Edinburgh Medical School, Edinburgh, Scotland.

and a surgical attack on these tumors is now much less common. With the steady accumulation of data for tumors of less aggressive biological behavior, such as carcinoma of the breast, necessarily involving longer periods of clinical "follow-up," it seems that the principle so clearly seen in carcinoma of the bronchus has wide, probably universal, applicability to malignant neoplasms. In a survey of 103 cases of breast carcinoma (Shivas and Douglas, 1972), with special reference to the prognostic significance of elastosis in this neoplasm, it was striking that, while those patients whose tumors showed marked elastosis enjoyed very long postoperative survivals, with a mean of almost 8 years and a maximum of about 20 years, they nevertheless succumbed ultimately to distant, blood-borne, metastases, the "seeds" of which must, therefore, have been present at the time of operation, *or even earlier.* Their fate was sealed just as surely and by the same mechanism as in those patients with nonelastotic tumors, whose survival was short, sometimes only a few months and with a mean value of under 3 years. All were identically treated; all died from metastatic disease, and the conclusion is thus inescapable that hematogenous dissemination at, or possibly before, the time of operation is the general rule, for all practical purposes. It would seem that the principle of "biological predeterminism," the innate biological aggressiveness of each individual tumor as the prognostic characteristic, determines the outcome *ab initio* in an inexorable way. Naturally, whether the course of a malignant disease be long or short, should it present to the clinician when a substantial part of it has already elapsed, the length of interval to the appearance of metastases is proportionately reduced. Large differences between individual survivals within a group are thus easily understood. Entirely in accord with the foregoing has been the failure to show that "early" or "earlier" diagnosis confers a better outlook in breast carcinoma. In short, a great weight of evidence points, in surgery for malignant diseases generally, to a strong analogy with "locking the stable door after the horse has bolted."

From this central concept there emerge practical considerations in principles of tumor management. It is clearly logical to excise malignant tumors locally, and the clinical features commonly dictate such a course; it remains equally logical to excise adjacent tissue at risk, as part of a "field change" which might subsequently give rise to local recurrence. The logical extent of such excision, however, may be very much more difficult to determine, and more radical procedures demand a most searching scrutiny of their justification. As in so many problems the real difficulty is not "how" but "how much." Where a long-established and generally accepted operation exists, such as local mastectomy, the problem may thereby be conveniently disposed of, if not solved. But other situations may pose much more searching questions. Where, for example, a diagnosis of malignant melanoma has been made in a skin lesion by frozen section histology, generally a fairly straightforward exercise, despite some statements to the contrary and an assurance of complete excision given by the pathologist, a surgeon will commonly proceed to excise a substantial further margin of surrounding skin. This frequently necessitates skin grafting, and it is thus mandatory to consider to what extent the procedure benefits the patient. In terms of its very well-documented biological behavior the malignant melanoma fits, perhaps best of all tumors, the concept outlined in the opening paragraph. Here we are dealing with the neoplastic analogue of the melanoblast, a cell whose *normal* biological behavior in the embryo involves *movement* in the tissues, and again in the formation of the benign pigmented nevus, which is, of course, a hamartoma and not a neoplasm of any kind. It is less than surprising that such cells, having undergone malignant transmutation, should exhibit very great potential for invasive growth and the establishment of metastases, both lymphatic and hematogenous. Such lesions are commonly visible from their earliest beginnings, being in a site easily accessible to observation by patient and surgeon alike, yet it is well known that, however small the lesion and early the surgical intervention, it is often too late as judged by the appearance of distant metastases, sometimes after a latent period of many years. In consequence, radical ablative surgery aimed at achieving a complete cure is performed much less today than formerly. It thus becomes very difficult to see any real value, where local excision of the lesion has been complete, in excising a further margin of skin. It is certainly impossible to set any logical limit on the extent of such a procedure. When the added problem of grafting is taken into account its validity becomes even more questionable. This is not to deny that in such further excisions a small nidus of tumor growth is very occasionally demonstrated histologically, with the implication of inevitable local recurrence. But equally, that finding in itself suggests that other deposits are present beyond the scope of even the second excision, and it can scarcely be claimed that the risk of local recurrence is thereby obviated.

Having referred to lymphatic and hematogenous dissemination of tumor it is appropriate to examine another long-cherished dictum of great significance to the surgeon. The notion that lymph node metastases in carcinoma occur "early," while blood-borne metastases appear "late," is at least as firmly established as the endeavor to achieve surgical removal of every tumor cell. By the same evidence which invalidates the one, the other is similarly invalidated. It is obvious that since tumor cells are commonly if not invariably present at distant sites at the time of operation, they may well be there when, on histological examination of lymph nodes from the excised specimen, there is no evidence of involvement, or perhaps microscopic foci only. It would appear that lymph node invasion may become evident sooner, but that it does not occur earlier. The ambiguities in clinical assessment of enlarged lymph nodes resulting from nonspecific "reactive" changes are too well known to require repetition. Distant, blood-borne metastases must reach substantial dimensions frequently before symptoms arise, and, indeed, must be of considerable size to permit demonstration by even the most modern scanning techniques.

The surgeon is faced with something of a dilemma in deciding upon his most useful contribution, for some of the factors influencing his conclusions are contradictory, or even diametrically opposed! In the examples so far considered it is clear that surgical cure, taken to mean the removal of every tumor cell, is scarcely a rational objective. It does not follow, however, in tumors of lesser biological aggressiveness, of relatively indolent behavior, such as squamous carcinoma of the skin, that cure by surgical excision is not possible; the more so since such lesions may be correctly diagnosed at what probably is, in reality, an early stage, due to their site. With other neoplasms, local excision, possibly with adjacent tissue which might constitute a "field of growth," is obviously logical, as mentioned previously, but beyond this point great uncertainties arise. Since no form of local or focal treatment will normally be successful once dissemination occurs, it follows that only systemic therapy, with the use of antitumor agents, can offer the prospect of long-term control or possibly cure. This might at first sight appear to indicate only minimal surgery, but it is generally agreed that the fewer the tumor cells to be treated, the greater the chance of success. Accordingly, the more extensive the surgery, provided that the tissue excised in addition to the tumor and any adjacent "field" *does* contain tumor, the better the prospect for the patient. Such material, however, will frequently comprise a dissection of lymph nodes and related connective tissue and another imponderable factor of immune mechanisms is then introduced. It is doubtful whether, at the time of writing, knowledge is sufficient to permit logical deduction; all that can be done is to point out that if lymph nodes which may harbor tumor cells must remain in the body to exercise a possible immune antitumor role, then the ideal requirements for systemic chemotherapy cannot also be met: The concepts are mutually exclusive.

Having examined the more practical aspects of metastatic tumor growth as they involve the surgeon, it is now appropriate to consider some of the more basic elements in this process. Every metastasis grows from a tumor embolus, yet not every tumor embolus becomes a metastasis. On the fate of those which fail to survive we are relatively well informed; most, apparently, are overwhelmed by thrombus formation. Regarding the survival of those which are later to become metastases, however, we are profundly ignorant. There can be no doubt that a metastasis can grow only if it acquires a blood supply, which itself must also grow *pari passu* with the neoplastic deposit. Since so many tumor emboli fail to make this biological transition, it must surely constitute the crucial point of metastatic tumor growth. It is well known that the distribution of metastases in the body in malignant diseases generally is not explicable on a purely anatomical basis, taking account of blood supply, characteristics of microcirculation, and such factors as the contractility of skeletal and cardiac muscle. Refuge is provided to some extent by the "seed and soil" theory, which is no more than a hypothesis to the effect that particular tissues provide favorable conditions of growth for particular tumor cells, an analogy derived largely from the culture techniques of microbiology. It may well have some validity, but it is at least equally possible that the facility with which circulatory connection is established may explain apparent anomalies of metastatic tumor distribution.

There is certainly good evidence that tumor circulation is abnormal, both morphologically and hemodynamically. The former provides the means whereby the diagnostic radiologist, using contrast medium, can commonly recognize the peculiarities of form of tumor vasculature; the latter is most easily and immediately grasped by considering the situation in intracranial tumors. No matter how high the intracranial pressure may become, the circulation to the neoplasm is never significantly embarrassed; it continues, if untreated, to grow, ultimately causing the death of the patient. This can only imply a considerable capillary/venous hypertension, however this may be mediated. Similarly, there is evidence that tumor growth is sensitive to the arterial pressure which must constitute the "input pressure" to tumor circulation. Autopsy studies in tissues having a dual circulation, the lungs and liver, both common sites of metastatic tumor growth, have shown that tumor deposits are vascularized almost entirely, if not exclusively, from the high-pressure arterial vessels—the bronchial and hepatic arteries, respectively. Experimentally, the Brown–Pearce carcinoma implanted in rabbit liver shows the same phenomenon; injection studies using neoprene latex yield a cast of the weird and bizarre tumor vessels when injection is through the hepatic artery, while the portal venous route gives only a "filling defect" at the site of the implanted tumor (Shivas and Gillespie, 1969). It would seem that tumor hemodynamics are dependent on high arterial "input" pressure and that the peculiarities of tumor circulation are as basic and integral a characteristic of the neoplastic state as any other of its biological modifications. At the clinical level, it may well be that much of the firmness on palpation, so typical a feature of tumor, is contributed by the turgidity associated with capillary/venous hypertension. Of course, the standard explanation of firm consistency is the high proportion of fibrous tissue found in scirrhous carcinoma of the breast, and indeed it may well be true of that specific example. But tumors having so large a component of fibrous tissue are otherwise rare. Experimentally, nodules of Brown–Pearce carcinoma, a tumor having minimal stroma, which are very firm on palpation at operation, are commonly much less easy to feel after death of the animal and arrest of the circulation. Some observers have noted a similar change occurring postmortem in the human subject.

There is little doubt that the concept of "stromal reaction" has not helped to stimulate inquiry into tumor circulation. It will be recalled that this concept holds the connective tissue component of tumors, which, of course, includes the vasculature, to be nonneoplastic and not an integral part of the tumor growth. The stroma of the tumor is regarded as some form of variable proliferative "reaction" by the normal connective tissues of the site of origin of the tumor to its presence there. Breast carcinoma has always been taken as the classical example, with "scirrhous" and "encephaloid" tumors illustrating the range of "reaction." There was thus no reason to suppose that any abnormality would exist in tumor circulation, and, indeed, every reason to suppose that it would be in all respects normal. For the concept of "stromal reaction," so long accepted as to have acquired axiomatic status, there has never been any real evidence, and there is now evidence that it is invalid.

Investigating the origins of the elastica so often a feature of breast carcinoma, using electron microscopy, it became clear that the material was derived from the tumor cells, i.e., the neoplastic epithelial cells, there being indeed no connective tissue cells which might otherwise account for its presence. More significantly, the elastica was found to show minor admixtures of collagen (Douglas and Shivas, 1974). This prompted examination of typical "scirrhous" carcinomata which were found to be completely devoid of any normal connective tissue, the material seen on light microscopy being an ill-organized heterogeneous mixture of elastica, collagen, reticulin, and other elements possibly representing precursors. Normal connective tissue cells such as fibroblasts were entirely absent, and the morphology, in any case, again indicated clearly the origin of these elements from the tumor cells (Shivas and Mackenzie, 1974). The evidence thus suggests very strongly that "stromal reaction" is a misconception and that both elements of a tumor, "parenchyma" and "stroma" alike, are integral parts of the neoplasm. A fundamental reappraisal of our ideas regarding epithelial tumor growth seems necessary, coupled with further, similar investigation of other tumors. In terms of basic tumor pathology, the elaboration of elastica and collagen by neoplastic epithelial cells can well be regarded as examples of "anomalous function" in tumor cells, differing from the earlier recognized endocrine and paraendocrine phenomena, only in that they give rise to a visible product. More basic still is the concept that under conditions of malignant neoplasia, the distinction between epithelial cells and connective tissue cells dwindles greatly, if not indeed to vanishing point. Returning to the matter of tumor vasculature it becomes clear that abnormal morphology and abnormal hemodynamics are allied to neoplastic cells of origin.

No consideration of tumor circulation could be deemed respectable without scrutiny of another long-cherished but equally dubious concept of traditional tumor pathology, namely that focal necrosis, so common a feature of malignancy, results from "the tumor outgrowing its blood supply." How this phenomenon is mediated is far from clear; of many experts asked, none has so far provided a satisfactory, or for that matter any explanation! Since it is so often a hemorrhagic necrosis, akin to that found in venous infarction, it seems most probably that it results from focal occlusion of venous return, possibly due to collapse of a vessel in what must surely be a precarious circulatory mechanism, if function in any way parallels morphology. Bearing in mind the apparent sensitivity to arterial "input" pressure of tumor growth it may well be that fluctuations, particularly hypotensive episodes, could precipitate these foci of necrosis. To conclude on an optimistic note, it seems not improbable that systemic hypotension, produced by the standard techniques of the anesthetist, might induce substantial foci of necrosis. Such a maneuver could scarcely be expected to result in cure of a tumor, but it might be possible to keep the volume of tumor tissue in check. Further, since it would amount only to an intensification of a process which occurs as a natural event, the acquisition of resistance to it by the tumor cells is unlikely. It would seem at least worth a trial. The trick, if it worked, could be repeated as necessary.

References

Douglas, J. G., and Shivas, A. A. (1974). The origins of elastica in breast carcinoma. *J. Royal Coll. Surg. Edinburgh* **19**:89–93.

Shivas, A. A., and Douglas, J. G. (1972). The prognostic significance of elastosis in breast carcinoma. *J. Royal Coll. Surg. Edinburgh* **17**:315–320.

Shivas, A. A., and Gillespie, W. J. (1969). The vascularisation of Brown-Pearce carcinoma implanted in rabbit liver. *Br. J. Cancer* **xxiii**:638.

Shivas, A. A. and Mackenzie, A. (1974). The origins of stromal reaction in breast carcinoma. *J. Royal Coll. Surg. Edinburgh* **19**:345–350.

Recommended Reading

(1) Willis, R. A. (1973). *The Spread of Tumours in the Human Body,* 3rd Ed. Butterworth, London.

(2) Walter, J. B., and Israel, M. S. (1974) *General Pathology.* 4th Ed. Churchill Livingstone, Edinburgh/London.

(3) Stuart, A. E., Smith, A. N. and Samuel, E. (1975). *Applied Surgical Pathology.* Blackwell, Oxford.

PATHOLOGICAL ASPECTS
SELECTED TOPICS IN TUMOR PATHOLOGY

ARNOLD LEVENE

The pathological background of surgical diseases is for the most part regional in its scope, especially in the context of malignant diseases. All those gross and microscopic changes which are productive of symptoms, signs, and operative findings are the province of surgical pathology which is par excellence a practical combination of the science and art of pathology and integral to sound surgical diagnosis and treatment.

The literature of the subject in English is ample,* but these sources of

---

*A basic library strongly leaning toward malignant diseases would contain a brief authoritative general text: Ackerman's *Surgical Pathology* is recommended, and must include the series of monographs issued by the American Armed Forces Institute of Pathology, the deservedly acclaimed *Atlas of Tumor Pathology* which, in continuation, is constantly kept up to date, successive issues often being completely rewritten, or at least extensively revised. They should be complemented by regular reading of the journal *Cancer* and the A.M.A. *Archives* in the various medical and surgical specialties among the general surgical literature. In Britain, there are useful contributions in the *Journal of Clinical Pathology* and occasionally in *The British Journal of Cancer*. As an introduction to the whole subject of neoplasia Willis's *Pathology of Tumours* is unrivaled for content, style, accuracy, and bibliography. For tumors of the head and neck, the textbook of that title by Batsakis is excellent. Other recommended texts are in the list of references.

Arnold Levene • Consultant Pathologist, The Royal Marsden Hospital, Fulham Road, London, SW3 6JJ, England.

knowledge are not enough. True comprehension comes from correlation of the operative findings with the subsequently dissected specimen and its histological study. Because of increasing demands on the surgeons' time a generation has emerged which with outstanding exceptions has acquired an uncertain grasp of surgical pathology in comparison with its teachers and cannot usefully study a microscopic preparation nor discuss or query a written pathology report. The remainder of this chapter, while no substitute for the reading of good standard texts or the practical study of the subject, is an attempt to circumvent a lamentable hiatus by dealing with some aspects of the surgical pathology of tumors which in the author's experience are generally misunderstood.

The relationship of surgeon and pathologist should be one of mutual education, and it is helpful if they study the tissue together, in clinic, operation theater, or laboratory whenever possible. For the well-being of the patient their roles must be complementary. By raising some issues not usually brought to the surgeon's attention, it is hoped that the following notes will heighten his understanding of the problems in which his colleague in the laboratory is involved.

(1) *The relevant history,* including the previous pathology reference number if available, and physical signs, briefly stated, should accompany the request for examination of a specimen. When the tissue has been irradiated this fact must be mentioned. No pathologist should be expected to provide a histological diagnosis in the absence of the clinical background. "A pathological diagnosis is not a mere matching of microscopic pictures, it involves the whole evidence of the case, the natural history of the disease, and the pathologist's judgement" (Fred Stewart).

(2) *Good fixation* is the key to good histological preparations. Poor or inadequate fixation may cause irreversible changes and render diagnosis impossible. Detailed histological examination demands fixation of tissue that is both rapid and productive of gentle coagulation of protein and arrest of autolysis, which begins immediately after the specimen is removed. (For specific instructions on fixation of tissue see Appendix.)

Drying of the specimen is deleterious. Preliminary photography is of little importance in the recording and study of a surgical specimen. It is not as informative as intelligently performed photography of the dissected specimen.

(3) *Squeezing of unfixed tissue* produces irreversible artifact of greater significance in some situations than others. Some tumors, oat cell carcinoma and the lymphomas, and some nonneoplastic changes in which numerous reticulo-endothelial cells are present, are notorious for exhibiting crush artifact in those very clinical situations in which such tissue damage is difficult to avoid, e.g., the punch or needle biopsy. All the more reason for the utmost delicacy to be employed in excising a lymph node for diagnostic purposes.

(4) In a good laboratory the senior technician is a knowledgeable, helpful colleague. When he is made to feel part of an important service the response will be measured by more thoughtful processing and preparation of the tissues. In general, elegant sections may be prepared from tissue fragments in say 24 hours. Allow 48 to 72 hours for lymph nodes and bulkier subjects and 4 to 5 days where bone is to be studied.

(5) *Rapid frozen section techniques* enable a histological section to be obtained in from 2 to 7 min and a report issued to provide guidance to the surgeon on the further conduct of the operation. Other uses of the technique, e.g., the pronouncement of prognosis to anxious relatives immediately after operation, are on occasion valuable, but to use it in order to bypass pathological studies carried out on paraffin sections, out of curiosity, from sheer impatience, or as a temporary report while a paraffin section is being prepared constitutes a misuse of the technique. To repeat, frozen section examination is used during operation to assist immediate decision making. The author prefers that rapid frozen section studies be carried out either in or adjoining the operating theater, so that the surgeon may see the histological appearances in the tissues he handles.

The indications for the use of frozen section technique are as follows:

(1) To ascertain that a piece of tissue selected for frozen section is indeed relevant to the clinical diagnosis and is not neighboring tissue of similar consistency, e.g., in the case of swellings in the parotid and thyroid glands, or soft tissue swellings of dubious nature.

(2) As an initial diagnostic procedure on a swelling where the surgeon considers that for certain malignancies a definitive radical procedure should be carried out immediately.

(3) For preliminary scouting, where the nature of the planned procedure is determined by the distribution of the tissue involved by tumor.

(4) For final assessment of the margin of clearance in an operative surgical specimen.

(5) For the diagnosis of any intraoperative tissue abnormality.

The absolute contraindications are:

(6) Its use as a substitute for examinations best carried out on paraffin-processed material.

(7) The investigation of heavily calcified or ossified tissue.

(8) Where the tissue specimen is unique and of small dimensions.

The reasons for the above categorization are as follows:

(1) There are situations, for example where a biopsy has been reported as being of unsatisfactory quality with respect to size or condition, or where normal or quasinormal tissue only has been removed, when at the repetition of the procedure the surgeon requires unequivocal assurance that the biopsy is satisfactory and representative. (In the case of bony tumors there is no substitute for generosity in tissue volume; see section 7 below).

(2) Though this is a standard procedure in the management of mam-

mary swellings, there is no reason why it should not be applied in the case of suspected melanoma (Davis and Little, 1974) and with many of the tumors arising in parotid and thyroid glands.

The difficulties inherent in the diagnosis are not a contraindication to attempting a frozen section approach, merely an inhibiting factor. Success is largely dependent on the fact that in the greater number of situations there is a sufficiently large difference in histological appearance between normal and abnormal, innocence and malignancy that a diagnosis may be made with confidence.

Two examples must suffice to illustrate difficulties experienced with small biopsies which would be quite adequate in amount for other situations.

(a) A drill biopsy on an undiagnosed sarcoma is not likely to provide a diagnosis because of the degree of crush artifact attendant on the procedure and the unrepresentative nature of such a small volume of tissue, inadequate for the study of growth patterns.

(b) Small thyroid acini separated by a diffuse lymphocytic infiltration is an appearance common to several entities including Hashimoto's thyroiditis, lymphosarcoma arising in this condition, or lymphosarcoma alone. It may be difficult to distinguish lymphoma from small cell carcinoma. Even in the large sections available from a thyroidectomy the most critical evaluation may be required, and in this situation a small biopsy fragment may prove inadequate quantitatively (see also section 6 below).

(3) A standard use of the technique in head and neck surgery is for the examination of tissues supposedly remote from the primary tumor, for the presence of malignant disease. This is not usually indicated in the virgin case, but where irradiation or chemotherapy has resulted in reparative fibrosis the tissue changes present may be difficult to assess by sight and touch alone. Furthermore, a preliminary selective biopsy of a lymph node may be informative when the extent of a dissection is being decided.

(4) For the pathologist to be of assistance in assessing the adequacy of clearance of a resected malignant tumor he must familiarize himself with the anatomy of the operation and possess an intimate knowledge of the behavior of the various types of tumor the surgeon deals with. A margin of clearance regarded as adequate for a well-differentiated squamous carcinoma is of a different order from that required for some melanomas or for a salivary adenoid cystic carcinoma. An obvious point of procedure is that *the resected specimen should be sent* to the pathologist for assessment of clearance. Too often the specimen is kept in the operating theater, or elsewhere, and instead, portions of tissue from the plane of excision are sent to the pathology department, a report of freedom from tumor being equated with adequacy of excision!

(5) When sight and touch are felt to be inadequate, frozen section may provide a sure guide. For example, after irradiation of melanoma of the intranasal and paranasal areas, blackening which appears in the mucosa may prove to be melanin tattooing, the result of macrophage activity, rather than tumor. Induration in the tongue may be pure fibrosis rather than scirrhous carcinoma; the firm polypoidal nodules in a colostomy may be granulation tissue and not recurrent colonic carcinoma, and so on.

(6) Since, along with accuracy, speed is of the essence in frozen section work a limitation on its use are those histological studies which are time consuming. These include the investigation of granulomatous or other complex tissue changes, and the lymphomas in particular. As mentioned (discussion on section 2) the possibility of success in frozen section work is based on the relative ease with which pathological patterns may be distinguished in sections not of the quality of the best paraffin preparations. In the case of squamous carcinomas, adenocarcinomas and inflammatory changes the contrast with normal tissues is striking. On the other hand, scirrhous polygonal cell carcinoma may, on occasion, not be readily distinguishable from scar tissue containing macrophages, the presence of lymphoma may not be apparent, and the precise allocation of a soft tissue sarcoma may remain in doubt. Such special histochemical investigations as searching for mucin, melanin, or intracellular fat, or appropriate bacteriological examination require considerable time both for their preparation, and perhaps interpretation. The pathologist is the arbiter in the decision to defer an opinion until paraffin sections are available for study.

(7) Tissue which requires decalcification before sections can be cut from it is clearly not susceptible to frozen section study. In addition, the distinction of the various types of bone tumor requires in general large sections and perhaps special staining for critical evaluation (Lichtenstein, 1972).

(8) The production of frozen sections is destructive of tissue and results in very few sections in comparison with the several which become available from paraffin studies, such serial and step sectioning being a procedure frequently resorted to in the study of biopsy fragments. For this reason undue loss of biopsy material* is to be avoided since the *whole* of

---

*Apropos—keeping the specimen whole. This is an important principle in the investigation of biopsy material. Confusion, resulting in harm to the patient has been brought about by the unscrupulous practice, not rarely adopted, of dividing a biopsy and sending each portion to different pathologists on the pretext that this is an added check on the accuracy of diagnosis. No pathologist of repute will knowingly involve himself in such unethical, harmful practices. The author has had experience of more than one instance where entirely contrary opinions were expressed by the pathologists involved, where no diagnosis at all could be reached, and one instance where the adequacy of excision of a tumor remained in doubt because each examiner only received a portion of the tumor.

the biopsy may require study in order to arrive at a definitive diagnosis.†

From a consideration of the foregoing, the limitations of the frozen section technique emerge. It is not an inferior method of tissue investigation, but improperly used, at the surgeon's behest, and with its limitations uncomprehended it may become a dangerous tool. For example, it plays little or no part in the investigation of an enlarged cervical lymph node, since the diagnosis of adenitis, lymphoma, or metastatic tumor provides no indication for further surgery, per se. Again, to ask whether the edge of a specimen is clear of tumor is the wrong question, which should have been: How great a clearance has been attained in the prevailing clinico-pathologic circumstance (discussion on section 4)?

The Examination of Lymph Nodes

The late Sir Francis Walshe used to say with regard to lumbar puncture that it was to be carried out purposefully, after the case had been "sucked dry clinically," and we could well apply this advice to any other

†Pathologists too, by thoughtless "routine" examination of surgical specimens may also be guilty of so destroying or distorting the histological picture available from a valuable specimen as to render the diagnosis uncertain. In the author's experience the following common practice is a significant source of uncertainty, and is described in detail only to be condemned.

In the cases of excision of skin blemishes, small ulcers and the like, the specimen consists of an ellipse of skin around the visibly diseased central area (Fig. 1). A block of tissue (B) selected thus will demonstrate histogenesis, histopathology, and depth of extension. Where the specimen is of small dimensions, 1 cm or less across, and the lesion is benign, all relevant information will be available in the section. Where malignancy exists, clearly the maximal margin of clearance *can* only be a few millimeters, but the surgeon rightly wishes to know whether the edges are clear, for which purposes the lines of excision on A and C may be studied. Where the diagnosis proves to be melanoma the margin of clearance on such an excision is an irrelevance; further adequate surgery is mandatory.

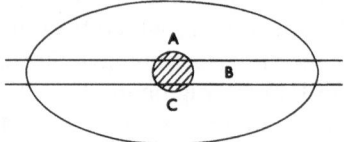 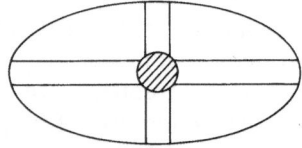

Figure 1   Figure 2

Recommended (Fig. 1) and poor (Fig. 2) block selection.

Now a routine method of treating such specimens (Fig. 2) is to quarter them, or worse, with the excuse that by such means margins of clearance are best assessed at four representative points. It often happens that the central area, the raison d'être of the whole operation, is not only partially destroyed by multiple incisions and by the inevitable histological techniques which follow, but it may render the interpretation of the changes present in the edge of four fragments highly uncertain, particularly when the diagnosis is melanoma versus melanotic nevus.

surgical diagnostic procedure. It frequently happens that the nature of a presumed enlarged lymph node in the neck remains obscure after taking a meticulous history and physical, hematological, serological, and radiological examinations have been carried out. The biopsy findings can be conclusive, yet (a) it may be carried out crudely; (b) a small node may have been removed instead of the largest available; (c) the node may have been fragmented or crushed in the process; (d) it may have been fixed immediately in formalin when a bacteriological swab of the sectioned surface and consigning half of the fresh node for animal inoculation would have been prudent; or (e) it may have been placed in an inadequate amount of fixative to irremediably conceal the evidence. The point cannot be overstressed that the management of a lymph node biopsy should be a planned procedure and not likened to the routine examination of a blood sample. It is always safe to send the node fresh in a sterile container directly to the pathologist.

Some Causes of Error in Diagnosis

There are numerous sources of error which may result in a false histological report. From the surgeon's viewpoint these sources are in the operation theater, in transit, or in the laboratory. In the operation theater there may be mislabeling of specimens and misleading information may be written on the pathology forms, but a further source of error results from the surgeon's not carrying out a brief examination of the tissue. This examination has two purposes. It may reveal a tissue change which is of special interest to him and can be appropriately indicated to the pathologist. Equally important, it may enable him to complete his own assessment of the pathological changes present, which is the only check he has on the validity of the report he receives from the laboratory. The following case illustrates the price which may be paid for neglect of this procedure.

A female age 25 had a lump removed from the breast and the surgeon neither incised it at the time nor sent it for frozen section examination in the pathology laboratory. Surprised at the report of scirrhous carcinoma on the paraffin section, he approached the junior assistant who had reported on the case, asked for the histology to be checked by the senior pathologist, was satisfied with the latter's agreement on the diagnosis, and ordered a radical mastectomy to be carried out. Only after this had been done did a laboratory technician draw the pathologist's attention to a double error which had occurred in processing; the label on a fibroadenoma had been attached to that of a carcinoma and vice versa. Immediate checking through the possible sources of the error revealed that the junior's gross description of the tissue was very poor indeed, that the reserve tissue in formalin was half of an encapsulated typical fibroadenoma, that the surgeon had not asked to examine it when he visited the laboratory, and that the pathologist had not reexamined the tissue either. Had the surgeon incised the specimen in the theater and made the diagnosis himself he would surely have prevented this tragedy.

Within the laboratory, mislabeling of specimens is a commonplace error in the processing of perhaps tens of thousands of tissue fragments each year, and when the various fail-safe mechanisms are bypassed, it is almost always detected by the intelligent diagnostician, the clue being in the lack of correspondence between the clinical history and naked-eye description on the one hand and the microscopic appearances on the other. Such technical faults are rapidly corrected. However, the worst source of error is that whose mode of action is through the goodwill of the pathologist, and that is the demand for haste in producing a report. Undue haste in tissue processing may so distort the tissue as to render it valueless or worse for diagnostic purpose. Undue haste on the part of the pathologist may lead to neglect of prudent technique which would clarify an obscure situation, most commonly (A) a neglect of long-considered thought, (B) the application of selective special stains, and (C) thorough exploitation of tissue by the cutting of further sections.

(A) The first is self-evident. Time for contemplation and for reference to the pathologist's extracerebral memory—his reference cabinet provides the right atmosphere for a considered opinion.

(B) The application of special stains may be desirable to demonstrate myofibrils in one sarcoma, collagen production in another, or finely divided intracellular lipoid material in a third. In a spindle cell, apparently epithelial tumor, one may need to search for intercellular bridges to confirm its squamous nature or the fine, dustlike silver-positive granules produced by melanin-producing cells. A tumor, apparently undifferentiated, may be seen to be freely mucin secreting, or the intercellular homogeneous material formed in a cervical tumor deposit may prove to be amyloid, but the possibilities must be considered and the appropriate staining techniques applied.

Social considerations should *never* be an indication for undue haste, with its abundant risks. A simple explanation from surgeon to pathologist will receive a sympathetic ear, and if necessary special processing of tissue separate from the laboratory routine is carried out with the saving of some hours if this is of therapeutic moment.

(C) The third merits special consideration. A paraffin block of a biopsy fragment can generate 250 sections/mm thickness of tissue. A solitary section in the superficial part of the block may not be representative. Failure to examine the residual, major portion of a biopsy is a neglect of technique which may result in failure to demonstrate quite gross pathological changes, including the overlooking of malignant disease.

It behooves a surgeon to have some acquaintance not only with the sources of error in histopathology, but also with those of uncertainty, a failing which on occasion may be inevitable. In pathology, as in any diagnostic service, one strives for the definitive and contemplates with dissatisfaction provisional, partial, or broad diagnoses; yet these are inevitable in certain circumstances. On such occasions the pathologist may be tempted to extrapolate, to offer refinement in diagnosis beyond that which is warranted by the demonstrable tissue changes. It must be realized that certain pathological appearances represent a final common path—the anaplastic sarcoma of uncertain histogenesis, the polygonal cell carcinoma with no demonstrable secretory activity, and nonspecific granulation tissue, to name three. Pressure for a refinement of diagnosis, when reasonably complete histological studies have been carried out, indicate ignorance of the fundamentals of histopathology.

Reviewing

A request for further evaluation of the tissue changes is quite another matter, and the querying of a report on sensible grounds can be beneficial. In a salivary gland biopsy reported as undifferentiated carcinoma, it is reasonable to ask if it could be a muco-epidermoid carcinoma or a malignant mixed tumor. It is reasonable to demand whether an adenocarcinoma could be an adenoid cystic carcinoma, whether a mixed salivary gland tumor is malignant, and so on. Clinical and histological similarity do not necessarily go hand in hand. Whereas, for example, keratinizing squamous carcinoma and lymphosarcoma of the tonsil bear some clinical resemblance to each other, there is none histopathologically. If an upper deep cervical nodule is reported as an adenolymphoma it is the merest fancy to suggest it to be reviewed to see if it has been confused with metastatic oat cell carcinoma.

Difficulties in diagnosis may arise from ignorance of the pathologist on the nature of evident tissue changes, but they are more likely to be due to inadequate or inappropriate biopsy material, or insufficient exploitation of the material. There are, however, situations notoriously productive of problematic pathology because of the sheer difficulty of interpreting the changes seen. Among these chordoma, verrucose squamous cell carcinoma, chronic destructive midline "granuloma," and some postirradiation tissue changes are examples. A correct diagnosis may not be made on the first biopsy, nor by the first pathologist examining the tissues!

The Difficulties of Giving a Second Opinion

It is of frequent occurrence that a senior pathologist is approached to give a second opinion on a pathological specimen when, for a number of reasons, there is disquiet or dissatisfaction with the initial report. This may have been equivocal, ill expressed, at great variance with the clinical assessment and totally unexpected or, on occasion, totally incomprehensible.

So far as the etiquette of the matter is concerned the request from a clinician that pathological material be made available to another pathologist should always be acceded to by the initial investigator, who should put at the disposal of the pathologist asked to give the second opinion all the relevant information he possesses. This must include (1) a clinical résumé, (2) a description of the gross specimen and the manner in which the tissue blocks were selected, and (3) a generous number of unstained sections or the paraffin block. The second pathologist would be unwise to give an opinion in the absence of this tripod. (Failure of the pathologist to familiarize himself with the clinical aspects of the case and failure to study representative blocks of tissue are high on the list of causes of error in judgment).

The expression of a dissident second opinion should always be firm, if not forthright, when it is requested by a surgeon, with none of the false modesty which might be considered proper when giving the same opinion to a fellow pathologist, whether peer or junior. Similarly, assent should be unequivocal and brief.

Classification and Nomenclature

For the surgeon a knowledge of the classification and nomenclature of tumors is indispensable to their proper management. Whenever possible the allocation of a tumor to a particular class and type should be as precise as possible and the use of such loose terms as "soft tissue sarcoma" other than in the most general context, or worse "solid tumor" is a retrograde step. Tumors are classified on the basis of their histogenesis and behavior principally, often with an essential qualification which has a regional flavor to it. For example, in a biopsy of the larynx, "squamous cell carcinoma of the vocal cord" conveys precisely its histogenesis (from squamous epithelium), behavior (malignancy), and locus of origin. A lymph node biopsy report of "metastatic, well-differentiated carcinoma of the thyroid" requires a different degree of awareness from the diagnostician not only in asserting that the tumor is secondary, but in pinpointing the organ of orgin. This latter facility is rather restricted since the majority of malignant tumors possess common growth patterns, for example squamous carcinomas, anaplastic carcinomas, visceral adenocarcinomas, and so on. Where fairly distinctive growth patterns are well-known features of tumors arising in particular organs, it behoves the pathologist to recognize them, e.g., certain tumors of breast, lung, kidney, liver, and so on.

Other limitations on the accuracy of tumor diagnosis are imposed (A) by the variable growth patterns exhibited by malignant neoplasms in comparison with their normal tissues of origin, and (B) by the degree of exploitation of the tissue in the laboratory:

(A) Malignant epithelial thyroid neoplasms exhibiting follicular and papillary growth patterns are regularly recognized for what they are when well differentiated and manufacturing colloid, but they are totally unrecognizable when undifferentiated and anaplastic. An intermediate degree of differentiation may lead to a *suggestion* that the thyroid gland is the primary source of a metastatic carcinoma. It is in such cases that the shrewd pathologist will review the case from the clinical presentation to assist in providing a sensible, working diagnosis for his colleague. Again, some tumors with a characteristic pattern have no normal histological counterparts. For example, mesothelioma of the pleura, synovial sarcoma, parvicellular scirrhous carcinoma of the breast, oat cell carcinoma of the lung, and chordoma must be recognized for what they are in the light of experience.

(B) Because it is technically easier to make histological preparations from small blocks of tissue, and fewer blocks naturally entail less labor for all in the laboratory, in some instances thorough examination of tissue is skimped. There is no substitute for the examination of adequate numbers of large blocks of tissue, the number required naturally varying from one situation to another. One good-sized block through the average mammary tumor thought to be a carcinoma is sensible, whereas 20 blocks may be reasonable from a large fibroadenoma in order to exclude sarcomatous change. Apart from examining an adequately sampled volume of tissue, there are a number of easily performed supplementary stains of the greatest value in bringing out, or confirming, the details of histology or cytoarchitecture only suspected in a hematoxylin and eosin preparation. Mucin, glycogen, amyloid, and melanin are examples of important chemical constituents whose presence will not be demonstrated or confirmed unless specific staining techniques are employed, and myofibrils, intercellular bridges, and reticulin patterns are examples of cytological and histological detail which would similarly remain unrevealed. The presence or absence of such chemical or structural features may be of decisive weight in the process of arriving at a clear-cut diagnosis. The differential diagnosis of some neoplasms includes granulomas of physico-chemical or infective origin. Adequate tissue examination of such cases will of necessity involve special stains for bacteria and fungi, or a simple examination under polarized light.

Grading and Staging

The grading and staging of tumors has a variable value depending on the current therapies available. In the grading of a tumor there is the assumption that the histological appearances give an indication of likely clinical behavior, including the response to certain treatments. Empirically it is found to be of greater value in some groups than in others. For example, knowledge of the grading of a squamous cell carcinoma based on its differentiation plays little part in general in the planning of treatment, though it may alert the clinician to the likely behavior of the tumor. In the case of fibrosarcoma the plan of treatment must take into account the grade of the tumor.

The parameters used in grading are usually related to differentiation for example in squamous and adenocarcinoma, or to a combination of growth patterns and stromal appearances in the case of mammary carcinoma.

Other tumors for different reasons are not graded, e.g., basal cell carcinoma, melanoma, oat cell carcinoma, osteosarcoma, acinic cell tumor of the parotid gland, adenoid cystic carcinoma of salivary gland. The further the histological appearances depart from those of the tissue in which the tumor has arisen, or which it simulates, that is to say the greater the anaplasia, the less differentiated it is said to be. The class of completely undifferentiated tumor is not susceptible of further refinement and histogenesis is then based on conjecture or experience of probabilities with a given clinical situation. If in an anaplastic tumor features of an epithelial origin only are retained it is justifiable to classify it as an undifferentiated carcinoma (synonyms: polygonal cell carcinoma, anaplastic carcinoma). In many instances though, the demonstration of intercellular bridges or mucin secretion will lead to such tumors being redesignated as poorly differentiated squamous carcinoma or adenocarcinoma, respectively.

In a biopsy the range of differentiation of a tumor may not be representative. It is common to find that a moderately well-differentiated rectal carcinoma on biopsy proves to be more anaplastic when the whole tumor is available for examination. Biopsies of a surface tumor are often obtained from its most accessible part, that is, the edge or surface which, in the case of rectal carcinoma for example, is not entirely representative.

Grading is not to be confused with *typing** and staging. The typing of a tumor is its accepted nomenclature(s) and where different types of tumor occur in the same organ (the breast is an example of an organ in which different tumor growth *patterns* are associated with different biological properties), by a loose mental association a tumor with a better prognosis is

---

*Recommended study is the series *International Classification of Tumors*, published by the World Health Organization.

called a lower-grade tumor than one which carried the worse prognosis. This is to use "grade" in a more general form, e.g., in the statement that "osteosarcoma is of higher grade malignancy than basal cell carcinoma," which is another way of saying that osteosarcoma is a more malignant tumor than basal cell carcinoma.

The staging of a tumor is by far the most important qualification a pathologist can add to the description of a tumor specimen. There is no uniform method applicable to tumors in the different body sites, but all effective staging systems must have a clinico-pathological sanction if they are to maintain their validity. Whether serial letters or numbers are used to give an abbreviated description of each stage is not as important as, nor a substitute for, an appreciation of the written description. After a pathologist has described a moderately well-differentiated adenocarcinoma of the rectum as having "infiltrated all coats of the bowel, metastasized to 4 of 17 lymph nodes sectioned including one near the inferior mesenteric pedicle, and infiltrated a tributary of the superior mesenteric vein," the request from a surgeon for a "Dukes classification" reveals total ignorance of that classification on the part of the questioner, since if the report had been understood, no amplification would have been necessary and to one familiar with Dukes's system, immediate assignation to the appropriate subdivision follows from the information provided.

For tumors arising on the body surface the larger the tumor, the greater the depth of invasion, and the presence of lymph node metastases, the worse the prognosis. But the purpose of staging is not only for prognostic purposes; it may be a factor involved in treatment planning.

To illustrate the relationship of tumor type, grade, and stage to prognosis and management, the author has chosen the divers group of tumors referred to as melanoma. By definition they are malignant tumors arising in melanocytes. When they arise within the eye or other part of the central nervous system, they are not usefully typed or graded and the stage of the disease is a clinical assertion. In skin, and probably in the mucous membranes, the histogenetic type of tumor carries an increasingly poor prognosis in the order (1) lentigo maligna melanoma, (2) superficial spreading melanoma, and (3) nodular melanoma. However, for all three types there is a second prognostic factor, the depth of invasion when first seen. For the first two there is an *in situ* phase, but for all of them four deeper levels are recognized, invasion of papillary dermis, the papillary–reticular interface, the reticular dermis, and the subcutaneous fat (level 5). Now, it is about level 3 and deeper that there is increasinging association with regional node metastasis. This system does not take into account interesting cellular features of the tumor, or local immunologic response, nor such significant matters as ulceration and vascular invasion, notorious for carrying a poor prognosis.

Irradiation may lead to alterations in cytology and histology of a nonneoplastic nature which yet simulate neoplasia. Their importance is such as to make it a rule to inform the pathologist when the specimen consigned to him for examination has had past irradiation. Immediate preoperative irradiation leads to no such problems, but days to years later a range of changes appear, some of which are a source of confusion when unrecognized. Irradiation fibroblasts are large cells with hyperchromatic atypical nuclei, recognizable for what they are by their being scattered in scar or inflammatory tissue usually, and not forming a coherent cellular grouping after the manner of a sarcoma. Pseudosarcomatous proliferation is principally found in the head and neck region and its adequate assessment requires both histological experience and a thorough knowledge of the clinical aspects. Pseudoepitheliomatous proliferation of mucous glands or their ducts is a change seen after irradiation of buccopharyngeal neoplasia. Scarring and tissue distortion may also be deceptive and their innocent nature not appreciated.

The criteria of malignancy vary from one tissue or organ to another. The well-differentiated astrocytoma may not be apparent on a small biopsy where it is indistinguishable from reactive gliosis. The normal placenta is a pleomorphic structure exhibiting mitotic activity and vascular invasion. Moles and melanomas, keratoacanthoma, and epidermoid carcinoma are all invasive, unencapsulated lesions. Endometrium, thyroid gland, and melanocytes in lymph nodes are not necessarily indicative of malignancy any more than is chorion or amnion in postpartum lung. Recurrence of one of the fibromatoses does not indicate neoplastic, malignant potential, nor failure of adamantinoma to metastasize, innocence. Occasionally special conditions are required for exceptional tumor behavior to become apparent; for example craniotomy for glioma and giant size in a basal cell carcinoma are prerequisites for metastasis to occur. In some situations even the neoplastic nature of progressive, ultimately fatal cellular proliferation may be in doubt, as in pseudomyxoma peritonei. There are several tumors whose biological status may not be determinable from the histological appearances alone, e.g., the acinic cell tumor of salivary gland, the Hürthle cell tumor of the thyroid, even the appendicular carcinoid. The histological differentiation of chondroma from chondrosarcoma is based on minimal changes in nuclear size and structure and cellular grouping in otherwise very similar tissue. Add to these the occasional cases of spontaneous regression in some tumors—melanoma and embryomas, e.g., neuroblastoma—and it will be recognized that the surgical pathologist, as does the surgeon, constantly studies his material with its distinctive regional origin in the forefront of his mind.

Consider the histological entity, squamous cell carcinoma. The malignancy of this tumor is entirely dependent on its organ of origin. When it arises in an actinic keratosis it is (rightly) managed as a tumor of the lowest grade malignancy since it rarely, if ever, proves fatal. It is a highly curable tumor when it occurs on the vermilion border of the lip, carries a worse prognosis in the larynx, even worse in the cervix uteri, and in the esophagus few are cured. There are some social, or anatomical factors at work in the production of this spectrum, but there are as yet unrevealed factors too. For example, carcinoma of the lower lip is eminently curable by irradiation when it has not spread to one or other of the commissures, but with involvement of the angle of the mouth response becomes very poor indeed.

To reiterate, the histological appearances, grade, and staging are only *some* of the factors to be taken into consideration in the assessment and management of a malignant tumor.

In situ malignancy is a term restricted to the epithelia which exhibit the cytological changes of malignancy without invasion of the underlying tissue. Allowance must be made for the inevitable differences in the appearance of a tumor which is growing without the molding and reactive effects of tissue, and one which is infiltrating. The appearances are not to be regarded as early malignancy nor as a precancerous change. These terms refer to a clinical stage in the former, and to a clinico-pathological entity in the latter. In the skin there are a number of chronic dermatoses, such as Bowen's disease which are characterized by the presence of intraepithelial malignancy. This phase may last for years or decades. Eventually a proportion of these chronic *in situ* malignancies are associated with the development of invasive, squamous cell carcinoma. Lentigo maligna whose duration may be measured in decades and another type of *in situ* melanoma termed superficial spreading with a duration of months or years are known to precede invasive melanoma, or they may undergo spontaneous regression, and *in situ* carcinoma of the cervix uteri is also well known to behave in a similar manner. In the breast, *in situ* carcinoma assumes different forms, intraduct carcinoma, intralobular carcinoma with a similar cytology, and *in situ* lobular carcinoma. It is known that mastectomy for this stage of mammary carcinoma is likely to be curative, and we may rightly assume they are stages in the development of mammary carcinoma in view of the frequency with which they are seen in association with established infiltrating carcinoma.

In view of the long, or unknown duration of these *in situ* phases it is clearly incorrect to call *early* cancer a change which may have been present as long as half a century. Certainly they are for the most part quite curable cancers. Earliness is a clinical term, properly related to staging. Clearly a tumor which is not fixed deeply is at an earlier stage than one which is, and a tumor with regional node metastases is at a later stage than one which is yet localized.

The histological appearances of a tumor which has been present for several years, and has not extended as far as one present for a few weeks or months only, are spatial manifestations of inherent growth properties, and of complex tumor/host relationships, rather than of an indication of a temporal relationship.

Precancerous is a term loosely applied to established *in situ* cancer— Bowen's precancerous dermatosis and precancerous melanosis of the conjunctiva which are examples of *in situ* squamous carcinoma and melanoma, respectively—but should be restricted in application to those tissue changes which in a significant proportion of cases are associated with the later development of histological malignancy. For example, in the skin chronic irradiation dermatitis, on the tongue certain of the histological types of leukoplakia, in the colon multiple polyposis, in bone Paget's disease. In many instances chronic irritation is associated with the sequence hyperplasia–metaplasia–*dysplasia–in situ* carcinoma–invasive carcinoma. An important duty of the pathologist and surgeon is to detect precancerous changes, in order to initiate appropriate supervision, prophylaxis, or definitive treatment of malignancy at its earliest detectable appearance.

Appendix on Fixation

The aim of fixation is to preserve tissue in as lifelike a manner as possible. In its absence tissue undergoes putrefaction and liquefaction. A 10% formalin solution is the best all-round fixative and should be used generously, 15–20 times the volume of the specimen being suggested. While this is practicable for small specimens, breasts, major amputations, and bulky tumors cannot be so managed since the rate of penetration of fixative into tissue falls off very rapidly with time. The optimum thickness of tissue blocks for fixation and processing is 3–5 mm. Such a block would be well fixed in 4 hours at room temperature. By the time formalin reaches the middle of a mymph node, 15-mm-thick central autolysis will have spoiled much of the node for critical histological evaluation.

The management of the larger specimens should be in three steps:

(1) Dissection of the fresh specimen, so that formalin may reach important areas of tissue to be studied, particularly tumor and regional nodes. With lung and bowel, inflation with formalin is recommended.

(2) Incision of these areas a few hours later when further penetration of fixative will be facilitated without the tissue distortion which would have followed had they been cut into thin slices when fresh.

(3) A final selection of blocks.

Incision of a specimen should be thoughtfully directed to yield the maximum of information, while at the same time not be such as to render it useless for possible later demonstration, or permanent preservation in a museum.

References

Ackerman, L. V. and Rosar, J (1974). *Surgical Pathology,* 5th Ed. C. V. Mosby, St. Louis.

The Atlas of Tumor Pathology. Armed Forces Institute of Pathology, Washington D.C.

Batsakis, J. G. (1974). *Tumors of the Head and Neck, Clinical and Pathological Considerations.* Williams & Wilkins, Baltimore.

Culling, C. F. A. (1974). *Handbook of Histopathological and Histochemical Techniques,* 3rd Ed. Butterworth, London.

Davis, N. C., and Little, J. H. (1974). The role of frozen section in the diagnosis and management of malignant melanoma. *Br. J. Surg.* **61**:505–508.

Lichtenstein, L. (1972). *Bone Tumors,* 4th Ed. C. V. Mosby, St. Louis.

Mackenzie, D. H. (1970). *The Differential Diagnosis of Fibroblastic Disorders.* Blackwell Scientific, Oxford/Edinburgh.

Morson, B. C., and Dawson, I. M. P. (1972). *Gastro-intestinal Pathology.* Blackwell Scientific, London.

Nakazawa, H., Rosen, P., Lane, N., and Lattes, R. (1967). Frozen section experience in 3000 cases: Accuracy, limitations, and value in residency training. *Am. J. Clin. Pathol.* **49**:41–51.

Spencer, H. (1968). *Pathology of the Lung,* 2nd Ed. Pergamon Press, Oxford.

Stewart, F. W. (1950). *Tumors of the Breast.* Armed Forces Institute of Pathology, Washington, D.C. p. 74.

Willis, R. A. (1967). *Pathology of Tumours,* 4th Ed. Butterworth, London.

Chapter 5

DEVELOPMENTAL BIOLOGY RELATED TO ONCOLOGY

WOLFGANG WECHSLER AND ADALBERT KOESTNER

Introduction

Research in perinatal tumor induction experienced a new impetus in past years through several important discoveries in experimental chemical and viral oncogenesis. The following discoveries probably had the greatest impact: (1) The experimental proof that leukemia tumor viruses can be transmitted in rodents by infection from animal to animal, i.e., horizontal transmission, but also by inheritance of the viral genome from generation to generation, i.e., vertical transmission. (2) The successful transplacental induction of various organ tumors in rodents by alkylating chemical carcinogens (Mohr and Althoff, 1964, 1965; Druckrey *et al.,* 1966). (3) The discovery of the high susceptibility of rat fetuses to the oncogenic effect of ethylnitrosourea (Ivankovic and Druckrey, 1968).

Perinatal cancer experiments demonstrated a dose-dependent latency period following exposure to the carcinogenic agent. If one extrapolates

Wolfgang Wechsler • Max-Planck-Institut für Hirnforschung, Abteilung für Allgemeine Neurologie, Ostmerheimer Strasse 200, D 5000, Köln 91, West Germany. **Adalbert Koestner** • Department of Veterinary Pathobiology. The Ohio State University, 1925 Coffey Road, Columbus, Ohio 43210. The research for this chapter was supported in part by Deutsche Forschungsgemeinschaft and National Institutes of Health Grant CA 11224.

latency periods observed in experimental tumor production in rodents to human life, estimates may range from a few months to decades. It is, therefore, not possible to exclude perinatal tumor induction of neoplasms expressed at different stages of human life, ranging from infancy to adulthood.

Stimulated by modern methods of molecular and experimental biology, animal models were established to unfold the relationship between development and neoplastic transformation. Such studies advanced the concept that ontogenetic development and cancer may be closely interrelated. In this chapter observations are discussed from clinical and experimental oncology with particular emphasis on neurooncology and its relationship to development and maturation. Tumors of the nervous system have been chosen as a specific example because of their importance in developmental pathobiology and because neurooncology is the authors' field of interest.

Childhood Tumors in Man: Current Concepts

While it is possible in experimental oncology to determine exactly the periods of induction, latency, and clinical tumor expression, in clinical oncology the grossly detectable tumor generally is the first determinable manifestation of a neoplastic disease. The etiologic agent, induction time, and latency period are usually unpredictable parameters of the neoplastic process with the exception of rare incidences of known exposure to a carcinogen, e.g., the atomic bomb incident in Hiroshima. In the context of this discussion, it is therefore desirable to concentrate on tumors which allow the determination of temporal parameters related to tumor induction, latency, and growth. Such examples in human oncology are neoplasms already present at birth or detectable in early infancy. With these neoplasms, intrauterine determinants responsible for neoplastic transformation are undisputable and closer temporal relationships between induction and tumor expression are more readily established.

There is now for the first time evidence in man of a causal relationship between maternal administration of a synthetic hormone and an increased rate of cancer in female offspring. Herbst et al. (1971a,b) and Greenwald et al. (1971) reported an increased incidence of vaginal clear cell adenocarcinomas in children whose mothers had been treated with stilbestrol during pregnancy. The tumor developed in girls and young women, 14 to 20 years of age, that is after an apparent latency period of two decades. This type of cancer is otherwise rare and does not occur so early in life.

Cancer is a major cause of death not only in adults but also in children. Unlike adults, leukemia and tumors of the nervous system occupy a prominent position in cancer statistics of children and adolescents. According to Peller (1960), leukemias are the most common type of neoplasia in children up to the age of 15 years (57% of all tumors). They are followed by tumors of the nervous system (25%), of which the majority occur in the brain (20%). Tumors are also observed in the autonomic nervous system (sympathetic neuroblastoma) and in the retina (retinoblastoma). The third most commonly affected organ in children is the kidney; the Wilms tumor represents 7% of all neoplasms in children. The remaining 11% of tumors arise in various other organs.

The best examples of neoplasms initiated and expressed during intrauterine life are those already present at birth, or clinically detectable during the first months postnatally (congenital tumors). In a survey by Miller (1973), neurogenic tumors responsible for the death of newborn children during the first 24 h surpass even leukemias in incidence (29% against 22%). During the first 4 weeks neurogenic tumors follow leukemias closely (45% compared with 42%) as the primary cause of death (Table 1).

These facts emphasize the importance of nervous system tumors in pediatric oncology and justify their selection for conceptual and pathogenetic analysis of mechanisms of perinatal tumor induction.

Childhood Tumors of the Nervous System

The salient features of the pathology of human tumors of the nervous system have been well described (Zülch, 1956, 1965; Rubinstein, 1972, etc.). Pediatric neurooncology has become of particular interest to oncolo-

TABLE 1. Neonatal Deaths from Congenital Tumors in the U.S.A. (1960–1967)[a]

Tumor types	24 Hours		1–28 Days	
	Number	Percentage	Number	Percentage
Leukemia	18	23.07	54	39.13
Neuroblastoma, sympathetic	19	24.35 ⎱ 30.75	23	16.66 ⎱ 27.52
Brain tumors	5	6.4	15	10.86
Kidney cancer	5	6.4	14	10.74
Hepatoma–hepatoblastoma	3	3.84	7	5.07
Teratoma	7	8.97	2	1.44
Rhabdomyosarcoma	3	3.84	2	1.44
Other	18	23.07	21	15.21
Total	78	100	138	100
Neurogenic tumors	24	30.8	38	27.5

[a]Modified according to Miller, 1973.

gists, because of the inherent unique implication (Wechsler 1971, 1972a, Wechsler and Zülch, 1974), but also to pediatricians, neurologists, and neurosurgeons because of the relatively high incidence of neurogenic tumors in infants (second to leukemia) in contrast to adults. In this chapter we shall restrict our discussion to problems of neurooncology as they relate to ontogenetic development.

The high incidence of neurogenic tumors in infants may indicate a high susceptibility for neoplastic transformation of cells of the nervous system during development and maturation. It must be noted, however, that only certain tumors develop preferentially in children, while others show similar preferences in adults. Tumors of the brain in infants and adolescents arise prominently adjacent to the ventricles or within the posteria or fossa. It is conceivable that precursor cells or differentiated cells in these areas have preferential susceptibility for neoplastic transformation.

According to the spectrum of cellular homogeneity or diversity and according to the degree of differentiation or anaplasia, nervous system tumors may be grouped into:

(1) *Differentiated neoplasms* of predominantly one cell type, e.g., spongioblastoma, choroid plexus papilloma, and neurinoma; or neoplasms composed of two or more cell types, e.g., mixed glioma (astrocytic and oligodenrocytic), subependymal ependymomas, and certain meningiomas.

(2) *Neoplasms composed of differentiated as well as anaplastic cellular elements* demonstrating varying degrees of differentiation or anaplasia of one or more cell types, e.g., malignant astrocytomas or oligodendrogliomas, and certain pineal tumors and gliosarcomas.

(3) *Anaplastic or primitive neoplasms,* in which it is often difficult to decide morphologically whether a mono- or polyclonal tumor type is present as exemplified in tumors such as neuroblastoma, retinoblastoma, medulloblastoma or medullo- and neuroepithelioma.

Tumors encountered most commonly in children are medulloblastomas, ependymomas, plexus papillomas, spongioblastomas, neuroblastomas of the sympathetic ganglia, and craniopharyngiomas. In addition, sarcomas, teratomas, gangliocytomas, pineal tumors, retinoblastomas, and a few other tumors have also been recognized. Tumors classified as glioblastoma, meningioma, or neurinoma occur only exceptionally before the age of 15 years. The incidence of various tumor types in infants within the first year of life is illustrated in Table 2 and is based on surveys by Koos and Miller (1971), and Jänisch and Schreiber (1970).

There are differences in growth behavior among the various tumor types, ranging from slow (e.g., benign differentiated spongioblastoma) to rapid (e.g., malignant anaplastic medulloblastoma) growth. In general, even the most malignant tumors of the nervous system do not metastasize to extraneural locations in contrast to malignant neoplasms of nonneural

TABLE 2. Classification and Incidence of Brain Tumors in Early Infancy

| Tissue of origin | Classification | Koos & Miller (1971) | | Jänisch & Schreiber (1970) | |
		Congenital	First year of life	First year of life	Total
Neuroectodermal	Medulloblastoma	1	1	11	13
derivatives	Spongioblastoma	—	1	7	8
	Astrocytoma	1	1	—	2
	Glioblastoma	—	1	—	1
	Ependymoma	2	1	17	20
	Plexus papilloma	—	1	17	18
	Unclassified	2	5	9	16
Mesenchymal derivatives	Meningeoma		1	4	5
	Sarcoma		4	7	11
	Unclassified	1		4	5
Ectodermal derivatives	Craniopharyngioma	1		4	5
	Dermoid cyst	1	1	5	7
Total number of tumors		9	17	80	111

organs. Exceptional cases of abdominal neuroblastomas may, however, metastasize, but other tumors of this type may become stationary or regress spontaneously (Everson and Cole, 1966).

The following conclusions may be drawn from present available data in neurooncology:

(1) There is undisputable evidence of prenatal tumor induction in man. Based on the incidence of various tumor types in early infancy, the developing nervous system seems preferentially susceptible to tumor induction, similarly to the hematopoetic system and the kidney. This relatively high rate of neurooncogenicity during early life contrasts with a relatively low rate in adulthood.

(2) Tumor development within the nervous system is mostly confined to certain preferential sites, e.g., during childhood to periventricular regions of the brain, the cerebellar cortex, the retina, and the abdominal sympathetic ganglia.

(3) Since the latency period between tumor induction and tumor growth is unknown, it is impossible to determine the time of neoplastic transformation for tumors recognized during various periods of human life. Two possibilities may be considered: (a) All neurogenic tumors are induced perinatally, and due to different latent periods neoplastic transformation and tumor growth occur throughout life, however, in different life periods, or (b) tumor induction occurs throughout life, i.e., from ontogeny to senescence. In reference to the first hypothesis, clinical tumor expression

would depend primarily upon different latency periods of various tumor types ranging from several months to decades. If such were the case, neoplasms with the shortest latency periods and fatal outcome would preclude the development of neoplasms with longer latency periods. If, for instance, the maximal latency period would be 20 years, a period estimated for various occupational tumors, neurogenic tumors in man could be induced during all periods of life. Evidence will be presented from animal experiments that latency periods for different tumor types of the nervous system vary greatly, and that tumor induction is possible both during development and in adulthood. If one extrapolates growth rates of neoplasms as judged by clinical and pathological experience, the range between the lowest and the highest rate would not explain the appearance of neurogenic tumors during infancy and senescence following solely prenatal induction. Both parameters, the latency period and the growth rate, support the hypothesis that neurogenic tumors may be induced at different periods of life, however, with different degrees of neurooncogenicity.

(4) In the context of perinatal carcinogenesis, precursor cells as well as differentiated cells are available as target cells for tumor induction and neoplastic transformation. Using the various neurogenic tumors as classified by Bailey and Cushing (1926), i.e., the cytogenetic principle of classification as a basis for the determination of the cell of origin, a pilocytic astrocytoma or so-called spongioblastoma would indicate a neoplastic transformation of a differentiated fibrillary bipolar glial cell, while a medullobastoma would point to a primitive cerebellar cell type as the cell of origin. While little is known about target cells for tumor induction in the developing human brain, it is striking that neither oligoydendrogliomas (well-differentiated type) nor glioblastomas (anaplastic glial cell type) are common tumors in infancy, although they have a relatively high incidence in adults.

(5) Several exogenous agents capable of cancer production in other organs are prevented from entering the brain because of its protected location within the body. Oncogenic viruses and chemical carcinogens may reach the central nervous system preferentially in case of a systemic distribution perhaps with the additional provision that the blood brain barrier be passed by the carcinogenic agents. Environmental chemical carcinogens have been recognized as causative agents for certain tumors in man, including tumors of the bladder (aniline dyes), of the lung (tars, asbestos, cigarette smoke), of the liver (vinyl chloride), and of the skin (soots, tars, oils). There is at present no indication, however, that environmental carcinogens are responsible for human neurogenic neoplasms, although neurogenic tumors have been produced experimentally in animals with several chemical compounds present in our environment as carcinogens or their precursors.

There are indications that some human tumors may be etiologically related to virus infections, such as Burkitts lymphoma (Epstein–Barr virus) and carcinoma of the cervix (herpes-II virus). SV-40-specific tumor antigens were recently demonstrated in a few human meningiomas (Weiss *et al.*, 1975), in addition, a relatively high reverse transcriptase activity, a possible biochemical fingerprint of RNA tumor viruses, was reported in association with human gliomas (Cuatico *et al.*, 1973; Birkmayer *et al.*, 1974). Furthermore, two types of human papova virus, the JC and the SV-40 PML virus strains recovered from patients with progressive multifocal leukoencephalopathy, a degenerative brain disease caused by a slow-virus infection, were shown to possess the capability to induce brain tumors in newborn hamsters (Walker *et al.*, 1973; Narayan and Weiner, 1974).

Since the etiology of human tumors of the nervous system is unknown and some of these tumors show age-, sex-, and family-dependent preferences, experimental neurooncology should address itself to the following specific subjects: (1) etiologic agents such as viruses and chemicals; (2) genetic factors determining susceptibility or resistence to tumor development; (3) tumor induction related to prenatal and postnatal periods of life; (4) organ susceptibility and resistence; (5) tumor growth within preferential sites of the nervous system; (6) ranges of latency periods for various tumor types and specific etiologic agents; (7) target cells for tumors and differentiation of tumors, and (8) contributory factors, such as hormones, nutrition, or the immune system.

Experimental Perinatal Oncology

General Principles of Tumor Induction

It is recognized today that tumor induction is ultimately based upon molecular changes of cellular constituents. Theoretically, two possibilities may be considered to explain the molecular biology of neoplastic transformation: (1) chemically induced DNA alteration or integration of exogenous viral DNA into the host-cell genome results in a mutation(s) responsible for transformation, and/or (2) biochemical alterations of macromolecules responsible for regulatory functions result in desuppression of normally suppressed DNA sequences (genes), or they may result in activation of vertically transmitted endogenous viruses, leading to neoplastic transformation.

Viral and Chemical Carcinogenesis

Exogenous Oncogenic Viruses. The discoveries by Baltimore (1970) and Temin and Mitzutani (1970) that the RNA of oncogenic viruses is enzymatically transcribed into DNA has led to the unifying concept of viral integration into cellular DNA. There is no longer a principle difference of action between DNA and RNA tumor viruses (Temin and Baltimore, 1972). Total viral nucleic acids or fragments of DNA tumor viruses become integrated into the genome of infected cells, or by encoding the reverse transcriptase retroviruses have evolved the ability to integrate themselves into the cell chromosomes as a provirus. In this context, the capability of some retroviruses to cause cancer is "today the most challenging and important attribute of these retroviruses and the one that will dominate future research efforts in this area" (Baltimore, 1976).

Endogenous Oncogenic Viruses. Based upon more recent studies the concept has been advanced that genes are present in the vertebrate DNA, perhaps incorporated during evolution, which are capable of coding for oncogenic viral information (Huebner and Todaro, 1969). It is assumed that these genes are suppressed under normal conditions but may be partially (oncogene) or fully (virogene) desuppressed spontaneously or by contact with exogenous agents, such as chemical carcinogens. Desuppression may result in neoplastic transformation associated with the appearance of C-type viral particles. The possible significance of prenatal expression of the virogene–oncogene for embryonal development and problems of immunological tolerance to RNA tumor virus expression was extensively discussed by Huebner *et al.* (1971). It is suggested that the virogene–oncogene is controlled by regulatory genes and perhaps by hormonal and immunological mechanisms during embryogenesis and early postnatal life. Genetic deficiencies in host-gene functions may result in failure of these mechanisms leading to neoplastic transformation of affected cells.

Chemical Carcinogens. Since the first demonstration that some human tumors are caused or promoted by chemical agents, e.g., the bladder carcinoma by aniline dyes and scrotal carcinomas by coal dust, chemical carcinogens and cocarcinogens have attracted much attention. Considering exposure and application, two types of carcinogens have been generally distinguished as *topical* and *systemic carcinogens*. The differences between the two will be illustrated by experimental results from neurooncology. The oncogenic potential of a great variety of chemical compounds has been tested in experimental animals and cell culture. Neoplastic transformation by chemical carcinogens is probably the result of the molecular interaction of the carcinogen or its metabolites with nuclear macromolecules leading to changes in the cellular genetic information or its expression. These inflicted changes must become permanently incorporated into the genome of the target cells to assure neoplastic growth (Miller, 1970; Miller and Miller, 1971; Heidelberger, 1973). Repair mechanisms may correct the changes inflicted by a carcinogen as was shown with some radiation experiments and with alkylating nitrosourea compounds, e.g., as demonstrated in experimental neurooncology (p. 107).

Chemical induction of tumors may be by direct application of the carcinogen to the target organ (topical carcinogenesis) or by systemic distribution of an administered carcinogen affecting organs distant from the application site (systemic carcinogenesis). Systemic carcinogenesis is mostly restricted to selected target organs. The reasons for selectivity may depend upon the selective activation of the carcinogen (availability of activating enzymes), organ of excretion, or differential repair capacities among different organs. Chemical tumor induction may occur during all phases of life including prenatal stages of development. The perinatal cancer induction is of particular importance for the present discussion and will be exemplified by recent achievements in experimental neurooncology.

Viral Tumor Genetics. The involvement of genetic factors in expression or suppression of the MLV (mouse leukemia virus) genome was summarized recently by Rowe (1973) and Lilly and Pincus (1973). Lymphomas in mice are considered to be a genetically determined infectious disease in the AKR mouse strain (high lymphoma incidence strain). The genetic link is stated by Rowe (1973) as follows: The 2V loci induce endogenous virus, the FV-2 locus regulates its spread, and the H-2 locus (or its immune response region) appears to be involved in some contributory manner.

In the analysis of this model it can be demonstrated that two principle genetic factors contribute to the neoplastic disease; the etiologic factor (oncogene–virogene) and factors responsible for expression or suppression of the oncogenes (regulatory genes). Similar principles may be operable with exogenous oncogenic viruses and chemical carcinogens. They may indicate desuppression of normally suppressed DNA sequences by interacting either directly with DNA or with regulatory nuclear proteins. Genetic factors may determine rates of susceptibility or resistence to any of the exogenous carcinogenic agents (Temin, 1972).

Experimental Neurooncology

Viral Neurooncology. The role of viruses in brain tumors has been subject to considerable research (Table 3). Rous sarcoma virus, an RNA virus, produces sarcomas and gliomas, following intracerebral injection into newborn hamsters (Burger *et al.*, 1973). The inoculation of 10^5 FFU of SR-RSV into the brain of 2-day-old inbred CDF rats is followed by a 96% incidence of usually multiple tumors within a period of 3 months (Wilfong *et al.*, 1973). Intracerebral injection of 2.5×10^5 FFU of the Bratislava 77 strain of avian Rous sarcoma virus into fetal, newborn, 3-, 10-, 30-, and 100-day-old CDF rats clearly indicates the decline in susceptibility with age. Apart from the demonstration of fetal production of neurogenic tumors, all newborn rats develop multiple tumors only (Copeland *et al.*, 1975). Adeno-

TABLE 3

Tumor viruses	Species	CNS tumors	PNS tumors
RNA viruses			
Rous sarcoma virus	Hamster Rat	Gliomas: astrocytoma Spongioblastoma Oligodendroglioma Sarcoma	None
DNA viruses			
SV-40	Hamster Mouse	Ependymoma Plexus papilloma Neurosecretory nerve Cell tumor line	None
Human papova virus (JC)	Hamster	Medulloblastoma Pinealis tumors Neuroblastoma Glioma Ependymoma Meningioma	None
Human papova virus (SV-40 PML)	Hamster	Plexus papilloma	None
Human papova virus (BK)	Hamster	Plexus papilloma	None
Human adenovirus-12	Mouse Hamster Rat	Primitive neuroepithelial tumors similar to med-ulloepithelioma, reti-noblastoma, or neuroblastoma	Primitive anaplastic tumors?

virus-12, a DNA virus, induces primitive neuroectodermal neoplasms, e.g., in the brain of mice, hamsters, and rats (Ogawa *et al.*, 1969), but also in the eye (Mukai and Kobayashi, 1973). Virus-induced brain tumors in experimental animals comprise a variety of different types, including sarcomas, gliomas, and primitive neuroectodermal tumors, while neuronal tumors are usually absent (Table 3). Recently, de Vitry *et al.* (1974) succeeded in producing a highly differentiated neuronal tumor after treatment of cultured fetal diencephalic mouse brain cells with SV-40 viruses. After *in vitro* transformation, cloning of a homogeneous neoplastic cell population was possible with morphological, biochemical, and immunological characteristics of a neurosecretory tumor cell type, capable of synthesizing specific hormones, i.e., vasopressin and neurophysin.

The JC-strain virus produces a high incidence of primitive brain tumors after intracerebral inoculation into newborn hamsters (Walker *et al.*, 1973). Narayan and Weiner (1974) demonstrated subsequently the oncogenic capacity of two strains of SV-40 PML viruses in cell culture experiments and in hamsters, but not in mice. The tumors developed subcutaneously as sarcomas and intracerebrally as choroid plexus papillomas. These observations are the first examples that viruses rescued from the human brain with a degenerative disease are oncogenic in animals. We are convinced that there are closer links between slow-virus infections of the nervous system and viral oncology than previously believed. Studies along these lines should be encouraged. Todaro (1974) reported an interesting observation that a recently isolated C-type virus from wild mouse embryos produced a slowly progressive neurologic disease either alone or together with lymphoma. The Marek-Herpes virus also produces neural lymphomatosis in some flocks of chickens and a chronic neuropathy in others (see Koestner, 1974). Such viruses bridge the gap between chronic progressive neurological diseases and neoplasia initiated by the same agent (Johnson and Narayan, 1974; Walker *et al.*, 1974).

Among the mammalian species there are those which are resistant to viral transformation of cells of the nervous system regardless of dose. Experiments with different animal species and strains indicate that the susceptibility or resistence to tumor induction are predetermined to a great extent by age and genetic factors. Transformation experiments in cell cultures by oncogenic viruses led to the conclusion that after integration of viral DNA into the host-cell genome at least one or more cell cycles are necessary in order to express molecular oncogenic information. This observation may explain the high preference for glial tumor types in contrast to the scarcity of neuronal neoplasms. Nerve cells lose their capacity for multiplication early during development in contrast to glial and meningeal cell elements, which remain in part replicating cells throughout life. There are exceptions to this observation, e.g., JC virus induces primitive tumors of the nervous system in hamsters, inclusive neuroblastomas, medulloblastomas, and pinealoblastomas (zu Rhein and Varakis, 1975; Varakis *et al.*, 1976a,b).

Chemical Neurooncology. Brain tumors were produced initially with polycyclic hydrocarbons (methylcholanthrene, dibenzanthracene, benzpyrine) implanted as pellets into the brain (Zimmerman, 1969). The discovery of a great variety of systemically applicable carcinogens was a major breakthrough in experimental cancer research (Druckrey *et al.*, 1967). Comparing topical and systemic carcinogens as model systems (Table 4) for naturally occurring tumors in man and animals, the advantage of the systemic carcinogens over the topically applied hydrocarbons is readily apparent since natural routes of exposure are more closely simulated. The differential organotropic effects of 65 alkylating nitrosamines and nitrosamides in rats described by Druckrey *et al.* (1967) were shown to be dependent upon the chemical structure of the carcinogen, the dose schedule, and the route of administration. Of all N-nitroso compounds, two have been shown to be particularly interesting for experimental neurooncology,

TABLE 4. Experimental Tumors of the Nervous System

Carcinogen	Species	CNS tumors	PNS tumors
Methylcholanthrene	Mouse Rat	Glioblastoma Astrocytoma Ependymoma Oligodendroglioma Mixed glioma Spongioblastoma Medulloblastoma Sarcoma (rare)	Fibrosarcoma
Alkylating agents MNU and ENU	Mouse	Oligodendroglioma Mixed glioma Medulloblastoma Meningioma	Neurinoma
	Hamster Rat Rabbit Dog	None Differentiated and ana- plastic gliomas and ependymomas	Neurinoma Differentiated and anaplastic neurinomas

i.e., *N*-methyl- and *N*-ethyl-*N*-nitrosourea (MNU and ENU). Extensive research has been accomplished with these two compounds in the past 10 years. While MNU had a greater neurooncogenic potency in adult animals, ENU had a particular neurooncogenic effect upon the fetus when administered to pregnant rats during the third period of gestation.

MNU Experiments in Adult Animals. Repeated applications of MNU to different animal species resulted in tumor production of the nervous system and other organs. There were species-dependent differences in susceptibility and tumor location (Table 5). If a total dose of 180 mg/kg was administered to different species, the mean survival time of animals with neurogenic tumors was about 270 days in mice (Denlinger *et al.*, 1974), 314 days in rats (Swenberg *et al.*, 1971), and approximately 3 years in boxer dogs (Koestner and Denlinger, unpublished data). These differences in survival time in mice, rats, and dogs should not necessarily be interpreted as differences in susceptibility to MNU carcinogenesis. Comparing the survival times with the life expectancy in these three species, they represent roughly one-third to one-fifth of the total lifetime of the individual species. If one extrapolates these figures to human life, a latency period of approximately 20 years would be estimated at a similar exposure, provided man is equally susceptible to this particular carcinogen. The incidence of neurogenic tumors in rats differed with routes of application, being the highest with intravenous administration (over 95%), followed by oral (52%), intraperitoneal (36%), and subcutaneous (12%) (Koestner *et al.*,

1972; Swenberg *et al.*, 1975). Immune suppression with antilymphocytic serum did not change the incidence and location of neurogenic tumors in rats, nor did it influence the survival time (Denlinger *et al.*, 1973).

ENU Experiments (Perinatal Exposure). The remarkable discovery by Druckrey and co-workers that a single exposure of pregnant rats during the fetal stage of gestation (12–22 days) results in a high incidence of neurogenic tumors in the offspring initiated a new phase in experimental oncology. It was found that under optimal conditions neurogenic tumors could be produced in all offspring and that fetuses were approximately 50 times more susceptible than adult rats (Ivankovic and Druckrey, 1968). A striking dose–response was demonstrated; with decreasing doses the tumor incidence diminished and the latency period was prolonged (Swenberg *et al.*, 1972). The mean survival time ranged from 211 days (50 mg/kg ENU) to 655 days (1 mg/kg) in this experiment. An extrapolation of these survival times to man would indicate a possible latency time range from 2 to 6 decades. Striking differences among species were demonstrated in ENU carcinogenesis particularly with regard to organ susceptibility (Table 6). While tumors of the central and peripheral nervous system were produced almost exclusively in rats (incidence close to 100%), only tumors of the peripheral nervous system were observed in hamsters, (Mennel and Zülch,

TABLE 5. MNU-Induced Tumors in Various Animal Species by Systemic Inoculation at (Optimal) Conditions Selected

Organ	Percentage				
	Rats	Mice	Hamsters	Rabbits	Dogs
Brain	77	10	0	50–70	0–40
Spinal cord	4	0	0	0– 4	0
Cranial nerve	3	0	0	0	0
Peripheral nerve	13	0	0	0	0–70
Total neurogenic	97	10	0	50–74	0–50
Lymphopoetic Hematopoetic	8	(15)[a]	0	0	30
Stomach (Carcinoma)	0	37	7–71	0	0
Lung (Carcinoma)	0	(45)[a]	2	0	1
Liver (Hepatoma)	0	(10)[a]	0	0	0
Inoculation site	0	0	50	0	0
Others	15	0	41–86	30	70 (Sarcomas)
Total nonneurogenic	23	37	60–86	30	70

[a]Not related to treatment.

TABLE 6. Organ Susceptibility to Perinatal ENU-Tumor Induction in Different Species

Organ	Mouse	Hamster	Rat	Rabbit
Brain	+[a]	0[b]	+++	0
Spinal cord	0	0	++	0
Nerves	++	++	+++	0
Nonneurogenic organs	+++	++	0	++

[a](+) Relative incidence of tumor growth.
[b](0) No tumors.

1972; Rustia, 1974). Different organ tumors including lymphohematopoetic neoplasms as well as tumors of the brain, the rare cerebellar medulloblastoma), the meninges, and cranial, spinal, or peripheral nerves were only produced in special inbred strains of mice (Searle and Jones, 1972; Denlinger et al., 1974; Diwan and Meier, 1974; Vesselinovitch et al., 1974; Wechsler et al., 1974). After transplacental exposure to ENU during fetal gestation, rabbit fetuses will receive a molecular program to develop kidney tumors similar to the Wilms tumors in children (Güthert et al., 1973; Stavrou et al., 1975).

Genetic factors must be responsible for the remarkable differences in tumor incidence and organ specificity among different rodent strains. The majority of tumors of the nervous system in rats are classified as anaplastic or malignant gliomas, ependymomas, and neurinomas. CNS and PNS tumors in mice appear better differentiated than in rats. In contradistinction to rats, the mice have a relatively high incidence of large and differentiated oligodendrogliomas and a small number of cerebellar medulloblastomas (Searle and Jones, 1972; Wechsler et al., 1974, 1976; Vesselinovitch et al., 1974). Opossums treated during early development may have tumors of the kidney, diagnosed as embryonal nephromas (Wilms tumor), and teratoid medulloepitheliomas of the eye and the brain (Jurgelski, 1976). Since all these tumors were produced perinatally by ENU, species-related factors must have determined the main tumor type in different species of animals, this species specificity is further modified by strain differences and may preclude the experimental production of certain tumor types known from human neurooncology. Transplacental, neonatal, and postnatal carcinogenesis have been reviewed recently in several articles (Ivankovic and Druckrey, 1968; Wechsler et al., 1969; Druckrey et al., 1972; Tomatis and Mohr, 1973; Rice, 1973; Koestner, 1974; Mennel and Ivankovic, 1975; Ivankovic, 1975, Kleihues et al., 1976).

How do these experimental findings relate to human cancer? There is at present no evidence that nitrosoureas are etiologically associated with human cancer. Since these substances are capable of producing tumors in different species of animals, man cannot be exluded as a possible target host. The fact that nitrosoureas may be synthesized intragastrically from harmless precursors present in our environment increases the hazard of human exposure (MNU precursors: Sander, 1970; Koestner *et al.*, 1975: ENU precursors: Ivankovic and Preussmann, 1970; Osske *et al.*, 1972; Ramadan and Wechsler, 1975; Koestner *et al.*, 1975).

Several attempts have been made to correlate carcinogenesis of these compounds with alkylation, i.e., with respect to MNU and ENU methylation or ethylation of nucleic acids, DNA in particular (see review by Kleihues *et al.*, (1976) on alkylation theory of cancer and neurooncology). Among the alkylation products of DNA, the relative extent of O^6-alkylation of guanine appears to be of importance for carcinogenesis as demonstrated with MNU (Lawley and Shah, 1972; Kleihues and Magee, 1973) or ENU (Goth and Rajewsky, 1972). More recently evidence has been presented that (specific) DNA damages exerted by the reactive intermediates of these carcinogens (carbonium ions) can be repaired. After application of ENU (Goth and Rajewsky, 1974) or of MNU (Kleihues and Margison, 1974; Margison and Kleihues, 1975) to newborn or adult rats, respectively, the rate of loss of O^6-alkylation from brain DNA, i.e., the principal target organ for tumor development was significantly lower than for nontarget organs. These observations suggest that different organs of an experimental animal vary in their capacity for excision of damaged DNA according to their oncogenic susceptibility or resistance. Thus, the alkylation theory of cancer has been linked with biological repair mechanisms, an attractive hypothesis which certainly will stimulate cancer research in perinatal and adult carcinogenesis.

If one further considers the multifold biochemical and biological actions of MNU and ENU, a special class of molecules among the alkylation agents, affecting nucleic acids and proteins, multipotential effects in the organism must be considered. We would like to mention only one possible way of thinking. MNU and ENU cause on a dose-dependent scale, changes of DNA which may be nullified or modified by repair mechanisms, but which also can become permanently integrated as an exogeneously induced error into the genetic program of the genome of somatic cells and germ cells. Therefore it is not surprising that MNU and ENU are not only potent carcinogens but also mutagens and teratogens.

Toxic effects depend—well known from basic principles in pharmacology—on both the chemical agent and the biological system involved. The oncogenic and teratogenic effects of MNU and ENU after perinatal exposure to rats have been summarized by Druckrey (1973) and Wechsler (1972b, 1973). More recently Druckrey (1974, 1975) has advanced the concept of "genotoxicology" and emphasized the possibility "that 'genotoxic' substances may be responsible also for certain disturbances of normal development, as proven by their teratogenicity, and for some diseases of unknown etiology." And he continues: "since neuronal cells are unable to divide, the question arose whether or not 'genotoxic' substances can induce mental disorders, which may be considered equivalent to 'malignant transformation'" (Druckrey, 1975). This hypothesis appears to be of particular importance to pathogenetic concepts for some chronic diseases of idiopathic nature which may manifest themselves after long latency periods, as it has been proven to be the case with experimental perinatal cancer induction but also with some degenerative diseases of the nervous system caused by slow-virus infections. Perinatal pathology, i.e., the exogeneous or endogeneous induction of a molecular disease program appears to be a new hypothesis not only valid for pediatric diseases but also diseases in adulthood. It is now well documented that developmental biology and oncology are interrelated, at least in special cases of human and experimental neoplasia.

References

Bailey, P., and Cushing, H. (1926). *A Classification of the Tumors of the Glioma Group on a Histogenetic Basis with a Correlated Study of Prognosis*, Lippincott, Philadelphia.

Baltimore. D. (1970). Viral RNS-dependent DNA polymerase. *Nature (London)* **226**:1209–1211.

Baltimore, D. (1976). Viruses, polymerases, and cancer. *Science* **192**:632–636.

Birkmayer, G. D., Miller, F., and Marguth, F. (1974). Oncorna-viral information in human glioblastomas. *J. Neural Transm.* **35**: 241—254.

Burger, P. D., Bigner, D. D., and Self, J. D. (1973). Morphologic observations of brain tumors in PD4 hamsters induced by four strains of avian sarcoma virus. *Acta Neuropathol. (Berlin)* **26**:1–21.

Copeland, D. D., Vogel, F. S., and Bigner, D. D. (1975). The induction of intracranial neoplasms by the inoculation of avian sarcoma virus in perinatal and adult rats. *J. Neuropathol. and Exp. Neurol.* **34**:340–358.

Cuatico W., Cho, J. R., and Spiegelman, S. (1973). Particles with RNA of high molecular weight and RNA-directed DNA polymerase in human brain tumors. *Proc. Nat. Acad. Sci. U.S.A.* **70**:2789–2793.

Denlinger, R. H., Koestner, A., and Wechsler, W. (1974). Induction of neurogenic tumors in C3HeB/FeJ mice by nitrosourea derivatives: Observations by light microscopy, tissue culture and electron microscopy. *Int. J. Cancer* **13**:559–571.

Denlinger, R. H. Swenberg, J. A., Koestner, A., and Wechsler, W. (1973). Differential effect of immunosuppression on the induction of nervous system and bladder tumors by *N*-methyl-*N*-nitrosourea. *J. Nat. Cancer Inst.* **50**:87–93.

Diwan, B. A., and Meier, H. (1974). Strain- and age-dependent transplacental carconogenesis by 1-ethyl-1-nitrosourea in inbred strains of mice. *Cancer Res.* **34**:764–770.

Druckrey, H. (1973). Chemical structure and action in transplacental carcinogenesis and teratogenesis. In *Transplacental Carcinogenesis* (Tomatis and Mohr, ed.), pp. 45–58. IARC Scientific Publ. No. 4, Lyon.

Druckrey, H. (1974). Krebserzeugung durch Inhalation. *Ärztliche Praxis* **Nr. 68**:2848–2852 and **Nr. 69**:2877–2878.

Druckrey, H. (1975). Chemical Carcinogenesis on *N*-Nitroso Dervatives. *Gann Monogr. Cancer Res.* **17**:107–132.

Druckrey, H., Ivankovic, S. and Preussmann, R. (1966). Teratogenic and carcinogenic effects in the offspring after single injection of ethylnitrosourea to pregnant rats. *Nature (London)* **210**:1378–1379.

Druckrey, H., Ivankovic, S., Preussmann, R., Zülch, K. J., and Mennel, H. D. (1972). Selective induction of malignant tumors of the nervous system by resorptive carcinogens. In *The Experimental Biology of Brain Tumors*, pp. 85–147. Thomas, Springfield, Ill.

Druckrey, H., Preussmann, R., Ivankovic, S., and D. Schmähl, D. (1967). Organotrope carcinogene Wirkungen bei 65 verschiedenen *N*-Nitroso-Verbindungen an BD-Ratten. *Z. Krebsforsch.* **69**:103–201.

Everson, T. C. and Cole, W. H. (1966). *Spontaneous Regression of Cancer.* W. B. Saunders, Philadelphia.

Goth, R. and Rajewsky, M. F. (1972). Ethylation of nucleic acids by ethylnitrosourea 1-^{14}C in the fetal and adult rat. *Cancer Res.* **32**:1501–1505.

Goth, R. and Rajewsky, M. F. (1974). Persistence of O^6-ethylguanine in rat brain DNA: Correlation with nervous system-specific carcinogenesis by ethylnitrosourea. *Proc. Nat. Acad. Scie. USA* **71**:639–643.

Greenwald, P., Barlow, J. J., Nasca, P. C., *et al.* (1971). Vaginal cancer after maternal treatment with synthetic estrogen. *N. Engl. J. Med.* **285**:390–392.

Güthert, H., Jäckel, E. M., and Warzok, R. (1973). Zur karzinogenen Wirkung von *N*-Äthyl-*N*-nitrosoharnstoff (ÄNH) bei Kaninchen. *Zbl. allg. Pathol.* **117**:461–471.

Heidelberger, C. (1973). Current trends in chemical carcinogenesis. *Fed. Proc.* **32**:2154–2161.

Herbst, A. L., Ulfelder, H., and Poskanzer, D. C. (1971a). Adenocarcinoma of the vagina: Association of maternal stilbestrol therapy with tumor appearance in young women. *N. Engl. J. Med.* **284**:878–881.

Herbst, A. L., Ulfelder, H., and Poskanzer, D. C. (1971b). Registry of clear-cell carcinoma of genital tract in young women. *N. Engl. J. Med.* **285**:407.

Huebner, R. J., and Todaro, G. J. (1964). Oncogenes of RNA tumor viruses as determinants of cancer. *Proc. Nat. Acad. Sci. Wash.* **64**:1087–1094.

Huebner, R. J., Sarma, P. S., Kelloff, G. J., Gilden, R. V., Meier, H., Meyers, D. D., and Peters, R. L. (1971). Immunological tolerance to RNA tumor virus genome expressions: Significance of tolerance and prenatal expression in embryogenesis and tumorigenesis. *Ann. N.Y. Acad. Sci.* **181**:246–268.

Ivankovic, S. (1975). *Handbuch der allgemeinen Pathologie, Bd. 6, Praenatale Carcinogenese*, pp. 941–1002. Springer-Verlag, Berlin Heidelberg New York.

Ivankovic, S., and Druckrey, H. (1968). Transplazentare Erzeugung maligner Tumoren des Nervensystems. I. Äthylnitrosoharnstoff an BD IX-Ratten. *Z. Krebsforsch.* **71**:320–360.

Ivankovic, S., and Preussmann, R. (1970). Transplazentare Erzeugung maligner Tumoren nach oraler Gabe von Äthylharnstoff und Nitrit an Ratten. *Naturwissenschaften* **57**:460.

Jänisch, W., and Schreiber, D. (1970). *Hirngeschwülste bei Neugeborenen und Säuglingen. Pädiatrische Neurochirurgie.* Verlag der Wiener Medizinischen Akademie, pp. 51–56.

Johnson, R. T., and Narayan, O. (1974). Experimental neurological diseases of animals caused by viruses. In *Models of Human Neurological Diseases* (H. L. Klawans, Jr., ed.), Excerpta Medica, Amsterdam, pp. 43–82.

Jurgelsky, W. (1976). Tissue differentiation and susceptibility to embryonal tumor induction by ethylnitrosourea in the developing opossum. *Conference on Perinatal Carcinogenesis, 19–21 January, 1976.* Tampa.

Kleihues, P., and Magee, P. N. (1973). Aklylation of rat brain nucleic acids by N-methyl-N-nitrosourea and methyl methanesulphonate. *J. Neurochem.* **20**::595–606.

Kleihues, P., and Margison, G. P. (1974). Carcinogenicity of N-methyl-N-nitrosourea: Possible role of excision repair of O^6-methylguanine from DNA. *J. Nat. Cancer Inst.* **53**:1839–1841.

Kleihues, P., Lantos, P. L., and Magee, P. N. (1976). Chemical carcinogenesis in the nervous system. *Int. Rev. Exp. Pathol.* **15**:153–232.

Koestner, A. (1974). Transplacental carcinogenesis. *Proc. Cancer Res. Canada,* 65–82.

Koestner, A., Denlinger, R. H., and Wechsler, W. (1975). Induction of neurogenic and lymphoid neoplasms by feeding threshold levels of methyl- and ethylnitrosourea precursors to adult rats. *Food Cosmet. Toxicol.* **13**:605–609.

Koestner, A., Swenberg, J. A., and Wechsler, W. (1972). Experimental tumors of the nervous system induced by resorptive N-nitroso-compounds. *Prog. Exp. Tumor Res. (Basel)* **17**:9–30.

Koos, W. T., and Miller, M. H. (1971). *Intracranial Tumors of Infants and Children.* Georg Thieme Verlag, Stuttgart.

Lawley, P. D., and Shah, S. A. (1972). Methylation of RNA by the carcinogens dimethylsulfate N-methyl-N-nitrosourea or N-methyl-N'-nitro-N-nitrosoguanidine: Comparison of analyses at the base and nucleoside levels. *Biochem. J.* **128**:117–132.

Lilly, F., and Pincus, T. (1973). Genetic control of murine viral leukemogenesis. *Adv. Cancer Res.* **17**:231.

Margison, G. P., and Kleihues, P. (1975). Chemical carcinogenesis in the nervous system. *Biochem. J.* **148**:521–525.

Mennel, H. D., and Ivankovic, S. (1975). *Handbuch der allgemeinen Pathologie, Bd. 6 Experimentelle Erzeugung von Tumoren des Nervensystems,* pp. 34–122. Springer-Verlag, Berlin Heidelberg New York.

Mennel, H. D., and Zülch, K. J. (1972). Zur Morphologie transplacentar erzeuger neurogener Tumoren beim Goldhamster. *Acta Neurpathol. (Berlin)* **21**:140–153.

Miller, E. C., and Miller, J. A. (1971). The mutagenicity of chemical carcinogens: correlations, problems and interpretations. In *Chemical Mutagens, Principles and Methods of Detection* (A. Hollaender, ed.), Vol. 1 pp. 83–119. Plenum Publishing Corp., New York.

Miller, J. A. (1970). Carcinogenesis by chemicals: An overview. *Cancer Res.* **30**:559–576.

Miller, R. W. (1973). Prenatal origins of cancer in man: Epidemiological evidence. In *Transplacental Carcinogenesis* (L. Tomatis and U. Mohr, eds.), pp. 175–180. Int. Agency for Research on Cancer, Lyon.

Mohr, U., and Althoff, J. (1964). Mögliche diaplacentar-carcinogene Wirkung von Diäthylnitrosamin beim Goldhamster. *Naturwissenschaften* **16**:515.

Mohr, U., and Althoff, J. (1965). Die diaplacentare Wirkung des Cancerogens Diäthylnitrosamin bei der Maus. *Z. Krebsforsch.* **67**:152–155.

Mukai, N., and Kobayashi, S. (1973). Extraocular orbital tumors induced by human adenovirus type 12 in hamsters. *Invest. Ophthalmol. (St. Louis)* **12**:185–192.

Narayan, O., and Weiner, P. L. (1974). Biological properties of two strains of simian virus 40 isolated from patients with progressive multifocal leukoencephalopathy. *Infect. Immun.* **10**:173–179.

Ogawa, K., Hamaya, K., Fuji, Y., Matsuura, K., and Endo, T. (1969). Tumor induction by adenovirus type 12 and its target cells in the central nervous system. *Gann* **60**:383–392.

Osske, G., Harzok, R., and Schneider, J. (1972). Diaplazentare Tumorinduction durch endogen gebildeten N-Äthyl-N-Nitrosoharnstoff bei Ratten. *Arch. Geschwulstforsch.* **40**:3, 244.

Peller, S. (1960). *Cancer in Childhood and Youth*. Wright, Bristol.

Ramadan, M. A., and Wechsler, W. (1975). Transplacental induction of neurogenic tumors in BD IX-rats by intragastric administration of ethylnitrosourea precursors. *Z. Krebsforsch.* **84**:177–187.

Rice, J. M. (1973). An overview of transplacental chemical carcinogenesis. *Teratology* **8**:113–126.

Rowe, W. P. (1973). Genetic factors in the natural history of murine leukemia virus infection. G. H. A. Clowes memorial lecture. *Cancer Res.* **33**:3061–3068.

Rubinstein, L. J. (1972). *Tumors of the Nervous System. Atlas of Tumor Pathology*. Armed Forces Institute of Pathology, Washington D.C.

Rustia, M. (1974). Multiple carcinogenic effects of the ethylnitrosourea precursors ethylurea and sodium nitrite in hamsters. *Cancer Res.* **343232–3244**.

Sander, J. (1970). Induktion maligner Tumoren bei Ratten durch orale Gabe von N, N'-Dimethylharnstoff und Nitrit. *Arzneim Forsch.* **20**:418–419.

Searle, C. E., and Jones, E. L. (1972). Tumors of the nervous system in mice treated neonatally with N-ethyl-N-nitrosourea. *Nature (London)* **240**:559–560.

Stavrou, D., Hänichen, T., and Wriedt-Lübbe, I. (1975). Oncogene Wirkung von Äthylnitrosoharnstoff beim Kaninchen während der pränatalen Periode. *Z. Krebsforsch.* **84**:207–215.

Swenberg, J. A., Koestner, A., and Wechsler, W. (1971). The induction of tumors of the nervous system in rats with intravenous methylnitrosourea. *J. Neuropathol. Exp. Neurol.* **30**:122.

Swenberg, J. A., Koestner, A., and Wechsler, W. (1972). The induction of tumors of the nervous system with intravenous methylnitrosourea. *Lab. Invest.* **26**:74–85.

Swenberg, J. A., Koestner, A., Wechsler, W., and Denlinger, R. H. (1975). Quantitative aspects of transplacental tumor induction with ethylnitrosourea in rats. *Cancer Res.* **32**:2656–2660.

Temin, H. M. (1972). The protovirus hypothesis and cancer. In: *RNA-Viruses and Host Genome in Oncogenesis*, (P. Emmelot and P. Bentvelzen, eds.) North-Holland, Amsterdam, pp. 351–363.

Temin, H., M. and Baltimore, D. (1972). RNA-directed DNA synthesis and RNA tumor viruses. *Adv. Virus Res.* **17**: 129–186.

Temin, H. M., and Mizutani, S. (1970). RNA-dependent DNA polymerase in virions of Rous sarcoma virus. *Nature (London)* **226**:1211–1213.

Todaro, G. T. (1974). Biology of RNA- and DNA-containing oncogenic viruses. In *Slow Virus Diseases,* (W. Zeman, E. H. Lennette, and J. G. Brunson, eds.). Williams & Wilkins, Baltimore.

Tomatis, L. and Mohr, U. (1973). *Transplacental Carcinogenesis*. Int. Agency for Research on Cancer, Lyon.

Varakis, J. N., Zimmerman, G. M., Padgett, B. L., and Walker, D. L. (1976a). Experimental (JC-virus induced) neuroblastomas in the Syrian hamster. *J. Neuropathol. Exp. Neurol.* **35**:314.

Varakis, J. N., ZuRhein, G. M., Padgett, B. L., Walker, D. L., and Quay, W. B. (1976b). Experimental pineocytomas: A morphlogical, virological and biochemical study. *J. Neuropathol. Exp. Neurol.* **35**:355.(b)

Vesselinovitch, S. D., Rao, K. V. N., Mihailovich, N., Rice, J. M., and Lombard, L. S. (1974). Development of broad spectrum of tumors by ethylnitrosourea in mice and the modifying role of age, sex, and strain. *Cancer Res.* **34**:2530–2538.

de Vitry, F., Camier, M., Czernichow, P., Benda, P., Cohen, P., and Tixier-Vidal, A. (1974). Establishment of a clone of mouse hypothalamic neurosecretory cells synthesizing neurophysin and vasopressin. *Proc. Nat. Acad. Sci. USA* **71**:3573–3579.

Walker, D. L., Padgett, B. L., zu Rhein, G. M., Albert, A. E., and Marsh, R. F. (1973). Human papovavirus (JC). Induction of brain tumors in hamsters. *Science* **181**:674–676.

Walker, D. L., Padgett, B. L., zu Rhein, G. M., Albert, A. E., and Marsh, R. F. (1974). Current study of an opportunistic papovavirus. In *Slow Virus Diseases* (W. Zeman and E. H. Lennette, eds.), pp. 41–58. Williams & Wilkins, Baltimore.

Wechsler, W. (1971). Zur Pathogenese der Tumoren des Nervensystems im Kindes- und Jugendalter. *Verh. Dtsch. Ges. Pathol.* **55**:305–310.

Wechsler, W. (1972a). Old and new concepts of oncogenesis in the nervous system of man and animals. In *Recent Advances in Brain Tumor Research.* (W. G. Bingham, Jr. ed.), pp. 219–278. S. Karger, Basel.

Wechsler, W. (1972b). Teratogenic and oncogenic effects of ethylnitrosourea on the developing nervous system of rats. In *CIBA Symposium on The Brain in Unclassified Mental Retardation* (Cavanagh, ed.), pp. 133–139. Churchill Livingstone, London.

Wechsler, W. (1973). Carcinogenic and teratogenic effects of ethylnitrosourea and methylnitrosourea during pregnancy in experimental rats. In *Transplacental Carcinogenesis* (Tomatis and Mohr, eds.), pp. 127–142. IARC Scientific Publ. No. 4, Lyon.

Wechsler, W., Kleihues, P., Matsumoto, S., Zülch, K. J., Ivankovic, S., Preussmann, R., and Druckrey, H. (1969). Pathology of experimental neurogenic tumors chemically induced during prenatal and postnatal life. *Ann. N.Y. Acad. Sci.* **159**:360–408.

Wechsler, W., Rice, J. M., Vesselinovich, S. D., and Arai, T. (1974). Perinatale Tumorinduktion mit Äthylnitrosoharnstoff. Ein Beitrag zur Frage der Organotropie alkylierender Resorptivkanzerogene bei verschiedenen Mäusestämmen. *Verh. Dtsch. Ges. Pathol.* **58**:546.

Wechsler, W., and Zülch, K. J. (1974). Pathology of neurogenic tumors in childhood and adolescence. In *Progress in Paediatric Neurosurgery* (Bushe, Spoerri, and Shaw, eds.), pp. 13–18. Hippokrates-Verlag, Stuttgart.

Wechsler, W., Rice, J. M. and Vesselinovitch, S. D. (1976). Transplacental and systemic induction of tumors of the nervous system in mice by ethylnitrosourea: a comparative evaluation. In: *Conference on Perinatal Carcinogenesis,* Tampa. 19–21 Jan.

Weiss, A., Portman, R., Fischer, H., Simon, J., and Zang, K. D. (1975). SV 40 related antigens in three human meningiomas with defined chromosome loss. *Proc. Nat. Acad. Sci. USA* **72**:609–613.

Wilfong, R. F., Bigner, D. D., Self, D. J., and Wechsler, W. (1973). Brain tumor types induced by the Schmidt-Ruppin strain of Rous sarcoma virus in inbred Fischer rats. *Acta Neuropathol. (Berlin)* **25**:196–206.

Zimmerman, H. M. (1969). Brain tumors. Their incidence and classification in man and their experimental production. *Ann. N.Y. Acad. Sci.* **159**:337–359.

Zülch, K. J. (1956). *Handbuch der Neurochirurgie. Biologie und Pathologie der Hirngeschwülste,* Vol. III, pp. 1–702. Springer, Berlin.

Zülch, K. J. (1965). *Brain Tumors, Their Biology and Pathology,* 2nd Ed. Springer, New York.

Zülch, K. J. (1971). *Atlas of the Tumors of the Nervous System.* Springer, Berlin.

Zülch, K. J., and Mennel, H. D. (1973). Recent results in new models of transplacental carcinogenesis in rats. In *Transplacental Carcinogenesis* (L. Tomatis and U. Mohr, eds.), pp. 29–44. Int. Agency for Research on Cancer, Lyon.

zu Rhein, G. M., and Varakis, J. (1975). Morphology of brain tumors induced in Syrian hamsters after inoculation with J.C. virus. A new human Papova virus. In *VIIth International Congress on Neuropathology,* pp. 479–481. Excerpta Medica, Amsterdam.

Chapter 6

BIOCHEMICAL ASPECTS

DENNIS V. PARKE

The Biochemistry of Cancer

Since the earliest observation of the London surgeon, Percivall Pott, in the eighteenth century that contact with soot was associated with scrotal skin cancer in chimney sweeps, a wide variety of agents causing cancer have been discovered. These include an extensive number and variety of organic chemicals, metals, oncogenic viruses, ultraviolet light, X-rays, and other ionizing radiations, which may singly and in various combinations result in malignancies of many different types. The epidemiology of cancer suggests that a high proportion of human malignancies are environmental in origin, as for example the lung cancer due to cigarette smoking, the bladder cancer of chemical workers using 2-naphthylamine or benzidine, and the liver cancer due to eating food contaminated with aflatoxins or nitrosamines. Furthermore, although the importance of radiations and oncogenic viruses in the causation of human cancer should in no way be discounted or minimized, it would seem nevertheless that chemicals comprise the major cause (Miller, 1970; Miller and Miller, 1971; Weisburger and Williams, 1975). These chemicals are both naturally occurring, such as the aflatoxins produced by the mold *Aspergillus flavus,* nitrosamines, formed by the interaction of food amines with nitrites, cycasin, present in the cycad nut, and the pyrrolizidine alkaloids of *Senecio, Crotolaria,* and other plant species; and man-made chemicals such as the polycyclic aromatic hydro-

Dennis V. Parke • Department of Biochemistry, University of Surrey, Guildford, Surrey, GU2 5XH, England.

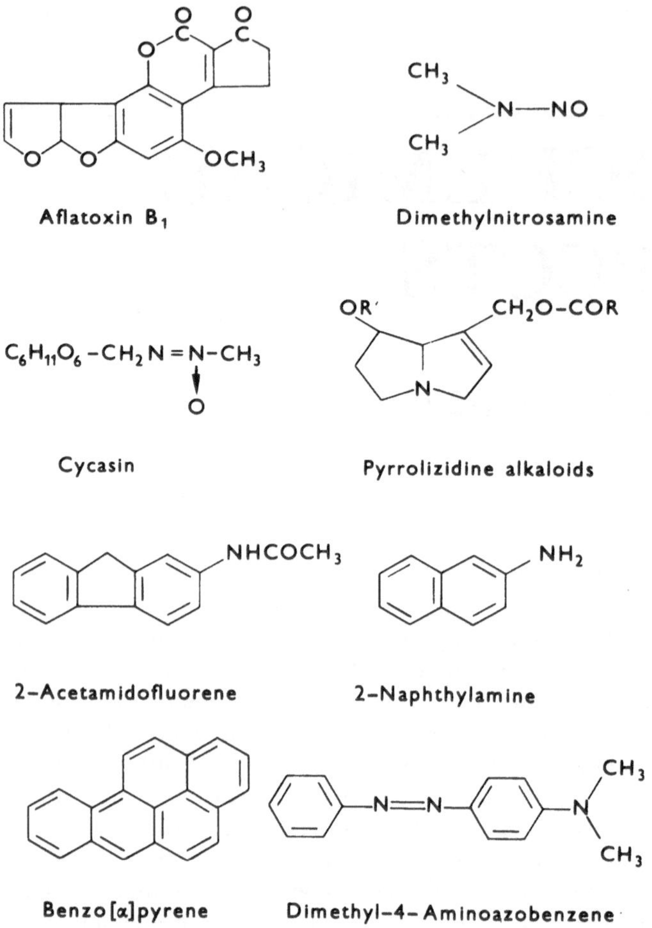

Figure 1. Some naturally occurring and man-made chemical carcinogens.

carbons (benzo[a]pyrene), aromatic amines (2-naphthylamine), polycyclic amides (2-acetamidofluorene), and azo dyes (N-methyl-4-aminoazobenzene) (see Figure 1).

Chemical Carcinogenesis

Apart from a few metallic compounds, such as the salts of nickel, cadmium, and chromium (Furst and Haro, 1969), chemical carcinogens are organic compounds, of diverse structure, including polycyclic aromatic hydrocarbons, amines, amides, nitrosamines, N-oxides, urethanes, lactones, ethyleneimines, etc. Most of these organic compounds are not carcinogenic per se but are activated by metabolism into the highly reactive proximate and ultimate carcinogens. In this way the reactive carcinogen is produced inside the biological cell whereby it evokes the most damage.

In contrast, there are a few chemicals which are active carcinogens per se, for example, β-propiolactone, propanesultone, N-acyl ethyleneimines, and the nitrogen mustards (see Figure 2). These substances are chemically highly reactive and interact with DNA and other cellular constituents by S_{N2} (biomolecular nucleophilic substitution) reactions resulting in alkylation or arylation of essential biological components. These alkylating agents possess an electrophilic (positive) atom which combines with nucleophilic (negative) centers in the DNA and other biological materials, but as they are initially reactive they interact with water and other extracellular nucleophilic materials before penetrating into the cell, and thus may not be carcinogens as potent as compounds which first have to be biologically activated within the cell.

The chemical carcinogens (procarcinogens) which have first to undergo metabolism to form the reactive proximate carcinogens are activated, mostly by enzymes of the endoplasmic reticulum, forming alkylating and arylating agents similar to the carcinogens active per se. It would seem, therefore, that the alkylation of DNA, and possibly other cellular constituents, is fundamental to the initiation of carcinogenesis. Indeed, it is this aspect of chemical carcinogenesis, the formation of the proximate carcinogen and its interaction and covalent binding to DNA, that has received the

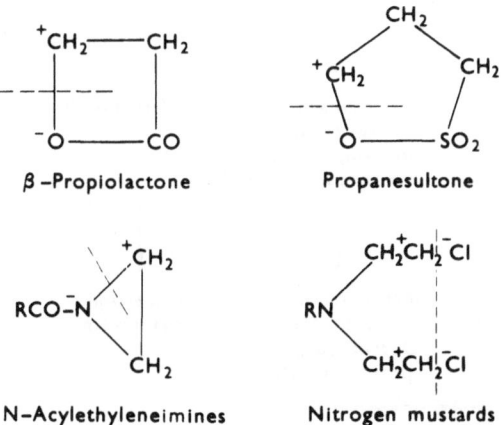

Figure 2. Carcinogenic alkylating agents which undergo scission as shown during the alkylation of biological molecules.

greatest attention from research workers in this field of study. Nevertheless, the development of a malignant neoplasm is a more complex, multistage process that involves not only the damage of the DNA of a cell (mutation) but also a reorientation of the cell's metabolism (initiation), comprising a period of rapid cellular growth and division (promotion), alteration of the cellular immune response (immunosuppression), and destruction of the host's normal tissues (invasion). These latter processes are not so well understood as are the formation of the proximate carcinogen and the damage to the DNA by alkylation, but recent studies have given the first glimpses of possible mechanisms whereby the proximate carcinogen may cause similar damage to other cellular components, namely the plasma membrane, the endoplasmic reticulum, the lysosomes, and the mitochondria. These further cellular changes probably result in the subsequent "initiation" processes of "promotion," "immunosuppression," and "invasion" which are essential to the establishment of a malignant neoplasm (see Figure 3).

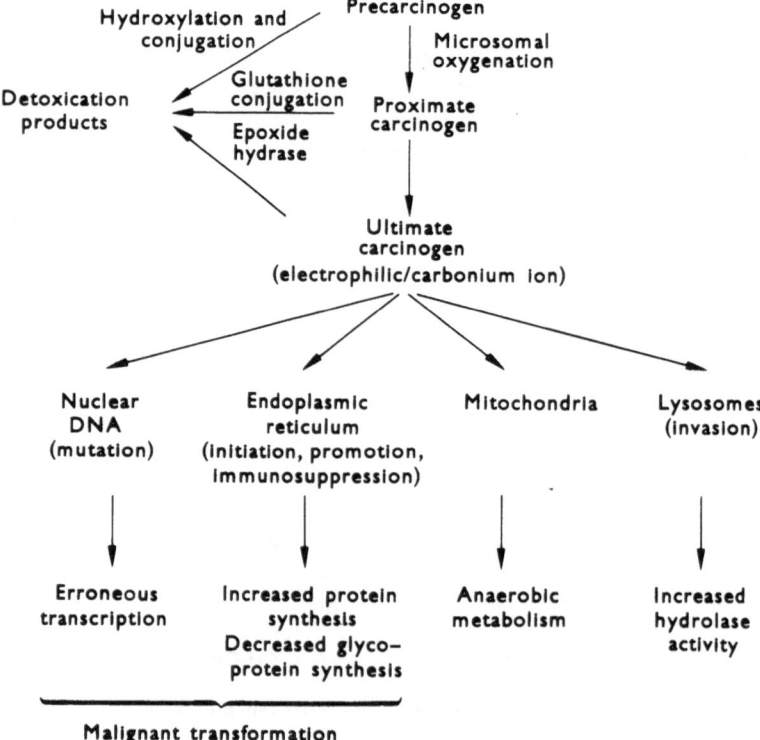

Figure 3. Hypothetical scheme for multifunctional initiation of chemical carcinogenesis.

Activation of Carcinogens

Despite the many structural differences of chemical carcinogens, they have a common property of being metabolized to highly reactive electrophilic compounds, the proximate carcinogens. Metabolism occurs primarily in the endoplasmic reticulum (microsomes) of the cells and is effected by the mixed-function oxidases, enzymes which also metabolize drugs and other foreign chemicals by processes of hydroxylation (oxygenation). These mixed-function oxidases require the coenzyme NADPH and molecular oxygen for activity, and transfer one atom of the oxygen molecule to the substrate (procarcinogen) to form the proximate carcinogen, while the other atom of oxygen is converted to water. The enzyme system has a number of components, including NADPH–cytochrome-c oxidoreductase, cytochrome P_{450} (the terminal oxygenase), and cytochrome P_{450} reductase (see Figure 4) and is found in many mammalian tissues including the liver, gastrointestinal tract, kidneys, lungs, skin, and gonads, which are, not unexpectedly, the more common sites of primary malignancies.

The enzymic processes involved in the activation of carcinogens include (a) epoxide formation, (b) N-hydroxylation, and (c) oxidative dealkylation, to yield the reactive nucleophiles. There is substantial evidence that the K-region epoxides, or arene oxides, of the polycyclic hydrocarbons may be the proximate carcinogens, reacting with nucleic acids and proteins both *in vivo* and *in vitro* (Van Duuren, 1969; Keysell *et al.*, 1973). The 5,6-oxide of benz[a]anthracene, the 5,6-oxide of dibenz[a,h]anthracene, and the 11,12-oxide of 3-methylcholanthrene are known metabolites of the corresponding polycyclic hydrocarbon carcinogens and are highly active in inducing malignant cell transformations

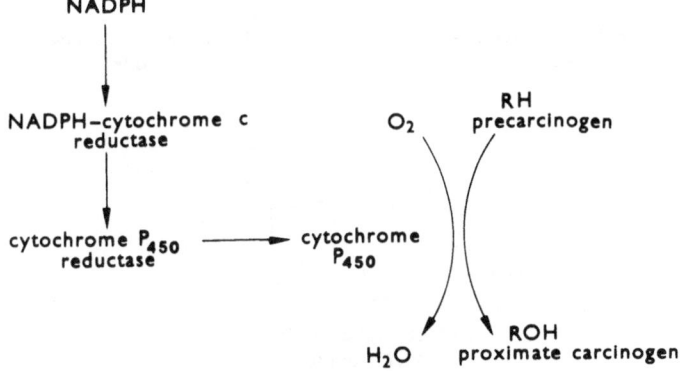

Figure 4. Mechanism of activation of precarcinogens.

(Figure 5). More recently, the rather elusive K-region epoxide of the ubiquitous carcinogen benzo[a]pyrene, namely, the 4,5-oxide, has been shown to be formed by the enzymes of rat liver microsomes (Kinoshita *et al.*, 1973). Other metabolic reactions can occur with these polycyclic hydrocarbons to produce noncarcinogenic metabolites. These alternative reactions include oxygenation to non-K-region epoxides, further metabolism to dihydrodiols by the enzyme epoxide hydrase, or metabolism to glutathione conjugates and mercapturic acids by glutathione transferase, all of which may be regarded as true detoxication reactions. Thus both activation to the proximate carcinogen epoxides and detoxication to dihydrodiols and glutathione conjugates are possible routes of metabolism for these carcinogenic polycyclic hydrocarbons (Figure 6), and as both pathways of metabolism appear to be catalyzed, at least in part, by the same enzyme system it is extremely important to our understanding of chemical carcinogenesis to learn what are the factors that affect and regulate these alternative and opposing processes.

Although the K-region epoxides have many properties that make them likely to be the ultimate carcinogens of the polycyclic hydrocarbons, in that they readily react with nucleic acids, induce malignant transformation in cell culture, and are mutagenic, this has not been proved unequivocally (Sims and Grover, 1974). More recently, it has been shown that the K-region epoxide of benzo[a]pyrene (Sims *et al.*, 1974) and

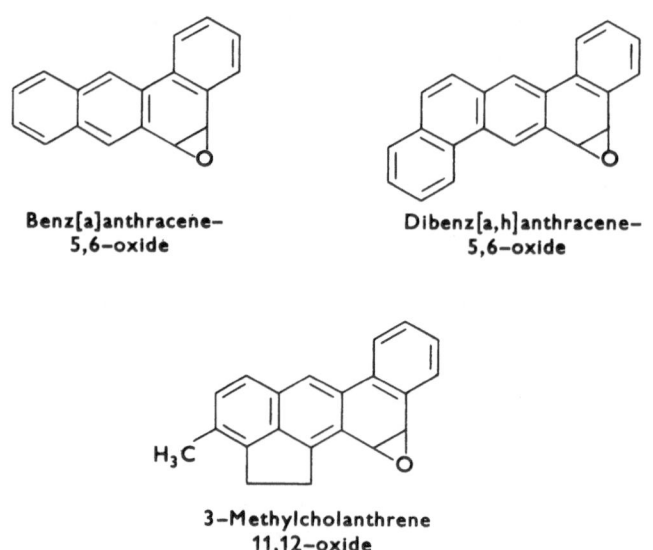

Benz[a]anthracene–
5,6–oxide

Dibenz[a,h]anthracene–
5,6–oxide

3–Methylcholanthrene
11,12–oxide

Figure 5. K-region epoxides of some carcinogenic polycyclic hydrocarbons.

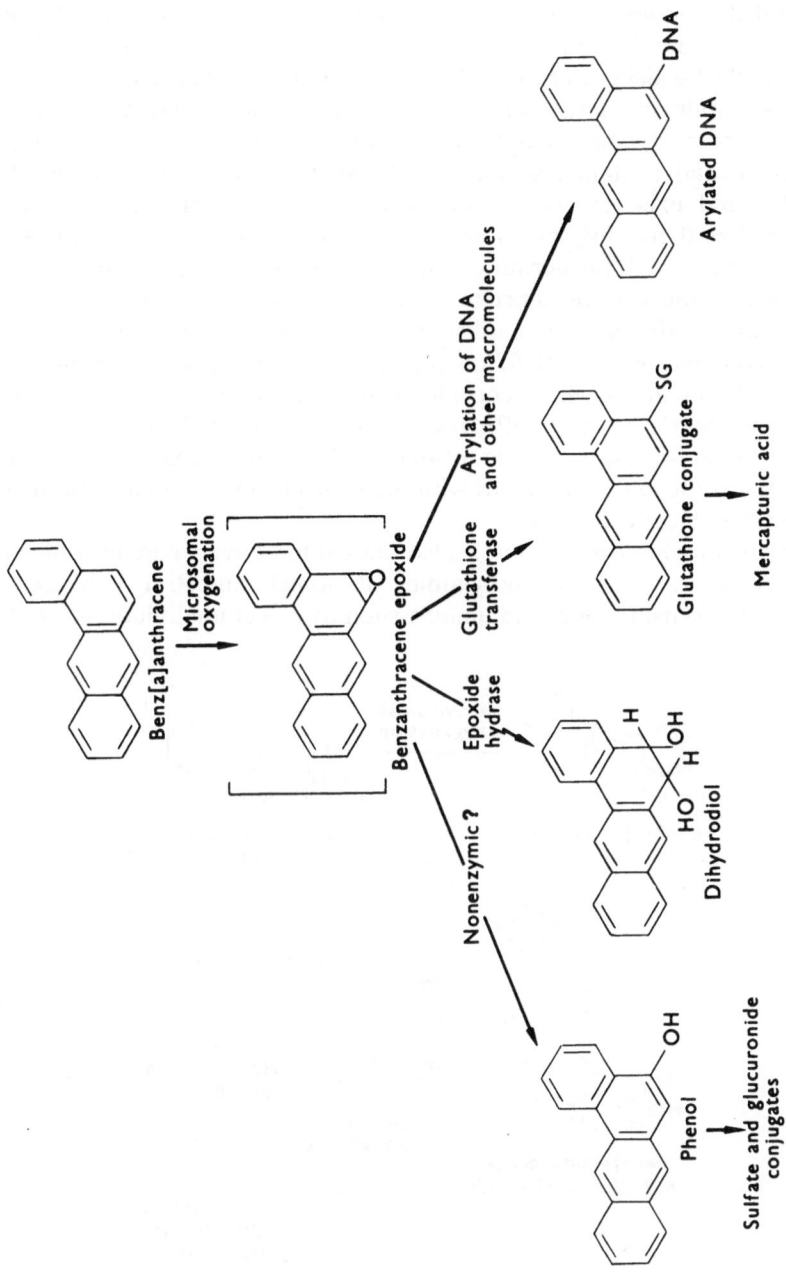

Figure 6. Metabolism of benz[*a*]anthracene.

benz[a]anthracene (Swaisland *et al.*, 1974b) are not the ultimate carcinogens and that more extensively oxygenated metabolites, namely the diol
epoxides, are implicated as the reactive metabolites that bind to DNA
(Sims, 1975; Swaisland *et al.*, 1974b) (see Figure 7). These diol epoxides
can form stabilized internal ion-pair compounds which will react as carbonium ions and may consequently react with DNA, even in the presence of
glutathione and proteins, so that no threshold concentration of the diol
epoxide need exist for DNA arylation (Hulbert, 1975). However, it is
possible that there may be more than one ultimate carcinogen for each
procarcinogen, and furthermore, different ultimate carcinogens may be
concerned in the various subcellular processes of carcinogenesis.

Similarly, the natural carcinogen aflatoxin B_1, on incubation with
human liver microsomes or following injection to rats, has been shown to
form a 2,3-epoxide which is considered to be the proximate agent of this
carcinogen (Swenson *et al.*, 1974) (see Figure 8), and evidence has recently
been obtained for the metabolic formation of a stilbene oxide (by epoxida-
tion of the stilbene double bond) with the transplacental carcinogen, diethylstilbestrol (Metzler, 1975).

Microsomal hydroxylation is also known to convert carcinogenic aromatic amines, such as 2-naphthylamine (Radomski and Brill, 1970; Deich-
man and Radomski, 1969) and amides such as 2-acetamidofluorene (Miller

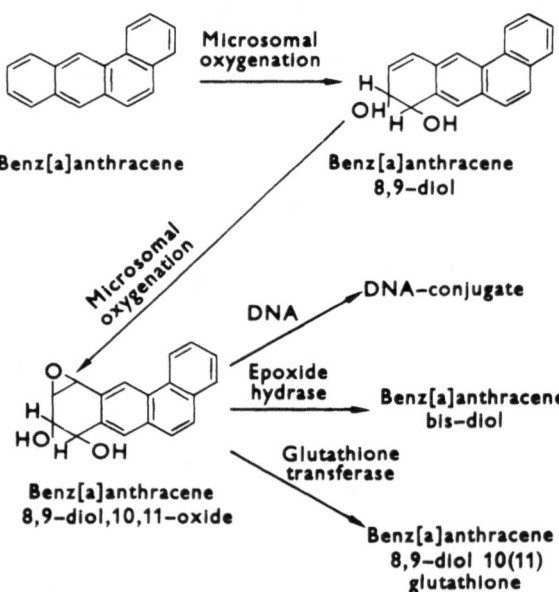

Figure 7. Formation of diol epoxide of benz[a]anthracene.

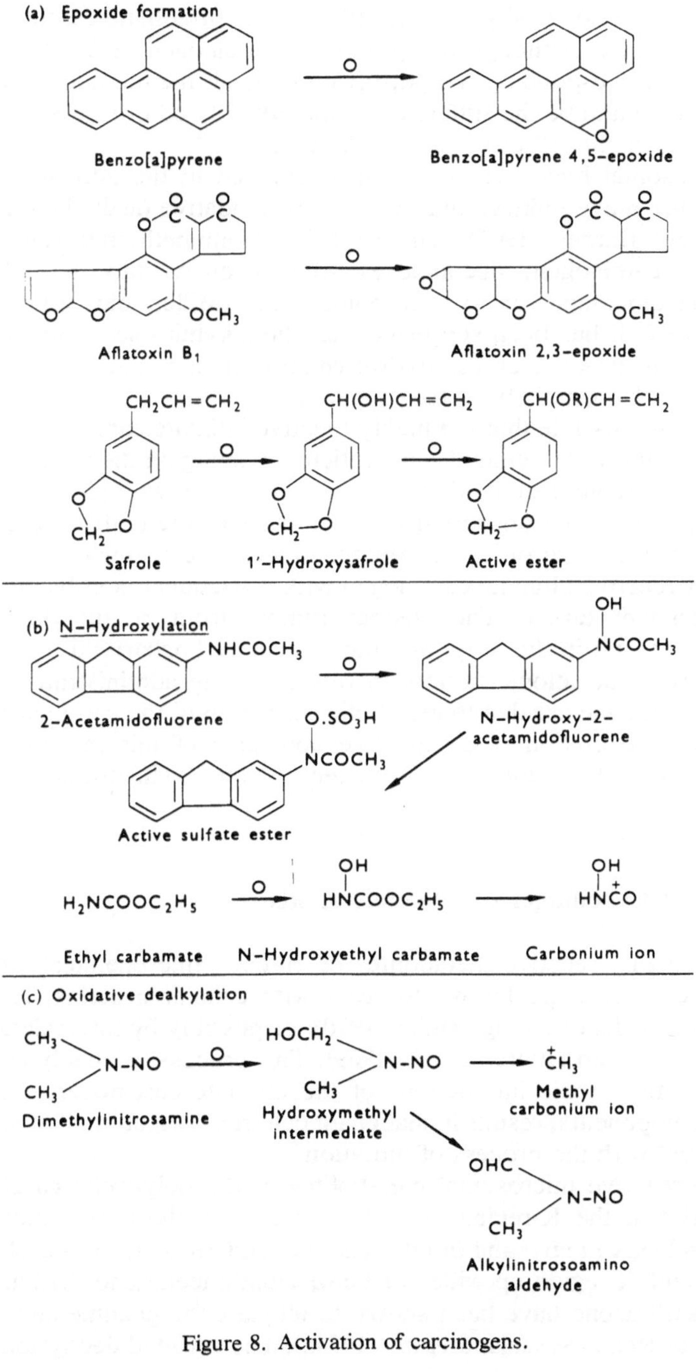

(a) Epoxide formation

Benzo[a]pyrene   Benzo[a]pyrene 4,5-epoxide

Aflatoxin B$_1$ Aflatoxin 2,3-epoxide

Safrole   1'-Hydroxysafrole   Active ester

(b) N-Hydroxylation

2-Acetamidofluorene   O.SO$_3$H   N-Hydroxy-2-acetamidofluorene

Active sulfate ester

$H_2NCOOC_2H_5$ $HNCOOC_2H_5$ $HN\overset{+}{C}O$

Ethyl carbamate   N-Hydroxyethyl carbamate   Carbonium ion

(c) Oxidative dealkylation

Dimethylinitrosamine   Hydroxymethyl intermediate   Methyl carbonium ion

Alkylinitrosoamino aldehyde

Figure 8. Activation of carcinogens.

and Miller, 1969; Weisburger *et al.*, 1972) to the proximate carcinogens by
N-hydroxylation. Although the proximate carcinogen of 2-acetamidoflu-
orene is the corresponding *N*-hydroxy compound, the ultimate carcinogen
has been shown to be the sulfate ester and possibly other esters, of this *N*-
hydroxy metabolite (Weisburger *et al.*, 1972).

   Microsomal hydroxylation is also involved in the activation of the
carcinogenic nitrosamines, and in this case oxidative dealkylation occurs
(Magee and Barnes, 1967). The resulting monomethylnitrosamine, the
proximate carcinogen, decomposes spontaneously into the alkylating
agent, diazomethane, or to a carbonium ion (Miller and Miller, 1965).
Alternatively, it has been suggested that the alkylnitrosoamino aldehyde,
the oxidation product of the hydroxymethyl metabolite, is the ultimate
carcinogen (Schoental, 1973) (see Figure 8).

   It is also possible that the highly reactive ultimate carcinogen, formed
by the enzymes of the endoplasmic reticulum acting on the precarcinogen,
may undergo rapid deactivation by conjugation, say with glucuronic acid,
then be excreted or transported to other parts of the body where hydrolases, such as β-glucuronidase, would hydrolyze the conjugate and liberate
the highly reactive ultimate carcinogen with consequent possible formation
of a malignant tumor. The bladder tumors from β-napthylamine are
believed to result in this way, and more recently Pozharisski *et al.* (1975)
have shown that colonic tumors in rats following administration of 1,2-
dimethylhydrazine are due to metabolic activation of the carcinogen in the
liver, biliary excretion of an inactive conjugate of this metabolite, and
reactivation to the ultimate carcinogen by the β-glucuronidase of the
intestinal microflora.

Binding of Carcinogens to Nucleic Acids

   The highly reactive metabolites of carcinogenic chemicals, the ultimate carcinogens, are known to react with cellular proteins, RNA and
DNA, by covalent binding (Miller, 1970), or possibly by intercalation with
nucleic acids (Van Duuren *et al.*, 1969). This process, probably accompanied by similar toxic interactions of the ultimate carcinogen with other
cellular components, results in malignant cell transformation. Alone, it may
be identical with the process of mutation.

   The reactive microsomal metabolites of the polycyclic carcinogenic
hydrocarbons, the K-region epoxides, react with the purine moieties of
RNA and DNA *in vivo* and *in vitro* (Grover and Sims; 1973; Kuroki *et al.*,
1971/2), and K-region epoxides of benz[*a*]anthracene and 7,12-dimethyl-
benz[*a*]anthracene have been shown to alkylate the guanine and adenine
moieties of RNA (Swaisland *et al.*, 1974a). The arylated deoxyribonucleo-

sides obtained from degradation of the DNA of mouse embryo cells cultured in the presence of benzo[a]pyrene differed from those obtained by treating DNA with benzo[a]pyrene 4,5-oxide, the K-region epoxide of the hydrocarbon (King et al., 1975). From these results it is inferred that the ultimate carcinogen of benzo[a]pyrene is not the K-region epoxide, but some other highly reactive microsomal metabolite.

Metabolites of aflatoxin B_1 also become bound to RNA and DNA, but whereas the binding of the carcinogen in vivo is reduced following treatment of the animals with phenobarbitone, the rate of formation of the 2,3-epoxide, which is considered to be the proximate carcinogen, is increased by this treatment (Garner, 1975).

The carcinogen 2-acetamidofluorene becomes covalently bound to liver DNA and transfer RNA when administered in vivo. The ultimate carcinogen is an ester of N-hydroxyacetamidofluorene and the primary target on the DNA and transfer RNA has been shown to be the 8-position of guanosine (Kriek, 1972; Fujimura et al., 1972). The proximate carcinogen, N-hydroxy-2-acetamidofluorene, has also been shown to bind covalently to the nuclear acidic proteins and histones (Jungmann and Schweppe, 1972) and may consequently alter the regulation of gene expression and function.

Similarly, the hepatocarcinogens N-methyl-4-aminoazobenzene and 4-dimethylaminoazobenzene react with hepatic DNA and RNA to bind at the 8-position of guanine. A suggested mechanism for this binding of the azo dyes again involves N-hydroxylation, esterification of the N-hydroxy derivative, and reaction of the electrophilic esters with DNA and RNA, as with 2-acetamidofluorene (see Figure 9) (Lin et al., 1975). The binding of 4-dimethylaminoazobenzene metabolites to nuclear DNA in rats was reduced by pretreatment with phenobarbital but increased by pretreatment with 3-methylcholanthrene, possibly due to the stimulation of different modes of metabolism of this azo dye carcinogen (De Cloitre et al., 1975).

The potent carcinogen, dimethylnitrosamine, is metabolized to a potent alkylating agent which methylates the bases of RNA and DNA, the position most heavily attacked being the 7-position of guanine (Engelse and Emmelot, 1971/72).

The carcinogenic triazene, 1-phenyl-3,3-dimethyltriazene, when administered to rats similarly results in the 7-methylation of guanine moieties of liver DNA and RNA, and also of brain and kidney RNA (Krüger et al., 1971). Methylation of the nucleic acids of liver and colon, as indicated by the formation of 7-methylguanine, was also observed in rats and mice treated with the carcinogen, 1,2-dimethylhydrazine (Hawks and Magee, 1974).

With the neuroselective carcinogen, N-methyl-N-nitrosurea, alkylation of the purine bases of DNA of brain exceeded that occurring in other tissues. Hydrolysis of the DNA yielded 3- and 7-methylguanine and O^6-

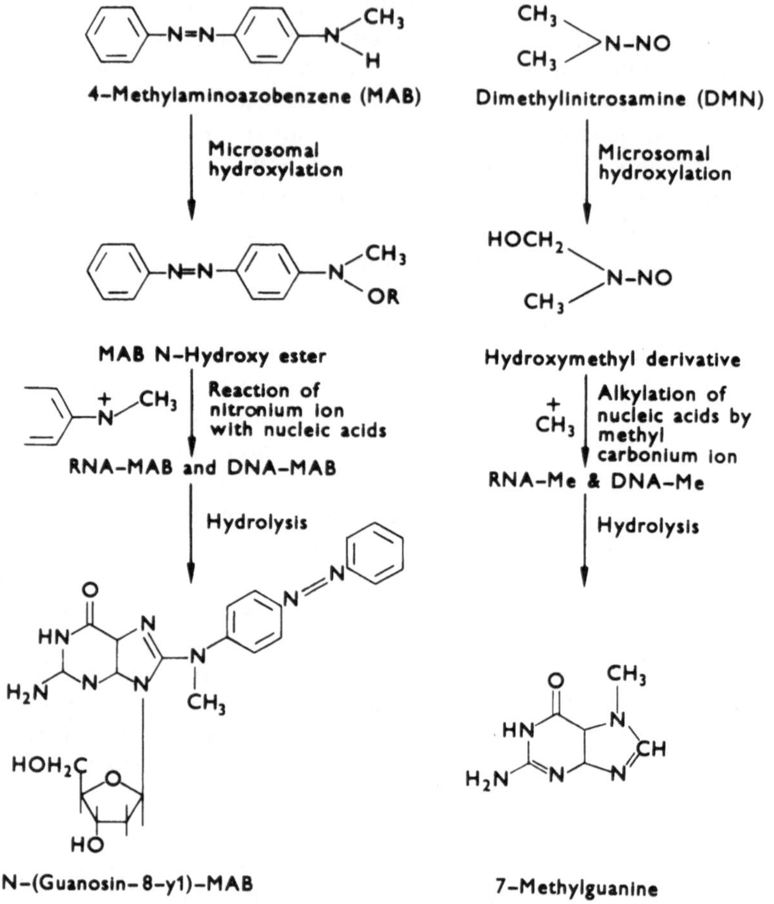

Figure 9. Postulated mechanism of alkylation and arylation of purine bases by ultimate carcinogens.

methylguanine, and the kinetics of formation showed that no mechanism exists in the brain to excise the methylated bases from DNA. This absence of a repair mechanism in the brain could be a determining factor in the selective induction of neurological tumors by this carcinogen (Margison and Kleihues, 1975).

It would thus seem that in the alkylation and arylation of the bases of DNA and RNA by the reactive ultimate carcinogens, guanine is a primary target and at least two different mechanisms are involved. The first, seen with dimethylnitrosamine, N-methyl-N-nitrosurea, and phenyldimethyltriazene results in alkylation at the N-7, the N-3, and the O-6 positions of guanine, while the second mechanism, which is involved in the arylation of DNA and RNA by 2-acetamidofluorene and methylaminoazobenzene derivatives, gives rise to C-8 complexes of guanine (see Figure 9).

The binding of carcinogens to DNA has been shown to be enhanced by vitamin A deficiency. The binding of the ultimate carcinogen of benzo[a]pyrene to DNA of hamster tracheal epithelium *in vitro* was four- to fivefold greater than normal in preparations from vitamin-A-deficient animals, and may involve an effect of the retinoid on the metabolic activation of the carcinogen (Genta *et al.*, 1974).

DNA Repair

Presumably all chemical carcinogens, or their reactive metabolites, interact with nuclear DNA to alkylate, arylate, or acylate certain of the component purine and pyrimidine bases of this genetic material with consequent erroneous transcription of messenger RNA and the synthesis of modified enzymic and structural proteins. The damaged DNA with its changes in base sequences, and therefore in genetic information, will propagate this false information during DNA replication, leading ultimately to the establishment of a clone of malignant cells from the original single cell transformed largely as the result of the damaged DNA. Natural mechanisms of DNA repair may interrupt this process by excising the damaged DNA before it can be replicated and so lead to the formation of a malignant clone. Treatment of rats with a variety of alkylating agents has been shown to give rise to increased urinary excretion of 7-methylguanine, deoxycytidine, and thymidine, which could result from portions of DNA excised during the repair process (Chu and Lawley, 1975).

Delayed repair of the DNA damage produced by carcinogens may lead to permanent changes in the DNA and suggests a relationship between DNA repair and cancer (Farber, 1975). If the target cells of the carcinogens are not actively engaged in replication, the DNA repair system obviously has a greater opportunity to eradicate the damage to the DNA before replication occurs, and similarly, any inhibition of the repair mechanism will potentiate the likelihood of the progression of a transformed cell into a malignant tumor. Consequently, the DNA repair mechanism has an essential role in the prevention or formation of cancer. In keeping with this view is the fact that partial hepatectomy greatly potentiates the occurrence of liver cancer following suboptimal doses of hepatocarcinogens (Warwick, 1969; Craddock, 1973; Farber, 1973). A single dose of dimethylnitrosamine administered to rats 24 h after partial hepatectomy induced a greater incidence of hepatocellular carcinoma than when administered 0–6 h after

surgery. The higher incidence of tumors following administration of carcinogen during the period of maximal DNA replication suggests that replication of the alkylated DNA before the abnormality is repaired is necessary
for the initiation of the cancer. The mechanism of carcinogenesis, therefore, concerns not only the interaction of the ultimate carcinogens with
genetic material, but also the rate of DNA synthesis and the state of the cell
at the time of injury (Craddock, 1975). There is, however, no evidence that
tumor-promoting agents, cocarcinogens, steroid-inducing agents, or DNA-
binding chemicals inhibit DNA repair (Cleaver and Painter, 1975).

Enzyme Induction and the Endoplasmic Reticulum

The coordination of the body's tissues is regulated by the hormones
and chalones, and the control of intermediary metabolism is similarly
regulated by these hormones acting on cell membranes and enzymes. The
regulation of enzymes may be effected by various means, including allo-
steric activation of enzymes and the increased synthesis of the enzyme, a
phenomenon known as enzyme induction. This induced synthesis of an
enzyme can be brought about by the action of hormones, by the presence of
high concentrations of the enzyme substrate, and in certain cases by
carcinogenic chemicals.

The microsomal enzymes of the liver (mixed-function oxidases) which
metabolize drugs and other chemicals present in our environment are
similarly subject to regulation by enzyme induction and may be induced
following exposure of the animal to a wide variety of drugs, pesticides, and
other chemicals such as the carcinogenic polycyclic hydrocarbons (Conney, 1967; Parke, 1975). The increased synthesis of these enzymes occurs
only when the inducing compounds are administered to the living animal,
are perfused through the isolated liver or other organs (Juchau et al., 1965),
or are added to cell cultures in vitro (Nebert and Gelboin, 1968a, b). The
drugs and other chemicals which induce the microsomal enzymes have
widely differing pharmacological activities, and the only features that they
would seem to have in common are that (a) they are lipid soluble and hence
become localized in the endoplasmic reticulum of the liver and other
tissues, and (b) they are substrates of, or become bound to, the microsomal
drug-metabolizing enzymes.

The essential enzyme of the microsomal mixed-function oxidase system is cytochrome P_{450}, the terminal oxygenase. This cytochrome, abundant in the liver, is also found in the adrenal mitochondria and many other
tissues which hydroxylate steroids and exogenous chemicals, including
carcinogens. In its reduced form the cytochrome forms a ligand complex
with carbon monoxide, which shows a characteristic absorption maximum

at 450 nm, hence the name of cytochrome P_{450} and the earlier synonym of "carbon-monoxide-binding pigment." This cytochrome requires NADPH and molecular O_2 for activity, is inactivated by CO, and when induced by treatment of animals with chemicals such as phenobarbital produces an increased synthesis of cytochrome P_{450} itself. Induction of the microsomal enzymes by carcinogenic polycyclic hydrocarbons, such as 3-methylcholanthrene, produces a cytochrome with a characteristic CO-difference absorption spectrum at 448 nm, instead of the usual 450 nm, from which it has been inferred that more than one distinct form of this cytochrome exists (Sladek and Mannering, 1966).

Considerable evidence has accumulated to show that cytochrome P_{448} is not merely a stable complex of cytochrome P_{450} with 3-methylcholanthrene or one of its metabolites (Fujita and Mannering, 1971; Shoeman, Vane and Mannering, 1973), as is known to occur with safrole and piperonyl butoxide (Franklin, 1972), but is a separate entity or a different conformational form of cytochrome P_{450}.

Soluble preparations of purified cytochrome P_{450} and P_{448} have been prepared by a sonication/sodium cholate method (Lu and Levin, 1972) and when reconstituted by addition of phospholipid and NADPH–cytochrome-c reductase, they catalyze the hydroxylation of a variety of substrates with exhibition of different substrate specificities (see Table 1) (Jacobson *et al.*, 1972). It has also been shown, from a study of the biosynthesis of the different microsomal cytochromes, that cytochrome P_{448} is formed after

TABLE 1. Difference in Substrate Specificity of Liver Microsomal Cytochromes from Rats Pretreated with Phenobarbital and 3-Methylcholanthrene

	Relative increase in specific enzyme activities[a]	
Substrate	Phenobarbital treated	Methylcholanthrene treated
Pentobarbital	1000	60
Benzphetamine	250	50
Ethylmorphine	100	100
Aniline	120	170
Benzo[*a*]pyrene	70	390
Testosterone		
6β-Hydroxylation	100	100
7α-Hydroxylation	100	200
16α-Hydroxylation	550	50

[a]The activities of cytochrome P_{450} from untreated (control) rats being 100 for all substrates.

treatment of animals with methylcholanthrene, even when the synthesis of new heme and protein are inhibited (Imai and Siekevitz, 1971). It would thus seem that during treatment with carcinogenic polycyclic hydrocarbons, conversion of cytochrome P_{450} to P_{448} occurs, and this may be a separate process from the subsequent synthesis of new hemoprotein. Other workers have shown that increased enzyme activity and spectral changes accompanying the transformation of P_{450} to P_{448} occur only 2 h after treatment of animals with 3-methylcholanthrene, and long before the increase in total hemoprotein becomes manifest (Alvares *et al.*, 1973). This suggests that the spectrally different microsomal cytochromes produced by phenobarbital and methylcholanthrene are two physically distinct forms of a single molecular species of hemoprotein and probably result from differences in their immediate environment in the microsomal lipoprotein membrane (Imai and Siekevitz, 1971).

Further evidence that the increase in enzyme activity produced by phenobarbital is due to increased enzyme synthesis, whereas that resulting from pretreatment with carcinogenic polycyclic hydrocarbons is due also to a change in the character of the enzyme, is provided by studies of enzyme kinetics. In the hydroxylation of benzo[*a*]pyrene by rat liver microsomes, pretreatment with methylcholanthrene reduced the K_m value, indicating that the enzyme had been modified to have a greater affinity for the substrate than normal (Alvares *et al.*, 1968). On the other hand, pretreatment with phenobarbital resulted in an increase of normal enzyme since for this hydroxylation there was an increase of V_{max} with no decrease of K_m.

A further difference in the enzyme induction by phenobarbital and carcinogenic polycyclic hydrocarbons is that whereas both inducing agents enhance the activity of benzo[*a*]pyrene hydroxylase of the endoplasmic reticulum, only the carcinogens increase the activity of the hydroxylase in the nuclear membrane. Furthermore, although treatment with phenobarbital and methylcholanthrene increase the benzo[*a*]pyrene hydroxylase of microsomes 2- and 10-fold, respectively, the methylcholanthrene-induced increase in hydroxylase activities of the nuclear membrane is some 20-fold of normal (Khandwala and Kaspar, 1973).

The treatment of young rats with carcinogenic polycyclic hydrocarbons such as 3-methylcholanthrene is generally followed by marked activation of the hepatic nuclear RNA-polymerase system resulting from an increased chromatin template efficiency (Bresnick and Mossé, 1969). Benzo[*a*]pyrene and several other carcinogens have been shown to react with the nonbasic regions of arginine-rich rat liver histones (Sluyser, 1968), an interaction which may be involved in the initiation of genomal activation by polycyclic hydrocarbon enzyme-inducing agents. This activation of the genome results in an increase in the rate of synthesis of RNA and also in qualitative changes in the types of RNA (Bresnick and Mossé, 1969; Yee and Bresnick, 1971). Furthermore, 3-methylcholanthrene reduces the activity of rat liver ribosomal ribonuclease, increasing the polysome stabilization (Pousada and Lechner, 1972) and protein synthesis, especially the microsomal hemoproteins, and reducing the rates of their degradation (Black et al., 1971; Lanclos and Bresnick, 1973).

Not all carcinogens produce this increase in transcription and enhancement of RNA-polymerase activity, and the mycotoxin, aflatoxin B_1 causes inhibition of RNA-polymerase activity in liver cell nuclei of rats dosed with this material (Edwards and Wogan, 1970). This has been presumed to be due to inactivation of the chromatin template, and more recently it has been shown that aflatoxin leads to the deacetylation of the nuclear histones of rat liver through an increased activity of the deacetylases (Edwards and Allfrey, 1973). Treatment with phenobarbital before administration of aflatoxin B_1 decreases the mycotoxin-induced inhibition of RNA synthesis and aflatoxin toxicity in the case of the rat, whereas with mice the reverse effect was observed, and the inhibition of transcription and toxicity of aflatoxin were both increased (Moulé et al., 1975). These are all the more anomalous since rats are normally much more susceptible than mice to the toxic and carcinogenic effects of aflatoxin.

The proximate carcinogen, N-hydroxy-2-acetamidofluorene, also drastically reduces transcription, and inhibition of hepatic RNA synthesis in rats treated with this compound is thought to be due to impairment of DNA template function (Zieve, 1973; Grunberger et al., 1973). More recent studies suggest that there are two mechanisms concerned, namely the direct inhibition of nucleoplasmic RNA polymerase resulting in inhibition of the synthesis of messenger RNA, and inhibition of ribosomal RNA resulting from the effects of the carcinogen on regulatory proteins of the nucleus (Glazer et al., 1975).

The microsomal mixed-function oxygenase, 3,4-benzo[a]pyrene hydroxylase, hydroxylates both carcinogenic and noncarcinogenic polycyclic hydrocarbons and is found in many tissues of various animal species. It is a highly inducible enzyme, the activity being increased up to 300-fold in certain tissues by treatment with polycyclic hydrocarbons and other environmental chemicals. This enzyme may be responsible for the activation of carcinogens to the proximate carcinogen, and yet may also be implicated in the hydroxylation system which leads to the detoxication of carcinogens. Its involvement in carcinogenesis by polycyclic hydrocarbons is evidenced by the following observations: (1) covalent binding of benzo[a]pyrene to DNA is catalyzed by this microsomal hydroxylase, (2) inhibition of the hydroxylase in mouse skin homogenates by 7,8-benzoflavone parallels the inhibition of 7,12-dimethylbenz[a]anthracene skin tumorigenesis, and (3) increased levels of benzopyrene hydroxylase parallel increased tumorigenesis (Gelboin et al., 1972).

The induction of benzo[a]pyrene hydroxylase is genetically controlled, and certain inbred strains of mice exhibiting high inducibility of this enzyme were more susceptible than other strains to the formation of skin tumors with 3-methylcholanthrene (Kouri et al., 1973). The inducibility of benzo[a]pyrene hydroxylase activity of human lymphocytes also shows a genetic variation and in a recent study of 50 patients with bronchial carcinoma a marked correlation was observed between the incidence of cancer and high levels of inducibility of this enzyme (Kellerman et al., 1973). Two types of benzo[a]pyrene hydroxylase have recently been distinguished in rat liver. One of these predominates in the male, occurs in neonates, is induced by phenobarbital, and is stimulated by 7,8-benzoflavone. The other predominates in the female, is induced by polycyclic hydrocarbons, and is inhibited by benzoflavone. The distribution of the two forms of this enzyme might well be a determinant in the susceptibility of an organism to polycyclic hydrocarbon carcinogenesis (Wiebel and Gelboin, 1975).

The role of enzyme-inducing agents in carcinogenesis may also involve enhancement of DNA synthesis and promotion of hyperplasia which would then facilitate rapid development of malignantly transformed cells before DNA repair can be effected. Marquadt and Heidelburger (1972) have shown that the K-region epoxide of benz[a]anthracene, possibly the proximate carcinogen, stimulates DNA synthesis and malignant transformation in hamster embryo cells. Inducing agents might also potentiate carcinogenesis initiated by other chemical carcinogens and by oncogenic viruses (Roe and Rowsen, 1968; Benedict et al., 1973). Simultaneous feeding of phenobarbital reduced the hepatocarcinogenic effect of the 2-acetamidofluorene in rats (Peraino et al., 1971), whereas the sequential feeding of acetamidofluorene followed by prolonged treatment (100 days) with phenobarbital markedly increased the incidence of hepatoma over treatment with carcinogen alone (Peraino et al., 1971, 1973). The enzyme-inductive effects of phenobarbital administered simultaneously would appear to result in enhanced detoxication of the carcinogen and a reduction of its oncogenic effects, whereas when given subsequently to the carcinogen the phenobarbital potentiates the stimulation of mitosis and DNA and protein synthesis, thereby establishing the malignant cell transformations effected by the acetamidofluorene. Similarly, the simultaneous administration of phenobarbital and diethylnitrosamine decreased the incidence and severity of the nitrosamine-induced hepatocellular carcinoma, whereas when phenobarbital was given subsequently to a limited period of treatment with diethylnitrosamine the carcinogenic effect was increased (Weisburger et al., 1975). In this study, the possibility of any immunosuppressive effect causing the enhancement of malignancy was eliminated since a purified gamma fraction of antilymphocyte serum was shown to have no effect.

In a similar manner, simultaneous administration of phenobarbital considerably reduced the appearance of malignant tumors in rats fed aflatoxin, probably the result of induction of the liver microsomal enzymes which metabolize aflatoxin to noncarcinogenic products (McLean and Marshall, 1971). Induction of the hepatic microsomal enzymes by the antioxidant, butylated hydroxytoluene (BHT), also reduces the carcinogenicity of 2-acetamidofluorene and of its more toxic metabolite, N-hydroxy-2-acetamidofluorene (Ulland et al., 1973) probably by increasing the detoxication of the carcinogen, particularly the rate of glucuronide conjugation (Grantham et al., 1973). Pretreatment of animals with enzyme inducers such as phenobarbital and chlordan also reduces the number of pulmonary tumors produced in mice following administration of urethane (Yamamoto et al., 1971). The effects of enzyme-inducing agents on chemical carcinogenesis may thus be either potentiation of inhibition, dependent on the nature of the inducing agent, the nature of the carcinogen, the enzymic pathways for activation and detoxication, and the relative times of administration of the enzyme-inducing agent and carcinogen.

Studies of the mechanisms of enzyme induction in isolated cell culture have the advantages of employing a homogeneous simplified system free from the complexities of hormonal regulation and distribution kinetics which occur in the intact mammalian organism. Detailed studies of the induction of benzo[a]pyrene hydroxylase in cultures of hamster fetal cells (Nebert and Gelboin, 1968a, b) and rat liver cells (Whitlock and Gelboin, 1974) have shown that the enhanced enzymic activity is related to the appearance of a new microsomal CO-binding cytochrome with an absorption maximum at 446 nm, suggesting that benzo[a]pyrene hydroxylase activity is related more to this new cytochrome (P_{448}) than it is to normal cytochrome P_{450} (Nebert, 1969). In the rat hepatocyte system, phenobarbital and carcinogenic polycyclic hydrocarbons represent two distinct classes of microsomal enzyme inducers, with additive effects (Gielen and Nebert, 1971); both inducers stimulate synthesis of new enzyme by increased transcription and translation, but the carcinogenic polycyclic hydrocarbons have the additional effect of converting cytochrome P_{450} to cytochrome P_{448}. In the induction of benzpyrene hydroxylase in cultures of fetal cells from various inbred strains of mice marked genetic differences have been observed (Nebert and Bausserman, 1970), due probably to differing rates of enhanced synthesis of CO-binding cytochrome together with differences in its character (absorption maximum at 448–9 instead of 446 nm) (Nebert and Bausserman, 1970). The occurrence in mouse of this ability to induce benzpyrene hydroxylase activity is expressed as a single autosomal dominant trait, possession of which is associated with a greater tendency to skin tumorigenesis (Nebert et al., 1972). As benzpyrene hydroxylase results in the metabolic formation of the toxic, proximate carcinogens of polycyclic hydrocarbons (probably arene oxides), the carcinogenicity of these chemicals may be greater in those strains in which the enzyme is highly inducible. This cell culture may, therefore, prove valuable in the evaluation of potential carcinogenicity of drugs and environmental chemicals by providing an *in vitro* system which reflects not only species difference but also genetic variations in response from the normal living organism *in vivo*.

Effects of Carcinogens on the Endoplasmic Reticulum and Protein Synthesis

The structural and functional integrity of a cell depends on, among other factors, the rate of synthesis and degradation of proteins (enzymes) and on the pattern of protein synthesis which is regulated, at least in part, by the ratio of "rough" to "smooth" endoplasmic reticulum. It has been suggested that the free ribosomes are responsible for the synthesis of those proteins which are to remain within the cell, while the ribosomes bound on the endoplasmic reticulum (rough endoplasmic reticulum) synthesize proteins that are secreted from the cell (Rolleston, 1974). The membrane–ribosome interaction, that is the movement of the ribosomes on to the "smooth" endoplasmic reticulum to form the "rough" membrane, is a dynamic equilibrium that shifts as the functional requirements of a cell demand (Ragnotti and Aletti, 1975). Thus the two classes of polyribosomes, "membrane-bound" and "free," are not functionally separate, even though they are morphologically distinct.

When an animal is treated with the microsomal enzyme-inducing agent phenobarbital, the rate of protein synthesis by the membrane-bound polyribosomes of rat liver is substantially increased, while that of the free polyribosomes is unchanged, due largely to the shift of ribosomal RNA on to the endoplasmic reticulum (Ragnotti and Aletti, 1975). The administration of most carcinogens *in vivo* causes degranulation of the rough endoplasmic reticulum, that is detachment of the polyribosomes bound to the endoplasmic reticulum. Characteristically, neoplastic cells generally have a low proportion of their polysomes bound to the membrane (Sunshine *et al.,* 1971).

Treatment of rats with the proximate carcinogen N-hydroxyacetamidofluorene results in disarray of the endoplasmic reticulum and disaggregation of the polyribosomes (Popp and Shinozuka, 1974). The natural carcinogen aflatoxin B_1 both *in vitro* and *in vivo* induces degranulation of the liver endoplasmic reticulum (Sunshine *et al.,* 1971), presumably with an altered pattern of protein synthesis. Similarly in HeLa cells, treatment with the carcinogens dimethylnitrosamine and thioacetamide results in fragmentation of the endoplasmic reticulum with a marked increase in the proportion of free ribosomes, their disaggregation, and a consequent shift in the metabolism of the cell to the synthesis of a greater proportion of endogenous proteins (Delaunay and Schapira, 1974). The potent carcinogen 1,2-dimethylhydrazine causes marked disaggregation of hepatic polysomes and inhibition of protein synthesis comparable to dimethylnitrosamine, whereas the weak carcinogens 1-methylhydrazine and 1,1-dimethylhydrazine have no similar effect (Hawks *et al.*, 1974).

Thus it appears that in cancer cells, possibly related to the actual process of malignant transformation, there is a loss of bound ribosomes from the endoplasmic reticulum with a concomitant increase in free ribosomes. This would imply a shift in the pattern of metabolism in a cancer cell towards the synthesis of intracellular proteins. As glycoproteins are synthesized by membrane-bound polyribosomes, the shift produced by carcinogens would result in impairment of glycoprotein synthesis, with all that this may imply in changes to the glycocalyx, and possibly also to the immune system.

Many steroid hormones affect the pattern of protein synthesis in their target tissues, probably by regulating the induction of enzyme synthesis and the balance between the free and membrane-bound polyribosomes. Degranulation of the rough endoplasmic reticulum has been shown to be effected by steroids, and in male rat liver (a marked sex difference has been demonstrated) cortisol, estrone, and cholesterol have been shown to cause degranulation, whereas corticosterone, estradiol, and pregnanediol protect against this (Sunshine *et al.*, 1971). It is probable that the pattern of intracellular/extracellular protein synthesis of a cell is regulated by the balance of the steroid hormones within the cell controlling the degree of degranulation. It also appears that the site of action of carcinogens on the endoplasmic reticulum is the same as that of the steroid hormones, since the two classes of chemicals appear to act in competition with each other. Carcinogens, like aflatoxin, may degranulate rough endoplasmic reticulum by displacing the activating steroid and then binding to the steroid specific site (Sunshine *et al.*, 1971).

The toxic changes afflicted on the endoplasmic reticulum by exposure to carcinogens, such as displacement of the ribosomes (degranulation), may constitute one of the most significant events in malignant cell transformation, possibly as fundamental to carcinogenesis as is the damage to the nuclear DNA. Since the endoplasmic reticulum is the intracellular site of enzymic activation of the carcinogens it is logical to expect that the endoplasmic reticulum may also be the site of greatest damage, for the proximate and ultimate carcinogens are highly reactive compounds likely to interact with adjacent molecules as soon as they are formed. Using the chemical biphenyl as a model substrate which is metabolized by liver microsomal preparations to both 2- and 4-hydroxybiphenyl, Creaven and Parke (1966) have shown that whereas phenobarbital and other drugs and

TABLE 2. The Effects of Carcinogenic Compounds on the 2- and 4-Hydroxylation of Biphenyl by Rat Hepatic Microsomes

Test compound[a]	Carcino-genicity	Percentage of change in activity relative to control values	
		Biphenyl 2-hydroxylation	Biphenyl 4-hydroxylation
3,4-Benzo[a]pyrene	+	+252	−9
22-Methylcholanthrene	+	+243	+8
20-Methylcholanthrene	+	+125	−4
2-Acetamidofluorene	+	+74	−9
Dimethylnitrosamine	+	+98	−18
Aflatoxin B_1	+	+87	+2
Safrole	+	+82	−34
Piperonyl butoxide	?	+62	−31
β-Naphthylamine	+	+198	+3
α-Naphthylamine	−	+17	−4
Phenobarbital	−	+16	− 8
1,2,3,4-Dibenzo[a]pyrene	−	+8	+4
Hexobarbital	−	+11	+2

[a]From McPherson *et al.*, 1974.

noncarcinogenic chemicals induce the 4-hydroxylation of biphenyl, carcinogens, and only carcinogens, induce the 2-hydroxylation of the substrate. More recently this observation has been developed into a simple *in vitro* test for potential carcinogenicity in chemicals (McPherson *et al.*, 1974). The suspected carcinogen is incubated with a fresh preparation of tissue microsomes (endoplasmic reticulum) in the presence of NADPH and O_2; after an interval of 10 to 30 min to allow maximum formation of the proximate carcinogen and subsequent damage of the endoplasmic reticulum, the substrate biphenyl is added to the incubation mixture, and after a further 5-min incubation the rate of formation of the 2-hydroxybiphenyl is determined spectrophotometrically. The carcinogenic potential of the chemical under test is indicated by the increase in the biphenyl-2-hydroxylase activity, relative to controls. Results obtained with this test using rat liver microsomal preparations to evaluate the potential carcinogenicity of a series of known carcinogens and noncarcinogenic chemicals is given in Table 2 (McPherson *et al.*, 1974). As this test measures the combined effects of (a) rate of formation of the reactive proximate carcinogen, and (b) extent of damage to the endoplasmic reticulum, it is likely to reflect species, genetic, and tissue differences in carcinogenesis. Although the test does not incorporate any measure of the covalent binding of the proximate carcinogen to DNA, it does appear to have a high degree of reliability in determining carcinogenic potential, with good correlation between chemical carcinogenicity and enhancement of biphenyl-2-hydroxylation. Indeed, this correlation may suggest that the two toxic processes measured by this test may be even more fundamental to carcinogenesis than binding to DNA though, of course, this latter process, with its alteration of genetic information, must surely be an essential prerequisite for malignant cell transformation.

This increase in biphenyl-2-hydroxylase activity resulting from treatment of animals with carcinogens, or from the incubation of endoplasmic reticulum with carcinogens *in vitro,* is not true enzyme induction for it occurs within a very short time period and is not inhibited by actinomycin D or other inhibitors of protein synthesis. Instead, it is a process of enzyme activation in which this particular form of hydroxylation by the cytochrome P_{450} system is fully revealed as a consequence of damage of the membrane of the endoplasmic reticulum by the proximate carcinogen. It is indeed likely that it is a quantitative expression of the loss of ribosomes from the endoplasmic reticulum, the removal of the ribosomes allowing a presentation of the substrate (biphenyl) to the cytochrome P_{450} system that is not possible when the ribosomes are attached (see Figure 10). This hypothesis

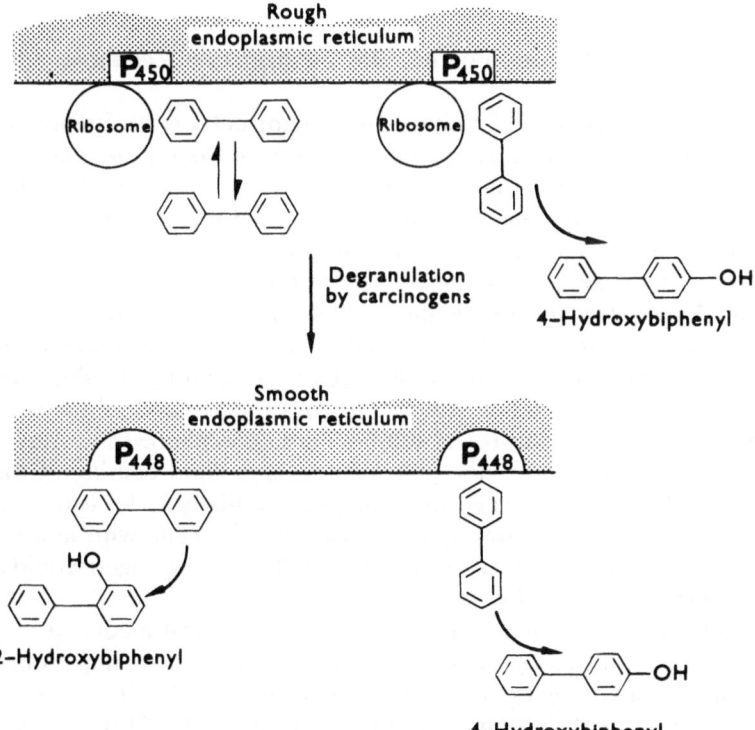

Figure 10. The effect of carcinogens on "degranulation" of the endoplasmic reticulum, cytochrome P450, and the hydroxylation of biphenyl.

is supported by the observations of Burke and Mayer (1975) that a reconstituted rat liver microsomal monooxygenase system consisting of NADPH–cytochrome-c oxidoreductase plus cytochrome P_{450} catalyzes only the 4-hydroxylation of biphenyl, whereas the oxidoreductase plus cytochrome P_{448} catalyzes both 2- and 4-hydroxylation. Furthermore, subfractionation of hepatic microsomes from rat and mouse have shown that the rough endoplasmic reticulum contains a cytochrome with the spectral characteristics of P_{450}, whereas the smooth endoplasmic reticulum contains cytochrome P_{448} (Mailman *et al.*, 1975), and it is now well established that carcinogens enhance degranulation of the endoplasmic reticulum and bring about a conversion of cytochrome P_{450} to P_{448}. Full validation of this relatively simple biphenyl test for determining the carcinogenic activity of chemicals is currently being pursued, but it does appear to have considerable potential and, in combination with similar *in vitro* and short-term tests for DNA binding and mutagenesis, it would seem to herald a new approach to carcinogenicity testing. Perhaps even more important, the elucidation of the mechanism involved would greatly enhance our understanding of the molecular and cellular mechanisms of carcinogenesis.

The Plasma Membrane and the Altered Immune Response

The development of a clone of malignant cells is an immunological paradox and must involve escape by the tumor of the normal immunological surveillance. A similar immunological situation is seen in the tolerance by the pregnant female mammalian to accept and nourish an antigenically "foreign" fetus, and it is probably not insignificant that malignant transformation results in reversion to the synthesis of many fetal-type enzymes and proteins. A recent review of the immunological escape of tumors suggests a multifactorial response and lists the following among the possible mechanisms: host nonreactivity, antigen deletion, cryptic antigens, blocking antibodies, and antigen shedding (Currie, 1975). In fact, many of the immunological and biological features of tumors may be explained in terms of the stability of the glycocalyx (the glycoprotein/glycolipid coating of the cell surface), and cells which shed their antigen are likely to be less immunogenic and more prone to develop mestastases than cells with more stable surface structures. Moreover, the released cell surface antigen would act as a smokescreen to defensive antibodies.

Evidence has been obtained for a reduced cell-mediated immune response, as measured by the lymphocyte transformation, in patients with malignant tumors of the breast (Knight and Davidson, 1975). Moreover, the plasma of these patients contained a factor which reduced the transformation of lymphocytes from a healthy donor, and a similar immunosuppressive peptide fraction, not present in normal subjects, has been isolated from the sera of patients with several different types of malignant tumor (Nimberg *et al.*, 1975). This peptide is very similar to the immunoregulatory α-globulin, an immunosuppressive peptide previously detected in trace amounts in normal subjects. The antiviral substance, interferon, has been demonstrated to inhibit the growth of spontaneous, transplanted, virally induced, and chemically induced neoplasms in mice, though the mechanism of this is as yet unknown (Salerno *et al.*, 1972). Degradation of immunoglobulins by the lysosomal enzymes of tumors has also been shown to occur (Keisari and Witz, 1973) and, since tumors are known to exhibit high lysosomal proteolytic activity and to release these enzymes extracellularly, this also may explain the reduced immune response.

The plasma membrane of a cell may be visualized as a fluid mosaic in which the polar carbohydrate chains of the component glycolipids (gangliosides) and glycoproteins, that is the glycocalyx, are oriented to the external surface from the more hydrophobic milieu of the membrane, forming a highly specific recognition system which is involved in cell–cell recognition, antigenicity, agglutination, and contact inhibition of growth. The transformation of mouse cells by oncogenic viruses, X-irradiation, or chemical carcinogenesis results in a reduction of the oligosaccharide chains of the gangliosides which is also associated with a decrease in the activities of the glycosyltransferases (Brady and Fishman, 1974). Although the consequences of these observations are not clear, it is possible that these changes in the carbohydrate moiety of the gangliosides may profoundly affect the antigenic and trophic characters of the plasma membrane and hence the relationship of the malignant cell to its cellular and immunological environment. Hakomori (1975), in a most lucid and comprehensive review of this complex field, has identified three categories of change in the glycolipids and glycoproteins of cell surface membranes associated with the malignant transformation of mammalian cells, namely (1) changes in glycolipid composition (ganglioside, neutral glycolipid, and fucolipid) associated with reduced activity of glycosyltransferase(s), (2) absence of cell-contact-dependent enhancement of glycolipid synthesis, and (3) deletion of a high molecular weight galactoprotein and a greater exposure of the glycolipid. It is possible that all three categories of change could be dependent on reduced activities of the glycosyltransferases.

Another modification of the glycocalyx observed in the malignant cell is the decrease in fucose-containing glycoprotein together with a higher content of sialic acid. The presence of extra sialic acid in the glycoprotein of malignant cells has been demonstrated in several different types of cell transformed either spontaneously, or by oncogenic viruses, or by a chemical carcinogen (van Beek *et al.*, 1973). These authors suggest that the transformed cell does not modulate the chemistry of its surface glycocalyx in the normal manner characteristic of the cell cycle and is blocked in a condition of increased sialyl extension. This results in the malignant cell resembling the normal mitotic cell in its surface characteristics which annuls the usual nonproliferative relationships that exist between cells. Other workers have suggested that the increased sialic acid of the malignant cell surface results from the attachment of serum glycoproteins having a high sialic acid content, the so-called "symbodies" (Kawasaki et al., 1974).

In carcinoma of the gastrointestinal tract, Filipe and Branfoot (1974) have shown that the mucus of the large intestine is characterized by an increase of sialomucins, and we have demonstrated that in gastric cancer there is a reduction in the rate of synthesis of mucus glycoproteins as indicated by a decreased rate of incorporation of N-acetyl[^{3}H]glucosamine and [^{14}C]galactose (Johnston et al., 1975).

The study of the chalones, tissue-specific glycopolypeptides and glycoproteins concerned with inhibition of mitosis, is possibly another view of the same phenomena. Mitosis of a cell is normally inhibited by the chalone of the epidermal cell and the cell only enters the division phase in the basal layer where the effect of the chalone is counteracted by a mesochymal factor produced in the dermis. The tumor cell contains abnormally low concentrations of chalone, due to loss of the chalone across an abnormal cell membrane (Bullough, 1974). As the tumor grows, the loss of chalone results in increased blood concentrations of the chalone, initially resulting in a reduced mitosis of the normal tissue of origin and later in increasing mitotic inhibition of the tumor itself (tumor growth plateaus or becomes lethal).

In an endeavor to stimulate the immune response to counter this reduced immunological surveillance characteristic of malignancy, BCG has been used therapeutically, usually in combination with cytotoxic drugs. Also, new chemical immunostimulants, such as levamisole and tilorone, which it is hoped will be even more effective than BCG, are currently being clinically evaluated.

Lysosomes

Lysosomes are ubiquitously distributed subcellular organelles, probably arising from endoplasmic reticulum and containing a diverse range of hydrolytic enzymes sequestered within them in latent form. The activation and release of these enzymes into phagocytic vacuoles, or into the cytosol of the cell, results in the digestion of ingested macromolecular material and may be responsible for regulation of the turnover of the normal cell constituents. An excessive labilization of the lysosomal membranes and excessive release of the hydrolases results in cell damage and tissue injury.

The corticosteroid hormones, cortisol and cortisone, and synthetic steroids, betamethasone, prednisolone, and prednisone, stabilize the lysosomal membranes and inhibit the release of hydrolases (Goldstein, 1975). In contrast, the steroid sex hormones, estradiol-17β, testosterone, and synthetic estrogen, diethylstilbestrol, at physiological doses to gonadectomized rats, produced a marked reduction in the structural latency (increased labilization) of these hydrolases in rat preputial glands, although for other tissues there is a sex-dependent specificity and selectivity of action (Szego et al., 1971). Rapid translocation of the labilized lysosomes to the nucleus may result in intranuclear liberation of hydrolases, including a variety of nucleases, which may be associated with hormonal-mediated derepression processes (Szego et al., 1971).

Lysosomal enzymes are also changed in cancer. β-Glucuronidase activity is increased in many malignant tissues and is similarly increased by androgens (Fishman et al., 1955). Liver tissue of patients with malignant renal tumor had raised levels of the lysosomal enzymes, β-glucuronidase, aryl sulfatase, and cathepsins (Scherstén et al., 1969). Similar increased levels of lysosomal enzymes in muscle tissue of patients with malignancies may be related to the development of cachexia of malignant disease (Scherstén and Lundholm, 1972). Lysosomal enzymes may also be involved in the regression of hormone-dependent tumors, since following ovariectomy and regression of estrone-induced mammary tumors in rats there is a general increase in the activities of acid phosphatase, β-glucuronidase, and cathepsins of the tumors (Cutts, 1973).

Lysosomes are also profoundly altered during chemical carcinogenesis, and increased numbers of lysosomes and increased activity of lysosomal enzymes have been observed in rat liver after treating these animals with the hepatocarcinogens aflatoxin and dimethylnitrosamine. Many carcinogens have been shown to destabilize the lysosomes, presumably by damage of the membrane, increasing the release of the hydrolases into the cytosol with a consequent increased rate of turnover of cell constituents (Allison, 1969).

The potent carcinogen aflatoxin B_1, when administered to rats produced a marked elevation of the liver cytoplasmic DNase, with a concomitant reduction of the enzyme remaining in the lysosomes, and also destabilized rat liver, lysosomal membranes in vitro. It is perhaps significant that the relatively weak carcinogen aflatoxin B_2 produced no similar effect (Pitout and Schabort, 1973). Feeding rats with 2-acetamidofluorene for several weeks has been shown to give rise to marked increased in total activities of lysosomal hydrolases, acid DNase and β-glucuronidase, in the hepatocytes, from which tissue the resulting hepatomas are derived, but not in the Kupfer cells (Berg and Christofferson, 1974). Furthermore, the increased enzyme activities were primarily associated with the nuclear fraction (80% increase), the cytosol (30–60% increase), and the mitochondrial fraction (20% increase), whereas the microsomal fraction showed no change and the lysosomal fraction exhibited a marked loss of activity (30–40% decrease). This increase of total hydrolase activity (40–60%) suggests an increased *de novo* synthesis of these enzymes after continuous administration of the carcinogen. The association of these enzymes with the nuclear fraction may suggest the formation of enlargened lysosomal particles or, if the enhanced membrane labilization is still apparent, a greater catabolic effect upon the nuclear material. The uptake of acid hydrolases by the nucleus has been proposed as an important step in chemical carcinogenesis (Allison, 1969) and could facilitate the process of genomal derepression, as has been proposed for the steroid hormones.

It is possible that these effects of carcinogens on the lysosomes are a further manifestation of the membrane-damaging effects of the highly reactive ultimate carcinogens, as has been demonstrated for the membranes of the endoplasmic reticulum and for the plasma membrane. Furthermore, just as the lysosomal destabilizing effects of the sex steroids in certain target tissues is associated with rapid cell proliferation, so may certain carcinogens lead to a similar program of cell division. It is also possible that cyclic AMP may regulate the amounts of lysosomal enzymes and be involved in tissue proliferation, for in these three types of activity there is a close parallelism following administration of 2-acetamidofluorene and partial hepatectomy, and during the perinatal period (Berg and Christoffersen, 1974).

Mitochondria

Compared with the extensive studies made of the effects of carcinogens on the nucleus and nuclear DNA, little attention has been directed to the effects of these agents on the mitochondria of the cell. However, following the administration of dimethylnitrosamine to rats, mitochondrial DNA was found to be more extensively alkylated than was the nuclear DNA (Wilkinson *et al.*, 1975). This may possibly be due to the closer proximity of the mitochondria, than the nucleus, to the endoplasmic reticulum, the site of generation of the carcinogenic alkylating agent. However, mitochondrial DNA is unlikely to be a more important target molecule than nuclear DNA in the initiation of malignant transformation.

Nevertheless, such changes in the mitochrondrial DNA are likely to result in profound changes in the function of this organelle and may be responsible for the shift of basal metabolism of the malignant cell towards increased glycolysis (Aisenberg, 1961), a process of energy production more dependent on enzymes of the cytosol than on mitochondrial enzymes.

Steroid Hormones and Carcinogenesis

The changes in cell function and morphology brought about by the action of steroid hormones in their respective target tissues have been extensively documented (Sluyser, 1975). Interaction of the steroids, namely estrogens (Jensen and De Sombre, 1972), androgens and progestogens (Aakvaag *et al.*, 1972; Terenius, 1972), and corticosteroids (Sluyser, 1975), with specific cytoplasmic receptor proteins leads to transfer of the steroid–receptor complex to the nucleus, interaction of the complex with chromatin, and consequent stimulation of RNA synthesis (King and Gordon, 1972). This in turn leads to an increase in synthesis of protein and enzymes and, in certain cases, also to DNA synthesis, cell growth, and tissue proliferation. In this respect the steroid hormones bear some resemblence to carcinogens.

Many tumors, at least in their initial stages of development while they still have some degree of differentiation, retain some of the original characteristics of the cells from which they were derived and respond similarly to hormonal stimulation. This is particularly true of tumors occurring in those tissues which exhibit a high degree of hormonal response, e.g., the breast, uterus, and prostate. Eventually the progressive dedifferentiation process, which occurs in all malignant tumors, results in the loss of this faculty. Nevertheless, the hormonal induction of enzyme systems in malignant tumors must play an important part in the development of the disease (Williams and Smethurst, 1975).

Hormonal stimulation of protein synthesis may lead to enhanced synthesis of DNA polymerase, and hence increased DNA synthesis. Indeed, DNA synthesis and polymerase activity have been shown to be dependent on protein synthesis induced in rat prostate by testosterone (Chung and Coffey, 1971), and testosterone and dihydrotestosterone have been shown to stimulate the DNA polymerase in human hyperplastic prostatic tissue, although not in neoplastic tissue (Harper *et al.*, 1970a,b). Conversely, estrogens such as diethylstilbestrol and estradiol inhibit induction of prostatic RNA polymerase (Davis *et al.*, 1972) and DNA polymerase of hyperplastic and neoplastic prostate tissue (Harper *et al.*, 1971).

The increased rate of glycolysis which is characteristic of cancer tissues may also involve induction of enzymes, namely, hexokinase, phosphofructokinase, and pyruvate kinase, which are also induced by steroid hormones in their respective target tissues (Santti and Villee, 1971). Similarly, glucose-6-phosphate dehydrogenase, a controlling enzyme in the direct oxidative pathway of carbohydrate metabolism, and an important regulator of ribose and RNA synthesis, may be induced by testosterone in seminal vesicles (Singhal and Ling, 1969) and by estradiol in uterine tissue (Barker, 1967). Induction of these enzymes also occurs in malignant tissues, e.g., glucose-6-phosphate dehydrogenase is elevated in carcinoma of the prostate but not in benign prostatic hypertrophy (Miller *et al.*, 1972); and it may also be accompanied by changes in isoenzyme pattern, e.g., type V isoenzyme of lactate dehydrogenase is predominant in malignant prostate, where anaerobic glycolysis is favored, and type I is predominant in benign prostate where aerobic glycolysis predominates (Oliver *et al.*, 1970). Thus, in many ways, carcinogens mimic the steroid hormones in their regulation of metabolism, cell growth, and division, possibly because of similar molecular interactions at the endoplasmic reticulum and other subcellular membranes.

The steroid hormones themselves have sometimes been seen to be carcinogenic, to have a potentiating effect on carcinogenesis, or even to have a carcinostatic effect. Continuous administration of estrogens produces a wide variety of cancers in experimental animals, especially rodents. Most occur in the estrogen target tissues and in type are characteristic of the animal rather than the estrogens. The dog appears to be an exception and although not subject to oncogenesis from estrogens is susceptible to the formation of mammary tumors following prolonged administration of certain progestogens. Primates are remarkably resistant to any carcinogenic effect of the sex steroids. In man, long-term administration of androgens or estrogen–progestogen combinations may give rise to benign hepatomas, while continuous estrogen administration may produce adenocarcinoma of the uterus and high doses of stilbestrol during pregnancy may result in benign adenosis and clear cell cancer of the vagina in female offspring in later life (for a recent review see Segaloff, 1975). Estrogen treatment of rats seems to potentiate the carcinogenic effects of ionizing radiation (Segaloff, 1975), but at high doses both estradiol and progesterone protect the rat from mammary tumor induction by 7,12-dimethylbenz[*a*]anthracene (Kledzik *et al.*, 1974). Prolactin also appears to play a role in the prevention of mammary tumor induction in rodents.

Adrenocorticoids are commonly used to prevent host vs. graft reactions following tissue or organ transplants, in which they possibly act to prevent local inflammatory reactions. Cortisone, cortisol, and dexamethasone admistered in high dosage reduce the clonogenic growth of allogeneic tumor cells transplanted into the rat, presumably by a similar inhibition of local inflammatory reactions which support survival and early growth of tumor cells (Van den Brenk *et al.*, 1974). In contrast, dexamethasone has been shown to stimulate the expression of murine mammary tumor virus in tissue cultures of cell lines developed from mouse mammary adenocarcinoma (Parks *et al.*, 1974).

These apparent anachronisms in the stimulating and inhibiting effects of steroid hormones on carcinogenesis would suggest that these steroid regulators of tissue growth and metabolism play a fundamental role in the initiation/prevention and development/regression of cancer, the direction of action being dependent primarily on the type of tissue concerned and the nature of its natural hormonal regulation, although other features such as dose, time of administration, and animal species obviously also play a part.

Biochemical Differences between Normal and Cancer Cells

From the extensive studies that have been carried out to determine differences between normal and cancer cells no consistent general alteration in the biochemistry has as yet been observed. As with normal cells, cancer cells exhibit a great chemical diversity, not only among cancers of different organs but also among the different forms of cancer than can arise from the same type of normal cell. Furthermore, like normal cells, cancer cells are capable of changing their own metabolism to enable them to adapt to new conditions of their environment. However, new, esoteric methods are becoming available that allow more refined analysis of subtle differences in the metabolism and enzyme characteristics of cancer and normal cells, the exploitation of which may give rise to yet new approaches in chemotherapy.

One such example of a difference that has already been exploited is the need of certain types of leukemia cell for an essential component of many cellular proteins, namely, the amino acid, L-asparagine. Unlike normal cells, these neoplastic cells are unable to synthesize this amino acid for themselves, at least in sufficient quantity. Consequently, the accelerated destruction of circulating asparagine, by administration of the enzyme asparaginase, deprives the leukemic cells of an essential nutrient and provides a useful therapeutic regimen for those patients with an "L-asparagine-dependent" leukemia.

Enzymes

The study of enzymes in cancer goes back to 1924 when Warburg and his associates found that malignant tissues exhibit a greater rate of aerobic glycolysis than do normal tissues (Aisenberg, 1961). Decreases have been observed in the pathways of lipid and carbohydrate biosynthesis with increases in the catabolism of carbohydrates. Parallel to this is an increase in the anabolic pathways of protein and nucleic acid synthesis, to provide the necessary materials for the rapid growth of the malignant cells (Weber and Lea, 1966). The enzymes from rat liver hepatomas have been shown to be similar in their characteristics and activities to those of fetal rat liver and to differ from those of normal adult liver. Many of these tumor enzymes, especially those concerned with glycolysis, such as aldolase, pyruvate, kinase, and lactate dehydrogenase, have been shown to have isoenzyme patterns similar to those in fetal tissue but different from the adult pattern (Farron *et al.*, 1972). These differences in enzyme patterns in neoplastic tissue have been reviewed by Knox (1967).

Recent work has shown that the enzyme γ-glutamyl transpeptidase (glutathionase) in rat hepatomas has activity comparable to that of fetal and neonatal rat liver, but 10–100 times that of normal adult rat liver (Fiala *et al.*, 1972). Furthermore, in the chemical induction of hepatic tumors in rats by a diverse range of carcinogens, the high activity of γ-glutamyl peptidase is associated, almost from the beginning, with the induction of carcinogenesis (Fiala and Fiala, 1973). The substrate specificities and isoenzyme patterns of the aminopeptidases and arylamidases in cancer tissue of human lung, liver, and stomach have been shown to differ from those of corresponding normal, healthy tissues (Tamura *et al.*, 1975). Another different enzyme anomaly of cancer tissues concerns the microsomal mixed function oxidase system which in rat Morris hepatoma has almost zero activity despite the relative abundance of the constituent cytochrome P-450 and flavoproteins (Miyaki *et al.*, 1974). The hepatic microsomal mixed function oxidases were found to be similarly reduced in rats bearing Guerin carcinoma and showed a greatly diminished response to induction by phenobarbital (Basu *et al.*, 1974).

The normal metabolic adaptation to dietary changes, manifested by induction of enzymes of carbohydrate metabolism, such as glucokinase, glucose-6-phosphate dehydrogenase, and 6-phosphogluconate dehydrogenase, was not observed in rats dosed with the hepatocarcinogens 2-acetamidofluorene or 3'-methyl-4-dimethyl aminoazobenzene (Poirier and Pitot, 1970a). Similarly, in rats treated with chemical carcinogens, several of the liver enzymes concerned with amino acid metabolism, such as serine dehydratase and histidase did not show the normal inductive response to dietary stimulus (Poirier and Pitot, 1970b). It would seem that this inhibition of the normal adaptive increase in enzyme activity by enzyme induction, whether to dietary (substrate) or hormonal stimuli, is common to a number of hepatocarcinogens and characteristic of the resultant hepatomas.

In addition to these intrinsic changes in the enzymes of tumor cells, malignancy may result in changes in the levels of enzymes present in the blood serum of the host. These changes may result from (a) alteration of cell membrane permeability allowing an increased leakage of soluble enzymes, e. g., acid phosphatase in carcinoma of the prostate, (b) enzyme induction by the tumor, e.g., alkaline phosphatase in osteogenic sarcoma, (c) enzyme induction in normal tissue due to the presence of the tumor, e.g., alkaline phosphatase and 5'-nucleotidase in metastatic carcinoma of the liver, and (d) blockage by the tumor of ducts through which the enzyme may be secreted or excreted, e.g., alkaline phosphatase in carcinoma of the liver or amylase in carcinoma of the pancreas. These raised serum enzyme levels can be a valuable guide to diagnosis, and also to the efficacy of treatment (Schwartz, 1973).

Fetal Proteins

The formation, by malignant cells, of enzymes and other proteins characteristic of the period of embryonic growth have been the subject of much study in recent years. Fetuin, an α-globulin present in abundance in neonatal calf serum has been demonstrated in elevated levels in human sera in carcinoma of the stomach, pancreas, biliary tract and liver, and prostate (Dustin, 1972; McIntire et al., 1975). Although α-fetoprotein appears to be a potential marker for tumor activity, especially in gastrointestinal cancer, it has also been found to be elevated in hepatitis and certain other proliferative nonmalignant conditions and, using a sensitive double-antibody radioimmunoassay, was not found to be raised in patients with esophageal or small-bowel carcinoma (McIntire et al., 1975). The formation of these fetal proteins in the adult are biochemical evidence of a state of dedifferentiation of mitotically active cells with reactivation of genes normally active only during the embryonic period, (Dustin, 1972). They are indicative of, though not necessarily specific for, malignancy and may appear in high concentration in the serum during the early stages of chemical carcinogenesis before there is any objective evidence of tumor formation (Okita et al., 1974). An interesting observation of Castro and his colleagues is that there may be some immunological affinity between fetal and malignant tissues (Castro et al., 1973) which may, in part, explain the poor immune response to malignancies.

Cyclic AMP

It has been suggested that many of the properties of malignantly transformed cells are due to low levels of cyclic $3',5'$-adenosine phosphate (Pastan et al., 1975). When transformed isolated cells or hepatoma cells in culture are treated with cyclic AMP, dibutyryl cyclic AMP, or agents that raise cyclic AMP in cells, the transformed cells change in appearance to more closely resemble normal cells and grow more slowly (Pastan, 1975; van Wijk et al., 1972). On the other hand, dibutyryl cyclic AMP has been shown to increase the frequency of cell transformation by oncogenic viruses (Smith et al., 1973), and chemical carcinogenesis is associated with an increased responsiveness of adenyl cyclase to hormonal control (Boyd et al., 1974), so that a cascade effect magnifying the malignant transformation could result, especially in stressful conditions when the circulating

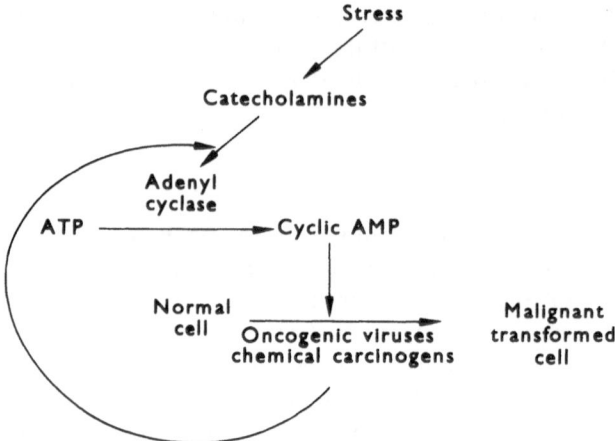

Figure 11. Possible cascade effect of chemical carcinogens and cyclic AMP on malignant cell transformation.

catecholamines are high (see Figure 11). Although the level of cyclic AMP of established tumors is always low and the hormonal responsiveness of their adenyl cyclase is not high (Boyd *et al.*, 1974) increased levels of cyclic AMP are characteristic of the initial malignant cell transformation. In keeping with this hypothesis is the observation that the tumor-producing phorbol esters, applied to mouse epidermis, also produce an initial increase in cyclic AMP followed by a marked depression, then a second period of elevation (Grimm and Marks, 1974). At the same time the hormonal regulation of adenyl cyclase is largely lost, indicating that the tumor promoters have resulted in damage of the cell membrane, the site of the β-adrenergic receptors of adenyl cyclase.

Recent work has suggested that the regulation of DNA synthesis and cell division is controlled by the ratio of cyclic AMP to cyclic GMP rather than by cyclic AMP alone. The tumor-promoting phorbol esters result in a marked increase in cyclic GMP, and conversely, cyclic AMP reduces the promoting effects of the phorbol esters. An increase of DNA synthesis, which follows a reduction of the cyclic AMP/cyclic GMP ratio, is considered to be the most important effect of the phorbol ester promoters, rather than inhibition of DNA repair mechanisms (Trosko *et al.*, 1975).

Conclusions

The key factor which determines the incidence of carcinogenesis following exposure to chemical carcinogens appears to be metabolism, namely the metabolic activation of the chemical, by the enzymes of the endoplasmic reticulum, in preference to alternative pathways of metabolism which result in detoxication. The direction of metabolism of a chemical carcinogen, namely, activation to a highly reactive proximate carcinogen, or deactivation to stable, readily-excreted metabolites, appears to be decided primarily by genetics, and also by other factors such as age, nutrition, and the presence of other environmental chemicals which may act as inhibitors or inducing agents of the microsomal enzymes catalyzing these processes (Weisburger and Williams, 1975). The genetically mediated differences in the inducibility of the activating enzyme, aryl hydrocarbon hydroxylase (benzpyrene hydroxylase), have been shown to correlate highly with potential to malignancy and have been suggested as the basis for a screening test. It has recently been shown (Sims, 1975) that in the case of certain polycyclic hydrocarbons the process of activation requires two oxygenations, and it is tempting to speculate that the first reaction may yield a proximate carcinogen which damages the endoplasmic reticulum, converting cytochrome P_{450} to cytochrome P_{448}, and thereby providing the required enzymic conditions for the second oxygenation to give the ultimate carcinogen.

Following the formation of the proximate and ultimate carcinogens, these short-lived and highly reactive chemical entities interact with the various chemical constituents and component structures of the cell, resulting in disruption of many normal cellular functions and intercellular regulatory systems. Because of the transcience and high reactivity of these proximate carcinogens it would appear most likely that they would produce their greatest damaging effect at, or near, the site of their formation, that is, the endoplasmic reticulum, and possibly also the nuclear membrane (Khandwala and Kasper, 1973). It is difficult to envisage how, if only produced in the endoplasmic reticulum, the proximate carcinogens could exert their major toxic effect on the DNA of the nucleus without simultaneously producing some damage, probably even greater damage, to other components of the cell. The damage of other components of the cell has therefore been considered in some detail. Among the most significant and fundamental would seem to be the action of proximate carcinogens on the integrity of the endoplasmic reticulum, leading to "degranulation" of the membranes and the resultant switch-over of protein metabolism from an extracellular to an intracellular economy, with its possible consequences of rapid cell growth and proliferation, loss of cell-recognition factors, and immune response mechanisms. Coupled with simultaneous damage to the nuclear DNA, and the resulting errors in genetic information, this mechanism would provide adequate explanation for the molecular action of chemical carcinogens. Additional damage to other cellular components, such as mitochondrial membranes and DNA, lysosomes, and the plasma membrane, would lead to even further disruption of cellular metabolism and intercellular economy, thereby exacerbating the malignant transformation.

Thus, the three critical steps in chemical carcinogenesis would seem to be: (1) metabolic formation of the proximate and ultimate carcinogens by enzymes of the endoplasmic reticulum; (2) irreversible degranulation of the endoplasmic reticulum leading to disruption of the normal regulation of cellular metabolism and a return to the embryonic state of tissue proliferation; and (3) covalent binding of the ultimate carcinogen to nuclear DNA, with consequent alteration of genetic information. The first two of these events may be monitored by the biphenyl hydroxylase test, described on p. 133, and the last, by a number of mutagenicity test systems. In view of the genetic variation in the metabolic activation of carcinogens, and hence the predictable wide species differences in susceptibility to chemical carcinogens, the validity of long-term animal carcinogenicity testing of potential chemical carcinogens should be questioned. Indeed, it would seem more meaningful, and would certainly be less expensive in time and money, to first examine potential carcinogens by a comprehensive series of short-term test systems which monitor the fundamental molecular events involved in carcinogenesis. If any of these tests are positive, long-term animal studies in a variety of species may then be justified.

The past quarter of a century has seen many exciting developments in the study of oncology but none more stimulating or rewarding than the study of the mechanisms involved in chemical carcinogenesis, for these are now beginning to lead to a unifying and revealing hypothesis of the cause of cancer which must result in a profound revision of attitude to the hazards of chemical carcinogens. The emphasis on preventive measures, possibly involving population screening for potential susceptibility, will undoubtedly increase, while treatment of this multifactorial disease, already involving multiple drug therapy, is likely to see the addition of even further dimensions reflecting the importance of the regulation of cell metabolism and the intercellular economy.

References

Aakvaag, A., Tveter, K. J., Unhjem, O., and Attramadal, A. (1972). Receptors and binding of androgens in the prostate. *J. Steroid Biochem.* 3:375–384.

Aisenburg, A. C. (1961). *The Glycolysis and Respiration of Tumors.* Academic Press, New York.

Allison, A. C. (1969). Lysosomes and cancer. In *Lysosomes in Biology and Pathology* vol. 2 (J. T. Dingle and H. B. Fell, eds.), pp. 178–204. North Holland, Amsterdam.

Alvares, A. P., Parli, C. J., and Mannering, G. J. (1973). Induction of drug-metabolism. VI. Effects of phenobarbital and 3-methylcholanthrene administration on *N*-demethylating enzyme systems of rough and smooth hepatic microsomes. *Biochem. Pharmacol.* **22**:1037–1045.

Alvares, A. P., Schilling, G. R., and Kuntzman, R. (1968). Differences in the kinetics of benzpyrene hydroxylation by hepatic drug-metabolizing enzymes from phenobarbital and 3-methylcholanthrene-treated rats. *Biochem. Biophys. Res. Commun.* **30**:588–593.

Barker, K. L. (1967). Cofactor induced synthesis of D-glucose-6-phosphate: NADP oxidoreductase in the uterus. *Endocrinology* **81**:791–797.

Basu, T. K., Parke, D. V., and Williams, D. C. (1974). Hepatic microsomal drug-metabolising enzymes in rats bearing Guerin carcinoma for various periods *Cytobios*, **11**:71–74.

Benedict, W. F., Considine, N., and Nebert, D. W. (1973). Genetic differences in aryl hydrocarbon hydroxylase induction and benzo(*a*)pyrene-produced tumorigenesis in the mouse. *Mol. Pharmacol.* **9**:266–277.

Berg, T., and Christoffersen, T. (1974). Early changes induced by 2-acetylaminofluorene in lysosomes in rat liver parenchymal cells. *Biochem. Pharmacol.* **23**:3323–3329.

Black, O., Cantrell, E. T., Buccino, R. J., and Bresnick, E. (1971). Effects of 3-methylcholanthrene administration on the proteins of endoplasmic reticulum. *Biochem. Pharmacol.* **20**:2989–2998.

Boyd, H., Louis, C. J., and Martin, T. J. (1974). Activity and hormone responsiveness of adenyl cyclase during induction of tumors in rat liver with 3'-methyl-4-dimethylaminoazobenzene. *Cancer Res.* **34**:1720–1725.

Brady, R. O., and Fishman, P. H. (1974). Biosynthesis of glycolipids in virus-transformed cells. *Biochim. Biophys. Acta* **355**:121–148.

Bresnick, E., and Mossé, H. (1969). Activation of genetic transcription in rat liver chromatin by 3-methylcholanthrene. *Mol. Pharmacol.* **5**:219–247.

Bullough, W. S. (1974). Chalone control mechanisms. *Life Sci.* **16**:323–330.

Burke, M. D., and Mayer, R. T. (1975). Inherent specificities of purified cytochrome P-450 and P-448 toward biphenyl hydroxylation and ethoxyresorufin deethylation. *Drug Metab. Dispos.* **3**:245–253.

Castro, J. E., Lance, E. M., Medawar, P. B., Zanelli, J., and Hunt, R. (1973). Foetal antigens and cancer. *Nature (London)* **243**:225–226.

Chu, B. C. F., and Lawley, P. D., (1975). Increased urinary excretion of nucleic acid and nicotinamide derivatives by rats after treatment with alkylating agents. *Chem. Biol. Interact.* **10**:333–338.

Chung, L. W. K., and Coffey, D. S. (1971). Biochemical characterization of prostatic nuclei. II. Relationship between DNA synthesis and protein synthesis. *Biochim. Biophys. Acta* **247**:584–596.

Cleaver, J. E., and Painter, R. B. (1975). Absence of specificity in inhibition of DNA repair replication by DNA-binding agents, cocarcinogens, and steroids in human cells. *Cancer Res.* **35**:1773–1778.

Conney, A. H. (1967). Pharmacological implications of microsomal enzyme induction. *Pharmacol. Rev.* **19**:317–366.

Craddock, V. M. (1973). Induction of liver tumours in rats by a single treatment with nitroso compounds given after partial hepatectomy. *Nature (London)* **245**:386–388.

Craddock, V. M. (1975). Effects of a single treatment with the alkylating carcinogens dimethylnitrosamine, diethylnitrosamine and methyl methanesulphonate, on liver regenerating after partial hepatectomy. II. Alkylation of DNA and inhibition of DNA replication. *Chem. Biol. Interact.* **10**:323–332.

Creaven, P. J., and Parke, D. V. (1966). The stimulation of hydroxylation by carcinogenic and non-carcinogenic compounds. *Biochem. Pharmacol.* **15**:7–16.

Currie, G. A. (1975). Immunological escape of tumours. In *Cancer and the Immune Response* (J. Turk, ed.), pp. 56–70. Edward Arnold, London.

Cutts, J. H. (1973). Enzyme activities in regressing estrone-induced mammary tumors of the rat. *Cancer Res.* **33**:1235–1237.

Davies, P., Fahmy, A. R., Pierrepoint, C. G., and Griffiths, K. (1972). Hormonal effects *in vitro* on prostatic ribonucleic acid polymerase. *Biochem. J.* **129**:1167–1169.

DeCloitre, F., Martin, M., and Chauveau, J. (1975). Comparative effect of phenobarbital and 3-methylcholanthrene on azo dye metabolism in rat liver. II. *In vivo* binding of metabolites to cellular macromolecules. *Chem. Biol. Interact.* **10**:301–307.

Deichmann, W. E., and Radomski, J. L. (1969). Carcinogenicity and metabolism of aromatic amines in the dog. *J. Nat. Cancer Inst.* **43**:263–269.

Delaunay, J., and Schapira, G. (1974). Ribosomes and cancer. *Biomedicine* **20**:327–332.

Dustin, P., Jr. (1972). Cell differentiation and carcinogenesis: A critical review. *Cell Tiss. Kinet.* **5**:519–533.

Edwards, G. S., and Allfrey, V. G. (1973). Aflatoxin B and actinomycin D effects of histone acetylation and deacetylation in the liver. *Biochim. Biophys. Acta* **299**:354–366.

Edwards, G. S., and Wogan, G. N. (1970). Aflatoxin inhibition of template activity of rat liver chromatin. *Biochim. Biophys. Acta* **224**:597–607.

Engelse, L. D., and Emmelot, P. (1971-72). Effects of feeding the carcinogen dimethylnitrosamine on its metabolism and methylation of DNA in the mouse, *Chem. Biol. Interact.* **4**:321–327.

Farber, E. (1973). Carcinogenesis—Cellular evolution as a unifying thread. *Cancer Res.* **33**:2537–2550.

Farber, E. (1975). Mechanisms by which chemicals initiate cancer, *J. Clin. Pharmacol.* **15**:24–28.

Farron, F., Hsu, H. H. T., and Knox, W. E. (1972). Foetal-type isoenzymes in hepatic and non-hepatic rat tumours. *Cancer Res.* **32**:302–308.

Fiala, S., and Fiala, E. S. (1973). Activation by chemical carcinogens of γ-glutamyl transpeptidase in rat and mouse liver, *J. Nat. Cancer Inst.* **51**:151–158.

Fiala, S., Fiala, A. E., and Dixon, B. (1972). γ-Glutamyl transpeptidase in transplantable, chemically induced rat hepatomas and spontaneous mouse-hepatomas, *J. Nat. Cancer Inst.* **48**:1393–1401.

Filipe, M. I., and Branfoot, A. C. (1974). Abnormal patterns of mucus secretion in apparently normal mucosa of large intestine with carcinoma. *Cancer* **34**:282–290.

Fishman, W. H., Artenstein, M., and Green, S. (1955). The renal β-glucuronidase response to androgens. *Endocrinology* **57**:646–657.

Franklin, M. R. (1972). Piperonyl butoxide metabolism by cytochrome P-450: Factors affecting the formation and disappearance of the metabolite–cytochrome P-450 complex. *Xenobiotica* **2**:517–527.

Fujimura, S., Grunberger, D., Carvajal, G., and Weinstein, I. B. (1972). Modifications of ribonucleic acid by chemical carcinogens. Modification of *Escherichia coli* formylmethionine transfer ribonucleic acid with *N*-acetoxy-2-acetylaminofluorene. *Biochemistry:* **11**:3629–3635.

Fujita, T., and Mannering, G. T. (1971). Differences in soluble P-450 hemoproteins from livers of rats treated with phenobarbital and 3-methylcholanthrene. *Chem. Biol. Interact.* **3**:264–265.

Furst, A., and Haro, R. T. (1969). Possible mechanisms of metal ion carcinogenesis. In: *The Jerusalem Symposia on Quantum Chemistry and Biochemistry. Physiochemical Mechanisms of Carcinogenesis* (E. D. Bergmann and B. Pullman, eds.), Vol. 1, pp. 310–320. Israel Academy of Sciences and Humanities, Jerusalem.

Garner, R. C. (1975). Reduction in binding of ^{14}C-aflatoxin B to rat liver macromolecules by phenobarbitone pretreatment. *Biochem. Pharmacol.* **24**:1553–1556.

Gelboin, H. V., Kinoshita, N., and Wiebel, F. J. (1972). Microsomal hydroxylases: Induction and role in polycyclic hydrocarbon carcinogenesis and toxicity. *Fed. Proc.* **31**:1298–1309.

Genta, V. M., Kaufman, D. G., Harris, C. C., Smith, J. M., Sporn, M. B., and Saffiotti, V. (1974). Vitamin A deficiency enhances binding of benzo(a)pyrene to tracheal epithelial DNA, *Nature (London)* **247**:48–49.

Gielen, J. E., and Nebert, D. W. (1971). Microsomal hydroxylase induction in liver cell culture by phenobarbital, polycyclic hydrocarbons, and *p,p'*-DDT. *Science (Washington)* **172**:167–169.

Glazer, R. I., Glass, L. E., and Menger, F. M. (1975). Modification of hepatic ribonucleic acid polymerase activities by *N*-hydroxy-2-acetylaminofluorene and *N*-acetoxy-2-acetylaminofluorene. *Mol. Pharmacol.* **11**:36–43.

Goldstein, I. M. (1975). Effects of steroids on lysosomes. *Transplant. Proc.* **7**:21–24.

Grantham, P. H., Weisburger, J. H., and Weisburger, E. K. (1973). Effect of the antioxidant butylated hydroxytoluene (BHT) on the metabolism of the carcinogens *N*-2-fluorenylacetamide and *N*-hydroxy-*N*-2-fluorenylacetamide. *Food Cosmet. Toxicol.* **11**:209–217.

Grimm, W., and Marks, F. (1974). Effect of tumour-promoting phorbol esters on the normal and the isoproterenol-elevated level of adenosine 3',5'-cyclic monophosphate in mouse epidermis *in vivo*. *Cancer Res.* **34**:3128–3134.

Grover, P. L., and Sims, P. (1973). K-region epoxides of polycyclic hydrocarbons: Reactions with nucleic acids and polyribonucleotides. *Biochem. Pharmacol.* **22**:661–666.

Grunberger, G., Yu, F. L., Grunberger, D., and Feigelson, P. (1973). Mechanism of *N*-hydroxy-2-acetylaminofluorene inhibition of rat hepatic ribonucleic acid synthesis. *J. Biol. Chem.* **248**:6278–6281.

Hakomori, S -I. (1975). Structures and organisation of cell surface glycolipids dependency on cell growth and malignant transformation. *Biochim. Biophys. Acta* **417**:55–89.

Harper, M. E., Fahmy, A. R., Pierrepoint, C. G., and Griffiths, K. (1970a). The effect of some stilboestrol compounds on DNA polymerase from human prostatic tissue. *Steroids* **15**:89–103.

Harper, M. E., Pierrepoint, C. G., Fahmy, A. R., and Griffiths, K. (1970b). The effect of prostatic metabolites of testosterone and other substances on the isolated deoxyribonucleic acid polymerase of the canine prostate. *Biochem. J.* **119**:785–786.

Harper, M. E., Pierrepoint, C. G., Fahmy, A. R., and Griffiths, K. (1971). The metabolism of steroids in the canine prostate and testis. *J. Endocrinol.* **49**:213–223.

Hawks, A., Hicks, R. M., Holsman, J. W., and Magee, P. N. (1974). Morphological and biochemical effects of 1,2-dimethylhydrazine and 1-methylhydrazine in rats and mice. *Brit. J. Cancer* **30**:429–439.

Hawks, A., and Magee, P. N. (1974). The alkylation of nucleic acids of rat and mouse *in vivo* by the carcinogen 1,2-dimethylhydrazine. *Brit. J. Cancer* **30**:440–447.

Hulbert, P. B. (1975). Carbonium ion as ultimate carcinogen of polycyclic aromatic hydrocarbons. *Nature (London)* **256**:146–148.

Imai, Y., and Siekevitz, P. (1971). A comparison of some properties of microsomal cytochrome P-450 from normal, methylcholanthrene-, and phenobarbital-treated rats. *Arch. Biochem. Biophys.* **144**:143–159.

Jacobson, M., Lu, A. Y. H., Sernatinger, E., West, S., and Kuntzman, R. (1972). The effect of altering liver microsomal CO-binding hemoprotein composition of pentobarbital-induced anesthesia. *Chem. Biol. Interact.* **5**:183–189.

Jensen, E. V., and De Sombre, E. R. (1972). Mechanism of action of the female sex hormones. *Ann. Rev. Biochem.* **41**:203–230.

Johnston, B., Lindup, W. E., Shillingford, J. S., Parke, D. V., and Smith, M. (1975). The pharmacological biochemistry of carbenoxolone. Its effects on gastric mucus. In *The Fourth Symposium on Carbenoxolone* (Sir Francis Avery Jones and Dennis V. Parke, eds.) pp. 3–24. Butterworth, London.

Juchau, M. R., Cram, R. L., Plaa, G. L., and Fouts, J. R. (1965). The induction of benzpyrene hydroxylase in the isolated perfused rat liver. *Biochem. Pharmacol.* **14**:473–482.

Jungmann, R. A., and Schweppe, J. S. (1972). Binding of chemical carcinogens to nuclear proteins of rat liver. *Cancer Res.* **32**:952–959.

Kawasaki, H., Nei, H., and Kimoto, E. (1974). Immunological demonstration of serum glycoprotein attached to carcinoma cell surface. *Gann* **65**:447–449.

Keisari, Y., and Witz, I. P. (1973). Degradation of immunoglobulins by lysosomal enzymes of tumours. 1. Demonstration of the phenomena using mouse tumours. *Immunochemistry* **10**:565–570.

Kellerman, G., Shaw, C. R., and Luyten-Kellerman, M. (1973). Aryl hydrocarbon hydroxylase inducibility and bronchogenic carcinoma. *N. Engl. J. Med.* **289**:934–937.

Keysell, G. R., Booth, J., Grover, P. L., Hewer, A., and Sims, P. (1973). The formation of ''K-region'' epoxides as hepatic microsomal metabolites of 7-methylbenz(*a*)anthracene and 7,12-dimethylbenz(*a*)anthracene and their 7-hydroxymethyl derivatives. *Biochem. Pharmacol.* **22**:2853–2867.

Khandwala, A. S., and Kasper, C. B. (1973). Preferential induction of aryl hydroxylase activity in rat nuclear envelope by 3-methylcholanthrene. *Biochem. Biophys. Res. Commun.* **54**:1241–1246.

King, H. W. S., Thompson, M. H., and Brookes, P. (1975). The benzo[*a*]pyrene deoxyribonucleoside products isolated from DNA after metabolism of benzo[*a*]pyrene by rat liver microsomes in the presence of DNA. *Cancer Res.* **34**:1263–1269.

King, R. J. B., and Gordon, J. (1972). Involvement of DNA in the acceptor mechanism for uterine oestradiol receptor. *Nature (New Biol.)* **240**:185–187.

Kinoshita, N., Shears, B., and Gelboin, H. V. (1973). K-region and non-K-region metabolism of benzo(*a*)pyrene by rat liver microsomes. *Cancer Res.* **33**:1937–1944.

Kledzik, G. S., Bradley, C. J., and Meites, J. (1974). Reduction of carcinogen-induced mammary cancer incidence in rats by early treatment with hormones or drugs. *Cancer Res.* **34**:2953–2956.

Knight, L. A., and Davidson, W. M. (1975). Reduced lymphocyte transformation in early cancer of the breast. *J. Clin. Pathol.* **28**:372–376.

Knox, W. E. (1967). The enzymatic pattern of neoplastic tissue. *Adv. Cancer Res.* **10**:117–161.

Kouri, R. E., Ratrie, H., and Whitmore, C. E. (1973). Evidence of genetic relationship between susceptibility to 3-methylcholanthrene-induced subcutaneous tumors and inducibility of aryl hydrocarbon hydroxylase. *J. Nat. Cancer Inst.* **51**:197–200.

Kriek, E. (1972). Persistent binding of a new reaction product of the carcinogen *N*-hydroxy-*N*-2-acetylaminofluorene with guanine in rat liver DNA *in vivo*. *Cancer Res.* **32**:2042–2048.

Krüger, F. W., Preussmann, R., and Niepelt, N. (1971). Mechanism of carcinogenesis with 1-aryl-3,3-dialkyltriazene. III. *In vivo* methylation of RNA and DNA with 1-phenyl-3,3-[^{14}C]dimethyltriazene. *Biochem. Pharmacol.* **20**:529–533.

Kuroki, T., Huberman, E., Marquardt, H., Selkirk, J. K., Heidelberger, C., Grover, P. L., and Sims, P. (1971-72). Binding of K-region epoxides and other derivatives of benz(*a*)anthracene and dibenz[*a,h*]anthracene to DNA, RNA and protein of transformable cells. *Chem. Biol. Interact.* **4**:389–397.

Lanclos, K. D., and Bresnick, E. (1973). Initiation factor activity in liver after 3-methylcholanthrene administration. *Drug Metab. Dispos.* **1**:239–247.

Lin, J -K., Miller, J. A., and Miller, E. C. (1975). Structures of hepatic nucleic acid-bound dyes in rats given the carcinogen *N*-methyl-4-aminoazobenzene. *Cancer Res.* **35**:844–850.

Lu, A. Y. H., and Levin, W. (1972). Partial purification of cytochromes P-450 and P-448 from rat liver microsomes. *Biochem. Biophys. Res. Commun.* **46**:1334–1339.

Magee, P. N., and Barnes, J. M. (1967). Carcinogenic nitroso compounds, *Adv. Cancer Res.* **10**:163–246.

McIntire, K. R., Waldmann, T. A., Moertel, C. G. and Go, V. L. W. (1975). α-Foetoprotein in patients with neoplasms of the gastrointestinal tract. *Cancer Res.* **35**:991–996.

McLean, A. E. M., and Marshall, A. (1971). Reduced carcinogenic effects of aflatoxin in rats given phenobarbitone, *Brit. J. Exp. Pathol.* **52**:322–329.

McPherson, F., Bridges, J. W., and Parke, D. V. (1974). *In vitro* enhancement of hepatic microsomal biphenyl hydroxylation by carcinogens, *Nature (London)* **252**:488–489.

Mailman, R. B., Tate, L. G., Muse, K. E., Coons, L. B., and Hodgson, E. (1975). The occurrence of multiple forms of cytochrome P-450 in hepatic microsomes from untreated rats and mice. *Chem. Biol. Interact.* **10**:215–228.

Margison, G. P., and Kleihues, P. (1975). Chemical carcinogenesis in the nervous system. Preferential accumulation of O^6-methylguanine in rat brain DNA during repetitive administration of N-methyl-N-nitrosurea, *Biochem. J.* **148**:521–525.

Marquardt, H., and Heidelberger, C. (1972). Stimulation of DNA synthesis in hydrocarbon-transformable hamster embryo cells by the K-region epoxide of benz(a)anthracene. *Chem. Biol. Interact.* **5**:69–71.

Metzler, M. (1975). Metabolic activation of diethylstilboestrol: Indirect evidence for the formation of a stilbene oxide intermediate in hamster and rat. *Biochem. Pharmacol.* **24**:1449–1453.

Miller, H. C., Rector, W., and Hilf, R. (1972). Preliminary enzymatic studies of human benign prostate hypertrophy and prostatic cancer. *Invest. Urol.* **10**:1–4.

Miller, J. A. (1970). Carcinogenesis by chemicals: An overview. *Cancer Res.* **30**:559–576.

Miller, J. A., and Miller, E. C. (1965). Metabolism of drugs in relation to carcinogenicity. *Ann. N.Y. Acad. Sci.* **123**:125–140.

Miller, J. A., and Miller, E. C. (1969). The metabolic activation of carcinogenic aromatic amines and amides. *Progr. Exp. Tumour Res.* **11**:273–301.

Miller, J. A., and Miller, E. C. (1971). Chemical carcinogenesis: Mechanisms and approaches to its control. *J. Nat. Cancer Inst.* **47**:v–xiv.

Miyake, Y., Gaylor, J. L., and Morris, H. P. (1974). Abnormal microsomal cytochromes and electron transport in Morris hepatoma, *J. Biol. Chem.* **249**:1980–1987.

Moulé, Y., Leasage, V., Darracq, N., and Rousseau, N. (1975). Opposite effects of phenobarbital treatment on aflatoxin B_1-induced inhibition of transcription in rat and mouse liver. *Biochem. Pharmacol.* **24**:1851–1854.

Nebert, D. W. (1969). Changes in aryl hydrocarbon hydroxylase activity and microsomal P-450 during polycyclic hydrocarbon treatment of mammalian cells in culture. *Biochem. Biophys. Res. Commun.* **36**:885–890.

Nebert, D. W., and Gelboin, H. V. (1968a). Substrate-inducible microsomal aryl hydroxylase in mammalian cell culture. I. Assay and properties of induced enzyme. *J. Biol. Chem.* **243**:6242–6249.

Nebert, D. W., and Gelboin, H. V. (1968b). Substrate-inducible microsomal aryl hydroxylase in mammalian cell culture. II. Cellular responses during enzyme induction. *J. Biol. Chem.* **243**:6250–6261.

Nebert, D. W., and Bausserman, L. L. (1970). Genetic differences in the extent of aryl hydrocarbon hydroxylase induction in mouse fetal cell cultures. *J. Biol. Chem.* **245**:6373–6382.

Nebert, D. W., Goujon, F. M., and Gielen, J. E. (1972). Aryl hydrocarbon hydroxylase induction by polycyclic hydrocarbons: simple autosomal dominant trait in the mouse. *Nature (New Biol.)* **236**:107–110.

Nimberg, R. B., Glasgow, A. H., Menzoian, J. O., Constantian, M. B., Cooperband, S. R.,
    Mannick, J. A., and Schmid, K. (1975). Isolation of an immunosuppresive peptide
    fraction from the serum of cancer patients. *Cancer Res.* **35**:1489–1494.
Okita, K., Gruenstein, M., Klaiber, M., and Farber, E. (1974). Localization of α-foetoprotein
    by immunofluorescence in hyperplastic nodules during hepatocarcinogenesis induced by
    2-acetylaminofluorine. *Cancer Res.* **34**:2758–2763.
Oliver, J. A., El Hilali, M. M., Belitsky, P., and MacKinnon, K. J., (1970). LDH isoenzymes
    in benign and malignant prostate tissues: The LDH V/I ratio as an index of malignancy.
    Cancer **25**:863–866.
Parke, D. V. (1975). Induction of the drug-metabolizing enzymes. In *Enzyme Induction*, (D. V.
    Parke, ed.), Vol. 6 of *Basic Life Sciences*, pp. 207–271. Plenum, London.
Parks, W. P., Scolnick, E. M., and Kozikowski, E. H. (1974). Dexamethasone stimulation of
    murine mammary tumour virus expression: A tissue culture source of virus. *Science*
    184:158–160.
Pastan, I. (1975). The role of cyclic AMP in malignant transformation. *Amer. J. Clin. Pathol.*
    63:669–670.
Pastan, I., Anderson, W. A., and Johnson, G. S. (1975). Role of cyclic nucleotides in growth
    control. *Ann. Rev. Biochem.* **44**:491–522.
Peraino, C., Fry, R. J. M., and Staffeldt, E. (1971). Reduction and enhancement by phenobar-
    bital of hepatocarcinogenesis induced in the rat by 2-acetylaminofluorine. *Cancer Res.*
    31:1506–1512.
Peraino, C., Fry, R. J. M., Staffeldt, E., and Kisieleski, W. E. (1973). Effects of varying the
    exposure to phenobarbital on its enhancement of 2-acetylaminofluorene-induced hepatic
    tumorigenesis in the rat. *Cancer Res.* **33**:2701–2705.
Pitout, M. J., and Schabort, J. C. (1973). Influence of aflatoxin B_1 and aflatoxin B_2 on rat liver
    lysosomal acid deoxyribonuclease. *Biochem. Pharmac.* **22**:1801–1805.
Poirier, L. A., and Pitot, H. C. (1970a). Metabolic adaptations during carcinogenesis: Dietary
    induction of some enzymes of carbohydrate metabolism during 3′-methyl- and 2-methyl-
    N,N-dimethyl-4-aminoazobenzene feeding. *Cancer Res.* **30**:1974–1979.
Poirier, L. A., and Pitot, H. C. (1970b). Dietary induction of some enzymes of amino acid
    metabolism following the acute administration of aminoazo dyes. *Cancer Res.* **30**:1980–
    1985.
Popp, J. A., and Shinozuka, H. (1974). Inhibition of protein synthesis and induction of helical
    polysomes in rat liver by *N*-hydroxy-2-fluorenylacetamide. *Chem. Biol. Interact.* **9**:37–
    43.
Pousada, C. R., and Lechner, M. C. (1972). Ribosomal and microsomal RNase activities in rat
    liver after methylcholanthrene administration. *Biochem. Pharmacol.* **21**:2563–2569.
Pozharisski, K. M., Kapustin, Y. M., Likachev, A. J., and Shaposhnikov, J. D. (1975). The
    mechnism of carcinogenic action of 1,2-dimethylhydrazine in rats. *Int. J. Cancer* **15**:673–
    683.
Radomski, J. L., and Brill, E. (1970). Bladder cancer induction by aromatic amines: Role of *N*-
    hydroxy metabolites. *Science* **167**:992–993.
Ragnotti, G., and Aletti, M. G. (1975). The effect of phenobarbitone on protein synthesis by
    liver polyribosomes in fed and starved rats. *Biochem. J.* **146**:1–12.
Roe, F. J. C., and Rowson, K. E. K. (1968). The induction of cancer by combinations of
    viruses and other agents. *Int. Rev. Exp. Pathol.* **6**:181–227.
Rolleston, F. S. (1974). Membrane-bound and free ribosomes. *Sub. Cell. Biochem.* **3**:91–117.
Salerno, R. A., Whitmire, C. E., Garcia, I. M., and Huebner, R. J. (1972). Chemical
    carcinogenesis in mice inhibited by interferon. *Nature (New Biol.)* **239**:31–32.
Santti, R. S., and Villee, C. A. (1971). Hormonal control of hexokinase in male sex accessory
    glands. *Endocrinology* **89**:1162–1170.

Scherstén, T., and Lundholm, K. (1972). Lysosomal enzyme activity in muscle tissue from patients with malignant tumor. *Cancer* **30**:1246–1251.

Scherstén, T., Wahlqvist, L., and Johansson, L. G. (1969). Lysosomal enzyme activity in liver tissue from patients with renal carcinoma. *Cancer* **23**:608–613.

Schoental, R. (1973). The mechanisms of action of the carcinogenic nitroso and related compounds. *Brit. J. Cancer* **28**:436–439.

Schwartz, M. K. (1973). Enzymes in cancer. *Clin. Chem.* **19**:10–22.

Segaloff, A. (1975). Steroids and carcinogenesis. *J. Steroid Biochem.* **6**:171–175.

Shoeman, D. W., Vane, F. H., and Mannering, G. T. (1973). Differences in P-420 hemoproteins from untreated and 3-methylcholanthrene-treated rats. *Drug Metab. Dispos.* **1**:40–44.

Sims, P. (1975). Epoxides as reactive intermediates in aromatic hydrocarbon metabolism. *Biochem. Soc. Trans.* **3**:59–62.

Sims, P., and Grover, P. L. (1974). Epoxides in polycyclic aromatic hydrocarbon metabolism and carcinogenesis. *Adv. Cancer Res.* **20**:165–274.

Sims. P., Grover, P. L., Swaisland, A. J., Pal, K., and Hewer, A. (1974). Metabolic activation of benzo(*a*)pyrene proceeds via a diol epoxide. *Nature (London)* **252**:326–328.

Singhal, R. L., and Ling, G. M. (1969). Metabolic control mechanisms in mammalian systems. IV. Androgenic induction of hexokinase and glucose-6-phosphate dehydrogenase in rat seminal vesicles. *Canad. J. Physiol. Pharmacol.* **47**:233–239.

Sladek, N. E., and Mannering, G. J. (1966). Evidence for a new P-450 hemoprotein in hepatic microsomes from methylcholanthrene treated rats. *Biochem. Biophys. Res. Commun.* **24**:668–674.

Sluyser, M. (1968). Interaction of carcinogens with histones *in vitro*. *Biochem. Biophys. Acta* **154**:606–609.

Sluyser, M. S. (1975). Mechanism of steroid hormone action at the cellular level. In *Enzyme Induction* (D. V. Parke, ed.) pp. 79–104. Plenum, London.

Smith, B. J., Defendi, V., and Wigglesworth, N. M. (1973). The effect of dibutyryl cyclic AMP on transformation by oncogenic viruses. *Virology* **51**:230–232.

Sunshine, G. H., Williams, D. J., and Rabin, B. R. (1971). Role for steroid hormones in the interaction of ribosomes with the endoplasmic membranes of rat liver. *Nature (New Biol.)* **230**:133–136.

Swaisland, A. J., Grover, P. L., and Sims, P. (1974a). Reactions of polycyclic hydrocarbon epoxides with RNA and polyribonucleotides, *Chem. Biol. Interact.* **9**:317–326.

Swaisland, A. J., Hewer, A., Pal, K., Keysell, G. R., Nooth, J., Grover, P. L., and Sims, P. (1974b). Polycyclic hydrocarbon epoxides: The involvement of 8,9-dihydro-8,9-dihydroxybenz(*a*)anthracene 10,11-oxide in reactions with the DNA of benz(*a*)anthracene treated embryo hamster cells, *FEBS Lett.* **47**:34–38.

Swenson, D. H., Miller, E. C., and Miller, J. A. (1974). Aflatoxin B_1-2,3-oxide: Evidence for its formation in rat liver *in vivo* and by human liver microsomes *in vitro*. *Biochem. Biophys. Res. Commun.* **3**:1036–1043.

Szego, C. M., Seeler, B. J., Steadman, R. A., Hill, D. F., Kimura, A. K., and Roberts, J. A. (1971). The lysosomal membrane complex. Focal point of primary steroid action. *Biochem. J.* **123**:523–538.

Tamura, Y., Niinobe, M., Arima, T., Okuda, H., and Fujii, S. (1975). Aminopeptidases and arylamidases in normal and cancer tissues in humans. *Cancer Res.* **35**:1030–1034.

Terenius, L. (1972). Specific progesterone binder in uterus of normal rats. *Steroids* **19**:787–794.

Trosko, J. E., Yager, J. D. Jr., Bowden, G. T., and Butcher, F. R. (1975). The effects of several croton oil constituents on two types of DNA repair and cyclic nucleotide levels in mammalian cells *in vitro*. *Chem. Biol. Inter.* **11**:191–205.

Ulland, B. M., Weisburger, J. H., Yamamoto, R. S., and Weisberger, E. K. (1973). Antioxidants and carcinogenesis: Butylated hydroxytoluene, but not diphenyl-*p*-phenylenediamine, inhibits cancer induction by *N*-2-fluorenylacetamide and by *N*-hydroxy-*N*-2-fluorenylacetamide in rats. *Food Cosmet. Toxicol.* **11**:199–207.

van Beek, W. P., Smets, L. A., and Emmelot, P. (1973). Increased sialic acid density in surface glycoprotein of transformed and malignant cells—A general phenomenon. *Cancer Res.* **33**:2913–2922.

Van den Brenk, H. A. S., Kelly, H., and Orton, C. (1974). Reduction by anti-inflammatory corticosteroids of clonogenic growth of allogeneic tumour cells in normal and irradiated tissues of the rat. *Brit. J. Cancer* **29**:365–372.

Van Duuren, B. L. (1969). Carcinogenic epoxides, lactones and halo-ethers and their mode of action. *Ann. N.Y. Acad. Sci.* **163**:633–651.

Van Duuren, B. L., Goldschmidt, B. M., and Seltzman, H. H. (1969). The interaction of mutagenic and carcinogenic agents with nucleic acids. *Ann. N.Y. Acad. Sci.* **153**:744–757.

van Wijk, R., Wicks, W. D., and Clay, K. (1972). Effects of derivatives of cyclic 3′,5′-adenosine monophosphate on the growth, morphology and gene expression of hepatoma cells in culture. *Cancer Res.* **32**:1905–1911.

Warwick, G. P. (1969). The covalent binding of metabolites of 4-dimethylaminoazobenzene to liver nucleic acids *in vivo*. The possible importance of cell proliferation in cancer initiation. In *Physico-chemical Mechanisms of Carcinogenesis* (E. D. Bergmann and B. Pullman, eds.), p. 218. Academic Press, New York.

Weber, G., and Lea, M. A. (1966). The molecular correlation concept of neoplasia. *Adv. Enzyme Regul.* **4**:115–145.

Weisburger, J. H., Madison, R. M., Ward, J. M., Vignera, C., and Weisburger, E. K. (1975). Modification of diethylnitrosamine liver carcinogenesis with phenobarbital but not with immunosuppresion. *J. Nat. Cancer Inst.* **54**:1185–1188.

Weisburger, J. H., and Williams, G. M. (1975). Metabolism of chemical carcinogens. *Cancer* **1**:185–234.

Weisburger, J. H., Yamamoto, R. S., Williams, G. M., Grantham, P. H., Matsushima, T., and Weisburger, E. K. (1972). On the sulphate ester of *N*-hydroxy-*N*-2-fluorenylacetamide as a key ultimate hepatocarcinogen in the rat. *Cancer Res.* **32**:491–500.

Whitlock, J. P., Jr., and Gelboin, H. (1974). Aryl hydrocarbon (benz(a)pyrene) hydroxylase induction in rat liver cells in culture. *J. Biol. Chem.* **249**:2616–2623.

Wiebel, F. J., and Gelboin, H. V. (1975). Aryl hydrocarbon (benz(a)pyrene) hydroxylases in liver from rats of different age, sex and nutritional status. Distribution of two types by 7,8-benzoflavone. *Biochem. Pharmacol.* **24**:1511–1515.

Wilkinson, R., Hawks, A., and Pegg, A. E. (1975). Methylation of rat liver mitochondrial DNA by chemical carcinogens and associated alterations in physical properties. *Chem. Biol. Interact.* **9**:157–167.

Williams, D. C., and Smethurst, M. (1975). Enzyme induction by steroid hormones with reference to cancer. In *Enzyme Induction* (D. V. Parke, ed.), pp. 143–168. Plenum, London.

Yamamoto, R. S., Weisburger, J. H., and Weisburger, E. K. (1971). Controlling factors in urethan carcinogenesis in mice: Effect of enzyme inducers and metabolic inhibitors. *Cancer Res.* **31**:483–486.

Yee, M., and Bresnick, E. (1971). Effect of administration of 3-methylcholanthrene on the salt-extractable chromatin proteins of rat liver. *Mol. Pharmacol.* **7**:191–198.

Zieve, F. J. (1973). Effects of the carcinogen *N*-acetoxy-2-fluorenylacetamide on the template properties of deoxyribonucleic acid. *Mol. Pharmacol.* **9**:658–669.

Chapter 7

STEROID HORMONES AND CANCER

D. C. WILLIAMS

Introduction

The mechanism of action of steroid hormones at a subcellular level remains one of the most fascinating and important problems in molecular biology. A great amount of effort has been expended, over the years, in an attempt to explain the wide range of morphological and biochemical effects which may be brought about by steroid hormones in experimental systems. Steroid analysis and, more recently, the analysis of the specific sites at which steroids function, has become an important part of clinical investigation. In spite of this the basic process of the steroid control of cellular function is still largely unexplained, so that any investigation of steroid participation in the cancer process must be based on certain assumptions as to the fundamental mechanism.

It has been postulated that steroid molecules react with a protein receptor molecule in the nucleus of the target cell and that a specific transport system is involved in achieving this.

Considerable attention has been given to explain how these steroid molecules achieve their specific responses and exhibit such striking organ selectivity. The presence of receptor proteins which specifically bind estradiol in estrogen-dependent target tissues was indicated in experiments using radioactive estradiol. It was demonstrated that particular organs have a striking affinity for this hormone resulting in the uterus, vagina, and

D. C. Williams • Head of Research Department, The Marie Curie Memorial Foundation, The Chart, Oxted, Surrey, England.

anterior pituitary taking up and retaining estradiol to reach concentrations considerably higher than that in the blood (Jensen and Jacobson, 1960). Subsequently, a two-stage system has been demonstrated in which the steroid binds to a cytoplasmic receptor protein which is later detected in the nucleus. This work has been extended by other workers who have shown the existence of specific receptor sites for androgen, progestagen, and corticosteroid hormones so that it would appear likely that these systems might represent a general pattern for steroid hormone action in mammalian cells (see review, Jensen and DeSombre, 1972).

The culmination of this interaction is a rapid stimulation in the synthesis of RNA, which the use of inhibitors of RNA synthesis has shown to be important in the hormonal regulation of protein synthesis and growth. Obviously, the induction of RNA synthesis and the transfer of RNA and ribonucleoprotein particles to the cytoplasm constitute a major basis for any gross change in the pattern of protein synthesis and enzyme induction that may occur with steroid hormones. Hence, the events leading to the activation of the genetic system represent an important aspect in the understanding of steroid hormone action.

Although much of the work on steroid receptors sites is based on experimental animal systems there is good evidence that human cells contain similar receptors, which appear to react with the steroid hormones in a similar manner, although further evidence of the distribution, and in particular the stability, of human receptor sites would appear to be desirable at the present state of our knowledge. It should also be remembered that receptor sites are generally estimated by combining them with appropriate steroid molecules labeled with radioactive atoms. Presumably only unoccupied receptor sites can be measured in this way so that the subject's previous steroid treatment is important in this context. A method for investigating total receptor capacity, both occupied and otherwise, would probably give a clearer picture of the steroid sensitivity of tumors, and several groups of workers are currently trying to develop such a system.

High endogenous circulating hormone levels already bound to some receptor sites may, therefore, play an important part in giving false-negative results in tumor specimens. Thus estimations of circulating hormones, or better, estimations of the hormone levels within the cell, should be examined at the same time as receptor sites are determined so that this factor may be taken into consideration. Such evidence as already exists suggests that amounts of endogenous circulating steroid are too small to play an important part in the system, but the relatively high levels of steroid or synthetic steroid blocking agent encountered during therapy are probably significant.

A nonsteroid method for quantitating or blocking available steroid receptor sites in tissues would be extremely useful at the present stage in our knowledge. A most promising approach to the problem appears to be the development of antisera against receptor sites. This technique will, however, require the separation and purification of receptor material in relatively large quantities, and the methods for doing so are not at present available.

Steroid-Sensitive Cancer

There are a number of cell types in the body which are normally under the complete or partial control of steroid hormones. These include the primary and secondary sex sites and, to a lesser extent and more conjecturally, liver, kidney, and epithelium. It is also often true that those organs which elaborate steroid hormones may sometimes be influenced by steroid treatment, presumably by some form of biochemical feedback.

In their initial stages, some human tumors which arise from hormone-sensitive tissues retain some of the steroid receptor capacity of the cells from which they were derived. Tumors arising from organs which are normally dependent upon hormones for growth and function may themselves be influenced by these substances until this facility is eventually lost by the normal dedifferentiation process which appears to be common to all malignant neoplasia.

Tumors sometimes retain their hormone sensitivity for a considerable period, although the sensitivity and hormonal stability of tumors arising from a particular site may vary widely, even in the same subject. During this period steroid hormone treatment, either by additive or ablative therapy, is often very valuable. Endocrine treatment appears most effective in those patients having slow-growing tumors. Tumors which have well-differentiated structures, sometimes a sign of retained hormone sensitivity, offer a better prognosis than do the rapidly metastasizing anaplastic tumors. There is much evidence in experimental animals, however, that the majority, if not all, of hormone-sensitive tumors consists of a mixed population of cells with varying hormonal responses so that altering the appropriate steroid levels eventually tends to encourage nonsensitive cells at the expense of the steroid-sensitive ones.

A long period between original diagnosis and recurrence of symptoms is also generally a good sign. Beyond these broad generalizations very little information can be gained, either from histological or clinical examination, as to the likely response of a particular tumor to therapy.

Steroid therapy has in the past been reserved for those tumors which have become difficult to treat surgically by virtue of their location or metastatic spread, so that the response figures, although rarely impressive, are generally related to advanced cases only.

Metastases arising from steroid-sensitive primary tumors have been treated with varying success by hormonal manipulation, either surgical or chemical. The two major problems in this form of therapy seem to be that it is very difficult to remove all sources of a particular hormone and that metastases may not have the same hormonal response as the primary tumor from which they arise, and in any case such tumors may quickly become autonomous.

A further perplexing clinical experience is that very occasionally the removal of a primary hormone-sensitive tumor causes a regression of its metastases. An experiment which may throw some light on the problem was performed recently in our laboratories (Bishun *et al.*, 1974). A transplantable mammary tumor was cloned using cytogenetic parameters, and it was found that both *in vitro* and *in vivo* some clones would not grow in the absence of others, but that by remixing the clones growth could then be mutually restored. This could be an example of an ectopic hormone being elaborated in one cell clone and acting on the other.

Estrogen-Sensitive Tumors

The most important site of human estrogen-sensitive carcinoma is the female breast; for this reason the majority of valid clinical evidence of antiestrogen therapy relates to this disease. Breast carcinoma is the most widespread malignancy in the female and may account for as much as 25% of total female cancer. There is, however, wide variation in its incidence in different countries. The extremes which are usually quoted are Japanese women, whose incidence is about 3.3/100,000 and British women at some 36.3/100,000 which, even when age adjustment is made for expectation of life in the two countries, represents a mortality of 6 to 1.

Carcinoma of the female breast is generally regarded as the first type of malignant tumor to have shown sensitivity to hormones. The proposal that oophorectomy should be used as a treatment for advanced breast cancer appears to have been made by Schinzinger in the 1880's. The assumption that estrogens were associated in some way with breast cancer was easily accepted since it could be effectively treated by the removal of the sources of estrogen in the body and it seemed logical that these cases should be typified by high levels of estrogen *in vivo*.

This in turn led to an interest in the synthesis and metabolism of estrogens in cancer patients. Most estrogen is produced in the ovary and varies in amount during the mentrual cycle. The metabolism of estrogen is shown in a simplified schematic form (Figure 1) Estradiol is the main estrogenic hormone but is in equilibrium with estrone, so that for clinical

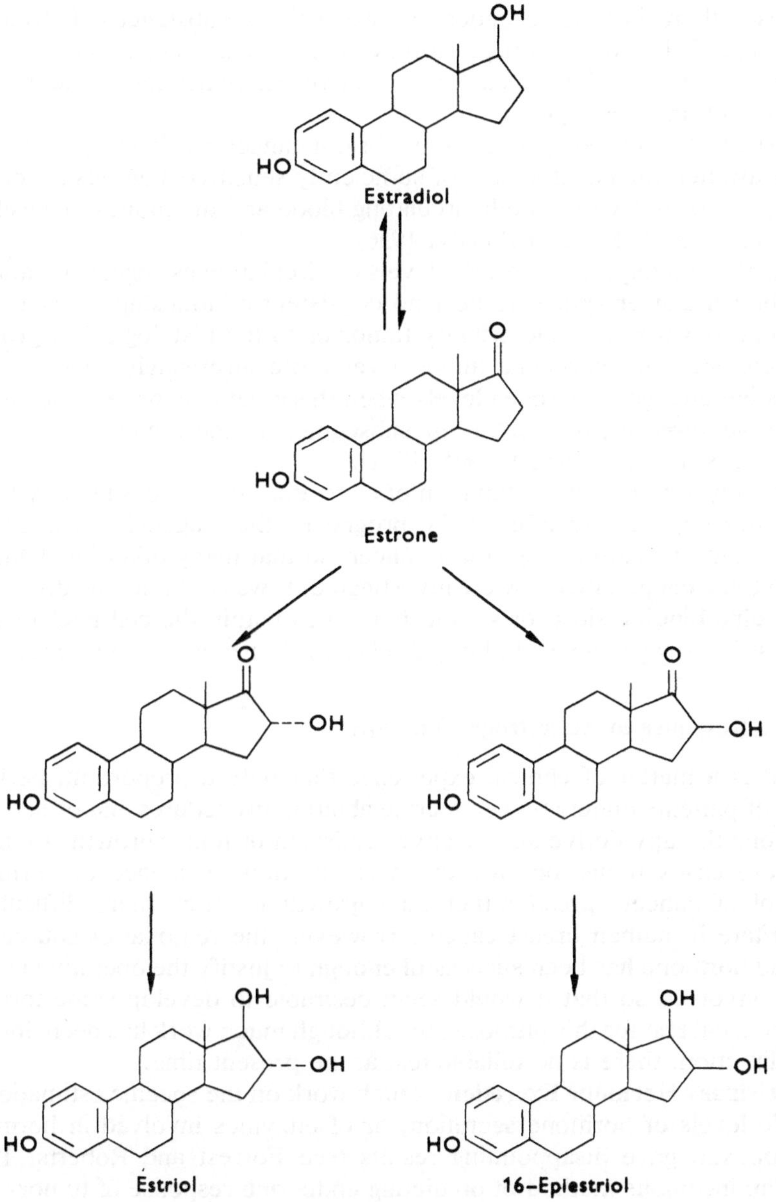

Figure 1. The relationship between the estrogens.

purposes there is little to choose between these substances. Estrone is often regarded as the "storage" form of the estrogen and estradiol as the "active" form, but this appears to be an over simplification of the mechanism of action of estrogens.

The testing of the hypothesis that breast cancer involved high estrogen levels awaited the development of sufficiently sensitive methods for determining estrogen levels in both circulating blood and the tissues themselves (Brown, 1955; Aitken and Preedy, 1956).

Unfortunately, however, the levels of circulating estrogens in patients with breast cancer appear to bear no consistent relationship either to the hormone sensitivity of the primary tumor or to the histological or growth characteristics of a particular tumor. Even more surprisingly, there was no consistent change in estrogen levels when these patients were subjected to endocrine surgery either before or subsequent to the removal of the primary breast tumor (Forrest, 1965, 1971).

It appeared that the estimation of estrogenic substances in body fluids or tissues had little to offer in the prognosis, the diagnosis, or even the assessment of treatment of breast cancer, so that many other biochemical and cytological parameters were investigated. It was not until the discovery of specific binding sites for steroid hormones within the cell nucleus that interest in estrogen levels in body fluids and tissues was reawakened.

Tumor Response to Antiestrogen Therapy

It is a matter of clinical experience that only a proportion, perhaps 40%, of patients undergoing endocrine ablation procedures and/or additive hormone therapy derive an objective remission of tumor growth. In many of these cases remissions are of short duration. Evidence of hormone control of cancer spread rather than growth is much more difficult to quantitate in human breast cancer. However, the removal of sources of steroid hormone has been successful enough to justify the operative procedures involved so that it would seem desirable to develop some form of biochemical test for this purpose but, although much work has been done in this direction, there is no reliable test at the present time.

Urinary Hormone Excretion. Much work on the specific estimation of simple levels of hormone secretion, or of enzymes involved in hormone metabolism, gave disappointing results (see Forrest and Roberts, 1973) until an ingenious method of predicting endocrine response of tumors, the discriminant factor, was evolved in the main by Bulbrook, Greenwood, and their colleagues. This predictive method depends upon the calculation of ratios between the quantities of specific urinary steroids, or groups of steroids, excreted by the cancer patient.

Thus Bulbrook *et al.* (1960), after testing many different combinations of excreted steroids, showed that the ratio of urinary etiocholanolone (derived from the metabolism of androgenic steroids and therefore an excretion product of testosterone, see Figure 2) to the total 17-hydroxycorticosteroid level (derived from the adrenal steroid metabolic pathway, see Figure 3) gave an index of the efficiency of hypophysectomy and possible adrenalectomy as forms of steroid ablation treatment. This has been confirmed by several other groups of workers, e.g., Juret (1968) and Atkins *et al.* (1968). The latter groups analyzed their results and concluded that: (1) Hypophysectomy was four times as likely to be effective in patients with a positive discriminant than in patients with a negative discriminant and that the survival period after hypophysectomy was, on the average, longer for the positive patient; and (2) the longer the period between removal of the primary tumor and the occurrence of secondary tumors the better the response to hypophysectomy of these patients with a positive discriminant.

Some workers, however, found difficulty in confirming this work, possibly due to differences in selection of patients. A number of attempts have been made to improve the effectiveness of the discriminant factor by the inclusion of other parameters, both biochemical and clinical. So far no clear advantage has been shown over the original factor, but studies on alternative systems continue.

Dao and his colleagues (1971) have developed a rather different approach to this problem and have shown that some breast tumors appear to have the capacity of enhancing the conjugations of certain steroids with sulfate. It has been suggested that those tumors possessing a high conjugation capacity give the best response, especially to adrenalectomy. They also suggest that those tumors giving the highest ratio of dehydroepiandrosterone (Figure 2) to estradiol (Figure 1) excreted as sulfate conjugates are likely to give the best response to therapy. These experiments again give rise to interesting speculation as to whether or not abnormal sulfate conjugation may be used as a screening technique and whether the effect is detectable at a premalignant level. If, on the other hand, steroid conjugation has a bearing on the initiation of the malignant process, may not lesions in other organs, especially perhaps the liver, affect the etiology of breast cancer?

Hormone Receptor Sites. All techniques which depend on the estimation of steroid hormones in the blood, urine, or tissues themselves suffer from a fundamental disadvantage. Simply because the hormone is present in the body fluids, or even within the cell, it does not follow that it is capable of affecting the metabolism of the cell. Many other factors such as protein binding, metabolic breakdown, conjugation, and steroid transport systems must play an important part in this process. The possibility of a

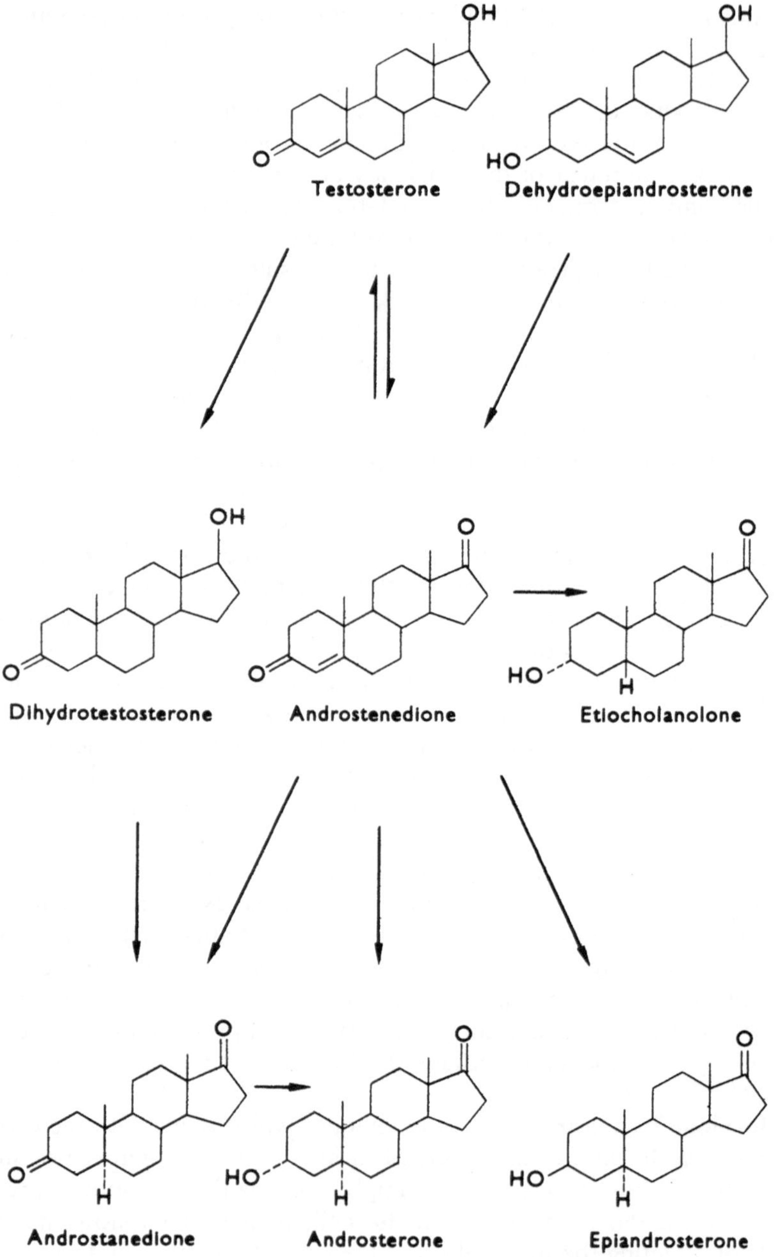

Figure 2. A simplified scheme for the metabolism of testosterone.

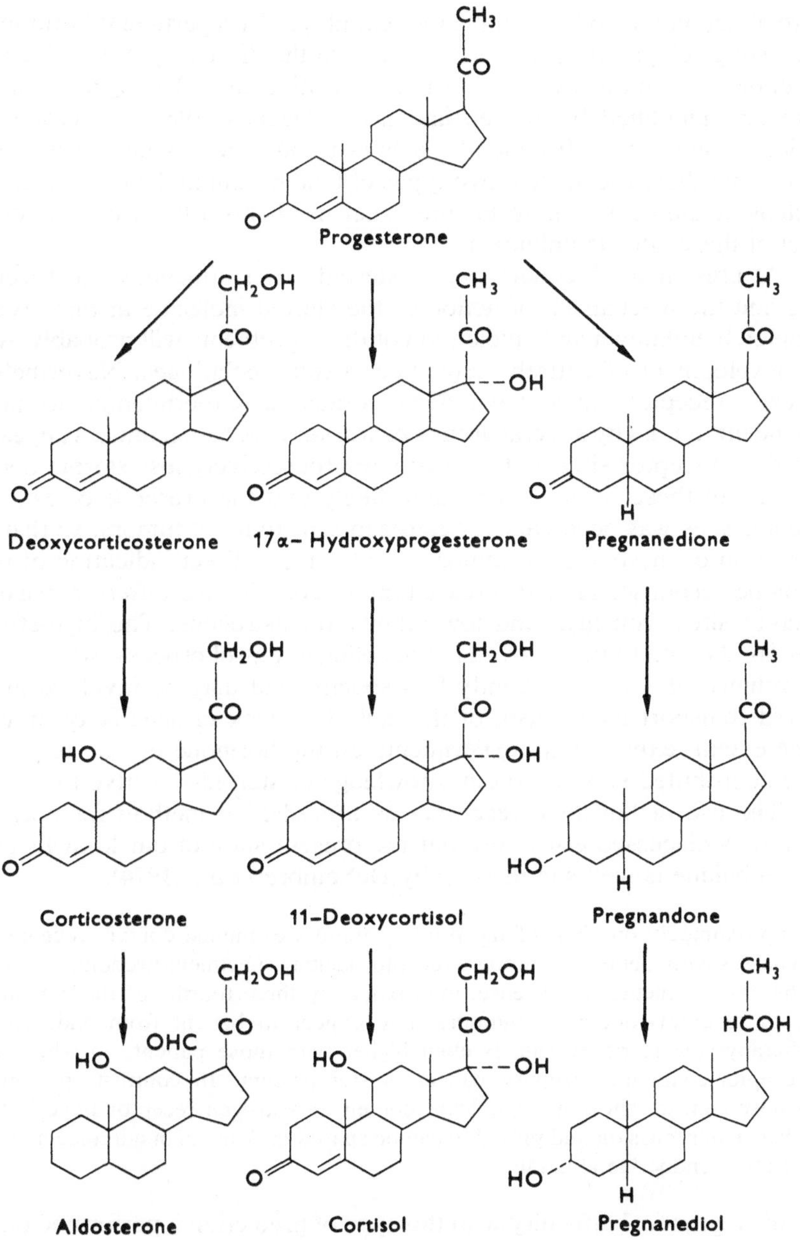

Figure 3. A simplified relationship between progesterone and the corticosteroids.

more direct method of estimating the part played by a particular hormone in controlling cell growth processes arose with the discovery of specific sites of action of hormones within hormone-sensitive cells. Estrogen receptors were first identified by Jensen and his colleagues (1967) in uterine and vaginal tissues and subsequently in breast and other tissues. It has been shown that there are at least two types of binding site in the cytoplasm and nucleus of the cells, but so far the exact mechanism by which estrogens react at these sites is unknown.

At present the biochemistry of steroids after attachment to receptor sites and the mechanism of action of the steroid molecule at that level is completely unknown and elucidation of these problems will probably await the development of entirely new experimental techniques. Nevertheless, estrogen receptors have been demonstrated in experimental hormone-dependent tumors by several groups of workers, and such tumors appear to lose their receptor sites as they become progressively less steroid dependent. From these results it appeared likely that the presence of estrogen receptor sites was necessary for estrogen sensitivity of tumors, so that the estimation of these sites in tumors should give a direct indication of their hormone response. Human breast tumors contain two different estrogen receptor sites with high and low affinity for estrogens. The high-affinity sites are thought to be involved in the cellular control process, whereas the low-affinity sites are apparently less specific and may be involved in the steroid transport mechanism of the cell. This lack of specificity may, to some extent, explain why experiments on the hormone uptake of tumors have contributed so little to our knowledge of steroid-sensitive tissues.

The use of hormone receptors as a predictive method for hormone therapy is discussed elsewhere but the present state of our knowledge of this technique is well summed up by DeSombre et al. (1974):

> Approximately one half of the primary tumors examined contain receptor, whereas with metastatic tumours receptor-lacking specimens predominate. In the case of metastatic disease, approximately three fourths of the patients with receptor-containing tumours may expect to benefit from endocrine therapy; the response rate is even higher with those patients in whom a receptor-containing primary cancer is still present. In contrast, patients whose cancers show no significant content of estrogen receptor have little chance of remission and probably can be spared the trauma of adrenalectomy or other endocrine ablation.

The main practical difficulty with this type of prediction if performed on the primary tumor is, therefore, that one must assume that the endocrine response of metastases is the same as that of the primary tumor from which they arise. This is certainly not always true in our experience of certain chemically induced animal tumors, and clinical experience suggests that neither is it true for human breast cancer. Recent research, however, shows the subject to be much more complicated and probably involves receptor proteins of other hormones such as progesterone and perhaps androgens (McGuire *et al.*, 1975a,b). The identification of specific sites for hormonal control of malignant cells, however, leads to the possibility of developing a cytotoxic drug which is receptor-site specific, possibly by modification of the appropriate steroid hormone, and perhaps eventually to the immunological blocking of the receptor site itself.

Steroid Stimulation *in Vitro*. The *in vitro* culture of malignant cells offers a further method of investigating steroid–tumor interactions and much effort has been expended on the tissue culture of tumors. It is only comparatively recently, however, that reproducible results have been obtained (Barber and Richmond, 1971; Bishun *et al.*, 1973, 1974) These cultures are viable over long periods and therefore give confidence that near normal growth rather than the slow death of cells has been achieved. Having established a healthy culture, it is possible to add appropriate hormones, or indeed almost any other drug, to the culture medium and to compare the growth rate of the tumor cells under various conditions (Figure 4). This method of predicting hormonal response of future metastatic growth has great potential value and, although this can only be established by long-term clinical studies, some interesting comparisons are already emerging with other predictive methods.

Tissue culture techniques suffer from a number of disadvantages which must be taken into account in evaluating results. In general, steroids are less well metabolized in culture than in the *in vivo* situation. This has the advantage of allowing steroid hormones to be added separately so that their effects can sometimes be separated. This technique is limited in that the tumor/host relationship, which is especially important to steroid elaboration, is absent, so that only an approximation to the *in vivo* state can be expected. A more realistic system would seem to be a mixed culture between the tumor and the tissue of the host to which it metastasized. This may be even more important when the host organ itself is known to play a part in steroid metabolism or conjugation. It seems likely, now that the culturing of human tumors is reasonably well understood, that the technique of mixed cultures will prove very useful in investigating the metastatic spread of breast tumors.

Androgen Therapy. Primary androgen therapy has been used as an alternative to castration, or other endocrine ablation, but results have almost always been inferior in spite of a marked reduction in estrogenic activity. This effect is probably mediated mainly by direct interference with estrogen synthesis, but competition for hormone receptor sites may also

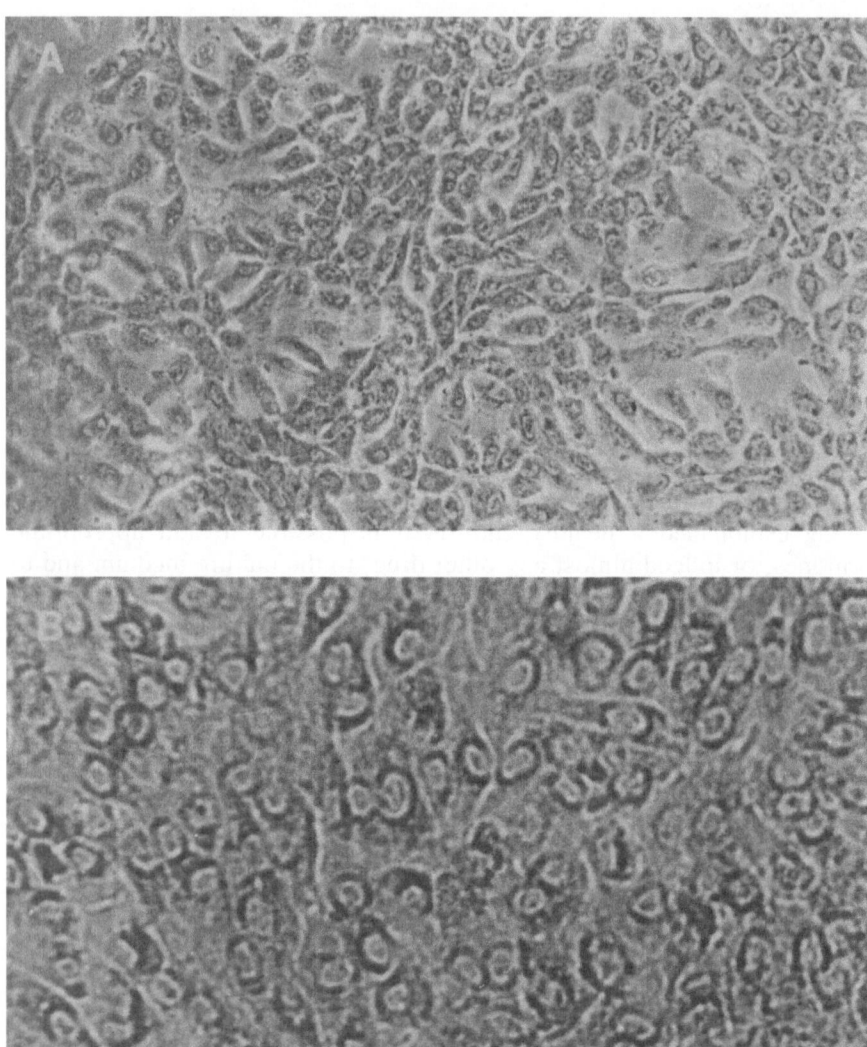

Figure 4. Human breast carcinoma in culture: (a) without added hormone; (b) after addition of estradiol.

play a small part. Androgens have, however, been used for the treatment of advanced metastatic disease mainly as a secondary control measure, especially for patients with bone metastasis.

The undesirable side effects of androgens are, again, hypercalcemia and fluid retention, as in estrogen treatment. Erythrocythemia is also produced since androgens increase erythropoiesis. Another undesirable side effect is virilization, and much work has been done in the hope of discovering a nonvirilizing androgen which has comparable therapeutic effects to testosterone. Among the most effective anticancer substances are testolactone (17-oxa-D-homoandrostra-1, 4-diene-3, 17-dione), fluoxymesterone (androst-4-en-3-one-9-fluro-11,17-dihydroxy-17-methyl), and the corresponding 3-one-4,5-dihydro-2-methyltestosterone or its propionate and several other testosterone derivatives. These compounds at optimal doses appear to have comparable activity to testosterone against breast cancer, but they have much lower virilizing activity and therefore, presumably, a modified mode of action. When comparisons were made between these drugs and estrogenic substances or adrenalectomy, the response to androgen was generally inferior to either of the other two.

Androgen-Sensitive Tumors

There are several tumors, generally arising from primary or secondary sex sites in the male, which are sensitive to androgens, and of these the most important is carcinoma of the prostate. Although the connection between the prostate and testicular function was well recognized, it was Berthold in 1849 who first postulated a "blood borne chemical effect" which was probably the first statement of hormone activity. It was not, however, until the classical work of Huggins and Clarke (1941), working on prostatic hyperplasia in dogs, that the tumors were shown to be androgen dependent and could be controlled by large doses of estrogen. These results were rapidly applied to human cancer and by 1946 Huggins published the 5-year results on the treatment of prostatic carcinoma by castration. The geographical distribution of this disease shows considerable variation; the lowest being approximately 1.4/100,000 in Japan and the highest, 21.3/100,000 males in the nonwhite population of the United States of America. In general, however, prostatic carcinoma appears to be one of the most common malignant tumors in men over the age of 60 years.

Prostatic carcinoma is a difficult disease to detect in its early stages as it is often associated with benign prostatic hyperplasia. The usefulness of radical prostatectomy as an initial treatment is still much discussed and depends on the stage of the disease. It is apparently only of value when the tumor is confined to its primary site. The successful castration performed by Huggins and others for advanced carcinoma raised the question whether this form of treatment was preferable to prostatectomy in early cases. This, coupled with the fact that there is a body of evidence to suggest that prostatic carcinoma can be disseminated during needle biopsy, or other exploratory surgery, has limited the clinical use of biochemical and histological diagnostic techniques. The most widely used diagnostic aid has been the raised serum acid phosphatase levels which are sometimes, but not always, found. A high serum acid phosphatase, however, generally indicates that the disease is advanced and has metastasized to bone or some other site.

A number of methods involving hormonal estimations in body fluids have been investigated in the hope of improving early diagnosis of prostatic carcinoma. These include androgen levels (either testicular or adrenal), gonadotrophin (follicle stimulating hormone, FSH, or interstitial cell stimulating hormone, ICSH) or urinary 17-ketosteroid output, but no consistent success seems to have been achieved with any such estimation.

Antiandrogen Therapy

Antiandrogen therapy, both additive and ablative, is widely used in the control of human prostatic carcinoma, but the biochemical basis for this treatment is not clear. One of the main problems in the experimental investigation is the lack of an animal tumor having properties sufficiently similar to the human disease to give meaningful comparison between them.

There is a large body of evidence that the action of testosterone, unlike that of estrogens, is dependent upon the metabolism of hormone (Fig. 2). It is therefore likely that the metabolism of testosterone is a necessary prerequisite for its hormone action. This evidence supports the observations of Anderson and Liao (1968) who showed that 5α-dihydrotestosterone is the main testosterone metabolite within the nucleus of the prostate cell and this substance appears to exert the major "androgenic" influence in prostatic carcinoma. It is clear, however, that metabolites may respond in different ways in various species (Table 1, Williams and Smethurst, 1975).

Many estrogenic compounds, both natural and synthetic, have been used in an attempt to suppress androgen, but the majority of patients have been treated with diethylstilbestrol, or some derivative of estradiol, and there still appears to be little to choose between the various forms of estrogen therapy on a statistical basis. Owing to the effectiveness of castration and the ease and relative safety of estrogen treatment, many patients have been treated by a combination of these methods of androgen suppression with a consequent difficulty in obtaining figures for these treatments separately.

The mechanism of action of antiandrogen therapy by estrogens is still not clearly understood but there are probably at least three possible modes of action: (1) Direct competition with androgen receptor sites in the pros-

TABLE 1. Biological Activity of Testosterone and Some of Its Metabolites on Rat and Dog Prostatic Tissue

Metabolite	Biological activity	
	Rat prostate	Dog prostate
Testosterone	Slight stimulation of RNA polymerase[a]	Slight stimulation of RNA polymerase[a]
	Maintains secretion[c]	Stimulation of DNA polymerase[b]
Dihydrotestosterone	Stimulation of RNA polymerase[a]	Stimulation of RNA polymerase[a]
	Hyperplasia[c]	
	Maintains secretion[c]	
5α-Androstane-3α,17β-diol	Stimulation of RNA polymerase[a]	No stimulation of RNA polymerase[a]
	Slight hyperplasia[c]	Stimulation of DNA polymerase[b]
5α-Androstane-3β,17β-diol	Stimulation of RNA polymerase[a]	Slight stimulation of RNA polymerase[a]
	Stimulates secretion[c]	No stimulation of DNA polymerase[b]
5α-Androstane-3α,17α-diol	No stimulation of RNA polymerase[a]	Slight stimulation of RNA polymerase[a]
		Stimulation of DNA polymerase[b]

[a]Davies *et al.*, 1972.
[b]Harper *et al.*, 1970.
[c]Robel *et al.*, 1971.

tate cell and by this means, suppression of the androgen-stimulated DNA synthesis; (2) interference with the normal metabolic process of testosterone within the cell which gives rise to "active" metabolites; and (3) interference of synthesis of androgens, of either testicular or adrenal origin, either by direct action on the gland or by suppression of gonadotrophin secretion by the pituitary gland.

The term estrogen is sometimes used in clinical practice to cover a wide variety of natural and synthetic substances which exhibit some "estrogenic properties." It is also used on occasion for antiandrogens and for other substances whose mechanism of action is not clear. There is a considerable and growing body of evidence that these drugs may exert their influence by a variety of very different biochemical effects and at different sites of action. These forms of treatment cannot, therefore, be regarded as simple alternatives, and the possibility of combination therapy must be considered.

Corticosteroid/Progesterone-Sensitive Cancers

Certain tumors arising from tissues which may not be sensitive to the stimulation of sex hormones may nevertheless be treated by other steroid hormones. In particular, considerable success has been claimed for both corticosteroid and progesterone treatment in a wide variety of tumors which appear to have very little in common. These forms of treatment may perhaps be considered together because they both appear to function by some form of feedback mechanism and may share a common synthetic and metabolic pathway (Figure 3).

Adrenocorticosteroid Treatment

The feedback mechanism of corticosteroids on the adrenal gland is well documented, and suppression of sex steroids of adrenal origin as well as of costicosteroids may be achieved in this manner.

It is reasonable, therefore, to expect that this form of treatment would produce effects similar to surgical adrenalectomy. Pearson et al. (1955) have shown that, in fact, remissions do occur in a considerable number of cases. However, these remissions are not of long duration, and the treatment is considerably less effective than adrenalectomy.

In order to separate chemical adrenalectomy from the hormonal effects of corticosteroids, a number of other substances have been tested in an attempt to produce adrenalectomy. The most effective drugs so far tested appear to be those related to the insecticide DDT. These include: DDD (1,1-dichloro-2,2-bis(p-chlorophenyl)ethane); Perthane (1,1-dichloro-2,2-bis(p-ethylphenyl)ethane); o,p-DDD (1,1-dichloro-2(o-chlorophenyl), 2-p-chlorophenylethane). These substances were carefully studied by Weisenfeld and Goldner (1962). Zimmermann et al. (1956) showed that some adrenal suppression could be obtained in patients with carcinoma of the breast or prostate by using DDD. Bergenstal et al. (1960) have obtained favorable results in adrenal cancer by using o,p-DDD, and this compound was also examined in Cushing's syndrome. It was concluded that these drugs decrease adrenal function in man, but that suppression of normal adrenal function does not occur uniformly and is not sufficient to be of value in treating metastatic breast or prostatic carcinoma. Although this treatment is never as effective as adrenalectomy, it is sometimes used after castration to depress the usual adrenal hypertrophy. The drug also has a place in treating patients who suffer from hypercalcemia and certain other conditions which are met with less often. The use of cortisone itself has been largely superseded by its derivatives hydrocortisone, prednisone, or prednisolone.

There appears to be little or no correlation between previous responsiveness to sex hormones and the corticosteroids so that this form of therapy is available to patients who do not respond to other forms of endocrine treatment. For patients not thoroughly treated by other endocrine therapy, corticosteroids may prolong life in the hypercalcemic syndrome.

The main problem in treating patients with corticosteroids is the development of Cushing's syndrome and other effects of hypercorticism. There is also the real danger of irreversible depression of the adrenal cortex or even of the pituitary by prolonged treatment with large quantities of adrenal hormone.

Some workers have obtained subjective response only in cases of disseminated prostatic carcinoma, but since this sometimes includes dramatic relief from pain the treatment seems worthwhile in late cases. Prednisone and prednisolone are usually used, especially in the management of advanced cases, where the obvious side effects may be tolerated.

Small-scale trial of prednisone by the Co-operative Group of the Cancer Chemotherapy National Service Centre showed no objective response with this drug. Corticosteroid therapy appears, therefore, to be useful only in the palliation of the final stages of prostatic carcinoma.

Corticosteroids have been used with some success in the treatment of acute lymphoblastic leukemia and with less effect in chronic leukemia. These treatments have largely been replaced by sequential combination chemotherapy in which prednisone is often a constituent, and it is in this direction that corticosteroid therapy appears to hold the greatest promise. It must, however, be remembered that the corticosteroids are suppressors of immune response so that their use, especially in early cancers, may even promote tumor spread rather than control growth.

Progestogen Treatment

There have been a few reports of treating patients with progesterone itself, but there is scanty evidence of any therapeutic advantage. Some progestogens were tested by the Co-operative Breast Cancer Group (1964a,b). This group found that progesterone does not cause regression in advancing breast carcinoma, even though such high oral doses of 2 g/day were given. However, the highly potent agents 17-ethyl-19-nortestosterone and 17-ethynyl-17-hydroxyestr-5, 10-en-3-one at 40 mg/day produced essentially the same rate of objective regression as testosterone propionate. This was so whether the results from testosterone propionate were reported separately by each investigator or by the group as a whole. Because of these regression rates other progestational hormones were studied: 17-acetoxy-6-methylprogesterone (medroxyprogesterone), 17-acetoxy-6-chloroprogesterone, and 17-hydroxyprogesterone caproate. Medroxyprogesterone appeared to produce a significant number of objective regressions as did 6-methyl-9-fluoro-17-acetoxy-21-deoxyprednisolone (Talley *et al.*, 1961).

Although the progestogen treatment of patients with prostatic carcinoma has produced favorable results in a proportion of cases over the years these have often been of a transient nature. The mechanism of action is not clear, although it is well known from both animal and human data that progestogens, in general, exert an antiandrogenic effect; there have also been reports of antiadrenal and antipituitary effects. These effects are associated in particular with some of the more potent synthetic progestational compounds which are available.

In the case of prostatic carcinoma, unlike breast carcinoma, medroxyprogesterone acetate gave no significant remission. Geller *et al.* (1967) reported successful treatment of patients with metastatic carcinoma of the prostate with hydroxyprogesterone caproate, chlormadinone acetate, and cyproterone acetate, all of which gave rapid relief of bone pain. The lack of toxic side effects and feminization led the authors to conclude that selected agents should be valuable in the long-term palliative therapy of prostatic carcinoma. Under certain favorable conditions, cyproterone acetate may be comparable with estrogen in its activity against primary carcinoma with no appreciable side effects. Unfortunately, it seems to have a variable effect against the metastatic disease, which may sometimes even be enhanced rather than decreased. It is obvious that more investigation of this drug is needed at both the biochemical and clinical levels, but the treatment of prostatic carcinoma, especially in its early stages with highly active progestational compounds, perhaps in sequential combination with a suitable estrogen, appears to have an interesting future.

Steroid Carcinogenesis

Since the early work of Lacassagne who demonstrated that mammary cancer could be induced by estrogen administration to mice, there have been a great number of experimental tumors produced in a wide range of animals by this means (see Segaloff, 1975). These results were mainly of academic interest, although it seemed curious that the effect was produced by estrogen only and not by androgen, or other steroid treatment. Within recent years, however, the clinical importance of possible steroid carcinogenesis has been brought into sharp focus by the use of high-dose therapy in pregnant women and long-term low-dose estrogen treatment as a form of oral contraception. The most dramatic demonstration of the carcinogenetic effect of estrogenic substances, but not of steroid hormones as such, on the human subject, is due to Herbst (1974, 1975) and his colleagues. These workers showed that when pregnant women were given very large doses of stilbestrol during the late stages of pregnancy for threatened spontaneous abortions, there was a definite risk of their female offspring developing clear cell tumors in the vagina and cervix. The tumors developed in the daughters over a period of some 14 to 22 years after the administration of the drug. It should perhaps be stressed that the doses used were very large compared with normal therapy, the risk is by no means as high for an individual case, and alternative therapy is available. On the other hand it must be said that, had not this type of tumor been extremely uncommon it is hardly likely that its cause would have been noticed on a statistical basis; so that other, similar effects may be produced at other sites, such as the breast. This is also one of the very few examples of human transplacental carcinogenesis available for study so that these unfortunate cases may provide valuable evidence in the future design of synthetic hormones.

Evidence for the carcinogenic hazard from long-term low-dose steroids is much more difficult to assess. There have been some suggestions that hepatomas and sometimes other tumors have been due to oral contraceptives in a very small number of cases (Davis *et al.,* 1975), but the evidence for this is by no means conclusive (Leonard, 1974). Evidence of the development of presumably benign breast nodules by oral contraceptives has been reported by Burn (1976). These nodules generally regress when oral contraceptives are discontinued, but nevertheless this situation is far from satisfactory and the effect warrants further study, especially in the relatively few cases which exhibit epithelial hyperplasia and do not readily regress.

The study of the effects of really long-term treatment with low doses of estrogen in women presents numerous complications. It appears likely, however, that malignancy arises from genetic dysfunction so that cytogenetic studies in women who have at sometime used oral contraceptives extensively and, in due course, of their offspring should provide a useful screening system for carcinogenic risk. Such a study is being carried out by Bishun and his colleagues (1975a) who have observed a slightly increased frequency of genetic abnormalities in mothers who had taken specific oral contraceptives and in their offspring. These studies are currently being extended to a much larger group of patients, but in any case there is as yet no conclusive evidence to link the type of genetic abnormality found with malignant growth.

References

Aitken, E. H., and Preedy, J. R. K. (1956). The estimation of urinary estrogens. *Biochem. J.* **62**:15.

Anderson, K. M. and Liao, S. (1968). Selective retention of dihydrotestosterone by prostatic nuclei. *Nature* **219**:277.

Atkins, H., Bulbrook, R. D., Falconer, M. A., Hayward, J. L., Maclean, K. S., and Schurr, P.

H. (1968). Ten years experience of steroid assays in the managment of breast cancer. *Lancet* **II**:1255.

Barber, J. R., and Richmond, C. (1971). Human breast carcinoma culture: The effects of hormones. *Brit. J. Surg.* **58**:732.

Berganstal, D. M., Hertz, R., Lipsett, M. B., and Moy, R. J. (1960). Chemotherapy of adrenocortical cancer with o,p′ DDD. *Ann. Int. Med.* **53**:672.

Bishun, N. P., Mills, J., Lloyd, N., and Williams, D. C. (1975a). Chromosomal examination of various cell clones (*in vitro*) derived from a D.M.B.A. induced male rat breast tumour. *Eur. J. Cancer.* **9**:865.

Bishun, N. P., Mills, J., Parke, D. V., and Williams, D. C. (1975b). A cytogenetic study in women who had used oral contraceptives and their progeny. *Mutat. Res.* **33**:299.

Bishun, N. P., Mills, J., Raven, R. W., and Williams, D. C. (1973). Culturing of human breast tumours. *Cytologia* **38**:651.

Bishun, N. P., Mills, J., Raven, R. W., and Williams, D. C. (1974). Culturing of breast tumours in the presence of hormones. *J. Surg. Oncol.* **6**:202.

Brown, J. B. (1955). A chemical method for the determination of oestriol, oestrone and oestradiol in human urine. *Biochem. J.* **60**:185.

Bulbrook, R. D., Greenwood, F. C., and Hayward, J. L. (1960). Selection of breast cancer patients for adrenalectomy or hypophysectomy by determining urinary 17-hydroxycorticosteroids. *Lancet* **I**:1154.

Burn, J. I. (1976). *Proc. R. Soc. Med.* (in press) and personal communications.

C.C.N.S.C. (1964). Report of the breast cancer group. *J. Amer. Med. Assn.* **188**:1069.

C.C.N.S.C. (1964). Report of the breast cancer group. *Cancer Chemother. Rep.* **41**:Supp. 1.

Dao, T. L. (1971). In *Proceedings of a Breast Cancer Workshop* (Dao, T. L., ed.) Chicago University Press, Chicago.

Davies, P., Fahmy, A. R., Pierrepoint, C. G., and Griffiths, K. (1972). Hormonal effects *in vitro* on prostatic ribonucleic acid polymerase. *Biochem. J.* **129**:1167.

Davis, M., Portman, B., Searle, M., Wright, R., and Williams, R. (1975). Histological evidence of carcinoma in hepatic tumour associated with oral contraceptives. *Brit. Med. J.* **4**:496.

DeSombre, E. R., Mohla, S., and Jensen, E. V. (1972). Hormonal response of breast cancer. *Biophys. Biochem. Res. Commun.* **48**:1601.

DeSombre, E. R., Smith, S., Block, G. E., Ferguson, D. J., and Jensen, E. V. (1974). Prediction of breast cancer response to endocrine therapy. *Cancer Chemother. Rep.* **58**:513.

Forrest, A. P. M. (1965). In *The Scientific Basis of Surgery* (Irving Livingstone, ed.) London.

Forrest, A. P. M. (1971) Hormonal influences in breast cancer. *Proc. R. Soc. Med.* **64**:509.

Forrest, A. P. M., and Roberts, M. M. (1973). Therapeutic choice for disseminated breast carcinoma. In *Modern Trends in Oncology* (R. W. Raven, ed.), Vol. 1, Butterworth, London.

Geller, J., Fruchtman, B., Newman, H., Roberts, T., and Silva, R. (1967). Effect of progestational agents on carcinoma of the prostate. *Cancer Chemother. Rep.* **51**:41.

Harper, M. E., Fahmy, A. R., Pierrepoint, G. G., and Griffiths, K. (1970). The effect of some stilboestrol compounds on DNA polymerase from human prostatic tissue. *Steroids.* **15**:89.

Herbst, A. L., Scully, R. E., and Robboy, S. J. (1975). Problems in the examination of the DES exposed female. *Obstet. Gynecol.* **44**:353.

Herbst, A. L., Robboy, S. J., Scully, R. E., and Poskanzer, D. C. (1974). Clear cell adenoma of the vagina and cervix in young females. *Am. J. Obstet. Gynecol.* **119**:713.

Huggins, C., and Clarke, P. J. (1941). The effect of castration on advanced carcinoma of the prostate gland in dogs. *Cancer Res.* **1**:293.

Jensen, E. V., and DeSombre, E. R. (1972). Mechanism of action of female sex hormones. *Annu. Rev. Biochem.* **41**:203.

Jensen, E. V., Desombre, E. R., and Jungblut, P. W. (1967). Estrogen receptors in hormone responsive tissues and tumors. In: *Estrogenous Factors Influencing Host-Tumour Balance* (Wissler, R. W., Dao, T. L. and Wood, S. Jr., eds.), p. 15. University of Chicago Press, Chicago.

Jensen, E. V., and Jacobson, H. I. (1960). Fate of steroid estrogens in target tissues. In *Biological Activities in Relation to Cancer* (Pincus, G., and Vollmer, E., eds.) p. 161. Academic Press, London and New York.

Juret, P. (1968). Urinary androgen excretion as a prognostic factor before hypophysectomy. In *Prognostic Factors in Breast Cancer* (Forrest, A. P. and Kunkler, P. B., eds.) p. 393. Longman, New York.

Leonard, B. J. (1974). *WHO Symposium—Pharmacological Models in Contraceptive Development, Geneva.* Briggs, M., and Diezfansy, S., eds. p. 34. Stockholm.

McGuire, W. L., Chamness, C. G., Costilow, M. E., and Richert, N. J. (1975). Steroids and human breast cancer. *J. Steroid Biochem.* **6**:723.

McGuire, W. L., Costolow, M. E., and Chamness, G. C., (1975a). Prolactin receptors in experimental breast cancer. Abstract of *Workshop on Human Prolactin Xth Acta Endocrinoligica Meeting,* Amsterdam.

McGuire, W. L., and Horowitz, K. B. (1975b) Steroid hormone receptors in human breast cancer. Abstract of *Workshop on Human Prolactin Xth Acta Endocrinologica Meeting,* Amsterdam.

Pearson, O. H., Li, M. C., McLean, J. P., Lipsett, M. B., and West, C. D. (1955). Endocrine therapy of metastatic breast cancer. *Ann. N.Y. Acad. Sci.* **61**:393.

Robel, P., Lasnitzki, I., and Baulieu, E. E. (1971). Testosterone metabolism in rat prostate gland grown in organ culture and hormone action. *Biochimie.* **53**:81.

Segaloff, A. (1975). Steroids and carcinogenesis. *J. Steroid Biochem.* **6**:171.

Talley, R. W., Kelly, J. E., Brennan, M. J., and Vaitkevicius, V. K. (1961). Clinical study of 6α-methyl- 9α-floro-17-acetoxy-21-deoxyprednisolone in human breast cancer. *Cancer Chemother. Rep.* **12**:59.

Weisenfeld, S., and Goldner, M. G. (1962). Treatment of advanced malignancy and Cushing's Syndrome with D.D.D. *Cancer Chemother. Rep.* **16**:335.

Williams, D. C., and Smethurst, M. (1975). Enzyme induction by steroid hormones with reference to cancer. In *Enzyme Induction* (D. V. Parke, ed.) Plenum Press, London and New York.

Zimmermann, B., Block, H. S., Williams, W. L., Hitchcock, C. R., and Hoelscher, B. (1956). The effect of D.D.D. on the human adrenal. *Cancer* **9**:940.

Chapter 8

CARCINOGENS AND CARCINOGENESIS

G. P. WARWICK

Introduction

The magnitude of the cancer problem and the years of life lost due to cancer mortality from different forms of cancer has been discussed recently (Murray and Axtell, 1974).

Chemicals, radiations, viruses, and sometimes combinations of these can produce cancer in experimental animals. Epidemiological studies and even shrewd observations by general practitioners have revealed a limited number of chemicals which have been proved to be carcinogenic for man. There is only suggestive evidence that viruses are involved in the etiology of any of the human cancers. Studies with experimental animals have shown that there are a large number of carcinogens, both naturally occurring and synthetic, and that many variables can influence the carcinogenic process. Since cancer research should have as a major aim the prevention of cancer in man, an urgent task is to evaluate the relevance of experimental data now available and to utilize it to help man.

As stressed by Farber (1973b), there is a need to understand in greater detail those processes and variables involved in carcinogenesis and whether or not there are common molecular and biological mechanisms underlying the production of cancer by chemicals, radiations, and viruses. An understanding of these details will hopefully provide means of cancer prevention and more subtle forms of cancer treatment. However, in such

G. P. Warwick • Institute of Cancer Research (Royal Cancer Hospital), Chester Beatty Research Institute, Fulham Road, London, SW3, England.

studies the danger of regarding cancer as a disease of cells, or even parts of cells should be avoided. The whole organism is involved, and even if cancer originates from the transformation of a single cell which gains a proliferative advantage, a whole range of host factors have probably influenced the initial transformation and the subsequent tumor development. This has presented one of the great difficulties to oncologists in their attempts to understand the genesis of cancer. It also stands clearly in the way of detecting carcinogens in the environment. When is a chemical or a virus truly a carcinogen? Experimental studies and observations of man have shown that one must qualify the definition. Thus a chemical which is able to produce cancer in one species possibly may not in another; or it may produce cancer at a particular site when given to a young animal, while an older animal may be refractory. Many variables exist which can modify the process of carcinogenesis at one stage or another: A far from exhaustive list includes species; strain; sex; method of absorption, metabolism, and excretion; hormonal status; immunological status; diet; proliferative activity of a tissue; and exogenous chemicals.

Neoplastic Development

It is now clear there is no entity which can be defined as a cancer cell, either in the morphological or biochemical sense, a point put forcibly by Smithers in his "attack on cytologism" (Smithers, 1962). He pointed out that cancer is a disease of the whole organism and should be regarded as resulting from the interplay of numerous variables and the breakdown of normal organismal homeostatic control mechanisms. It is thus not definable as a disease of cells per se, but there is a reasonable basis for supposing that at some stage in the genesis of cancer heritable changes in cells have occurred. That the change is not necessarily similar in each case can be deduced from the widely differing properties of cells, even within a given malignant neoplasm, and certainly when comparing different malignant neoplasms. An obvious example is the range of transplantable hepatocellular carcinomas induced by different means, some of which are highly differentiated and maintain many of the properties of normal liver, while others such as the Novikoff hepatoma are unlike normal liver in almost every respect, gross morphological and biochemical changes having been introduced within the cells. Tumor progression, which has been beautifully described by Foulds (1969), enhances this point. The carcinogenic process *in vivo* is thus one involving many stages, the interplay of numerous biological variables, and the operation of something at least akin to natural selection. But since there are, at one point in the spectrum of changes, obvious cellular derangements which largely satisfy the criteria of heritable alterations, it is not surprising that many workers have concentrated their investigations on cellular changes and the mechanisms by which these are brought about, in their studies of chemical, virus, and radiation carcinogenesis. Such studies are valid provided that they are made within the context of the process as it affects the whole organism. The extreme example of such studies at the cellular level is *in vitro* transformation and the subsequent ability of certain transformed cells to produce malignant neoplasms when inoculated into suitable recipients (Heidelberger, 1973). It seems reasonable to extend such studies to the intracellular level, so as to deduce the molecular changes which have been brought about in the process of transformation. There is now ample evidence that certain chemicals can produce malignant neoplasms in man. If these same chemicals or their metabolites produce transformation of cells *in vitro,* then one reasonable deduction, in the absence of spontaneous transformation, is that the chemical or its derivative has by some chemical (molecular) means brought about these cellular alterations. In the broadest sense one must consider the effects of the chemical or its metabolite on the host itself. There is evidence that chemicals, radiations, and viruses can produce adverse effects on those immune mechanisms which could reject neoplastic or preneoplastic cells (Baldwin, 1973; Outzen and Prehn, 1973). Waynforth and Magee (1974) and Currie (1973) have discussed the importance of immunological competence in the context of human cancer. Carcinogens influence to a greater or lesser degree the hormonal status of an organism, causing changes which can alter regulatory mechanisms at many levels such as rates of cellular proliferation, rates of macromolecular synthesis, and the concentration, or activity, of drug-metabolizing enzymes. The process of neoplastic development, therefore, can and should be studied using diverse techniques concomitantly. Part of such a multidisciplinary study can legitimately involve the action of carcinogens on cellular integrity.

The Latent Period

One of the most interesting and baffling facets of the process of formation of a morphologically visible malignant tumor is that named the latent or lapsed period. This can vary between many months for small animals to many years for man, and it is the period between the beginning of exposure to a carcinogen and the time of emergence of a visible cancer. It is a further representation of the complexity of the carcinogenic process. *In vitro* studies have suggested that many division cycles may be necessary to complete transformation (Berwald and Sachs, 1963; Williams *et al.,* 1973; Heidelberger, 1973), and studies with urethane *in vivo* have suggested that transformed epithelial cells, for example, can remain in a state of apparent equilibrium with normal cells for long periods. Malignant tumors can be made to appear even months later by applying various chemicals named promoters (Roe *et al.,* 1972), for example, croton oil. Such events suggest that experimental cancer production by chemicals involves at least two stages, one a rapid, largely irreversible and termed initiation, and the other a relatively slow, complex and termed promotion (Berenblum, 1969; Van Duuren, 1969). Thus, some chemicals are "initiators," some "promoters," and others "complete carcinogens." Urethane can apparently exert a dual function since, while it is only an initiator for mouse skin, it is able to produce a variety of tumors when administered to newborn animals. Current information on the mechanism of action of promoters in experimental animals is described later.

Precancerous Changes Observed in Animals

The various stages of the carcinogenic process can be followed more adequately in experimental animals than in man, and careful experimentation has produced valuable information concerning precancerous changes, processes of initiation and promotion, and the latent period. Such changes for a variety of sites in the rat have recently been well documented (Turusov, 1973). In no case does cancer emerge suddenly from a normal tissue background, but early changes such as irregular hyperplasia followed by nodular proliferation and later by papillomas and adenomas from which cancers can emerge is the usual sequence. Progressive changes in the liver during treatment with hepatocarcinogens have been described in detail by Farber (1973a). He views the process as a "cellular or micro-evolution" in which the hepatocarcinogen performs various functions including changing the information content of certain cells, thus "creating an environment which exerts selection pressure for certain types of cells but not for others," i.e., an environment which will eventually allow neoplastic cells to gain a proliferative advantage.

Similar early changes to those seen in experimental animals treated with carcinogens are frequently observed in man, for example, in the esophagus as leukoplakia, in the larynx as endophytic growth of epithelium by pachydermia, and in the cervix uteri as epidermoid-sinking growth reaching the glands by nonhealing erosio cervicus (Shabad, 1973). The author stresses that each cancer has its own precancer, and that since cancer is often multicentric, precancerous lesions are often multiple and "greater in number than the tumors developing from them."

Lesions in Man Including Congenital Malformation Often Associated with Subsequent Development of Cancer

The importance of "precancerous lesions" cannot be overemphasized, not only in helping to elucidate mechanisms of carcinogenesis, but in opening up new possibilities of cancer control and prevention. Precancerous changes in man often progress over a long period of time, and in some cases at least these early lesions are dependent for their continued existence and their progression upon the host organism. It is well established that continued growth, or regression, of certain lesions such as mammary fibroadenomas depends on the current hormonal status of the host. To quote some examples, oral cancer is preceded by a morphologically related group of squamous epithelial changes termed dyskeratosis. Conditions which can be associated with or lead to dyskeratosis include leukoplakia and buccal erythroplasia. Bowen's disease (Howarth, 1935) is often a precursor of cancer of the mesopharynx.

The possible importance of pernicious anemia, peptic ulcer, achlorphydria, gastric polyps, atrophic gastritis, hypertrophic gastritis, and benign tumors of the stomach in connection with development of cancer of the stomach have been discussed in detail by Raven (1967a). The author (Raven, 1967b), in discussing preventive measures for cancers of the small intestine, summarized current views concerning congenital anomalies of the duodenum such as diverticula and aberrant pancreatic tissue, Meckel's diverticulum, Peutz–Jeghers syndrome, celiac disease, and benign tumors of the small intestine. Bussey and Morson (1967) produced detailed information concerning familial polyposis coli and ulcerative colitis in the context of colon cancer.

Further research has clearly portrayed the progressive stages leading to carcinoma of the cervix uteri.

There is an excess of leukemia in children with Down's syndrome which is determined through meiotic nondisjunction. It is, therefore, possible these leukemias are determined prezygotically. Nearly all groups with a high risk of leukemia carry cytogenic abnormalities (Miller, 1967) such as those with Franconi's aplastic anemia, Bloom's syndrome, polycythemia vera, or those previously exposed to radiation or benzene. Lymphoma, on the other hand, is associated with inborn immunological deficiencies (Gatti and Good, 1971) such as congenital thymic alymphoplasia and Wiskott–Aldrich syndrome. Wilm's tumor, adrenal cortical neoplasia, and primary hepatocellular carcinoma in childhood are associated with certain congenital growth excesses (Miller, 1968). Of considerable interest for research workers is the rare human hereditary disease xeroderma pigmentosum, characterized by skin which is extremely sensitive to radiation of short wavelength from the sun. The cancers which develop on the unexposed areas do so during the early years of life and include basal and squamous cell carcinomas, melanomas, angiosarcomas, fibrosarcomas, and keratoacanthomas. The disease is inherited as an autosomal recessive gene without obvious chromosomal abnormalities. The particular sensitivity to uv light is related to impaired DNA repair mechanisms (Cleaver, 1973).

The problem of diseases with and without an apparently variable chromosome pattern in the context of carcinogenesis and certain forms of cancer has recently been extensively discussed (Rowley, 1974).

It is against the background of early and progressive lesions which often precede cancer, whether these are inherited or induced by some other means, that carcinogenesis should be studied.

Etiological Agents and Cancers in Man

Chemicals

The etiology of most cancers is still essentially unknown. A significant exception is bronchogenic lung carcinoma which has been attributed beyond reasonable doubt in the majority of cases to cigarette smoking. Again, approximately 10–20% of all bladder carcinomas in Western Europe were estimated at one time to be due to occupational exposures, such as to β-naphthylamine and benzidine (Clayson, 1962). A causative correlation exists between exposure to certain forms of asbestos and the development of mesothelioma of the lung and carcinomas of the lung.

The problem of respiratory carcinogenesis in relation to exposure to occupational and environmental agents including metals, radioactive materials, mustard gas, oils and tars, and others, has been reviewed (Hueper, 1966). A relatively small proportion of leukemia and other neoplasms may result from exposure to ionizing radiation.

Our knowledge of environmental cancers in man has been derived mainly from studies of occupational groups with high cancer rates. To the older list mentioned above may be added the recent discovery that vinyl chloride used in the production of the plastic PVC and as a propellant in some aerosol products can produce the rare tumor angiosarcoma of the liver and liver fibrosis.

Apparently vinyl chloride can produce nephroblastomas, liver angiosarcomas, and sometimes other tumors in rats after long-term exposure. This is one example, therefore, of an animal experiment from which the carcinogenicity of a chemical for man could have been predicted. In general, those chemicals which have been suspected of being carcinogenic for man can produce cancers in experimental animals, an exception possibly being arsenic. The difficulty of finding an appropriate test species for a particular chemical is exemplified by the fact that only in the dog does β-naphthylamine produce bladder cancer. The rat appears to be rather resistant, and liver tumors are produced in the mouse only after prolonged administration.

A risk which is being increasingly investigated is the possible carcinogenicity of drugs taken by pregnant women. That drugs can be teratogenic has been tragically demonstrated, but until recently transplacental carcinogenesis was known to be a real phenomenon only in experimental animals and only suspected in man. However, it is now reasonably established that stilbestrol given to pregnant women is a transplacental carcinogen and increases the risk of producing carcinoma of the vagina, a normally rare tumor in young women (Herbst *et al.*, 1971, 1972).

There are recent comprehensive reviews of experimental transplacental carcinogenesis (Tomatis, 1973; Tomatis and Mohr, 1973) and its implications for man. In the case of stilbestrol it is salutary that it had been shown to produce cancer in experimental animals in the 1950's. It has been estimated that 10,000 to 16,000 persons were exposed to stilbestrol between 1960 and 1970 (Lanier *et al.*, 1973).

In experimental systems a large number of chemicals of different structure are transplacental carcinogens for different animal species. They include chemicals which do and do not require prior enzymatic activation to reactive electrophiles (p. 196). Such chemicals produce tumors at various sites in offspring depending on the species, the chemical structure, and the time during pregnancy when administered. These facts assume important significance when considered with the fact that malignant tumors are one of the main causes of mortality among children under 15 in the majority of the industrialized countries. There is also a suspicion that the exposure of children to carcinogens *in vitro* or in very early life through the maternal milk might be significant in less-developed countries, such as in parts of Africa and Asia, where adult populations are known to be exposed to food-borne toxins as aflatoxin B_1 (Peers and Linsell, 1973; Shank *et al.*, 1972). A list of suspects could be added including nitrosamines, which are discussed in the next section.

Nitrosamines and Nitrosamides

The nitrosamines and nitrosamides are among the most likely candidates as environmental carcinogens (see Figure 1). They are multipotent carcinogens when tested in a range of animal species (Magee and Barnes, 1967), and are transplacental carcinogens (Tomatis and Mohr, 1973; Tomatis, 1973). They can be highly site-specific depending on species, dose, and nitrosamine structure. They have been found as contaminants of human food (Fong and Chan, 1973) and can be transferred through maternal milk (Mohr and Althoff, 1971). They can be produced by bacterial action *in vivo* (IARC Publications, No. 3, 1972; Lancet Editorial, 1973; Hill *et al.*, 1973) from nitrite or nitrate (following reduction) and secondary amines and amides (Mirvish and Chu, 1973). Nitrosamines could be produced by the interaction of nitrous acid and drugs *in vivo* (Lijinsky, 1974), or by the action of nitrite with certain agricultural chemicals (Elespuru and Lijinsky, 1973).

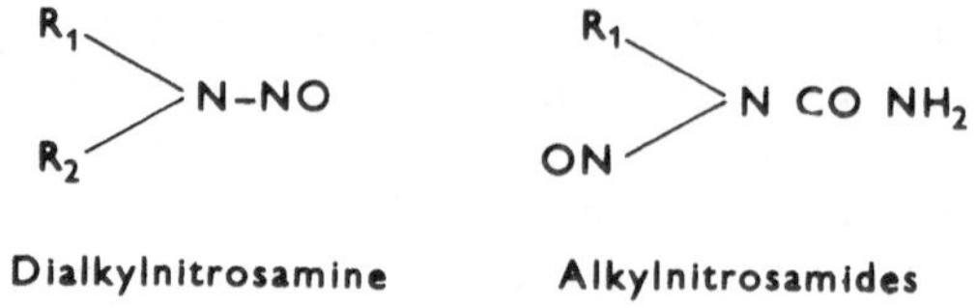

Dialkylnitrosamine   Alkylnitrosamides

Figure 1

Mycotoxins

The mycotoxins, characterized particularly by aflatoxin B_1, were discovered in Britain in 1962 as a result of an outbreak of disease among young turkeys which had ingested imported moldy groundnut meal. Aflatoxin B_1 is the most toxic of the products elaborated by *Aspergillus flavus*. There followed detailed investigations of the toxicity and carcinogenicity of aflatoxin B_1 in different species (Warwick, 1976). It transpires to be the most potent hepatocarcinogen yet discovered for some species. Even greater impetus was given to the study of aflatoxin B_1 and other mycotoxins by the discovery that *Aspergillus flavus* is a contaminant of cereals and groundnuts in many parts of the world, including some in which the incidence of hepatocellular carcinoma is moderate to high (Warwick, 1976).

Recent comprehensive food surveys have revealed a statistical correlation between the ingestion of aflatoxin B_1 in foodstuffs and the incidence of primary hepatocellular carcinoma. One survey was in Thailand and Hong Kong (Shank *et al.*, 1972), one was in the Muranga district of Kenya (Peers and Linsell, 1973), and another was in Mozambique (Van Rensburg *et al.*, 1974). These studies imply the importance of aflatoxin B_1 as an etiological agent in primary hepatocellular carcinoma in man in some parts of the world. The importance of other dietary factors in aflatoxin B_1 hepatocarcinogenesis has been studied by Rogers and Newberne (1971) who demonstrated a greater carcinogenic action in animals maintained on a diet marginally deficient in lipotropes, a finding possibly of great relevance to man in those areas where multiple dietary deficiencies are common. Animal experiments have also shown that aflatoxin B_1 can be ingested through maternal milk (Grice *et al.*, 1973). The toxicity and carcinogenicity of fungal metabolites has been reviewed by Enomoto and Saito (1972). It is not possible at present to dissociate the relative importance of aflatoxin B_1 and hepatitis-associated antigen (see p. 188) as etiological agents in the genesis of primary hepatocellular carcinoma in man.

Asbestos

Certain types of asbestos cause mesotheliomas and squamous carcinoma of the lung. All commercial types appear to be hazardous except anthophyllite. Recent evidence suggests that the dimensional range of fibers is critical for the production of mesotheliomas, rather than the chemical composition of the fiber. Thus fine long fibers of durable materials containing no asbestos such as glass and alumine, but within certain limits of diameter and length, can produce cancer in experimental animals (Bogovski *et al.*, 1973; Stanton, 1974). The question raised by Stanton is the level of the risk that such fibers may hold currently, or with the general increase in the use of fibrous materials.

Tests for Chemical Carcinogens

A valuable approach to cancer prevention is the screening of chemicals for carcinogenic potential in experimental animals, before exposing man to them. It is also a method employed to test the potential dangers of suspected chemicals already in use or present in the environment. Such tests are essential, but disagreement exists as to the best test systems to use. The usual tests include skin painting, oral administration, and subcutaneous injection using mice and rats (Grasso, 1970). Less common tests include bladder implantation, endotracheal insufflation and vaginal application, treatment of newborn mice, and multigeneration studies in rats and mice. However, most of the tests appear to have shortcomings and difficulties of interpretation (Grasso, 1970; Roe, 1968; Grasso and Crampton, 1972). There has been particular uncertainty about the use of newborn mice as test animals (Grasso and Crampton, 1972), but from a recent literature survey (Tomatis *et al.*, 1973) it was concluded that on the basis of the data obtained by the investigation of 58 chemicals, a positive correlation seemed to exist between the capacity of chemicals to induce liver tumors in the mouse and their capacity to induce tumors at any site in the rat and hamster, implying that this method of testing is of potential value.

Screening tests in chemical carcinogenesis have recently been reviewed (Montesano *et al.*, 1976) including mutagenic systems *in vitro*. Well-known substances banned in some parts of the world as a result of their carcinogenicity in one or more animal species include DDT and the sweetener cyclamate. The continued popularity of the cigarette-smoking habit despite the proven association with lung cancer and other conditions poses an interesting psychological problem.

Viruses

There is increasing suggestive evidence from many areas of the world that some human cancers may have a viral etiology, or at least that some viruses may play a vital role in neoplastic development. Some of the early leads came from studies of cancer in developing countries such as some areas of Africa and Asia. Important opportunities are offered by epidemiological and etiological research and by the suggestive cancer patterns seen in such emergent and developing areas. Within Africa, for example, dramatic variations in the frequency of particular cancers often occur within short distances, or with variations in altitude, and some of the most important information suggesting the role of viruses in the development of some cancers come from studies of Burkitt's lymphoma, primary hepatocellular carcinoma, nasopharyngeal carcinoma, and Kaposi's sarcoma in Africa and parts of Asia. However, in the following discussion it is hoped to draw attention to the complexity of the relationships.

Hepatitis-Associated Antigen (Australia Antigen) (HAA) and Primary Hepatocellular Carcinoma

The discovery of HAA has led to research on its possible role in different forms of hepatitis and in the development of cirrhosis and primary hepatocellular carcinoma. A reasonable standardization in techniques for measuring the level of the antigen has led to meaningful comparative studies from different areas. It is now generally agreed that the antigen is associated with serum of long-incubation hepatitis. It transpires that the antigen is surprisingly common in apparently healthy people (males more than females) in Kenya (Bagshawe and Nganda, 1973). HAA has been detected in high frequencies in adult Africans from Senegal, Ghana, Nigeria, Ethiopia, and Mozambique, and from some other tropical areas. It has been found to be associated with a significant number of cases of cirrhosis and hepatocellular carcinoma in Uganda (Vogel *et al.*, 1970; Maynard *et al.*, 1970), in Kenya (Bagshawe *et al.*, 1971), and elsewhere. These findings have led to the suggestion that HAA, which in many respects has viral-like properties, is in some way involved as a causative factor in cirrhosis and hepatocellular carcinoma in some parts of the world. The relationship between cirrhosis and hepatocellular carcinoma in man is complex, which is further illustrated by the fact that hepatocellular carcinoma can emerge from a noncirrhotic liver in man (Vogel *et al.*, 1970), and in experimental animals some of the most potent chemical hepatocarcinogens such as aflatoxin B_1 and diethylnitrosamine can produce hepatocellular carcinoma with little or no cirrhosis (Warwick, 1971a). If HAA is involved in a causative role in the development of hepatocellular carcinoma in man in some tropical countries, then because of the high frequency with which it is found in blood donors and apparently healthy people in countries such as Kenya and Nigeria, other variables must also be involved, otherwise the incidence of cirrhosis and hepatocellular carcinoma would be higher. In any case it is well known that people react differently to the presence of HAA, thus the antigen can disappear rapidly, or it can just persist. If it persists, a healthy carrier state may develop, or chronic liver disease such as chronic aggressive hepatitis can supervene, possibly because of inappropriate immunological reactions.

The role played by the immunological status in developing tropical countries is probably of great importance since not only could exposure to HAA occur and probably recur early in life, but the possibility that immunity is impaired by malnutrition (Geefhuysen *et al.*, 1971) should be considered as contributing towards the development of a carrier state. The development of liver damage could result from the situation in which the immune response would not be adequate to delete virus, but enough to produce immunologically mediated damage to hepatocytes.

It is very thought-provoking to consider the mechanism of the development of hepatocellular carcinoma in those areas where exposure to HAA and aflatoxin B_1 (see p. 195) can occur simultaneously from an early age.

Herpes Viruses

Two human herpes viruses, the Epstein–Barr virus (EBV) and herpes simplex II have recently been studied intensively because of the increasing evidence that they are associated with human cancers; Burkitt's lymphoma and nasopharyngeal carcinoma with the former and carcinoma of the cervix uteri with the latter. A more tenuous relationship exists between Hodgkin's disease and EBV than between Burkitt's lymphoma and EBV.

Burkitt's Lymphoma (BL). Following the demonstration of a relatively frequent occurrence of a juvenile lymphosarcoma in the population of central Africa, Burkitt (1967, 1972) developed his twofold theory of a viral etiology combined with an anthropod vector. The virus (EBV) has been found to be closely associated with the tumors in Africa and in many ways it fulfills the role of an oncogenic virus. Thus it can be found in cell cultures of BL cells which contain the virus-specific DNA associated with cellular DNA. Clones of somatic cell hybrids carry the virus genome which can be induced to replicate by iododeoxyuridine (in tissue culture). However, the virus alone cannot be involved, since antibodies to it are common in areas of high and low incidence, and in Africa the distribution of the lymphoma is apparently related to the endemicity of malaria. The relationship between malaria and BL has not been clarified, and it is still being questioned as to whether malaria, or EBV infection, comes first; the problem is made more difficult by the fact that two virtually ubiquitous diseases have had to be evoked, each with complex and variable effects on the host. These problems and others concerned with time–space clustering, socioeconomic factors, etc., have recently been summarized (Morrow, 1974) and discussed in subsequent papers at the Symposium.

Nasopharyngeal Carcinoma (NPC). The association between EBV and NPC is not as strong as that between EBV and BL. NPC is a disease which afflicts mainly Cantonese Chinese wherever they live in the world. The various aspects of the disease have recently been reviewed (Ho, 1972). There have been suggestions that a genetic factor is involved, but this appears less certain now on the basis of studies of the effect of migration on risk (Buell, 1974). EBV is the most interesting etiological factor to emerge and virtually 100% of NPC cases have elevated antibody titers to EBV. The EBV genome has been demonstrated by nucleic acid hybridization in NPC biopsies, but it is not clear whether the EBV genome is present in the epithelial carcinoma cells or in the lymphoid tissue associated with the tumor (de-Thé and Geser, 1974). The question as to whether EBV is just a passenger—it is commonly found in lymphoid tissue of the nasopharynx— also remains unresolved. On the other hand, EBV can transform lympho- cytes which can be maintained in culture for long periods, unlike normal lymphocytes, and etiological association has been found between the herpes group and naturally occurring tumors in animals.

In Africa NPC is common, particularly in Tunisia and Algeria. In Kenya where BL is also common and associated with EBV, the tumors are seen often in different tribes in different locations. Thus, in Africa an explanation is needed to account for the different geographical distributions of BL and NPC if EBV is a common etiological factor.

Cancer of the Cervix Uteri. There is good evidence that carcinoma of the cervix uteri originates in a regenerating epithelium which is thought by some to be relevant to some of the epidemiological findings concerning this cancer. Various etiological agents have been proposed as possible causa- tive agents including nitrosamines, hormones, smegma (and circumcision), sperm, trichomonas, syphilis, gonorrhea, mycoplasma chlamydia, and cytomegalovirus. The time of first intercourse and the number of sexual partners have also been considered (Alexander, 1973).

Recently, many studies have been carried out to investigate the possi- ble involvement of herpes simplex II as a causative factor, and it appears that the virus is associated with a significant number of cases with carci- noma of the cervix uteri. The current status of knowledge is summarized in two recent symposia (Cancer Research 1973, **33**, 1345–1563; 1974, **34**, 1090–1145). Recently Gentry (1974) has proposed a role for genital myco- plasma, a common inhabitant of the genital tract, in stimulating herpes- simplex-II-mediated carcinogenesis based on the assumption that part of the viral genome must be integrated into the host-cell genome in a preexist- ing single-strand DNA nick (Stich *et al.,* 1972). The endonuclease activity of *Mycoplasma hominis* could provide more such nicks, and it was there- fore of interest that endonuclease action in cell cultures doubly infected with herpesvirus and *Mycoplasma* was marked, compared with either agent alone.

Studies of the Mechanism of Action of Chemical Carcinogens in Experimental Systems

Studies with experimental systems have revealed hundreds of chemicals with diverse chemical structures, both organic and inorganic, which produce cancer in experimental animals or transform mammalian cells *in vitro*. Some of these are either known to be, or suspected of being, carcinogenic for man. Chemical carcinogens include those which are chemically reactive towards nucleophiles, those which are apparently inert but which are converted enzymatically or hydrolytically into reactive chemicals, and those which are inert and apparently are not activated. Included are synthetic chemicals or naturally occurring chemicals such as those mined or produced by plants and fungi, other environmental pollutants, and inorganic chemicals. Some chemicals produce cancer in animals following a single administration, others must be applied or fed for prolonged periods, and others are carcinogenic only if combined with other treatments such as with the promoter croton oil.

As mentioned later, studies with chemicals have provided valuable information about the morphological changes which occur during carcinogenesis. The reader is referred to these references for detailed discussions (p. 195).

Relationship to Age

The carcinogenicity of chemicals can often be influenced by the age of an animal at the time of administration and the site at which tumors are formed is often age dependent (see also p. 195). Thus, for example, urethane is hepatocarcinogenic for the rat when treatment is given *in utero*, or at a very young age, while its activity is low for adults. It is hepatocarcinogenic for young mice, but not for adults unless given soon after partial hepatectomy. However, the ability of urethane to produce lung adenomas, Harderian gland tumors, and ovarian tumors in mice was similar whether treatment was at 4 weeks or at 25 weeks. Urethane is a skin carcinogen only if it is applied during rapid DNA synthesis following application of croton oil (Pound, 1968) or if croton oil is given, often much later, following urethane application.

Studies of transplacental carcinogenesis have revealed the particular sensitivity of different body sites to particular carcinogens at different times during development. For example, ethylnitrosamine administered to pregnant BD IX rats on day 15 of gestation produced a high yield of tumors of the brain, cranial nerves, spinal cord, and the peripheral nervous system. The most sensitive period for the development of neurogenic malignancies was between day 18 and birth. No tumors were produced when the dose was given before day 12. When given on day 15 malignant neurinomas were produced easily, and on a dose basis the sensitivity of the nervous system to ethylnitrosourea was about 50 times greater than for the adult rat. However, no tumors of the olfactory bulbs were found, although these are easily produced in adults. For references and more detailed discussions of carcinogenesis in relation to age see Tomatis (1973) and Warwick (1973).

The variations in carcinogenic activity found with age are probably associated with many variables including degree of differentiation, cellular proliferative activity, the level and activity of drug-metabolizing enzymes, immunological and hormonal status, and others.

The likely relevance of these findings for man is illustrated in the recently discovered carcinogenicity of stilbestrol for the offspring of pregnant women (p. 185).

Relationship to Cell Proliferation

There is increasing evidence that resting cells, at least in some sites of the body, are less vulnerable targets for carcinogens than cells in cycle. The literature up to 1971 has been reviewed (Warwick, 1971b). The evidence is based on findings including the fact that some chemicals which are not hepatocarcinogenic for adult animals can produce tumors, sometimes after a single injection, when given during the wave of restorative hyperplasia following two-thirds partial hepatectomy. Likewise, certain chemicals produce hepatomas following partial hepatectomy in doses which are subcarcinogenic for normal adults (Craddock, 1973).

Skin is a sensitive target for some carcinogens when they are applied during the hyperplastic response following croton oil painting.

There is suggestive evidence that the high sensitivity of newborn animals, or animals *in utero,* to the carcinogenic effects of certain chemicals is related to the relative proliferative activities of cells at the affected sites compared with adults.

Studies of cell transformation in culture (Bertram and Heidelberger, 1973) showed that N-methyl-N'-nitro-N-nitrosoguanidine induced malignant transformation of synchronized C3H mouse fibroblasts at a specific stage in the cell cycle just prior to the onset of DNA synthesis.

These remarks are not intended to imply that cell division is important only in cancer initiation. There is evidence that many cell divisions are required to complete the process of transformation, and cell division must obviously occur in the phases of progression towards neoplasia.

The concept has far-reaching implications for cancer production in man, since tumors in man often emerge from areas of high proliferative activity such as hyperplastic nodules, cirrhotic nodules, leukoplakia, tropical ulcer, and other lesions. The cervix uteri appears to be most vulnerable to the action of carcinogens at times characterized by rapid cell division, and one role of hormonal stimulation of mammary neoplasia is probably related to stimulated cell division. Exposure *in utero,* or during formative years after birth, to carcinogens takes on a new significance when thought of in terms of carcinogenesis as related to cell division.

Effect of Diet

Dietary composition can alter the toxic effects of exogenous chemicals including their ability to produce cancer (Basu and Dickerson, 1973; Warwick, 1973; McLean, 1973). There is no one factor involved, but there are a number of ways in which dietary composition could influence the carcinogenic process.

Interactions between diet and chemical carcinogens may be responsible for many of the geographic variations in frequency of different cancers throughout the world, and the importance of considering these aspects has recently been stressed (Crawford, 1971; Warwick and Harington, 1973).

For example, vitamins such as riboflavin and vitamin A are directly involved in maintaining the integrity of certain types of epithelium. Vitamin A deficiency causes squamous metaplasia of epithelial tissue and several authors have reported its inhibiting effects on the development of experimentally induced tumors. Likewise, a deficiency of riboflavin, a common deficiency in man, accelerates skin tumor development in mice following dimethylbenz [α]anthracene treatment. Riboflavin deficiency causes deleterious effects on the integrity of stratified keratinizing epithelium in baboons as evidenced by gross morphological changes in facial and other skin, and a marked increase in mitotic rate of the skin, buccal, and esophageal mucosa. Riboflavin protects rat liver against the carcinogenic effects of butter yellow, probably by altering the manner in which the carcinogen is metabolized by its effects on the relative activity of different microsomal enzymes. By their effects on hormonal levels certain vitamins could again indirectly affect the route of metabolism of carcinogens. There is evidence that both vitamin E and ascorbic acid can influence the metabolism of exogenous chemicals (Basu and Dickerson, 1973).

Deficiencies of trace minerals are known in some cases to cause morphological lesions, since adequate quantities of many of them are essential for the normal development of most species. A zinc deficiency is thought to be responsible for dwarfism is some areas and the production of hyperkeratosis and parakeratosis of the skin and esophagus in animals.

An interesting view of the direct effects of dietary composition on the development of a particular tumor is that of Burkitt (1973) who provides evidence that the environmental factor most closely linked with cancer and other noninfective diseases of the large bowel . . . is the quantity of unabsorbable fibre in food. The hypothesis that the faecal arrest associated with fibre deficiency is responsible for bacterial proliferation and their degradation of bile salts to carcinogens is consistent with all available epidemiological evidence.

One might add to this the possibility of nitrosamine production from precursor nitrites and amines by bacteria (Hill *et al.*, 1973) and the dehydration of the steroid nucleus by human gut bacteria to produce possible colon carcinogens (Goddard and Hill, 1973). Epidemiological evidence has indicated a correlation between dietary fat intake and the incidence of colon cancer; this is of added interest in view of the recent finding of a correlation between beef intake and large bowel cancer in Hawaiian Japanese (Haenszel *et al.*, 1973). Beef has a higher proportion of saturated fat than other sources of animal protein.

Ingestion of a diet marginal in lipotropes enhances hepatocarcinogenesis in rats by aflatoxin B_1 (Rogers and Newberne, 1971) and nitrosamines (Rogers *et al.*, 1974).

The level of dietary protein influences the toxicity and carcinogenicity of chemicals such as hepatocarcinogens (Warwick, 1971a), and Cyzgan *et al.* (1974) have shown that dietary protein deficiency can affect the ability of isolated hepatic microsomes to alter the mutagenicity of primary and secondary carcinogens. However, uncertainty has always existed about the importance of malnutrition in neoplastic development in man. There is evidence that protein-calorie malnutrition per se does not lead to the production of cancer at any site and that it may even be protective (Jose and Good, 1973), but there is no reason to doubt that nutritional status influences the carcinogenic process in more than one way.

Because of the extent of malnutrition of diverse types in many parts of the world, further studies of the relationship between specific deficiencies or groups of deficiencies and cancer need to be carried out urgently. Changes in eating habits of populations, such as quantitative levels of dietary fiber intake such as have occurred in Britain (Robertson, 1972) need to be monitored.

Synergism

The importance of modifying influences such as age, species, diet, cell population, hormonal status, and immunological competence (Kersey *et al.*, 1973) has been discussed in other sections.

There are always many examples of both accelerating and retarding the effects of exogenous chemicals on the carcinogenicity of other chemicals, and some of these have recently been listed (Warwick, 1973). In general, retardation is related to effects on the metabolism of the carcinogen, leading to lower effective levels of enzymatically produced "ultimate carcinogen"; while chemical enhancement appears in some cases to be related to stimulation of cell division in the target tissue, for example, in the sequential feeding of acetylaminofluorene and phenobarbital (Peraino et al., 1971) or in carbon tetrachloride enhancement of dimethylnitrosamine hepatocarcinogenesis (Pound et al., 1973). Montesano et al. (1974) have reported an additive effect in the induction of kidney tumors in rats treated with dimethylnitrosamine and ethyl methanesulphonate.

There is increasing evidence that certain chemicals, including carcinogens and mutagens, can enhance transformation of mammalian cells by viruses (Ledinko and Evans, 1973; Castro et al., 1974; Castro and DiPaolo, 1973). In this context it has recently been shown that carcinogens such as N-methyl-N'-nitro-N-nitrosoguanidine, acetoxyacetylaminofluorene, 4-nitroquinoline-N-oxide, and benzpyrene significantly enhanced the frequency of transformation of human foreskin cells by SV-40 virus, by pretreatment of cells up to 24 hr before adding virus or 2 hr after virus adsorption. Inhibition rather than promotion was found with dimethylbenz[α]anthracene and methylcholanthrene, findings apparently related to differences in damaging effects to DNA and subsequent repair.

These results suggest the possibility that in some cases both chemicals and viruses could act synergistically in man to produce cancer (see p. 189).

The classical example of promotion of skin cancer by croton oil is still being intensively studied. Stimulation of cell proliferation alone provides an insufficient mechanism for the phenomenon (Raick, 1972). Thus Raick (1973) has suggested that promoters produce their effect by altering the normal pathways of differentiation enabling "expression of the neoplastic phenotype," and they produce a variety of changes in skin, not all of which are related to preparation for hyperplasia. Some type of gene activation is suggested by the stimulation of the phosphorylation of mouse epidermal histones by tumor-promoting agents (Raineri et al., 1973) and of the faster onset of DNA synthesis in initiated cells following croton oil treatment (Frankfurt and Raitcheva, 1973). A further suggestion is that promoters interfere with DNA repair mechanisms (Teebor et al., 1973) or with the integrity of cell membranes (Kubinski et al., 1973). The mechanism of this type of biological change is obviously complex when examined at the molecular level.

Morphological and Biochemical Changes Produced by Carcinogens

It is outside the scope of this chapter to discuss these aspects in detail, and the reader is referred to the following reviews (Turusov, 1973; Foulds,

1969; Farber, 1973b; Shabad, 1973; Warwick, 1971a, 1973; Weber, 1971; Weinhouse, Emmelot, 1971; Svoboda and Higginson, 1968; Farber, 1968; Bergmann and Pullman, 1969; Potter, 1964). Suffice it to mention that carcinogens produce a spectrum of changes which can range at the morphological level from cell death to subtle changes which can be determined only at the ultrastructural or biochemical level, chromosomal abnormalities, delay in the onset of cell division, and others. Likewise, they differ in their ability to produce biochemical changes such as inhibition of DNA, RNA and protein synthesis, or the inhibition or stimulation of the activity of microsomal and lysosomal enzymes. No clear-cut relationships exist (Warwick, 1971a, 1973).

It is now generally accepted that the diverse changes produced in target tissues by chemical carcinogens result from the carcinogen or its metabolite combining covalently, or sometimes possibly physically, with cell constituents such as nucleic acids and proteins. Studies of the mechanism of action of chemical carcinogens at the molecular level have advanced far during the past decade (Miller, 1970; Magee and Barnes, 1967; Lawley, 1973). It is now clear that many chemically inert compounds are converted enzymatically or hydrophobically *in vivo* to electrophiles which can react by S_N1, S_N2, or radical mechanisms with macromolecules (Lawley, 1973). The extent and site of reaction are determined by the chemical structure of the electrophile and its half-life. The alkylating agents which are reactive per se can react by S_N1, S_N2, or mixed mechanisms and react extensively with the N-7 atom of guanine (Lawley, 1973) (see Figure 2) and less with other sites. The ability to react with the O-6 atom of guanine residues (Loveless, 1969) may be of great importance both in mutagenesis and carcinogenesis since O^6-methylguanine in DNA is a miscoding base in the Crick–Watson sense. It is thus of interest and instructive that compounds such as dimethylnitrosamine and *N*-methyl-*N*-nitrosourea which probably methylate through a common intermediate represented by the tautomers monomethylnitrosamine or methyldiazohydioxide, or the derived methyldiazonium ion, and which will tend to react by the S_N1 mechanism, show a different pattern of methylation of bases from agents such as dimethyl sulfate and methyl methanesulfonate which are S_N2 reactors (Lawley, 1973). This difference is even more important when considered in relation to the different biological properties of the two groups of compounds. Compounds such as acetylaminofluorene are converted to their *N*-hydroxy derivatives and hydroxyesters, the latter being considered the ultimate carcinogenic species (Weisburger and Weisburger, 1973). While reaction occurs at more than one site in nucleic acids, the major point of attack is apparently the C-8 of guanine residues. This applies also to the *N*-hydroxy derivative of the carcinogen acetylaminobiphenyl.

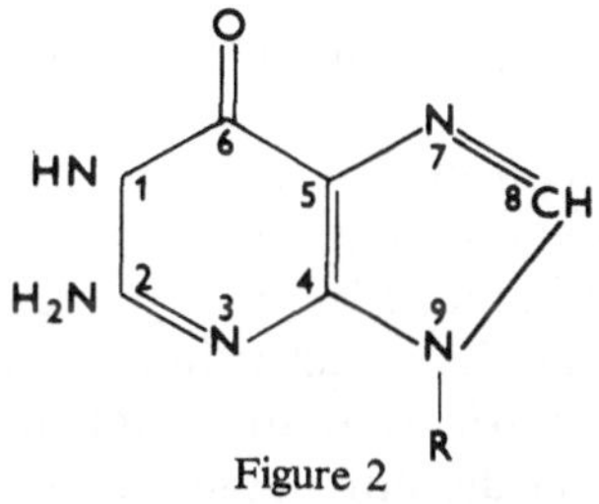

Figure 2

While the polynuclear aromatic hydrocarbons were the first purified chemical carcinogens discovered, their mechanism of action is still not clear. They are converted to reactive derivatives *in vivo* (Brookes and Lawley, 1964) and epoxides have been positively identified as products from *in vitro* systems (Grover *et al.*, 1972). However, the chemical identity of the reaction products of hydrocarbons such as 7-methylbenz[α]-anthracene with DNA *in vitro* remains to be established (Baird *et al.* 1973).

In the case of aflatoxin B_1, the potent hepatocarcinogen, there is increasing evidence that it is converted *in vitro* into a reactive metabolite, possibly an epoxide derived from the olefin-like double bond (Garner, 1973; Miller and Miller, 1976). This would be in keeping with variations in its toxicity and carcinogenicity for different species and the fact that hypophysectomy reduces its biological activity.

From the foregoing brief discussion it is clear that a variety of carcinogens owe their activity to metabolic conversion *in vivo* to reactive chemicals. That such conversions occur and are often dependent on the concentration and activity of drug-metabolizing enzymes can help to explain many of the properties of carcinogens such as site specificity and variations in carcinogenic potency found as a function of sex, age, hormonal status, dietary status, etc.

Viewed as a dynamic process, the mechanism of cancer initiation *in vivo* is complex and dependent on many variables including those just mentioned and probably the stage in the cell cycle when chemical interaction between carcinogen and cellular receptors occurs. One other very important variable is the ability of the cell to *repair* damage to its chemically modified DNA (Howard-Flanders, 1973). If, for example, reaction with the O-6 atom of guanine is a reaction potentially capable of leading to mutation, then whether or not this will occur will depend largely on the ability of the cell to repair this lesion by excision and replacement, a process probably requiring an endonuclease, an exonuclease, and a ligase (Roberts, 1976).

A recent report (O'Connor *et al.*, 1973) which compared the methylation products of DNA from rat liver following the administration of dimethylnitrosamine, a hepatocarcinogen, and methyl methanesulfonate which is not hepatocarcinogenic, showed not only interesting differences—for example, only the former yielded O-6 methylguanine—but evidence was obtained that this lesion was to some extent enzymatically excisable. In a further study of hepatic damage induced by methyl methanesulfonate and dimethylnitrosamine *in vivo,* and its repair (Mulivor *et al.,* 1974), it was found that the processing of depurination sites and the repair of single strand breaks was much slower in the nitrosamine-treated liver.

In a study of the rejoining of single-strand breaks following treatment of mouse fibroblasts with *N*-methyl-*N'*-nitro-*N*-nitrosoguanidine (Peterson *et al.,* 1974) at different times in the cell cycle it was concluded there was no direct correlation between DNA repair and susceptibility to transformation or lethality.

A recent attractive hypothesis suggested by Farber (1973b) is that hepatocarcinogens are those which cause double, rather than single strand breaks in liver DNA. This idea would be consistent with the behavior of hepatocarcinogens, including their apparently greater activity when cells in cycle are exposed to them, and that damage can remain latent for long periods of time as shown by the appearance of chromosomal abnormalities in dividing hepatocytes months after carcinogen or radiation treatment.

The problem of DNA repair in relation to uv-light-induced carcinogenesis in xeroderma pigmentation in man was mentioned earlier (p. 183). There is now evidence of a defect in DNA repair mechanisms in Fanconi's anemia (Poon *et al.,* 1974), a rare congenital disorder leading to bone marrow deficiencies and other abnormalities. There is an increased incidence of leukemia and an abnormally high frequency of chromosome aberrations which might be related to defects in repair mechanisms.

While carcinogens or their metabolites can react covalently with many intracellular sites, there is a growing consensus of opinion that reaction with nuclear DNA represents one important stage in the carcinogenic process, although it is not intended to underestimate the possible contribution of reaction at other sites, such as with one or more forms of RNA, or with certain key proteins to interface with processes of differentiation, for example.

However, since DNA viruses can become incorporated into nuclear DNA, RNA viruses via reverse transcriptases can produce DNA which could also be incorporated, and chemical and radiation carcinogens can also react with RNA in a variety of ways to produce changes including mutations (the first alternative is appealing) and could provide the basis for a broadly similar mechanism of action of all carcinogens. Any all-embracing theory has, however, to take account of plastic film carcinogenesis and asbestos (and other fiber) carcinogenesis. The problem of mutation in relation to human cancer has recently been discussed (Knudson, 1973).

References

Alexander, E. R. (1973). Possible etiologies of cancer of the cervix other than herpesviruses. *Cancer Res.* **33**:1485.

Bagshawe, A. F., Parker, A. M., and Jindani, A. (1971). Hepatitis-associated antigen in liver disease in Kenya. *Br. Med. J.* i:88.

Bagshawe, A., and Nganda, T. N. (1973). Hepatitis B antigen in a rural community in Kenya. *Trans. R. Soc. Trop. Med. Hyg.* **67**:663.

Baird. W.. Dipple. A.. Grover. P. L.. Sims. P.. and Brookes. P. (1973). Studies on the formation of hydrocarbon-deoxyribonucleoside products by the binding of derivatives of 7-methylbenz[α] anthracene to DNA in aqueous solution and in mouse embryo cells in culture. *Cancer Res.* **33**:2386–2392.

Baldwin, A. (1973). Immunological aspects of chemical carcinogenesis. *Adv. Cancer Res.* **18**:1.

Basu, T. K., and Dickerson, W. T. (1973). Inter-relationships of nutrition and the metabolism of drugs. *Chem. Biol. Interact.* **8**:193.

Berenblum, I. (1969). A re-evaluation of the concept of co-carcinogenesis. *Prog. Exp. Tumor Res.* **11**:21.

Bergmann, E. D., and Pullman, B., eds. (1969). Physicochemical mechanisms of carcinogenesis. In *The Jerusalem Symposia on Quantum Chemistry and Biochemisty*. Israel Academy of Science and Humanities, Jerusalem.

Bertram, J. S., and Heidelberger, C. (1973). Cell-cycle dependency of chemical oncogenic transformation in culture. *Proc Am. Assoc. Cancer Res.* Abs. No. 273.

Berwald, Y., and Sachs, L. (1963). *In vitro* cell transformation and chemical carcinogens. *Nature (London)* **200**:1182.

Bogovski, P., Gilson, J. C., and Wagner, J. C., eds. (1973). *Proceedings of the Conference on Biological Effects of Asbestos*. Int. Agency for Research on Cancer, Lyon.

Brookes. P. and Lawley. P. D. (1964). Alkylating agents. *Brit. Med. Bull.* **20**:91.

Buell, P. (1974). The effect of migration on the risk of nasopharyngeal cancer among Chinese. *Cancer Res.* **34**:1189.

Burkitt. D. P. (1967). African lymphoma. Epidemiological evidence suggested a viral aetiology. In *Racial and Geographic Factors in Tumor Incidence* (Shiva, ed.). Edinburgh Univ. Press, Edinburgh.

Burkitt, D. P. (1972). The trail of a virus—A review. In *Oncogenesis and Herpesviruses* (P. M. Biggs, G. de-Thé, and L. N. Payne, eds.), p. 343. Agency for Research on Cancer, Lyon.

Burkitt, D. P. (1973). Carcinoma of the colon and rectum. In *Modern Trends in Oncology* (R. W. Raven, ed.), Vol. 1, p. 227. Butterworth, London.

Bussey. H. J., Wallace. M. H., and Morson, B. C. (1967). Metachronous carcinoma of the large intestine and intestinal polyps. *Proc. Roy. Soc. Med.* **60**:208.

Castro. B. C. and DiPaolo. J. A. (1973). Virus, chemicals and cancer. *Prog. Med. Virol.* **16**:1.

Castro, B. C., Pieczynski, W. J., and Di Paolo, T. A. (1974). Enhancement of adenovirus transformation by treatment of hamster embryo cells with diverse chemical carcinogens. *Cancer Res.* **34**:72.

Clayson, D. B. (1962). *Chemical Carcinogenesis*. Churchill, London.

Cleaver, J. E. (1973). Xeroderma pigmentosum, DNA repair and carcinogenesis In *Current Research in Oncology* C. B. Anfinsen, M. Potter, and A. N. Schechter, eds.). Academic Press, New York.

Craddock, V. M. (1973). Induction of liver tumors in rats by a single treatment with nitroso compounds given after partial hepatectomy. *Nature (London)* **245**:386.

Crawford, M. A. (1971). Epidemiological interactions. In *Mycotoxins in Human Health* (I. F. H. Purchase, ed.) p. 231. Macmillan, London.

Currie, G. A. (1973). Human cancer and immunology. In *Modern Trends in Oncology* (R. W. Raven, ed.), Vol. 2. Butterworth, London.

Czygan, P., Greim H., Garro, A., Schaffer, F., and Popper, H. (1974). The effect of dietary protein deficiency on the ability of isolated hepatic microsomes to alter the mutagenicity of a primary and a secondary carcinogen. *Cancer Res.* **34**:119.

Elespuru, R. K., and Lijinsky, W. (1973). The formation of carcinogenic nitroso compounds from nitrite and some types of agricultural chemicals. *Food Cosmet. Toxicol.* **11**:807.

Emmelot, P. (1971). Some aspects of the mechanism of liver carcinogenesis. In *Liver Cancer*, pp. 94–109. IARC Publications No. 1.

Enomoto, M., and Saito, M. (1972). Carcinogens produced by fungi. *Annu. Rev. Microbiol.* **26**:279–311.

Farber, E. (1968). Biochemistry of carcinogenesis. *Cancer Res.* **28**:1859.

Farber, E. (1970). Studies on the molecular mechanisms of carcinogenesis. Homologies in enzymes and metabolic pathways. In *Cancer* (W. J. Whelan and J. Schultz, eds.). North Holland, Amsterdam.

Farber, E. (1973a). Chemical carcinogenesis in current research. In *Oncology* (C. B. Anfinsen, M. Potter, and A. N. Schechter, eds.) Academic Press, New York.

Farber, E. (1973b). Carcinogenesis—Cellular evolution as a unifying thread *Cancer Res.* **33**:2537.

Fong, Y. Y., and Chan, W. C. (1973). Dimethylnitrosamine in Chinese marine salt fish. *Food Cosmet. Toxicol.* **11**:841.

Foulds, L. (1969). *Neoplastic Development.* Academic Press, New York/London.

Frankfurt, O. S., and Raitcheva, E. (1973). Fast onset of DNA synthesis stimulated by tumor promoter in mouse epidermis at the initiation stage of carcinogenesis. *J. Nat. Cancer Inst.* **51**:1861.

Garner, R. C. (1973). Microsome-dependent binding of Aflatoxin B_1 to DNA, RNA, polyribonucleotides and protein *in vitro. Chem. Biol. Interact.* **6**:125.

Gatti, R. A., and Good, R. A. (1971). Occurrence of malignancy in immunodeficiency diseases. A literature review. *Cancer* **28**:89.

Geefhuysen, J., Rosen, E. V., Katz, J., Ipp, T., and Metz, J. (1971). Impaired cellular immunity in Kwashiorkor with improvement after therapy. *Br. Med. J.* **4**:527.

Gelboin, H. V. (1967). Carcinogens, enzyme induction and gene action. *Adv. Cancer Res.* **10**:1.

Gentry, G. A. (1974). Herpesviruses, mycoplasma and malignancy. *Proc Am. Assoc. Cancer Res.* **15**:567.

Goddard, P., and Hill, M. J. (1973). The dehydrogenation of the steroid nucleus by human-gut bacteria. *Biochem. Soc. Trans.* **1**:1113.

Grasso, P. (1970). Carcinogenicity testing and permitted lists. *Chem. Brit.* **6**:17.

Grasso, P., and Crampton, R. F. (1972). The value of the mouse in carcinogenicity testing. *Food Cosmet. Toxicol.* **10**:418.

Grice, H. C., Moodie, C. A., and Smith, D. C. (1973). The carcinogenic potential of aflatoxin or its metabolites in rats from dams fed aflatoxin pre- and postpartum. *Cancer Res.* **33**:262.

Grover, P. L., Hewer, A., and Sims, P. (1972). Formation of K-region epoxides as microsomal metabolites of pyrene and benzo (α) pyrene. *Biochem. Pharmacol.* **21**:2713.

Haenszel, W., Berg, J. W., Segi, M., Kurishara, M., and Locke, F. B. (1973). Large-bowel cancer in Hawaiian Japanese. *J. Nat. Cancer Inst.* **51**:1765.

Harington, J. S., Nunn, J. R., and Irwig, L. (1973). Dimethylnitrosamine in the human vaginal vault. *Nature (London)* **241**:49.

Heidelberger, C. H. (1973). Chemical oncogenesis in culture. *Adv. Cancer Res.* **18**:317.

Hennings, H., Michael, D., and Patterson, E. (1973). Enhancement of skin tumorigenesis by a single application of croton oil before or soon after initiation by urethan. *Cancer Res.* **33**:3130.

Herbst, A. L., Ulfelder, H., and Poskanzer, D. C. (1971). Adenocarcinoma of the vagina: association of maternal stilbestrol therapy with tumour appearance in young women. *N. Engl. J. Med.* **284**:878.

Herbst, A. L., Kurman, R. J., Scully, R. E., and Poskanzer, D. (1972). Clear-cell adenocarcinoma of the genital tract in young females. *N. Engl. J. Med.* **287**:1259.

Hill, M. J., Hawksworth, G., and Tattersall, G. (1973). Bacteria, nitrosamines and cancer of the stomach. *Brit. J. Cancer* **28**:562.

Ho, J. H. C. (1972). Nasopharyngeal carcinoma. *Adv. Cancer Res.* **15**:57.

Howard-Flanders, P. (1973). DNA repair and recombination. *Br. Med. Bull.* **29**:226.

Howarth, W. (1935). Precancerous epitheliomatosis (Bowen's disease) of palate and fauces. *J. Laryng. & Otol.* **50**:28.

Hueper, W. G., and Conway, W. D. (1964). *Chemical Carcinogenesis and Cancers.* CC Thomas., Springfield, Ill.

Hueper, W. C. (1966). *Recent Results in Cancer Research. Occupational and Environmental Cancers of the Respiratory System.* Springer-Verlag, New York;

Jose, D. G., and Good, R. A. (1973). Quantitative effects of nutritional protein and caloric deficiency upon immune responses to tumors in mice. *Cancer Res.* **33**:807.

Kannerstein, M. and Churg, J. (1972). Pathology of carcinoma of the lung associated with asbestos exposure. *Cancer,* **30**(1):14-21.

Kersey, J. H., Spector, B. D., and Good, R. A. (1973). Immunodeficiency and cancer. *Adv. Cancer Res.* **18**:211.

Knudson, A. G. (1973). Mutation and human cancer. *Adv. Cancer Res.* **17**:317.

Kubinski, H., Strangstalein, M. A., Baird, W. M., and Boutwell, R. K. (1973). Interactions of phorbol esters with cellular membranes *in vitro. Cancer Res.* **33**:3103.

Lancet Editorial (1973). Environmental nitrosamines. **2**:1243.

Lanier, A. P., *et al.* (1973). Cancer and stilbestrol. A follow-up of 1,719 persons exposed to estrogens in utero and born 1943–1959. *Mayo Clin. Proc.* **48**:793.

Lawley, P. D. (1973). The interaction of reactive metabolites with components of mammalian cells. *Biochem. Soc. Tran. (544th Meeting)* 7.

Ledinko, N., and Evans, M. (1973). Enhancement of adenovirus transformation of hamster cells by N-methyl-N'-nitro-N-nitrosoguanidine, caffeine and hydroxylamine. *Cancer Res.* **33**:2936.

Lijinsky, W. (1974). Reaction of drugs with nitrous acid as a source of carcinogenic nitrosamines. *Cancer Res.* **34**:255.

Loveless, A. (1969). Possible relevance of O-6 alkylation of deoxyguanosine to the mutagenicity and carcinogenicity of nitrosamines and nitrosamides. *Nature* **223**:206.

MacDonald, W. C., Brandborg, L. L., Taneguchi, L., and Rubin, C. E. (1963). Esophageal exfoliative cytology: A neglected procedure. *Annu. Intern. Med.* **59**:332.

Magee, P. N. and Barnes, J. M. (1967). Carcinogenic nitroso compounds. *Advances Cancer Res.* **10**:163.

Maynard, E. P., Sadikali, F., Anthony, P. P., and Barker, L. F. (1970). Hepatitis-associated antigen and cirrhosis in Uganda. *Lancet* **II**:1326.

McLean, A. E. M. (1973). Diet and chemical environment as modifiers of carcinogenesis. In *Host Environment Interactions in the Etiology of Cancer In Man* (R. Doll and L. Vodupuja, eds.). I.A.R.C. Scientific Publ. No. 7.

Miller, R. W. (1967). Persons at exceptionally high risk of leukemia. *Cancer Res.* **27**:2420.

Miller, J. A. (1970). Carcinogenesis by chemicals: An overview. *Cancer Res.* **30**:559.

202   G. P. Warwick

Miller, R. W. (1968). Relation between cancer and congenital defects: An epidemiologic
    evaluation. *J. Nat. Cancer Inst.* **40**:1079.
Miller, J. A., and Miller, E. C. (1976). The metabolic activation of chemical carcinogens—
    recent results with aromatic amines, safrole and aflatoxin B₁. In *Screening Tests in
    Chemical Carcinogenesis* R. Montesano, H. Bartsch, and Tomatis, eds. I.A.R.C. Publ.
    No. 12.
Mirvish, S. S., and Chu, C. (1973). Chemical detection of methylnitrosourea and ethylnitrosou-
    rea in stomach contents of rats after intubation of alkylureas plus sodium nitrite. *J. Nat.
    Cancer Inst.* **50**:745.
Mohr, V., and Althoff, J. (1971). Carcinogenic activity of aliphatic nitrosamines via the
    mother's milk in the offspring of Syrian golden hamsters. *Proc Soc. Exp. Biol. Med.*
    136:1007.
Montesano R., Bartsch, H., and Tomatis, L., eds. (1976). *Screening Tests in Chemical
    Carcinogenesis.* I.A.R.C. Publ. No. 12.
Montesano, R., Mohr, V., Magee, P. N., Hilfrich, J., and Haas, H. (1974). Additive effect in
    the induction of kidney tumours in rats treated with dimethylnitrosamine and ethylme-
    thanesulphonate. *Br. J. Cancer* **29**:50.
Morrow, R. H. (1974). Introduction: Burkitt's lymphoma in Africa. *Cancer Res.* **34**:1211.
Mulivor, R. A., Abanobi, S. E., and Sarma, D. S. R. (1974). Hepatic DNA damage induced by
    methyl methanesulfonate and dimethylnitrosamine *in vivo* and its repair. *Proc. Am.
    Assoc. Cancer Res.* **15**:337.
Murray, J. L., and Axtell, L. M. (1974). Impact of Cancer: Years of life lost due to cancer
    mortality. *J. Nat. Cancer Inst.* **52**:3.
Outzen, H. C., and Prehn, R. T. (1973). Alteration of cell-mediated immunity in the mouse
    following administration of 4-nitroquinoline-1-oxide. *Cancer Res.* **33**:408.
O'Connor, P. J., Capps, M. J., and Craig, A. W. (1973). Comparative studies of the
    hepatocarcinogen N,N-dimethylnitrosamine *in vivo*. Reaction sites in rat liver DNA
    and the significance of the relative stabilities. *Br. J. Cancer* **27**:153.
Peraino, C., Fry, R. J. M., and Staffeldt, E. (1971). Reduction and enhancement by pheno-
    barbital of hepatocarcinogenesis induced in the rat by 2-acetylaminofluorene. *Cancer Res.*
    31:1506.
Peterson, A. R., Bertram, J. S., and Heidelberger, C. (1974). Cell cycle-dependent rejoining of
    single-strand breaks in transformable mouse fibroblasts treated with *N*-methyl-*N*'-nitro-
    N-nitrosoguanidine. *Proc. Am. Assoc. Cancer Res.* **15**:59.
Poon, P. K., Parker, J. W., and O'Brien, R. L. (1974). Defect in DNA repair in Franconi's
    anaemia. *Proc. Amer. Assoc. Cancer Res.* **15**:75.
Potter, V. R. (1964). Biochemical perspectives in cancer research. *Cancer Res.* **24**:1085.
Pound, A. W. (1968). Carcinogenesis and cell proliferation. *New Zealand Med. J.* **67**:88.
Pound, A. W., Lawson, T. A., and Horn, L. (1973). Increased carcinogenic action of
    dimethylnitrosamine after prior administration of carbon tetrachloride. *Br. J. Cancer*
    27:451–459.
Raick, A. N. (1972). Studies on the mechanism of skin tumor promotion. The role of cell
    proliferation and epidermal hyperplasia. *Proc. Am. Assoc. Cancer Res.* **13**:39.
Raick, A. N. (1973). Ultrastructural, histological and biochemical alterations produced by 12-
    O-tetradecanoyl-phorbol-13-acetate on mouse epidermis and their relevance to skin
    tumor promotion. *Cancer Res.* **33**:269.
Raineri, R., Simsiman, R. C., and Boutwell, R. K. (1973). Stimulation of the phosphorylation
    of mouse epidermal histones by tumor-promoting agents. *Cancer Res.* **33**:134.
Raven, R. W. (1967a). The stomach.—Experimental and clinical considerations. In *The Pre-
    vention of Cancer* (R. W. Raven and F. J. C. Roe eds.), ch. 14, Butterworth, London.
Raven, R. W. (1967b). The small intestine. In *The Prevention of Cancer* (R. W. Raven and
    F. J. C. Roe eds.), ch. 18, Butterworth, London.

Robertson, J. (1972). Changes in the fibre content of the British diet. *Nature (London)* **238**:290.

Roe, F. J. C. (1968). Carcinogenesis and sanity. *Food Cosmet. Toxicol.* **6**:485.

Roe, F. J. C., Carter, R. L., Mitchley, C. V., Peto, R., and Hecker, E. (1972). On the persistance of tumour initiation and the acceleration of tumour progression on mouse skin tumorigenesis. *Int. J. Cancer* **9**:264.

Rogers, A. E., and Newberne, P. M. (1971). Diet and aflatoxin B_1 toxicity in rats. *Toxicol. Appl. Pharmacol.* **20**:113.

Rogers, A. E., Sanchez, O., Feinsod, F. M., and Newberne, P. M. (1974). Dietary enhancement of nitrosamine carcinogenesis. *Cancer Res.* **34**:96.

Rowley, J. D. (1974). Do human tumors show a chromosome pattern specific for each etiologic agent? *J. Nat. Cancer Inst.* **52**:315.

Saffiotti, V., and Shubick, P. (1963). Studies on promoting action in skin carcinogenesis. *Nat. Cancer Inst. Monogr.* **10**:489.

Setala, K. (1960). Progress in carcinogenesis, tumor-enhancing factors. A bio-assay of skin tumor formation. *Prog Exp. Tumor Res.* **1**:225.

Shabad, L. M. (1973). Precancerous morphologic lesions. *J. Nat. Cancer Inst.* **50**:1421.

Shank, R. C., Gordon, J. E., Wogan, G. N., Nondasyte, A., and Sunhamari, B. (1972). Dietary aflatoxins and human liver cancer. III. Field survey of rural Thai families for ingested aflatoxins. *Food Cosmet. Toxicol.* **10**:71.

Shimkin, M. B., and Triolo, V. A. (1969). History of chemical carcinogenesis: Some prospective remarks. *Prog. Exp. Tumor Res.* **11**:1.

Smithers, D. W. (1962). Cancer: An attack on cytologism. *Lancet* **1**:493.

Stanton, M. F. (1974). Fiber carcinogenesis: Is asbestos the only hazard? *J. Nat. Cancer Inst.* **52**:633.

Stich, H. F., Hammerberg, O., and Casto, B. (1972). The combined effect of chemical mutagen and virus on DNA repair, chromosome aberrations, and neoplastic transformation. *Can. J. Genet. Cytol.* **5**:911.

Svoboda, D., and Higginson, J. (1968). A comparison of ultrastructural changes in rat liver due to chemical carcinogenesis. *Cancer Res.* **28**:1703.

Teebor, G. W., Duker, N. J., Ruscan, S. A., and Zachary, K. J. (1973). Inhibition of thymine dimer excision by the phorbol ester, phorbol myristate acetate. *Biochem. Biophys. Res. Commun.* **50**:66.

de-Thé, G., and Geser, A. (1974). Nasopharyngeal carcinoma (NPC). Recent studies and outlook for a viral etiology. *Cancer Res.* **34**:1196.

Tomatis, L. (1973). Transplacental carcinogenesis. In *Modern Trends in Oncology* (R. W. Raven, ed.), vol. 1, p. 99. Butterworth, London.

Tomatis, L., Partensky, P., and Montesano, R. (1973). The predictive value of mouse liver tumour induction in carcinogenicity testing—A literature survey. *Int. J. Cancer* **12**:1.

Tomatis, L., and Mohr, V. eds. (1973). *Transplacental Carcinogenesis.* I.A.R.C. Publ. No. 4.

Turusov, V. S., ed. (1973). *Pathology of Tumours in Laboratory Animals,* Vol. 1, *Tumours of the Rat.* I.A.R.C. Scientific Publ. No. 5.

Van Duuren, B. L. (1969). Tumor-promoting agents in two stage carcinogenesis. Prog. Exp. Tumor Res. **11**:31.

Van Rensburg, S. J., Van der Watt, J. J., Purchase, I. F. H., Coutinho, L. P., and Markham, R. (1974). Primary liver cancer rate and aflatoxin intake in a high cancer area. *S. Afr. Med. J.* **48**:2508a.

Vogel, C. L., Anthony, P. P. Mody, N., and Barker, L. F. (1970). Hepatitis-associated antigen in Ugandan patients with hepatocellular carcinoma. *Lancet* **II**:621.

Warwick G. P. (1976). Some illustrative systems of chemical carcinogenesis: (4) aflatoxin and some other naturally occurring carcinogens. In *Scientific Foundations of Oncology* (T. Symington and R. L. Carter, eds.) (pp. 302–309). William Heinemann Medical Books.

Warwick, G. P. (1973). Newer aspects of carcinogenesis. In *Modern Trends in Oncology* (R. W. Raven, ed.) Vol. 1, p. 61. Butterworth, London.

Warwick, G. P. (1971a). Metabolism of liver carcinogens and other factors influencing liver cancer induction. I.A.R.C. Publ. No. 1:121.

Warwick, G. P. (1971b). The effect of the cell cycle on carcinogenesis. *Fed. Proc.* **30**:1760.

Warwick, G. P., and Harington, J. S. (1973). Some aspects of the epidemiology and etiology of esophageal cancer with particular emphasis on the Transkei Cape Province. *Adv. Cancer Res.* **17**:81.

Waynforth, H. B., and Magee, P. N. (1974). Immunosuppressive activity of *N*-nitroso-*N*-methylurea and dimethylnitrosamine. *Brit. J. Cancer.* **29**:92.

Weber, G. (1971). *Biochemistry of Liver Cancer.* I.A.R.C. Scientific Publ. No. 1, p. 69.

Weinhouse, S. (1971). Isozymes in cancer. *Cancer Res.* **31**:1166.

Weisburger, J. H., and Weisburger, E. K. (1973). Biochemical formation and pharmacological, toxicological and pathological properties of hydroxylamines and hydroxamic acids. *Pharmacol. Rev.* **25**:1.

Williams, G. M., Elliot, J. M., and Weisburger, J. H. (1973). Carcinoma after malignant conversion *in vitro* of epithelial-like cells from rat liver following exposure to chemical carcinogens. *Cancer Res.* **33**:606.

Wogan, G. N. (1973). Aflatoxin Carcinogenesis. In *Methods in Cancer Research* (H. Busch, ed.). Vol. 7, p. 309. Academic Press, New York.

Chapter 9

EPIDEMIOLOGY

DENIS BURKITT AND MICHAEL HUTT

General Principles

Genes and Environment

It is generally conceded that the cancer pattern in a population is determined to a large extent by its physical, biological, and human environment and that most racial differences are the result of these external factors. Some rare tumors, such as the squamous cell carcinoma that develops in the skin of individuals with xeroderma pigmentosa or the adenocarcinoma of the large bowel in patients with familial polyposis, clearly have a strong genetic component. Genetic factors may also play a role in determining which individuals in a population develop a tumor when exposed to a specific environmental hazard. Solar keratosis and squamous cell carcinoma of the skin which occurs as a result of ultraviolet irradiation is closely related to the degree of skin pigmentation. The albino African represents the highest risk, while the normal dark skinned African is completely immune from solar cancer except for his conjunctiva which is not protected by pigment (Templeton, 1967). Europeans show a spectrum of susceptibility according to their pigmentation. In an indirect way genetic factors may influence the liability of an African to develop Burkitt's lymphoma. Individuals of hemoglobin genotype AS which confers some protection against malaria have a significantly lower incidence of the tumor than those with the normal genotype AA (Morrow *et al.*, 1971). Evidence is also accumulating that genetically determined enzymes may play a role in determining

Denis Burkitt and Michael Hutt • Geographical Pathology Unit, Department of Morbid Anatomy, St. Thomas' Hospital Medical School, London, S.E.I., England

the susceptibility of individuals to some specific carcinogens (Brit. Med. J., 1974).

The dominance of environmental factors in the production of cancer distribution patterns has been emphasized by the study of migrant populations or populations exposed to the rapid changes in the environment which are a feature of this century (see below). Recognition of the magnitude of environmental influences in the production of cancer underlines the importance of studying distribution patterns of particular tumors in any search for etiological factors.

Cancer Registration

During the last 30 years cancer registries have been established throughout the developed world and also in many developing countries. In an ideal situation there should be a high rate of case detection with precise histological diagnosis and accurate registration which includes sufficient associated information for general analysis. The recorded cases should be derived from a population of known age and sex structure so that each tumor can be expressed as age- and sex-specific incidence rates. In some developing countries such rates are available from localized areas, usually around the capital city where medical facilities are good and widely used, but more frequently reliance has to be placed on proportional rates (relative frequency). Although crude, such frequencies have proved remarkably valuable in practice, and the various types of bias in such figures are usually similar in the different rural areas under consideration. Factors which influence case detection include age, sex, cultural practices, availability of health care, and appropriate facilities and methods for diagnosis. It is often possible to make corrections for some of the factors that produce bias (Templeton and Bianchi, 1972). A more accurate picture of the cancer pattern in developing countries can be obtained by inclusion of all clinical cases. The frequency of tumors based solely on a histological diagnosis will always tend to overestimate the incidence of superficial tumors and the odd lesions that defy diagnosis at the expense of deep tumors whose origin can often be clinically suspected (Burkitt et al., 1968).

Varieties of Distribution Patterns

Intercontinental. The marked and obvious variations in the frequency of some cancers between different continents have often led to unjustifiable generalizations such as the comment that "cancer is a disease of civilization" or that cancer of the liver is common throughout Africa. It is now apparent that the total incidence of all malignant tumors is almost as high in the developing countries of the world as in the developed, though the distribution of tumors varies considerably. The high frequency of liver cell carcinoma is limited to the rural areas of sub-Saharan Africa and for this reason is a problem of the indigenous African of various ethnic groups. By contrast, cancer of the colon has a low incidence throughout the whole of Africa except in those people, mostly whites, who live a western style of life. Kaposi's sarcoma is common in the indigenous population in many, but not all, parts of sub-Saharan Africa, and the statement that it is common in all Africans is misleading and may hide important clues to etiology.

Interterritorial and Intraterritorial. Many studies of cancer distribution have been based on comparisons between the total incidence or relative frequency of particular tumors on a national or territorial basis. Centralization of data, particularly in developing countries, may fail to reveal important variations in cancer patterns on a more localized geographical scale. Moreover, these variations rarely, if ever, correspond to political boundries which usually do not coincide with physical, biological, or cultural changes. The all-important "contour" lines of disease frequency are determined by the overall ecology of man (Hutt and Burkitt, 1965).

In the developing countries of the world man lives in closer contact with his natural physical and biological environment and also tends to retain his cultural patterns. The most useful information can often be obtained by studying cancer patterns in adjacent rural geographical areas independent of political boundaries (Cook and Burkitt, 1971). The very low incidence of Burkitt's lymphoma in southwest Uganda and in the adjacent country of Rwanda, both of which are over 6,000 ft, formed the starting point for the recognition of the relationship between tumor distribution, climatic factors, and malaria (Figure 1) (Burkitt, 1962).

By contrast, effects of natural environment are largely eliminated by man's activities in the industrial West, and carcinogenic hazards are increasingly those of his own making.

Patterns within Communities. Comparisons of the frequency of a particular tumor within a community living in the same place may show differences which are related to socioeconomic factors, cultural practices, or specific industrial hazards. For example, the pattern of cancer in the Parsi community of Bombay more closely resembles that of the West than that in other Indian groups living in that city; this is due to a combination of socioeconomic and cultural factors (Jussawalla et al., 1970).

More specifically, retrospective and case-control studies may show a relationship between a particular cancer and an environmental agent. Prospective cohort studies can then be utilized to see whether there is a significant difference in the incidence of the cancer in those exposed to varying doses of the suspected carcinogen. The clear relationship between cigarette smoking and certain types of lung cancer was shown by these classical methods (Doll and Hill, 1953, 1964). The relationship between

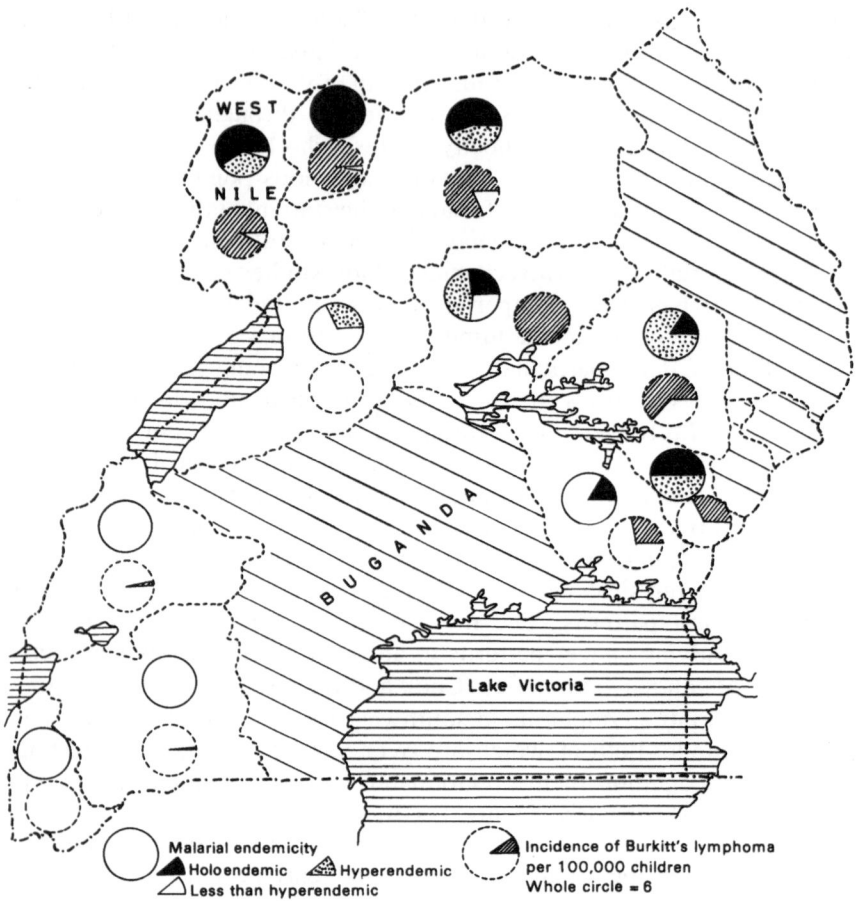

Figure 1. The coinciding geographical distribution of Burkitt's lymphoma and holoendemic and hyperendemic malaria in Uganda (from the *International Journal of Cancer*, Vol. 6, pp. 1–9, 1970).

bladder cancer and an occupational history of exposure to dyes or other substances containing 2-napthylamine, benzidene, or 4-aminodiphenyl is well established, and bladder cancer is now recognized as an occupational disease. Exposure to certain types of asbestos which are needed in a variety of industrial processes is associated with the development of mesothelioma. This agent may also have a synergistic effect with tobacco smoking in the development of lung cancer. There is a high incidence of cancer of the nose and nasal sinuses in some woodworkers and of angiosarcoma of the liver in workers using vinyl chloride polymers (Heath *et al.*, 1975).

The possible carcinogenic effect of drugs or other therapeutic substances is causing some alarm in the medical profession. The development of adenomas of the liver in women taking long-term contraceptive pills has been reported (Baum *et al.*, 1973), though these substances do not appear to increase the risk of developing breast or cervical cancer. The administration of diethystilbestrol to women during pregnancy may be associated with an increased risk of vaginal adenocarcinoma in their exposed female offspring (Herbst *et al.*, 1972).

The role of diagnostic or therapeutic irradiation has been the subject of much investigation. Treatment of ankylosing spondylitis by high-voltage X-ray therapy to the spine was shown to be associated with a tenfold increase in the incidence of leukemia in those exposed, as compared with a normal population.

Diagnostic radiology in pregnancy has also been shown to be associated with a significant rise in the incidence of leukemia and certain other tumors in the child (Court Brown *et al.*, 1960; Stewart *et al.*, 1958.; Mole, 1974).

Chronological Changes

Changes in the incidence of a particular tumor may be detected not only between geographical locations or different sections of a community, but also in the same community with the passage of time. Examination of such secular changes may provide important clues to etiology. The rapid rise in the incidence of bronchial cancer in men throughout the western world during the period 1920 to 1950, followed at a later date by a rise in women, fits well with the known pattern of cigarette consumption.

Cancer of the large bowel is both geographically and chronologically related to modern western civilization. Forty or more years ago this tumor was much less common in black as compared to white Americans (Lawrence, 1936; Quinland and Cuff, 1940); today the incidence is similar in both races (Doll, 1969).

On the other hand, the frequency of some forms of cancer falls with time. Gastric carcinoma, for example, is decreasing in most western countries, though the reasons for this are obscure.

In Uganda, examination of the records of one of the earliest mission hospitals, established before there was any western influence, revealed a pattern of tumors in 1900 very similar to that found today in the same area. This finding emphasizes that in a search for the carcinogenic factors for cancer in rural Africa one must look primarily at the physical, biological, and cultural environment rather than at Western exogenous influences (Davies *et al.*, 1964).

Changes Following Migration

The migration of sufficiently large numbers of people from one environment to another affords opportunities to study changes in cancer incidence in relation to specific environmental factors. Some of the classical studies have been conducted on Japanese who have migrated to Hawaii and other parts of the U.S.A.(Stemmermann, 1970; Wynder *et al.*, 1969). In Japan, there is a very high incidence of gastric cancer and a comparatively low incidence of large bowel cancer. Migration is associated with a decreasing rate of gastric cancer and an increase in colon cancer; these changes may not be great in the first generation and are more marked in their progeny. The rates may still remain slightly abnormal, even in the second generation, in relationship to the U.S.A. (Buell and Dunn, 1965). This suggests that some environmental, probably cultural, factors may be retained for a time but are gradually lost. The incidence of carcinoma of the large bowel has also been shown to increase in Jews who emigrated to Israel from North Africa and the Yemen (Steinits, 1974) and in Africans who have migrated from their rural homelands to urban Johannesburg (Robertson *et al.*, 1971).

European migrants to Western Australia have a greatly increased risk of developing skin cancer as a result of the increased exposure to sunlight.

Studies on Chinese migrants to the U.S.A. have also revealed interesting information. In women, the high rate for chloriocarcinoma rapidly decreases following immigration (Shanmugaratnum *et al.*, 1971), though the low rate for breast cancer and the high rate for adenocarcinoma of the lung persist (Fraumeni and Mason, 1974). In Chinese men the risk of nasopharyngeal carcinoma but not that of liver cell carcinoma decreases following emigration to America.

The Importance of Low-Incidence Rates

As Doll has put it, there is "no cancer that is common anywhere that is not rare somewhere else" (Doll, 1974). The occurrence of a very low incidence of a tumor in a geographical area or in a particular group of people may be of greater epidemiological significance than its high frequency in other areas. Yet reports of an unusually low incidence of any disease are rarely recorded.

In the epidemiological studies of lung cancer, one of the important clues was its rarity among Seventh Day Adventists who are a nonsmoking community (Wynder *et al.*, 1959). The high incidence of breast cancer and the low incidence of cervical cancer among nuns is another example of observations in a special group.

One of the important early clues in the study of Burkitt's lymphoma was its rarity in the densely populated mountainous region of the Nile-Congo Watershed, just south of the equator (Burkitt, 1962, 1969).

The Inclusion of Benign Lesions

One of the most neglected opportunities in the field of cancer epidemiology has been the importance of associations in frequency between one disease and another. When two or more diseases are always closely associated with one another epidemiologically it may at least be suspected that some causative factor may be common to each (Burkitt, 1970).

There is often a close association between the distribution of benign and malignant tumors in the same organ. This has been shown for adenomatous polyps and adenocarcinoma of the large bowel (Bremner and Ackerman, 1970; Hutt and Templeton, 1971; Burkitt, 1973a) fibrocystic disease and carcinoma of the breast, and macronodular cirrhosis and liver cell carcinoma. These associations suggest that there are common etiological factors and they may also give clues to the pathogenesis of the tumors. Associations between a malignant disease and a nonmalignant condition may also prove valuable as, for example, the observation that Burkitt's lymphoma did not occur in nonmalarious areas in Central Africa (Kafuko and Burkitt, 1970) (Figure 1).

Epidemiology of Specific Tumors

The presentation of cancer incidence rates on a geographical basis has been the result of the coordination of work done in many countries. These figures have been gathered together by the UICC and published as *Cancer Incidence in Five Continents* (Doll *et al.*, 1966, 1970). In these surveys tumors have been presented according to the WHO classification. The observations on rates from cancer registries can be supplemented by relative frequencies of tumors which are now available from many parts of the developing world. A detailed histopathological breakdown of tumors at different sites may uncover unusual patterns not evident from total figures (Templeton and Hutt, 1973).

Oral and Oropharyngeal Tumors

The most common form of cancer in many parts of India and also among Indian migrants in Malaysia, Fiji, and South America is squamous cell carcinoma of the buccal cavity. This is due to the social habit of chewing "quid" which contains various ingredients such as lime, tobacco, and betel nut. The quid is often held for long periods in the mouth, even during sleep (Tansurat, 1961; Paymaster, 1962). The development of carcinoma is often preceded by a leukoplakic type of lesion, and the high incidence of this cancer could be prevented by abandoning the habit of quid chewing.

A high incidence of squamous cell carcinoma in the region of the hard palate has recently been reported from India in women who smoke chuttas in reverse, with the lighted end of their cigarette in their mouths (Reddy, 1974).

Nasopharyngeal Tumors

These tumors are common among the Chinese in many parts of the Far East where rates may reach 100 times that in Europe (Muir and Shanmugaratnam, 1967). The high rates appear to be declining in many Chinese who have migrated to the U.S.A. (Fraumeni and Mason, 1974). Local areas of moderately high incidence are also found in parts of the Kenya Highlands (Clifford, 1967, 1970) and in the Sudan (el Hassan et al., 1967). Smoke from opium or from fires in closed huts has been suggested as an environmental factor. There is an association between this tumor and antibodies to Epstein–Barr virus both in Asian and Kenyan groups (Henle et al., 1970), but it is not clear whether the virus plays a pathogenic role. It seems probable that this is a tumor of multifactorial etiology, the factors varying in different areas (Clifford, 1970).

Esophageal Tumors

This tumor exhibits some of the greatest variations in incidence known in tumor epidemiology. These are probably in excess of 200-fold (Ahmed and Cook, 1969). The areas of very high incidence are geographically unrelated, and it seems probable that different etiological factors may be operating in each region.

In the Transkei district of South Africa esophageal carcinoma is the most common malignant tumor in man (Burrell, 1962). A survey of cancer patterns of Africans admitted to Baragwanath Hospital, Johannesburg shows that between the early 1950's and the 1960's the relative frequency of esophageal cancer had risen in men from 10.3 to 27.5% of all cancers, and in women from 0.8 to 4.7% (Robertson, et al., 1971). This increase was mainly evident in tribal groups from certain areas, including the Transkei. A high frequency of esophageal cancer has also been reported from Rhodesia (Skinner, 1967), Malawi (Borgstein, personal communication, 1975), and Western Kenya (Ahmed and Cook, 1969) (Figure 2). There is some evidence that the frequency is increasing in eastern Uganda (Templeton *et al.*, 1972), though throughout most of Uganda and Tanzania it is uncommon. The tumor is also rare in the Nile-Congo Watershed (Cook and Burkitt, 1971) and in West Africa.

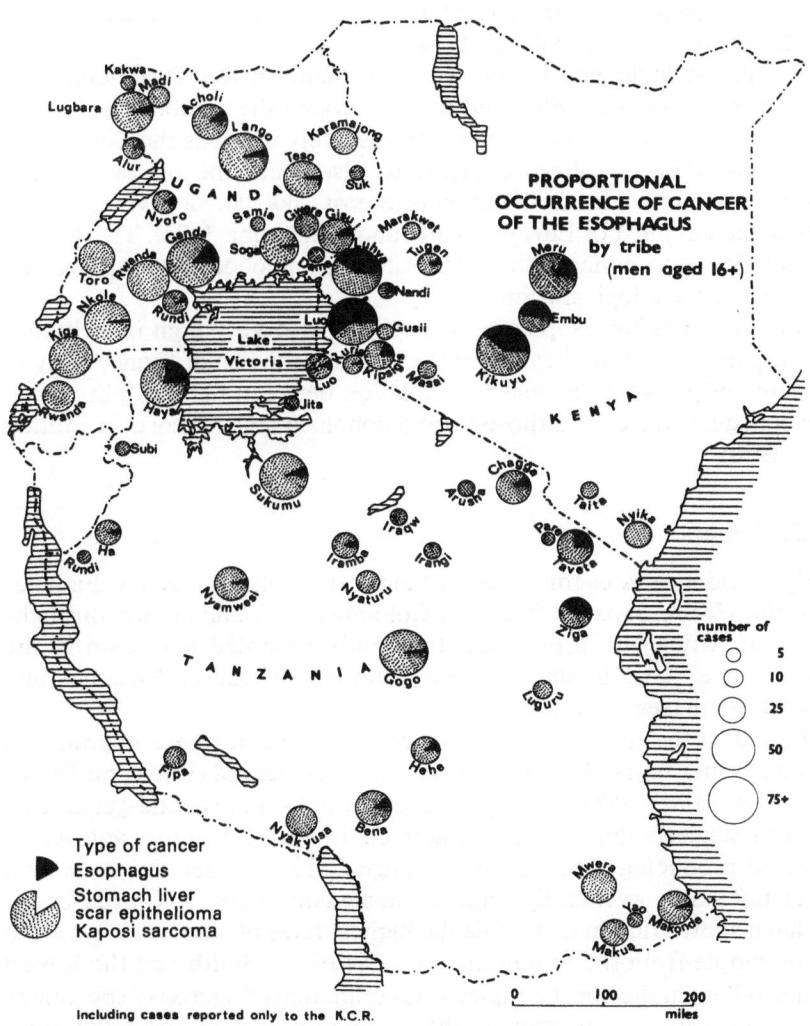

Figure 2. The geographical distribution of esophageal cancer related to that of some other forms of cancer in East Africa (from the *British Medical Bulletin*, Vol. 27, pp. 14–20, 1971).

The temporal as well as geographical changes in the frequency of this tumor in Africa suggest that it is related to changes in the environment. Many suggestions have been made as to possible factors, including fungal contamination of plants due to molybdenum deficiency in the soil, smoking, contamination of home-brewed alcohol, and the presence of nitrosamines in drink and of an unknown carcinogen specifically associated with maize beer (Cook, 1971). There is, as yet, no definite evidence to incriminate any of these factors, but a recent study in Johannesburg has shown a closer relationship between the tumor and tobacco consumption than alcohol intake (Bradshow and Schonland, 1974).

The highest incidence in the world is found in the Turkmenia and Kazakstan region of the USSR and in Iran around the southern border of the Caspian Sea. This high rate falls progressively towards the Southwest along the coastline. In sharp contrast to elsewhere the tumor is more common in women, with an incidence rate of 200/100,000, which is 200 times that seen in most of Europe (Kmet and Mahboubi, 1972). There is no definite evidence to connect this high rate with alcohol or tobacco or to point to another etiological agent.

Mortality rates for esophageal cancer are also very high in Brittany, particularly in men where they are twice those for the rest of France (Tuyns and Massé, 1973). There is also a correlation between the mortality rates from esophageal cancer and those from alcoholism and cirrhosis in France (Tuyns, 1970).

Stomach Tumors

High incidence rates for stomach cancer are found in Iceland, Finland, parts of the USSR, Japan, Chile, and Colombia. It is uncommon through-out most of Africa but is the most frequently recorded neoplasm in the region of Lake Kivu in the adjacent countries of Zaire, Rwanda, and Burundi (Clemmesen et al., 1962).

The fall in the incidence of stomach cancer in Japanese migrants to Hawaii and other parts of the U.S.A. is well documented (Buell and Dunn, 1965; Correa et al., 1973). The frequency in first- and second-generation immigrants suggests that the responsible environmental factors act over a long period producing precancerous changes which, under the same or a different influence, eventually undergo malignant changes. Correa et al. (1970) have shown that in Colombia the highest rates of stomach cancer are found in people from the mountainous areas of the South and the lowest rates in dwellers in the coastal regions. Examination of necropsy specimens of the stomach from individuals in these two groups who died from other causes shows a much higher frequency of chronic atrophic gastritis in those who come from the high cancer incidence areas. The importance of chronic atrophic gastritis in the pathogenesis of gastric carcinoma has also been shown by gastric biopsy studies in susceptible populations in Finland (Siurala *et al.*, 1972). One possible etiological factor is the nitrate content of the soil which is very high in the mountainous areas of Colombia. In England there appears to be an increased frequency of stomach cancer in Worksop which has a high nitrate content in the water (Hawksworth and Hill, 1971) in comparison with the country as a whole. The high rate in Japan has been attributed to contamination of rice by talc (Matsudo *et al.*, 1974).

Large Bowel Tumors

No form of cancer is more closely related to economic development and the western way of life than is adenocarcinoma of the large bowel. These tumors have their highest incidence in North America and Western Europe and their lowest in rural communities in developing countries. The geographical distribution of adenomatous polyps of the large bowel is similar to that of carcinoma. Moreover, there is a close association between large bowel cancer and several other diseases characteristic of economic development, including diverticular disease of the colon, hiatus hernia, acute appendicitis, and cholelithiasis (Burkitt, 1973b). Diverticular disease is a relatively new disease in the West and appears to be due to the change in our diet which is characterized by an increase in fat and a change in the character of the carbohydrate eaten. Fiber-depleted diets appear to be the significant factor in this condition. They result in loss of stool bulk, increased viscosity of feces, and lengthening of bowel transit time (Painter, 1964, 1967). It has been shown that the fecal bacterial flora differs between communities with a high or low incidence of large bowel cancer and that some of the anaerobes which are more numerous in high risk communities have the property of degrading the primary bile acid cholate into the potentially carcinogenic deoxycholate (Aries *et al.*, 1969; Hill *et al.*, 1971). There is also an increased content of steroids in the stools of high-risk groups (Hill and Aries, 1971). The change in bowel flora appears to be closely related to an increased fat content in the diet (Hill, 1971), but changes in the fiber content may also play a role in the pathogenesis by altering the output of the substrate bile on which bacteria act. Changes in stool bulk and transit time also affect the contact and concentration of carcinogenic substances with the bowel mucosa (Burkitt, 1973a).

Liver Tumors

Liver Cell Carcinoma. This is the most frequently recorded tumor in large areas of rural sub-Saharan Africa (Payet, 1957; Higginson and Oettlé, 1960; Davies and Steiner, 1957; Edington and MacLean, 1965). A very high frequency is reported from Senegal, and in Mozambique rates of over 260/

100,000 are found in men (Prates and Torres, 1965). Liver cell carcinoma is also common in many parts of the Far East (Simons *et al.,* 1971) and in Southern India. The condition is not common in the U.S.A. and Europe but appears to be increasing.

In both high- and low-incidence areas liver cell carcinoma is associated, in a large majority of cases, with cirrhosis, usually of the macronodular pattern (Anthony, 1973a). The increased frequency of liver cancer in cases of hemochromatosis suggests that cirrhosis per se may give an increased risk, but it is possible that the agent causing the cirrhosis may also play a direct role in the development of the tumor.

In most high incidence areas of liver cell carcinoma there is a high frequency of Australia antigen (HAA) in the sera of normal populations (Bagshawe and Nganda, 1973; Payet *et al.,* 1971) and a significantly higher frequency in patients with cirrhosis and liver cell carcinoma than in comparable groups in Europe (Vogel *et al.,* 1972). These and certain pathological observations suggest that viral hepatitis may play a role in the etiology of cirrhosis in high-incidence areas, and possibly also of liver cell carcinoma.

The epidemiological features of liver cell carcinoma correspond closely to conditions which predispose to fungal contamination of foodstuffs. Aflatoxin, a product of *Aspergillus flavus,* a contaminant of ground nuts and other cereals, has been shown to be one of the most powerful known carcinogens. The discovery suggested that this or another fungal toxin might be an important agent in the etiology of liver cell carcinoma (Wogan, 1966; Newberne and Butler, 1969). Epidemiological studies on foodstuffs in storage or from "plate sample" in Uganda, Kenya, South Africa, and Thailand have shown a close relationship between the presence of aflatoxin contamination and liver cell carcinoma (Keen and Martin, 1971; Shank *et al.,* 1972; Alpert *et al.,* 1971; Peers and Linsell, 1973).

A combination of aflatoxin and viral hepatitis has been shown to produce liver cell carcinoma in marmosets (Lin *et al.,* 1974). It seems possible that both hepatitis virus and aflatoxin may be involved in the etiology of liver cell carcinoma in very-high-incidence areas.

(b) **Bile Duct Carcinoma.** This is one of the few carcinomas clearly related to a living agent, the parasite *Clonorchis sinensis* (Gibson, 1971). The presence of this parasite induces changes in the bile ducts, particularly in the intrahepatic branches, which predispose to cancer (Chou and Gibson, 1970). Clonorchiasis was found twice as frequently in cases of cholangiocarcinoma than in control groups in a necropsy series from Hong Kong (Liang and Tung, 1959).

Respiratory Tract Tumors

The demonstration of the association between smoking and cancer of the lung is one of the classics of cancer epidemiology, (Doll and Hill, 1953,

1964), though regretably this knowledge has led to little decrease in smoking except in certain groups. This association has been demonstrated by the close relationship between smoking habits and the incidence of lung cancer in various situations. This has been shown in communities living in different geographical regions, with changes in smoking habits within communities, by careful case-control studies, and in particular by prospective cohort studies. These have shown not only a close relationship between the total consumption of tobacco and the risk of developing lung cancer, but also a lowering of this risk after smoking has been abandoned. Cancer of the lung is increasing in frequency in the urbanized African (Robertson *et al.*, 1971) and other urbanized groups in tropical countries. The association with smoking is most closely related to certain histological types, particularly epidermoid carcinoma. There is no relation between smoking and adenocarcinoma of the lung.

Breast Tumors

In general, the incidence of breast carcinoma is much higher in the western world thàn in developing countries, though breast cancer is also uncommon in Japan. It has been known for many years that the incidence is higher in the unmarried and the nulliparous and that some families appear to have an increased genetic susceptibility. A number of factors have been investigated to determine the role of fertility, the number of pregnancies, and the amount of breast feeding in the etiology of this condition. The studies of McMahon *et al.* (1970) in the U.S.A. suggest that the age of the individual at the time of the first pregnancy is a crucial factor. Women who have their first child after the age of 30 years have a significantly increased risk of developing breast carcinoma than those who have their first child before the age of 20. Recent studies do not support the concept that a horizontal transmitted virus plays any role in the development of breast carcinoma, though they suggest that maternal or parental genetic factors probably operating through some hormonal mechanism may be important (Henderson *et al.*, 1974). The geographical differences in the incidence of breast carcinoma are difficult to explain entirely on hormonal terms, and it has been suggested that dietary factors may play a role.

Tumors of the Female Genital Tract

Tumors of the Cervix Uteri. Carcinoma of the cervix uteri is the second most common tumor in women in the western world and is the most common tumor in women in the developing world, where the absolute rates are higher than in the West. The condition is significantly less common in Jewesses and in nuns and in unmarried or nulliparous women.

There is increasing evidence that the incidence is related to age at the time of first intercourse, frequency of intercourse, and change of partners

(Elliott, 1964; Malhotra, 1971). For these reasons it is closely related to the frequency of venereal disease. A low standard of hygiene associated with lack of circumcision in the male play a role, and smegma or penetration of cervical tissues by spermatozoa have been suggested as possible agents. Herpes genitalia infection has been suspected following a study of antibody titers against this virus in the sera of patients (*Brit. Med. J.,* 1970).

Tumors of the Corpus Uteri. There appears to be an inverse relationship between cancer of the cervix uteri and that of the corpus uteri. Ratios of up to 20:1 are found in some developing countries, while in some groups of Jewesses the ratio may be reversed 1:2. These differences are probably due to real changes on both sides of the equation. Infertility, obesity, hypertension, and diabetes mellitus have all been related to its high incidence.

Choriocarcinoma

This condition and its precursor hydatidiform mole is declining in frequency in western countries, but has a very high incidence in parts of the Far East and a moderately high incidence in many parts of Africa (James *et al.,* 1973). In Uganda it is more common than cancer of the corpus uteri. There is some evidence to suggest that the incidence may be related to the number and frequency of pregnancies and the age at the time of the first. The high rates in Chinese women are lost in those who migrate to the U.S.A.

Male Genitalia

Penis. There is a higher incidence of penile cancer in lower socioeconomic groups, in the developing countries, and in those who are not circumcised (Dodge and Kaviti, 1965). In East Africa, considerable differences have been shown between tribal groups who are ethnically and geographically closely related and who do not practice circumcision (Schmauz and Jain, 1971). This suggests that other factors, possibly specific types of infection such as herpes genitalis, may play an important role and that lack of hygiene and retention of the prepuce merely aggravate or initiate the etiological processes.

Tumors of the Kidney

It appears that nephroblastoma is one of the few tumors which has a similar incidence in all parts of the world (Davies, 1973).

Renal cell carcinoma has an unusually low incidence in Africa (Anthony, 1973b).

Tumors of the Bladder

The association between cancer of the bladder and specific industrial carcinogens has already been discussed. Cigarette smoking is also said to have a significant correlation with bladder cancer. The great majority of bladder cancers in Europe and the U.S.A. are transitional in type, whereas in Uganda 59% are squamous carcinomas and 20% are adenocarcinomas (Anthony, 1973b). These differences in histological type probably reflect a different etiology. Bladder cancer, often squamous in type, has a high frequency in Egypt where it has a clear association with schistosomiasis (Hashem, 1961). However, infection by *Schistosoma haematobium* is not prevalent throughout most of Uganda, so this cannot explain the preponderance of squamous cell carcinoma. It has been suggested that the high frequency of the squamous variant of carcinoma both in Egypt and Uganda may be the result of urinary stasis and infection, due to schistosomiasis in the former and urethral stricture in the latter (Dodge, 1964; Anthony, 1973b). Infection and stasis result in the presence of increased amounts of β-glucuronidase in the bladder which could release active carcinogens from inactive glucuronides.

Skin Tumors

The first established relationship between cancer and environmental influences were made by Percival Pott in 1775, who recognized that patients with cancer of the scrotum shared the common experience of having been chimney sweeps when young. A similar observation revealed that mulespinners cancer was related to contamination of the skin of workers in cotton mills. Many decades later these forms of cancer were related to the carcinogenic properties of hydrocarbons. Other agents, such as heat, were related to the "Kangri cancer" of the skin of the abdominal wall and thighs which results from carrying a pot of burning charcoal under the outer garments as a form of portable central heating.

Reference has been made to solar cancers due to the effect of ultraviolet irradiation (Urbach, 1969). Skin cancer may also result from irradiation, as in the early radiologists and from prolonged arsenical administration. The high incidence in darkly pigmented races in some tropical countries is mainly due to the development of cancers in depigmented scars, or ulcers, particularly those following tropical ulcer or burns (Iversen and Iversen, 1973).

Melanoma

The distribution and degree of pigmentation in different racial groups may determine the site of development of these tumors. The great majority of malignant melanomas in Africans occur on the sole of the foot and develop from preexisting nevi in this nonpigmented area of the skin (Lewis, 1967). The predeliction to the foot may be accentuated by the fact that rural dwellers often do not wear shoes. The highest incidence of malignant melanoma in the world is found in Queensland (Davis *et al.*, 1966), particularly among people of Celtic descent. The suggestion that this is due to the effect of ultraviolet light has been confirmed by Elwood *et al.* (1974) who have shown a close relationship between the age-standardized mortality rates in different parts of the U.S.A. and Canada and the geographical latitude; this in turn correlates with ultraviolet exposure and other skin cancers (Elwood *et al.*, 1974).

Tumors of the Eye

Africans in Equatorial Africa have a unusually high incidence of squamous cell carcinoma of the conjunctiva which appears to be solar induced. They have a low incidence of intraocular malignant melanoma (Templeton, 1967).

Tumors of the Thyroid

In Cali, Colombia, cancer of the thyroid shows an increased frequency as great as tenfold compared with some other areas. This is associated with a high prevalence of parenchymatous goiter (Correa and Llanos, 1966). High incidences have also been reported from other volcanic areas (Doll *et al.*, 1970).

Tumors of the Connective Tissues

There is some evidence to suggest that soft tissue tumors as a group have a higher frequency in sub-Saharan Africa than in Europe, but there is no doubt that Kaposi's sarcoma occurs in an unusually high frequency through much of sub-Saharan Africa. This tumor is rare in North Africa and less common in West than in East and Central Africa, where it frequently is the highest in western Uganda, Rwanda, Burundi, and eastern Zaire (Cook and Burkitt, 1971). This tumor, which has a male dominance of between 10–20:1, is uncommon in U.S. negroes and is likely to be realted to some unidentified environmental agent possibly modified by an endogenous factor.

Lymphoreticular Tumors

A recent survey of the relative frequency of lymphomas collected by the UICC (Correa and O'Conor, 1973) revealed five different geographical patterns: (1) tropical countries with epidemic proportions of Burkitt's lymphoma; (2) tropical countries where Burkitt's tumor was not excessive, with high proportions of Hodgkin's disease in children and low proportions in young adults; (3) tropical and subtropical countries with features of the second group, but with additional high proportions of Hodgkin's disease in young adults and high frequencies of the nodular sclerosis subtype; (4) affluent societies with a low incidence of Hodgkin's disease in children, a predominance of nodular sclerosis, and a high frequency of multiple myeloma, and (5) oriental countries with a low frequency of Hodgkin's disease and a high frequency of reticulum cell sarcoma.

A well-characterized syndrome of intestinal lymphomas has also been described in Israel, Iran, and Lebanon (Rappaport et al., 1972). In Iran there is strong evidence to relate this to severe infective stress in early infancy which leads to sprue-like atrophy of the bowel mucosa (Dutz et al., 1971). The evidence that immunosuppression may result in an increased incidence of malignant lymphoma suggests that the lymphoma in Iran may be associated with the immunodeficiency resulting from malnutrition (Dutz et al., 1971).

Burkitt's Lymphoma

The hypotheses postulated for the cause of this tumor have been the direct result of epidemiological observations. It was the pattern of geographical distribution that indicated a dependence on climatic factors, and this in turn seemed to implicate some biological agent (Burkitt, 1962). The first outcome was the vectored virus hypothesis, but the abundance of insect vectors in areas of low tumor prevalence and the ubiquitous nature of the most closely associated virus, the Epstein–Barr virus, discredited this theory. Moreover, there is no evidence that this virus is insect transmitted. Further scrutiny of the geographical distribution indicated the close relationship between the areas in which this tumor is endemic and those in which malaria is hyperendemic (Kafuko and Burkitt, 1970). It was thus realized that malaria was the factor that was delineated by the geographically limited climatic factors, and the current hypothesis is that hyperendemic malaria and the Epstein–Barr or other viruses are cofactors in the pathogenesis of this disease (Burkitt, 1969). Experimental evidence derived from the study of oncogenic viruses in mice suggests that malaria may produce its effect by immunodepression (Wedderburn, 1970).

Leukemia

There appears to be some decrease in frequency in leukemia in developing countries, but the problems of underdiagnosis may play an important role in these apparent figures. Nevertheless, it is generally agreed that acute lymphoblastic leukemia in children has a significantly lower incidence rate than in developed countries and that this is not just a failure of diagnosis.

The Role of Epidemiology in Forming Hypotheses

Since environmental influences play a major role in the causation of cancer, the identification and, subsequently, protection from those factors must be the fundamental aim in cancer research.

Epidemiological studies enable the formation of hypotheses which postulate the incrimination of certain environmental factors. These hypotheses can then be tested experimentally. Whether they prove to be right or wrong, or in need of modification, steps will have been taken toward the discovery of the cause of the tumor.

Testing the carcinogenic potential of different substances at random in the absence of any incriminating evidence is much less likely to give fruitful results than is the testing of specific hypotheses.

The process is akin to the construction of a jigsaw puzzle from a mass of heterogeneous fragments, each representing a piece of available data. As many pieces as possible are fitted together and then the imagination must be used to formulate a hypothesis as to what the completed picture might be. An attempt is then made to fit the remaining fragments into this picture. If the formulated hypothesis is inconsistent with any data, then it must be modified or abandoned rather than the factual data ignored; not until the picture is complete does the hypothesis become a fact.

References

Ahmed, N., and Cook, P. (1969). The incidence of cancer of the oesophagus in West Kenya. *Br. J. Cancer* **23**:302.

Alpert, M. E., Hutt, M. S. R., Wogan, G. N., and Davidson, C. S. (1971). Association between aflatoxin content of food and hepatoma frequency in Uganda. *Cancer* **28**:253.

Anthony, P. P. (1973a). Primary carcinoma of the liver: A study in 282 cases in Ugandan Africans. *J. Pathol.* **110**:37.

Anthony, P. P. (1973b). Malignant tumors of the kidney, bladder and urethra. In *Tumours in a Tropical Country.* (A. C. Templeton, ed.), p. 145. Heinemann Medical Books, London.

Aries, V., Crowther, J. S., Drasar, B. S., Hill, M. J., and Williams, R. E. O. (1969). Bacteria and the aetiology of cancer of the large bowel. *Gut* **10**:334.

Bagshawe, A., and Nganda, T. N. (1973). Hepatitis B antigen in a rural community in Kenya. *Trans. Soc. Med. Hyg.* **67**:663.

Baum, J. K., Holtz, F., Bookstein, J. J., and Klein, E. W. (1973). Possible association between benign hepatomas and oral contraceptives. *Lancet* **2**:926.

Bradshaw, E., and Schonland, M. (1974). Smoking, drinking and oesophageal cancer in African males in Johannesberg, South Africa. *Br. J. Cancer* **30**:157.

Bremner, C. G., and Ackerman, L. V. (1970). Polyps and carcinoma of the large bowel in the South African Bantu. *Cancer* **26**:991.

British Medical Bulletin (1971). **27**:14–20.

British Medical Journal (1970). Genital herpes and cervical cancer. **4**:256.

British Medical Journal (1974). Susceptibility to carcinogens in man. **1**:169.

Buell, P., and Dunn, J. E. (1965). Cancer mortality among the Japanese Issei and Nisei of California. *Cancer* **18**:656.

Burkitt, D. P. (1962). Determining the climatic limitations of a children's cancer common in Africa. *Br. Med. J.* **2**:1019.

Burkitt, D. P. (1969). Etiology of Burkitt's lymphoma. *J. Nat. Cancer Inst.* **42**:19.

Burkitt, D. P. (1970). Relationship as a clue to causation. *Lancet* **2**:1237.

Burkitt, D. P. (1973a). Carcinoma of the colon and rectum. In *Modern Trends in Oncology* (R. W. Raven, ed.), p. 227. Butterworth, London.

Burkitt, D. P. (1973b). Some diseases characteristic of modern western civilization. *Clin. Radiol.* **24**:271.

Burkitt, D. P., Hutt, M. S. R., and Slavin, G. (1968). Clinicopathological studies of cancer distribution in Africa. *Br. J. Cancer* **22**:1.

Burrell, R. J. W. (1962). Oesophageal cancer among the Bantu in the Transkei. *J. Nat. Cancer. Inst.* **28**:495.

Chou, S. T., and Gibson, J. B. (1970). The histochemistry of biliary mucins and the changes caused by infestation with *Clonorchis sinensis*. *J. Pathol.* **101**:185.

Clemmesen, J., Maisin, J., and Gigase, P. (1962). *Cancer in Kivu and Ruanda-Urundi*. Institut de Cancer, Université de Louvain.

Clifford, P. (1967). Malignant disease of the nasopharynx and paranasal sinuses in Kenya. In *Cancer of the Nasopharynx* (C. S. Muir and K Shanmugaratnam, eds.), Vol. 1. UICC Monograph Series, Munksgaard, Copenhagen.

Clifford, P. (1970). On the epidemiology of nasopharyngeal carcinoma. *Int. J. Cancer* **5**:287.

Cook, P. (1971). Cancer of the oesophagus in Africa. *Br. J. Cancer* **25**:853.

Cook, P., and Burkitt, D. P. (1971). Cancer in Africa. *Brit. Med. Bull.* **27**:14.

Correa, P., and Llanos, G. (1966). Morbidity and mortality from cancer in Cali, Colombia. *J. Nat. Cancer Inst.* **36**:717.

Correa, P., and O'Conor, G. T. (1973). Geographic pathology of lymphoreticular tumours. *J. Nat. Cancer Inst.* **50**:1609.

Correa, P., Cuello, C., and Duque, E. (1970). Carcinoma and intestinal metaplasia of the stomach in Colombian migrants. *J. Nat. Cancer Inst.* **44**:297.

Correa, P., Sasano, N., Stemmermann, G. N., and Haenszel, W. (1973). Pathology of gastric carcinoma in Japanese populations: Comparisons between Miyagi Prefecture, Japan and Hawaii. *J. Nat. Cancer Inst.* **51**:1449.

Court Brown, W. M., Doll, R., and Bradford Hill, A. (1960). Incidence of leukaemia after exposure to diagnostic radiation *in utero*. *Br. Med. J.* **2**:1539.

Davies, J. N. P. (1973). Childhood tumours. In *Tumours in a Tropical Country* (A. C. Templeton, ed.), p. 306. Heinemann Medical Books, London.

Davies, J. N. P., Elmes, S., Hutt, M. S. R., Mtimavalye, L. A. R., Owor, R., and Shaper, L. (1964). Cancer in an African Community, 1897–1956. An analysis of the records of Mengo Hospital, Kampala, Uganda. *Brit. Med. J.* **1**:259.

Davies, J. N. P., and Steiner, P. E. (1957). Cirrhosis and primary liver carcinoma in Ugandan Africans. *Brit. J. Cancer* **11**:523.

Davis, N. C., Herron, J. J., and McLeod, G. R. (1966). Malignant melanoma in Queensland. *Lancet* **2**:407.

Dodge, O. G. (1964). Tumours of the bladder and urethra associated with urinary retention in Uganda Africans. *Cancer* **17**:1433.

Dodge, O. G., and Kaviti, J. N. (1965). Male circumcision among the peoples of E. Africa and the incidence of genital cancer. *E. Afr. Med. J.* **42**:98.

Doll, R. (1969). The geographical distribution of cancer. *Brit. J. Cancer* **23**:1.

Doll, R. (1974). Quoted in: Cancer in Chinese migrants. *Lancet* 1:1027.

Doll, R., and Hill, A. B. (1953). Bronchial carcinoma: Incidence and aetiology. *Brit. Med. J.* 2:521–585.

Doll, R., and Hill, A. B. (1964). The mortality of doctors in relation to their smoking habits. *Brit. Med. J.* 1:1451.

Doll, R., Muir, C. S., and Waterhouse, J. A. H., eds. (1970). *Cancer Incidence in Five Continents*, Vol. II. UICC, Springer-Verlag, Berlin/Heidelberg/New York.

Doll, R., Payne, P. and Waterhouse, J. A. H., eds. (1966). *Cancer Incidence in Five Continents*, Vol. I. UICC, Springer-Verlag, Berlin/Heidelberg/New York.

Dutz, W., Asvadi, S., Sadri, S., and Kohout, E. (1971). Intestinal lymphoma and sprue: A systematic approach. *Gut* 12:804.

Edington, G. M., and MacLean, C. M. U. (1965). A cancer rate survey in Ibadan, Western Uganda. *Brit. J. Cancer* 19:471.

el Hassan, A. M., Nilosev, B., Daoud, E. H., and Kashan, A. (1967). Malignant diseases of the upper respiratory tract in the Sudan. In *Cancer in Africa* (P. Clifford, C. A. Linsell, and G. L. Timms, eds.), p. 307. East African Publ. House.

Elliott, R. I. K. (1964). On the prevention of carcinoma of the cervix. *Lancet* 1:231.

Elwood, J. M., Lee, J. A. H., Walter, S. D., Mo, T., and Green, A. E. S. (1974). Relationship of melanoma and other skin cancers to latitude and ultraviolet radiation in the United States and Canada. *Int. J. Epidemiol.* 3:325.

Fraumeni, J. K., and Mason, T. J. (1974). Cancer mortality among Chinese Americans, 1950–69. *J. Nat. Cancer Inst.* 52:659.

Gibson, J. B. (1971). *Parasites, Liver Disease and Liver Cancer*, p. 42. I.A.R.C. Scientific Publ. No. 1., Lyon.

Hashem, M. (1961). The aetiology and pathogenesis of bilharzial bladder cancer. *J. Egypt. Med. Assoc.* 44:857.

Hawksworth, G. M., and Hill, M. J. (1971). Bacteria and the N-nitrosation of secondary amines. *Brit. J. Cancer* 25:520.

Heath, C. M., Falk, H., and Creech, J. L. (1974). Characteristics of cases of angiosarcoma of the liver among vinyl chloride workers in the United States. *Annu. N.Y. Acad. Sci.* 246:231–236.

Henderson, B. E., Powell, D., Rosario, I., Keys, C., Hanisch, R., Young, M., Casagrande, J., Gerhms, V., and Pike, M. C. (1974). An epidemiologic study of breast cancer. *J. Nat. Cancer Inst.* 53:609.

Henle, W., Henle, G., Ho, H. C., Burtin, P. Cachin, Y. Clifford, P., DeSchryver, A., de Thé, Q., Diehl, V., Klein, G. (1970). Antibodies to Epstein–Barr virus in nasopharyngeal carcinoma. *J. Nat. Cancer Inst.* 44:225.

Herbst, A. L., Kurman, R. J., Scully, R. E., and Poskanzer, D. C. (1972). Clear cell adenocarcinoma of the genital tract in young females. *N. Engl. J. Med.* 287:1259.

Higginson, J., and Oettlé, A. G. (1960). Cancer incidence in the Bantu and cape coloured races of South Africa: Report of a cancer survey in the Transvaal (1953–55). *J. Nat. Cancer Inst.* 24:589.

Hill, M. J. (1971). The effect of some factors on the faecal concentration of acid steroids, neutral steroids and urobilins. *J. Pathol.* 104:239.

Hill, M. J., and Aries, V. C. (1971). Faecal steroid composition and its relationship to cancer of the large bowel. *J. Pathol.* 104:129.

Hill, M. J., Drasar, B. S., Aries, V. C., Crowther, J. S., Hawksworth, G. M. and Williams, R. E. O. (1971). Bacteria and aetiology of cancer of the large bowel. *Lancet* 1:95.

Hutt, M. S. R., Burkitt, D. P. (1965). Geographical distribution of cancer in East Africa. *Brit. Med. J.*, 2:719.

Hutt, M. S. R., and Templeton, A. C. (1971). The geographical pathology of bowel cancer and some related diseases. *Proc. R. Soc. Med.* 64:962.

International Journal of Cancer (1970). **6**:1–9.

James, P. D., Taylor, C. W., and Templeton, A. C. (1973). Tumours of the Female Genitalia. In *Tumours in a Tropical Country*. (A. C. Templeton, ed.), p. 101. Heinemann Medical Books, London.

Jussawalla, D. J., Deshpande, V. A., Haenszel, W., and Natekar, M. V. (1970). Differences observed in the site incidence of cancer between the Parsi Community and the total population of Greater Bombay. *Brit. J. Cancer* **24**:56.

Kafuko, G. W., and Burkitt, D. P. (1970). Burkitt's lymphoma and malaria. *Int. J. Cancer* **6**:1.

Keen, P., and Martin, P. (1971). Is aflatoxin carcinogenic in Man? The evidence in Swaziland. *Trop. Geogr. Med.* **23**:44.

Kmet, J., and Mahboubi, E. (1972). Oesophageal cancer in the Caspian Littoral of Iran. *Science* **175**:846.

Iversen, U., and Iversen, O. H. (1973). Tumours of the skin. In *Tumours in a Tropical Country* (A. C. Templeton, ed.), p. 180. Heinemann Medical Books, London.

Lawrence, J. C. (1936). Gastrointestinal polyps. *Amer. J. Surg.* **31**:499.

Lewis, M. G. (1967). Malignant melanoma in Uganda. *Brit. J. Cancer* **21**:483.

Liang, P. C., and Tung, C. (1959). Morphologic study and etiology of primary liver carcinoma and its incidence in China. *Chinese Med. J.* **79**:336.

Lin, J. J., Lin, C., and Svoboda, D. J. (1974). Long term effects of aflatoxin B_1 and viral hepatitis in marmosets. *Lab. Invest.* **30**:267.

Malhotra, S. L. (1971). A study of the uterine cervix with special reference to causation and prevention. *Brit. J. Cancer* **15**:62.

Matsudo, H., Hodgkin, N. M., and Tanaka, A. (1974). Japanese gastric cancer. Potentially carcinogenic silicates (talc) from rice. *Arch. Pathol.* **97**:366.

McMahon, B., Cole, P., Lin, T. M., Lowe, C. R., and Mirra, A. P. (1970). Age at first birth and breast cancer risk. *Bull. WHO* **43**:209.

Mole, R. H. (1974). Antenatal irradiation in childhood cancer. *Br. J. Cancer* **30**:199.

Morrow, R. H., Pike, M. C., Smith, P. G., Ziegler, J. L., and Kisuule, A. (1971). Burkitt's Lymphoma: A Time-space cluster of cases in Bwamba County of Uganda. *Br. Med. J.* **2**:491.

Muir, C. S., and Shanmugaratnam, K. eds. (1967). *Cancer of the Nasopharynx*, Vol. 1. UICC Monogr. Series, Munksgaard, Copenhagen.

Newberne, P. M., and Butler, W. H. (1969). Acute and chronic effects of aflatoxin on the liver of domestic and laboratory animals. *Cancer Res.* **29**:236.

Painter, N. S. (1964). The aetiology of diverticulosis of the colon with special reference to the action of certain drugs on the behaviour of the colon. *Ann. R. Coll. Surg. Eng.* **34**:98.

Painter, N. S. (1967). Diverticulosis of the colon—Fact and speculation. *Am. J. Dig. Dis.* **12**:222.

Payet, M. (1957). Primary cancer of the liver: Statistical anatomical and aetiological considerations. *Acta Un. Int. Cancer* **13**:860.

Payet, M., Saimot, G., Couland, J. P., et al. (1971). L'antigène Australie chez l'Africain. *Presse Méd.* **79**:52.

Paymaster, J. C. (1962). Some observations on oral and pharyngeal carcinomas in State of Bombay. *Cancer* **15**:578.

Peers, F. G., and Linsell, C. A. (1973). Dietary aflatoxins and liver cancer—A population based study in Kenya. *Br. J. Cancer* **27**:473.

Prates, M. D., and Torres, F. O. (1965). A cancer survey in Lourenço Marques, Portuguese East Africa. *J. Nat. Cancer Inst.* **35**:729.

Quinland, W. S., and Cuff, J. R. (1940). Primary carcinoma in the negro. *Arch. Pathol.* **30**:393.

Rappaport, H., Ramot, B., Hulu, N., and Park, J. K. (1972). The pathology of so-called Mediterranean abdominal lymphoma with malabsorption. *Cancer* **29**:1502.

Reddy, C. R. M. (1974). Carcinoma of the hard palate in India. *J. Nat. Cancer Inst.* **53**:609.

Robertson, N. A., Harington, J. S., and Bradshaw, E. (1971). The cancer pattern in Africans at Baragwanath Hospital, Johannesberg. *Br. J. Cancer* **25**:378.

Schmauz, R., and Jain, D. K. (1971). Geographical variations of carcinoma of the penis in Uganda. *Br. J. Cancer* **25**:25.

Shank, R. C., Bhamarapravati, N., Gordon, J. E., and Wogan, G. N., (1972). Dietary aflatoxins and human liver cancer. *Foods Cosmet. Toxicol.* **10**:171.

Shanmugaratnum, K., Muir, D. S., Tow, S. H., *et al.* (1971). Rates per 100,000 births and incidence of choriocarcinoma and malignant mole in Singapore Chinese and Malays. Comparisons with Connecticut, Norway and Sweden. *Int. J. Cancer* **8**:165.

Simons, M. J., Yu, M., Chew, B. K., Tan, A. Y. O., Yap, Y. E. H., Sea, C. S., Fung, W. P., and Shanmugaratnam, K. (1971). Australia antigen in Singapore Chinese patients with hepatocellular carcinoma. *Lancet* **1**:1149.

Siurala, M., Kekki, M., Varis, K., Isokoshi, M., and Ihmaki, T. (1972). Gastritis and Gastric Cancer. *Br. Med. J.* **3**:530.

Skinner, M. E. G. (1967). Malignant disease of the gastro-intestinal tract in the Rhodesian African. *Nat. Cancer Inst. Monogr.* **25**:57.

Steinitz, R. (1974). Communication to UICC Conference in Florence.

Stemmermann, G. N. (1970). Patterns of disease among Japanese living in Hawaii. *Arch. Environ. Health* **20**:266.

Stewart, A., Webb, J., and Hewitt, D., (1958). A survey of childhood malignancies. *Br. Med. J.* **1**:1495.

Tansurat, P. (1961). Cancer of the oral cavity and oesophagus in Thais and Chinese. *Acta Univ. Int. Cancer* **17**:877.

Templeton, A. C. (1967). Tumours of the eye and adnexa in Africans of Uganda. *Cancer* **20**:1689.

Templeton, A. C., and Bianchi, A. (1972). Bias in an African Registry. *Int. J. Cancer* **10**:186.

Templeton, A. C., Buxton, E., and Bianchi, A. (1972). Cancer in Kayadondo County, Uganda, 1968–1970. *J. Nat. Cancer Inst.* **48**:865.

Templeton, A. C., and Hutt, M. S. R. (1973). Distribution of tumours in Uganda. In *Tumour in a Tropical Country* (A. C. Templeton, ed.), p. 1. Heinemann Medical Books, London.

Tuyns, A. J. (1970). Cancer of oesophagus: Further evidence of the relation to drinking habits in France. *Int. J. Cancer* **5**:152.

Tuyns, A. J., and Massé, L. M. F. (1973). Mortality from cancer of the oesophagus in Brittany. *Int. J. Epidemiol.* **2**:241.

Urbach, F. (1969). Geographical pathology of skin cancer. In *The Biological Effects of Ultraviolet Irradiation* (F. Urbach, ed.). Pergamon Press, London.

Vogel, C. L., Anthony, P. P., Sadikali, F., Baker, L. F., and Peterson, M. R. (1972). Hepatitis-associated antigen and antibody in hepatocellular carcinoma. *J. Nat. Cancer Inst.* **48**:1583.

Wedderburn, N. (1970). Effect of concurrent malarial infection on development of virus-induced lymphoma in Balb/c mice. *Lancet* **2**:1114.

Wogan, G. N. (1966). Chemical nature and biological effects of aflatoxin. *Bacteriol. Rev.* **30**:460.

Wynder, E. L., Kajitani, T., Ishikawa, S., Dodo, H., and Takano, A. (1969). Environmental factors of cancer of the colon and rectum. *Cancer* **23**:1210.

Wynder, E. L., Lemon, F. R., and Bross, I. J. (1959). Cancer and coronary artery disease among Seventh-Day Adventists *Cancer* **12**:1016.

Chapter 10

ENDOCRINOLOGY

D. Y. WANG AND R. D. BULBROOK

Hormones and Neoplasia

Introduction

The possibility that humoral agents might control the growth of tumors was recognized as early as 1889 when Schinzinger suggested a relationship between ovarian function and breast cancer. It was not until 1896, however, that Beatson described the beneficial effects of oophorectomy in two patients with advanced breast cancer. Not for the first time, an observation of fundamental importance had been made by a practicing clinician on what would be considered today a totally inadequate number of patients. It was nearly 20 years later that basic biological work started in earnest. In 1916, Lathrop and Loeb demonstrated that oophorectomy reduced the incidence of breast cancer in a strain of mice that had a high spontaneous incidence of this disease. Murray (1928) reinforced this finding by reporting that in castrated male mice, mammary cancer could be induced by ovarian grafts. At this time vigorous work was going on in many laboratories to isolate and identify the ovarian hormones, culminating in the discovery of estrone by Doisy, Veler, and Thayer (1929) and Marrian's isolation of estriol in 1930. The new estrogens were available in minute amounts, but the French workers were able suddenly to produce relatively large quantities of estrone when Girard and Sandulesco (1936) devised a method for isolating methyl ketones. It was at last possible to investigate the role of the estrogens in mammary cancer using a pure standard hormone. Shortly afterwards, Lacassagne (1932) showed that the injection of estrone ben-

---

D. Y. Wang and R. D. Bulbrook • Department of Endocrinology, Imperial Cancer Research Fund Laboratories, Lincoln's Inn Fields, London, WC2A 3PX, England.

zoate into male mice led to the development of mammary tumors, and since this date literally hundreds of papers have appeared on the same subject. Such was the impact of these findings that investigation of the involvement of pituitary hormones in mammary carcinogenesis was relegated to a relatively minor role. One of the earliest indications of the importance of the pituitary gland was the demonstration by Kortweg and Thomas (1939) that the mammary cancer incidence in mice was diminished by hypophysectomy.

This early work established that hormones were of vital importance in the genesis of breast cancer, but the general impression was that once the malignant transformation had occurred, the process was irreversible and tumors were autonomous. In 1941, Huggins, Stevens, and Hodges published a study of human prostatic cancer. In their introduction they stated:

> All known types of adult prostatic epithelium undergo atrophy when androgenic hormones are greatly reduced in amount or inactivated. . . . Evidence is presented that significant improvement often occurs in the clinical condition of patients with far advanced cancer of the prostate after they have been subjected to castration. Conversely, the symptoms are aggravated when androgens are injected. We believe that this work provides a new concept of prostatic cancer.

From these findings the concept of hormone dependence was developed, where it was realized that all tumors are not necessarily autonomous but might retain some of the properties of the parent tissue from which they had developed. This concept was implicit in Beatson's findings of 1886. It was also obvious that some tumors were not hormone dependent and grew inexorably, whatever alterations were made in their hormonal milieu. With the passage of time, it was appreciated that regressions of tumors brought about by endocrine manipulations were invariably transient and the terms "hormone dependent" and "hormone independent" have been replaced by "hormone responsive" and "hormone unresponsive."

Finally, the introduction of adrenalectomy (Huggins and Bergenstal, 1952) and hypophysectomy (Luft and Olivecrona, 1953) for the treatment of breast and prostatic cancer followed as a logical consequence of the preceding results.

In this brief introduction there are two implied functions for the hormones. The first is their possible role as carcinogens; that is, as compounds that are directly responsible for the transformation of normal into malignant cells. It seems improbable that the hormones are true carcinogens in this sense. Their most likely function is to prepare the targets for such a transformation, either by simply increasing the number of cells at risk, or by altering irreversibly the biochemical processes in the target cells. Once a malignant transformation has taken place, the second function of the hormones is to act as mitogens, controlling the rate of cell division. In this role, the hormones may be very powerful agents, and while it may not be correct scientifically to think of the hormones as carcinogens, in operational terms such a concept may not be too far from the mark. This topic has been discussed extensively (Shimkin, 1957).

Hormones and Tumor Induction in Animals

The bulk of the evidence concerning the role of hormones in neoplasia has come from studies on laboratory animals. This evidence is outlined below for a variety of tumor sites.

Breast. As mentioned in the introduction, the close association between mammary tumorigenesis and ovarian hormones was established as early as 1916 by Lathrop and Loeb and reinforced by Murray in 1928. Blair *et al.* (1960) showed that the incidence of spontaneous mammary tumors in AC mice increased with the number of pregnancies. Thus, while in this strain virgin females rarely developed mammary tumors, the incidence ranged from 17 to 71% in mice that had had one to three litters, respectively. The prevention of suckling appeared to be protective; however, Mühlbock (1956) noted the opposite effect in that those mice permitted to lactate showed a considerably lower percentage of tumors.

There have been many confirmatory reports (see Noble, 1964) since the original report of Lacassagne (1932) of induction of mammary tumors in mice by prolonged administration of estrogen. These investigations show that certain strains of mice are more susceptible than others and that large doses of estrogen can give rise to a lower incidence and smaller tumors compared with mice given smaller quantities (Gardner, 1941). The induction of mammary tumors by the administration of estrogens appears to depend on the presence of mouse tumor virus, although there appear to be exceptions (Heston and Deringer, 1954; Mühlbock, 1956).

Prolonged administration of estrogens has resulted in mammary tumors in guinea pig (Podilcak, 1961) and in rats (Dunning and Curtis, 1952, 1954; Dunning *et al.*, 1949, 1950, 1951, 1953; Eisen, 1942; Geschickter, 1942; McEuen, 1938; Mackenzie, 1955; Mark and Biskind, 1941). As in mice, certain strains of rats were more susceptible to estrogen in producing tumors (Dunning *et al.*, 1953). Androgens have been reported to reduce the number of estrogen-induced tumors in mice (Heiman, 1944; Jones, 1941; Loeser, 1941; Nathanson and Andervont, 1939), while progesterone has been claimed to increase (Symeonidis, 1948), decrease (Heiman, 1945), or leave unaltered the incidence (Burrows and Hoch-Ligeti, 1946).

For more detailed information on hormonal tumorigenesis the reader is referred to the reviews of Bittner (1958), Bonser *et al.* (1961), Dmochowski (1953), Mühlbock (1956), and Shimkin (1945).

There have been many studies on the hormonal factors governing the growth of established tumors in laboratory animals. Foulds (1947, 1949a,b) studied the effect of repeated pregnancies on the growth of spontaneous mammary tumors in mice. He observed that on the basis of their growth behavior tumors could be divided into two categories. One category which he termed "unresponsive tumors," grew steadily irrespective of pregnancy. The other type, the so-called "responsive tumors," were influenced by pregnancy; these grew during pregnancy and ceased growing or regressed after parturition. This pattern was repeated in subsequent pregnancies. Foulds observed also that responsive tumors could become hormonally unresponsive. This transformation was unpredictable and did not relate to growth, size, or duration of the tumor. Also, progression of a tumor from a responsive to nonresponsive state occurred independently of other tumors in the same animal. Foulds observed also that responsive tumors were transplantable only in female hosts whereas unresponsive tumors could be transplanted into either male or female hosts.

Similar results have been obtained in the rat using transplantable mammary fibroadenomas. An increased growth of these tumors was observed during pregnancy, and growth ceased after parturition. It was noted also that successful transplantation occurred only in female rats, but that after successive transplantations this sex difference was abolished as the tumor became autonomous (Emge, 1934; Emge and Murphy, 1938; Grauer and Robinson, 1932; Heiman and Krehbiel, 1936; Millar and Noble, 1954a).

Inhibition of growth of transplanted mammary tumors in rats has been observed after the administration of either androgens or high amounts of estrogens (Glenn et al., 1959a, 1959b, 1960; Huggins and Mainzer, 1957; Huggins et al., 1958; Millar and Noble, 1954b). However, the growth of some spontaneous tumors has been observed to be stimulated by testosterone (Dunning, 1960).

The dimethylbenzanthracene (DMBA)-induced mammary tumor in the Sprague–Dawley rat has proved to be an interesting model system. Pearson and his colleagues (1969) have carried out a series of elegant experiments which implicate prolactin as the hormone responsible for the maintenance and growth of mammary tumors. They have shown that the effects of estrogen on tumor growth are mediated by stimulating prolactin release. Administration of estrogen to a hypophysectomized tumor-bearing rat did not prevent tumor regression. The evidence that prolactin production by pituitary isografts or prolactin administration results in an increased incidence of mammary tumors in mice supports this view (Boot, 1970; Mühlbock and Boot, 1959). A recent finding is that progesterone acts synergistically with prolactin in causing tumor growth (Röpcke and Boot, 1972).

There is further circumstantial evidence concerning the importance of prolactin. For example, the incidence of tumors after DMBA treatment is dependent upon the endogenous level of prolactin (Boyns *et al.*, 1973a). Canine mammary cancers are associated with increased pituitary prolactin levels (Saluja *et al.*, 1974).

In flat contradiction to these findings are the observations of Hilf *et al.* (1971) who showed that administration of fluphenazine to rats bearing the R 3230 AC tumor (a treatment that should increase prolactin secretion; Turkington, 1972) led to rapid breast growth and tumor regression. Also, increased prolactin levels before administration of DMBA appear to be protective against mammary tumors (see Gala and Loginsky, 1973).

Finally, measurements of the actual peripheral concentrations of prolactin brought about by various endocrine manipulations might help to clarify the situation. In some cases, one might expect levels of prolactin to be several hundred times higher than normal and this may not be a useful model system.

Pituitary Gland. Prolonged treatment of rats and mice with estrogen results in an initial hypertrophy of the anterior lobe of the pituitary gland and eventually in the appearance of chromophobe adenomas (Burrows, 1936; Cramer and Horning, 1936; Zondek, 1936). Reduction of thyroid activity and increased TSH release have also been claimed to induce such tumors (Gorbman, 1949). Griesbach and Purves (1960) reported that gonadectomy in rats resulted in basophil adenomas. It has been reported that androgens protect against estrogen-induced pituitary tumors in rats, but the role of progesterone is not clear since it has been claimed that this steroid may either protect against or enhance the effect of estrogens (Albert and Selye, 1942; Segaloff and Dunning, 1945; Selye, 1940, 1944).

Thyroid Gland. Treatment with antithyroid drugs or prolonged iodine deficiency has been reported to result in thyroid adenomas or adenocarcinoma in the rat, mouse, and hamster (Axelrad and LeBlond, 1955; Bielschowsky, 1953; Fortner *et al.*, 1960; Isler *et al.*, 1958; Leiken *et al.*, 1952; Napalkov, 1959; Purves and Greisbach, 1946, 1947). The administration of goitrogens to rats is also associated with an increased incidence of thyroid tumors and so is the transplantation of TSH-producing pituitary tumors (Greisbach *et al.*, 1945; Furth and Clifton, 1958; Harran-Ghera *et al.*, 1960).

Adrenal Gland. Castration in mice (Smith *et al.*, 1949) or prolonged treatment with growth hormone (Moon *et al.*, 1950) have been claimed to produce tumors of the adrenal medulla. Adrenocortical tumors have been found to follow gonadectomy in mice, rats, guinea pigs, and hamsters (Gardner, 1953; Smith *et al.*, 1949). These tumors were frequently accompanied by growth of mammary tumors (Woolley and Little, 1946). Administration of androgens or estrogens may prevent the induction of adrenal tumors by gonadectomy; and ovarian transplants inhibit the formation of carcinomas from adrenal adenomas (Tullos *et al.*, 1961).

Ovary. Ovarian tumors have been induced in rats and mice by transplanting the ovaries in such a way that the venous return enters the portal system (Biskind and Biskind, 1944, 1945). The rationale underlying this procedure is that hepatic metabolism results in a deficiency of circulating estrogen and hence an increased gonadotrophin production (Gardner, 1961). The administration of antigonadotrophic serum has been claimed to prevent tumor formation (Ely, 1956). However, estrogens themselves may also induce ovarian tumors since the administration of stilbestrol resulted in ovarian tumor development in seven out of eight dogs (Jabara, 1959, 1962). The hormonal responsiveness of ovarian tumor transplants appears to be variable since the growth of such tumors has been claimed to be stimulated by androgens, estrogens, or progestins, although gonadotrophins appear to be ineffective (Bern *et al.*, 1958; Clifton, 1959; Clifton and Pan, 1948; Gardner, 1958; Green, 1956; Mühlbock *et al.*, 1958). Also, hypo- or hyperthyroidism or hypophysectomy inhibited the successful formation of tumors from such transplants (Gardner, 1958; Fels and Foglia, 1960 a,b; Kullander, 1956). Gasparri (1958) noted an interesting relationship between hysterectomy and the subsequent incidence of ovarian cancer. He studied 358 women who had undergone hysterectomy for benign uterine conditions where one or both ovaries were preserved. Of 22 cases in which he was able to examine the ovaries, carcinoma was found subsequently in ten, and nine had benign tumors or cysts.

Uterus. Tumors of the uterine cervix have been reported in mice treated with estrogens (Allen and Gardner, 1941; Franks, 1958; Gardner and Allen, 1939; Pan and Gardner, 1948; Suntzeff *et al.*, 1938), although the rat and rabbit appear to be less susceptible to estrogen-induced cervical cancer (Loeb, 1948; McEuen, 1938; Pierson, 1937). The concurrent administration of androgens does not appear to be protective (Gardner and Allen, 1939).

Chronic estrogen administration and estrogen implanted directly into the uterus of guinea pigs or rabbits have resulted in fibromas of the uterine body (Lipschutz, 1950, 1957; Lipschutz and Vargus, 1941; Meissner *et al.*, 1957; Podilcak, 1959). The induction of these tumors has been claimed to be inhibited by administering progesterone, deoxycorticosterone or testosterone (Lipschutz *et al.*, 1939; Mardones *et al.*, 1954). The administration of testosterone to mice has resulted in the occurrence of metastatic uterine tumors (Homburger *et al.*, 1957; Van Nie *et al.*, 1961). Hamster uterine cancers have been reported after treatment with testosterone and stilbestrol combined (although not if given singly) (Kirkman, 1957; Rivière *et al.*, 1960). Some strains of rabbit have particularly high incidences (75%) of spontaneous uterine tumors which in some cases are metastatic (Burrows, 1940; Burrows and Boyland, 1938; Greene, 1941; Greene and Newton, 1948). Such spontaneous tumors have been found to be associated with mammary gland hyperplasia or cancer, and may indicate estrogenization (Greene and Newton, 1948; Greene et al., 1947; Selye, 1940).

Other Tumors. The chronic administration of estrogen to certain strains of mice has resulted in the appearance of vaginal (Gardner, 1959) and testicular tumors. In the latter case, gonadotrophins have been implicated since antiserum in gonadotrophins may prevent induction of the tumor (Ely, 1953). Progesterone has also been claimed to retard the induction of testicular tumors (Andervont et al., 1960). It is of interest that spontaneous testicular tumors in mice or rats have been observed to be associated with mammary and pituitary tumors (Athias, 1945; Athias and Furtado Dias, 1941; Guérin, 1954). The hormonal induction of prostatic tumors has proved difficult and the dog appears to be the only species, other than man, in which spontaneous cancers occur to any great extent (Roth, 1939; Schlotthauer and Millar, 1941).

Hormonal imbalance has also been reported to produce tumors in a variety of nonendocrine tissues. Thus, estrogen treatment resulted in hepatomas in mice (Schenken and Burns, 1943), kidney cancers in hamsters (Horning, 1954, 1956a,b; Horning and Whittick, 1954; Jolles, 1962; Kirkman, 1957, 1959; Kirkman and Bacon, 1950, 1952a,b; Matthews et al., 1947), bladder cancer and papillomas in rats (Angrist et al., 1960; Dunning et al., 1947), and lymphoid tumors in mice (Bischoff et al., 1942a,b; Gardner, 1937, 1942; Gardner and Dougherty, 1944; Gardner et al., 1944; Gardner et al., 1940; Lacassagne, 1937; McEndy et al., 1944; Murphy and Sturm, 1944; Shimkin and Wyman, 1946; Silberg and Silberg, 1945, 1949). Hepatomas in rats can be induced also by treating alternately with estrogen and androgen (Konoplev, 1959). The administration of estrogen together with testosterone, deoxycorticosterone, or progesterone has been claimed to prevent kidney tumors (Horning, 1954, 1956a,b; Horning and Whittick, 1954; Jolles, 1962; Kirkman, 1957, 1959; Kirkman and Bacon, 1950, 1952a,b; Matthews et al., 1947). Testosterone and cortisone have also been claimed to decrease the incidence of spontaneous or transplanted lymphoid tumors, while adrenalectomy increased it (Gardner et al., 1944; Heilman and Kendall, 1944; Kaplan et al., 1951; Law, 1948; Murphy and Sturm, 1949; Rudali et al., 1959; Woolley, 1951). For a more complete review of this subject the reader is referred to the excellent review of Noble (1964).

General Conclusions Concerning Hormones and Tumor Induction in Animals. There can be no possible doubt that alterations of the hormonal milieu in the majority of species of laboratory animals lead to an increased incidence of tumors of the breast, pituitary, thyroid, adrenal gland, ovary, cervix uteri, endometrium, testis, vagina, and a variety of other tissues.

Two important principles emerge from experimental data described above. The first is the generalization that "hormonal imbalance" is the common factor leading to carcinogenesis in animals in a wide variety of sites. The second was put forward by Hertz (1968) as follows:

All known carcinogenic agents for man have been shown to be also carcinogenic in animals and frequently in the same site. Hence common pathogenic factors are clearly involved in the development of cancer in man and in animals.

With the clues provided by the work with laboratory animals and with these principles in mind, we should now look at analogous situations in man.

Hormone Imbalance and Neoplasia in Man

Induced Imbalance. It is ethically impossible to induce experimentally in man conditions of gross hormonal imbalance, so the only source of evidence is derived from what might be termed adventitious data.

The effects of administration of steroid hormones (or stilbestrol) and pituitary hormones on the incidence of various cancers in man are summarized in Table 1. It is apparent immediately that steroidal hormones are remarkably poor "carcinogens" in these situations. Where there is an increase in incidence, it is so small that the patients can probably be numbered in tens: The decrease in incidence outweighs this by several orders. Even where tumors are induced, they occur only in bizarre circumstances.

As far as pituitary hormones are concerned, there is little evidence for a strong effect, even from drugs known to produce very large increases in the concentration of prolactin in the plasma. The results given in Tables 1, however, should be considered with caution since many of them were derived from retrospective studies, often without proper controls, or from very small series of patients in which only a catastrophic carcinogenic effect would have been detected. Furthermore, the subjects in whom hormonal imbalance was induced can hardly be considered as a representative sample of the normal population (with the exception of the studies on the women using steroidal contraceptives). Induced hormonal imbalance appears to be an effective method for tumor induction in many species of nonprimates and an extremely weak factor in monkeys and in man. The reasons for this discrepancy may be concerned with the fact that in many of the experiments with animals the degree of imbalance induced was of great severity whereas in man, imbalance might be almost within the normal range.

Endogenous Hormones and Neoplasia in Man. The question now arises about the role of endogenous hormone production and the induction of neoplasia in man. As far as breast cancer is concerned the results derived

TABLE 1. Induction of Cancers by Hormone Imbalance in Man

Agent	Subjects	Tumor site and effect on incidence	References
Steroid hormones			
Estrogen	Women with menopausal symptoms	Incidence of breast cancer lowered	Wallach and Henneman (1959); Wilson and Brevetti (1963)
Estrogen	Women with osteoporosis	Incidence of breast cancer lowered	Mustacchi and Gordon (1958).
Stilbestrol	Pregnant women with threatened abortion	Vaginal cancer in daughters	Herbst et al. (1971); Greenwald et al. (1973).
Estrogen	Gonadal dysgenesis	Endometrium	Cutler et al. (1972)
Estrogen	Male transvestites	Breast cancer	Symmers (1968)
Estrogen	Men with prostatic cancer	Breast cancer?	Graves and Harris (1952)
Estrogen	Pregnant women	Clear cell adenoma of cervix in daughters	Noller et al. (1972)
Contraceptive steroids	Normal premenopausal women	Protective against benign breast disease Protective against breast cancer?	Vessey et al. (1971, 1972a,b)
Pituitary hormones			
Phenothiazine	Women in mental hospitals	Breast cancer incidence doubled?	Ettigi et al. (1973).
Tranquilizers?	Women in mental hospitals	No change in breast cancer incidence	Katz et al. (1967)
Reserpine	Hypertensives	Breast cancer incidence doubled	Boston Collaborative Drug Surveillance Program (1974); Armstrong et al. (1974); Heinonen et al. (1974).
Antihypertensive agents other than reserpine	Hypertensives	No effect on breast cancer incidence	Boston Collaborative Drug Surveillance Program (1974); Armstrong et al. (1974); Heinonen et al. (1974).

from investigations in laboratory animals indicate that the ovarian hormones and prolactin are of prime importance, and from the late 1950's, great efforts were made to determine the estrogenic status in patients with the disease. In 1971, when methods became available for the determination of prolactin in plasma, attention was focused on this hormone (Bryant *et al.*, 1971; Guyda *et al.*, 1971; Jacobs *et al.*, 1971). The results of these and other studies are summarized below.

Urinary and Blood Estrogens. Measurements of the amounts of estrone, estradiol, and estriol excreted in the urine by women with breast cancer have led to contradictory results. It has been variously reported that the urinary estrogens in such patients are higher than (Brown, 1958; Nissen-Meyer and Sanner, 1963), the same as (Hellman *et al.*, 1967; Jull *et al.*, 1963), or lower than (Bacigalupo and Schubert, 1966; Lemon *et al.*, 1966; Schweppe *et al.*, 1967) those of normal women.

New methods for the determination of blood estrone and estradiol have not led to any clarification of the situation. Using single plasma specimens, Wang and Swain (1974) found no abnormalities in plasma estrone and estradiol levels in patients with breast cancer at the time of mastectomy. On the other hand, Skinner *et al.* (1974), who have taken serial samples of blood throughout complete menstrual cycles, claim there have been patients whose blood estrogen levels are raised significantly.

When all the results are considered, they do not support the concept that an increased secretion and raised blood level of estrogens is a factor in the etiology of human breast cancer. There has been some reluctance to accept these unpalatable experimental findings in man in view of the evidence from early work on animal models. However, the thesis that an increased secretion of ovarian hormones (or of adrenal precursors of plasma estrogens) is important in the development of malignancy is not in accord with the data shown in Table 1. Administration of relatively large amounts of estrogens to both pre- and postmenopausal women has not led to a discernible increase in breast cancer and, in some instances, may have led to a decrease in incidence (Vessey *et al.*, 1971, 1972a,b).

Prolactin. The first study on prolactin levels in the plasma of women with breast cancer and controls indicated that the plasma levels were elevated (Murray *et al.*, 1972). This finding was not confirmed in three subsequent studies (Boyns *et al.*, 1973a; Franks *et al.*, 1974; Mittra *et al.*, 1974); but a recent abstract from workers in Australia describes again a moderate elevation of prolactin levels in breast cancer patients (Murray and Sarfaty, 1974). Stimulation tests using TRF showed no convincing differences between patients and controls.

Epidemiological findings that pregnancy at an early age affords lifelong protection against breast cancer (MacMahon *et al.*, 1970a), and that the incidence of the disease is low in countries where prolonged lactation occurs (MacMahon *et al.*, 1970b) are hard to reconcile with the concept that prolactin is "carcinogenic," since in both situations elevated blood prolactin concentrations would be found. In the established disease, prolactin does not maintain or promote the growth of tumors since stalk section, which leads to a large increase in the circulatory concentration of prolactin, may lead to remission (Bowers *et al.*, 1971; Ehni and Eckles, 1959). Conversely, inhibition of prolactin release with ergot alkaloids (Besser and Edwards, 1972) is not effective in the treatment of advanced breast cancer (EORTC Breast Cancer Group, 1972).

It has also been reported that pregnancy following mastectomy may delay recurrence of the disease (Bond, 1967; Peters, 1968).

Gonadotrophins. Studies on the possible relationship between gonadotrophin excretion and response to treatment of breast cancer in postmenopausal women have led to equivocal results. Loraine, Strong, and Douglas (1957) studied 47 women with advanced breast cancer before treatment with stilbestrol. They reported that patients classified as "worse" after treatment had a higher mean level of excretion than that of the remainder of the group, or of 37 women with noncancerous diseases. Boyland *et al.*, in 1958, supported this claim by observing that high concentrations of urinary gonadotrophins were found in patients not responding to pituitary gland irradiation. However, the results of the studies of Segaloff *et al.* (1954) were in disagreement with the latter conclusions. Hayward, Bulbrook, and Greenwood (1961) estimated urinary gonadotrophins in 41 patients with advanced breast cancer and found no significant differences between patients who were responsive or nonresponsive to adrenalectomy or hypophysectomy; they did, however, observe that responsive patients tended to have higher gonadotrophin excretion. But Martin (1964) observed that women who responded to endocrine therapy had significantly lower gonadotrophin excretion. Beck *et al.* (1966) were unable to correlate gonadotrophin excretion with response to treatment because of the large between-patient variation which may well explain the divergence in results described above. Results in this laboratory from measurements of blood concentrations of LH and FSH revealed no significant differences between these levels in postmenopausal women with breast cancer and normal healthy controls.

Thyroid Hormones. There have been various reports over the years relating thyroid function and breast cancer. In 1952, Repert reported that the incidence of thyroid disease was ten times greater than expected in 305 women with breast cancer. Subsequently, Loeser (1954) and Wynder, Bross, and Hirayama (1960) published results in accord with those of Repert. These authors observed that breast cancer was more common in hypothyroid patients and that hyperthyroidism was more prevalent in a control group of women compared with women with breast cancer.

Epidemiological studies have also revealed a possible thyroid-linked reason for differences in incidence of breast cancer. Bulbrook, Thomas, and Utsunomiya (1964) and Bulbrook *et al.* (1967) found evidence from the pattern of urinary androgen metabolites that normal Japanese women may have a greater thyroid activity than normal British women, the latter having a much higher incidence of breast cancer.

In the established disease it has been reported that thyroid function appears to be normal in women with breast cancer in its early stages, but a decreased thyroid function and increased serum PBI occurs in the advanced disease (Carter *et al.*, 1960; Edelstyn *et al.*, 1958). Sommers (1955) reported histological evidence that thyroid atrophy may occur in patients with disseminated breast cancer. More recently, Mittra and Hayward (1974) have reported a significant increase in plasma TSH concentrations in women with both early and advanced breast cancer. The latter paper also reviews the epidemiological evidence for the involvement of thyroid function in the etiology of breast cancer.

Incidentally, it is of interest to note that the releasing factor (TRH) responsible for controlling TSH release also stimulates pituitary prolactin release (Bowers *et al.*, 1971). Thus, some patients with primary hypothyroidism also suffer from galactorrhea (Bayliss and Van't Hoff, 1969).

It is possible to overcome the latter by treatment with ergot alkaloids which act, presumably, by preventing or reducing prolactin secretion (Besser and Edwards, 1972; Forsyth *et al.*, 1971).

Androgens and Corticoids. The most intensively examined hormones in breast cancer studies are probably the urinary metabolites of ^{19}C neutral steroids. In regard to women with advanced metastatic breast cancer, there is general agreement that the amount of 11-deoxy-17-oxosteroids (11-DKS) excreted in the urine is lower than in normal women (Bulbrook *et al.*, 1962a; Juret, 1968; Kumaoka *et al.*, 1968; Marmorston, 1966). Cameron *et al.* (1970) found that this was true for women with locally advanced disease but not for patients with distant metastases. Similarly, results have been observed for the blood concentration of 11-DKS (Brownsey *et al.*, 1972; Deshpande *et al.*, 1965; Wang, 1969; Wang *et al.*, 1974).

There is some controversy as to the relative level of excretion of urinary 11-DKS in the early disease (around the time of mastectomy). Bulbrook *et al.* (1962b) found a subnormal excretion of androgen metabolites in women 10 days after mastectomy, an observation which was subsequently confirmed by other workers (Bacigalupo and Lingk, 1968; Gutierrez and Williams, 1968; Marmorston, 1966), although Cameron *et al.* (1970) were unable to detect such a difference in their study. The confusion probably arises from the time at which urine samples are taken, since the urinary levels of 11-DKS are significantly higher 1 day before mastectomy than 10 days after operation. Similar findings have been observed for circulating levels of plasma 11-DKS (Wang *et al.,* 1974). The reason for this difference between pre- and postoperative patients is unknown. However, it should be borne in mind that from the time a diagnosis of breast cancer is made, a number of uncontrolled variables affect the results of any investigations made on the endocrine status of such patients. Among these are emotional stresses and the effects of surgery (Chou and Wang, 1939; Hardy *et al.,* 1953; Katz *et al.,* 1970; Tanaka *et al.,* 1970; Thorn *et al.,* 1953; Zumoff *et al.,* 1971).

To complicate the situation still further, it has been suggested that the androgen levels are mainly important in their relationship with corticosteroids, and that a subnormal androgen excretion is part of a syndrome including a raised corticosteroid production (see Saez, 1971). Deshpande *et al.* (1967) have claimed that abnormalities in the relative secretion rates of androgens and cortisol, and hence abnormalities in plasma and urinary levels, can be traced back to abnormalities in adrenal steroidogenesis.

Summary of Results of Measurements of Hormonal Status in Patients with Breast Cancer. One of the aims of the work described above was an attempt to delineate an abnormal endocrine profile in patients with breast cancer in the hope that the abnormalities might have preceded the clinical appearance of the disease and might, therefore, provide clues concerning etiology. For example, if plasma and urinary estrogen levels had been found to be consistently raised in patients, it would have been a reasonable assumption that the same abnormality had existed for some years before diagnosis and was an important factor in the genesis of the disease in man, as it appears to be in rodents.

With the exception of the subnormal androgen production, in patients with breast cancer, no convincing abnormalities in endocrine function have been consistently demonstrated. The tentative conclusion is that if endocrine abnormalities are important, they must have occurred many years before the tumor was found.

Endogenous Hormones in Cancers other than of the Breast. We have detailed the increase in the incidence of cancers of the pituitary, ovaries, uterus, etc. which follow endocrine imbalance in laboratory animals and have described the sporadic occurrence of tumors of the vagina, endometrium, and cervix uteri in women in whom imbalance has been induced. The literature on endogenous hormone secretion in patients with endocrine-related tumors other than breast is sparse. The reader is referred to work by De Waard *et al.* (1968), Grattarola (1970, 1972), and Brush *et al.* (1974) on endometrial cancer and Marmorston *et al.* (1965), Bulbrook *et al.* (1956), Kent and Young (1964), Young and Kent (1968), and Farnsworth (1971) on prostatic cancer.

Prospective Studies. The so-called protective effects of a first pregnancy below the age of 25 indicate that early events have a profound influence on the subsequent incidence of breast carcinoma. There are great difficulties in the interpretation of studies on patients when a tumor has been diagnosed, since so many extraneous variables may affect hormone production. The ideal solution to these difficulties would be to carry out prospective studies in which endocrine function is measured in a young normal population who would then be followed-up for the next 30 years to see whether the incidence of a particular cancer correlated with previous endocrine function.

Two prospective studies have been carried out. The first of these was started in 1961 in the Island of Guernsey. Urine specimens were collected from 5,000 normal women. Urinary androgen and corticosteroid metabolites were measured in women who subsequently developed breast carcinoma and in appropriate controls. Current results indicate that a subnormal excretion of androgen metabolites is associated with an increased risk of breast carcinoma and that this abnormality may precede the clinical appearance of the disease by up to 9 years (Bulbrook et al., 1971).

Another prospective study in Holland, the so-called "Kamperfoelie project" (which is translated as "Honeysuckle"), was commenced in 1964. At present over 7,000 postmenopausal women have volunteered and have been followed-up for an average of 5.4 years. The study was to test the hypothesis that altered hormonal homeostasis, related to overnutrition, is the major determinant in the majority of postmenopausal patients who developed breast cancer. This hypothesis was based on the observations that breast cancer patients tend to be more overweight than normal women, and that there is a higher frequency of estrogenic smears in women who are obese, hypertensive, or diabetic. These smears were obtained from the urinary sediment and show reactions to estrogenic stimuli that are very similar to vaginal smears (De Waard and Halewijn, 1969). The results of this study so far indicate that the greatest risk of breast cancer results in the tallest and heaviest women (De Waard and Halewijn, 1974).

The conclusion from the Dutch and British prospective trials is that hormonal abnormalities do precede the onset of breast cancer. Whether these aberrations are causal or are reflections of other changes which are responsible for mammary tumorigenesis is unknown.

Epidemiological Results. Epidemiological studies with respect to breast cancer have been brilliantly reviewed by MacMahon, Cole, and Brown (1973), and these studies provide persuasive evidence that ovarian function is an important factor in the etiology of breast cancer. Early menarche and late menopause are associated with increased risk. Oophorectomy is associated with diminished risk. However, if these risk factors are related to ovarian hormone production, it is difficult to see why early pregnancy is protective.

Cole and MacMahon (1969) have attempted to resolve this paradox by postulating that estriol, which is produced in large amounts during pregnancy, is protective. Lemon (1969) had already claimed that the ratio of estrone and estradiol was lower in patients with breast cancer than in controls and had suggested that estriol might block the action of estradiol. Estriol apparently blocks the tumorigenic effect of DMBA in Sprague–Dawley rats (Terenius, 1971).

Measurements of urinary estrogen metabolites have shown that young Japanese women excrete relatively more estriol than comparable North American women. This finding is supported by other studies. Gross (1973) studied European and Yemenite women in Israel and Briggs (1972) studied African, European, and Indian women in Lusaka, Zambia. In both cases the higher estriol ratios were found in the groups with lower risk of breast cancer. In a more recent study, MacMahon et al. (1974) extended their findings by reporting essentially similar results for European women from Boston and Vancouver, and Asian women from Hong Kong, Taipei, and Shirakawa Gifu (Japan). Lastly, MacMahon and his colleagues (1970a) have shown that the protective effect of pregnancy is age related; thus women who have had their first child before the age of 20 have only about one-third of the risk of women who are either nulliparous or who have had their first child after the age of 35. They suggest that the protective effect is conferred by high estriol levels since urinary estriol increases dramatically during pregnancy. This particular suggestion needs to be viewed with caution since, for example, estradiol constitutes about 50% of unconjugated estrogens in maternal blood from the first trimester to full term, estriol contributing about 25%. On the other hand, about 78% of unconjugated estrogens in fetal plasma is accounted for by estriol (Shutt et al., 1974). Despite a very high ratio of estriol, newborn children can exhibit marked signs of mammary gland development, which suggests that in this particular instance estriol is not impeding the action of mammotrophic hormones. Another reservation about this theory is, as previously mentioned, that oral contraceptives have not increased the incidence of breast cancer, although Hertz (1968) comments on the latent period and that the age at which women commence taking oral contraceptives should be borne in mind.

A review of epidemiological findings has been published for endometrial cancer (MacMahon, 1974).

Hormones and Treatment

The results obtained when patients with hormone-related tumors are treated either by administration of hormones or by removal or destruction of endocrine organs have been reviewed extensively elsewhere (Hayward, 1970; Stoll, 1972; Heuson, 1974). In the following sections a brief summary of the major findings is given, together with the results obtained with some of the newer treatments. The main interest here is what information can be obtained about the basic biology of hormone-related cancers from the results of various therapies.

Breast Cancer

Androgens. In 1939, Lacassagne and Raynaud, and Nathanson and Andervont showed that testosterone propionate diminished the incidence of breast cancer in R3 and C3H mice. The compound was used clinically in the same year (Loeser, 1939; Ulrich, 1939), and subsequently massive trials have established the usefulness of androgen therapy in bringing about remissions in patients with advanced breast cancer. The overall remission rate is about 20%.

Estrogens. In 1941, Huggins and Hodges showed that diethylstibestrol might be a useful compound for the treatment of prostatic cancer. This finding, coupled with experimental data showing that hydrocarbon derivatives of the ethylene series inhibited the growth of the Walker 256 tumor in the rat led Haddow and his colleagues (1944) to test the clinical usefulness of synthetic estrogens in postmenopausal patients with advanced breast cancer. The beneficial effects of these treatments have been shown repeatedly, and an overall result in 1,037 patients gave an objective remission rate of 30%.

Progestins. Early reports on the usefulness of progestational agents yielded conflicting results (in some cases no remissions were found), but the introduction of more powerful agents such as norethisterone and norethynodrel have led to reports of remission rates of the same order as those found for the androgens.

Corticosteroids. Corticosteroids were first given to answer the question as to whether the replacement doses used after adrenalectomy or hypophysectomy played any part in inducing remissions of the disease. Later they were administered in the hope that their effects on adrenal suppression would be strong enough to effect a "medical adrenalectomy." As with the progestins, there are conflicting reports on their usefulness. Much of the confusion probably stems from the fact the dose appears to be critical. Remission rates vary from 0% to 21%. In 392 patients from six series the average was 8%.

Oophorectomy. Nissen-Meyer reviewed the literature in 1965 and reported that some 30% of 2,221 patients with metastatic breast cancer treated by oophorectomy obtained an objective remission of their disease. Additional treatment with thyroid hormone does not appear to increase the remission rate (O'Bryan *et al.*, 1974) and there is doubt about the use of corticosteroids (Nissen-Meyer and Vogt, 1961; Meakin *et al.*, 1974).

There is controversy over the benefits of prophylactic oophorectomy carried out at the time of mastectomy. Nissen-Meyer (1967) and Cole (1968) found it a useful therapy: Ravdin *et al.* (1970) did not. Similarly, oophorectomy in postmenopausal women rarely causes remission (Barlow *et al.*, 1969) but Nissen-Meyer (1967) disagrees.

Adrenalectomy and Hypophysectomy. Many series have been reported. The remission rate is about 30%. It has been claimed that the remission rate is increased if the operations are carried out at the first signs of recurrence (Dao and Nemoto, 1965), but no additional benefit was found by Atkins *et al.* (1966).

A controversial question is whether hypophysectomy carries a higher remission rate than adrenalectomy. Hayward *et al.* (1970) found hypophysectomy superior to adrenalectomy (in a controlled clinical trial). Retrospective investigations from a wide variety of centers showed no difference between the operations (Joint Committee on Endocrine Ablative Procedures, 1961).

Recent Treatments. Five new drugs used in the treatment of breast cancer should be mentioned. The first of these is CB154 (2-*Br*-α-ergocryptine), an antiprolactin agent. This compound lowers but does not abolish plasma prolactin. It appears to be ineffective in the treatment of advanced breast cancer (EORTC Breast Cancer Group, 1972), but further trials would be desirable.

A second drug that inhibits prolactin secretion is L-dopa. There are reports that objective remissions can be obtained (Murray *et al.*, 1972; Frantz *et al.*, 1973), but other workers have not confirmed these findings (Engelsman *et al.*, 1974). The antiprolactin drugs have been disappointing thus far, but until prolactin levels are reduced to zero by specific antiprolactin agents, it is impossible to know whether the existing compounds are ineffective because of their inefficiency in accomplishing this, or because abolition of production alone is not sufficient to induce remission.

Two antiestrogens have been tried, with encouraging results. These are tamoxifen (ICI 46474) and nafoxidine (U 11 100A). The former led to objective remissions in 36 of 114 patients (32%) and the latter in 35 of 114 patients (31%). Tamoxifen is reported to have remarkably few side effects (Heuson, 1974).

Finally, an interesting new compound is calusterone (17β, 17α-dimethyltestosterone) which is claimed to be the most effective antitumor steroid thus far identified (Gordon *et al.*, 1973). However, Falkson *et al.* (1974) have severe reservations about its clinical use.

Summary and Conclusions. In spite of decades of intensive work in searching for new agents for administrative therapy, for new techniques for the removal or destruction of endocrine glands, or in the use of combinations of hormonal agents (such as estrogen combined with progesterone) it has not been possible to increase the objective remission rate much above 30%. Expectation of life following various forms of endocrine therapy has also remained constant. The inescapable conclusion is that only some 30% of patients with advanced metastatic breast cancer have tumors that are responsive to endocrine manipulations.

The mechanism whereby hormonal treatment brings about regressions of tumors in the breast remains a mystery. These can be induced by androgen, estrogens, progestin, corticoids, or by removal of the glands producing these hormones. Some patients may have a remission following treatment and, upon relapse, may enjoy another remission from a different endocrine treatment. Cases have been documented where objective remission occurs after withdrawal of a hormonal agent. The simple concept that these treatments are effective in that they remove estrogen from the circulatory blood will not hold. Remissions have been reported in patients whose estrogen production is almost zero, and remissions have been noted in patients who continue to produce estrogen after endocrine ablation. Additive therapy with large doses of estrogens is also effective.

Similarly, stalk section of the pituitary may bring about remissions in spite of causing a large increase in prolactin secretion.

The complexity of the mechanism of hormone action at the biochemical level is admirably described by McKerns (1974). The probability is that until more is known about this subject, we shall remain in ignorance about the basic physiological processes that occur when a widely disseminated breast cancer rapidly regresses following treatment.

One of the most urgent problems in the field of endocrine therapy is the need to find methods for the selection of responsive patients. This subject has recently been reviewed (Bulbrook, 1974). A most promising test appears to be the measurement of estrogen receptor sites within the tumors. In the hands of Sarfaty et al. (1973), measurements of urinary androgen and corticosteroid metabolites appear to provide an estimate of the probability of remission after adrenalectomy for individual patients and an estimate of their survival time. This must surely be the ideal objective in any predictive test.

Endometrial Cancer

Since it was believed that endometrial cancer resulted from a prolonged and unopposed action of estrogens it was argued that progesterone might be useful in treatment. In 1961, Kelley and Baker reported that 17α-hydroxyprogesterone caproate administration led to remissions in 32% of patients with disseminated endometrial cancer.

Subsequent reports in which a variety of synthetic progestogens have been used have amply confirmed these results in that about 35% of patients with advanced disease responded (see Briggs *et al.*, 1967). Also, the observation that pulmonary metastases respond well to progesterone therapy has been observed by several workers (Kelley and Baker, 1961; Bergsjö, 1965; Nilsen and Kolstad, 1973).

There have been promising results from the use of intrauterine progestogen therapy which provides a means of presenting a very high concentration of steroid near the tumor (Truscott, 1964). Remissions obtained by this method of administration for the early phases of endometrial cancer suggest that such therapy might be of value preoperatively. With respect to the preinvasive disease, Nilsen and Kolstad (1973) claim that stage 0 patients responded favorably to 17α-hydroxyprogesterone caproate. Patients were treated with an initial dose of 1,000 mg followed by 500 mg weekly. Histological examination revealed that in 19 out of 24 patients the lesions had disappeared in a 12-week course of therapy. Adenomatous hyperplasia persisted in 3 patients, and 2 were found to have invasive endometrial cancer.

The general evidence suggests that the administration of massive amounts of progesterone fulfills a useful role in the treatment of metastatic endometrial cancer (see Brush *et al.*, 1973; Kennedy, 1968; Kistner, 1972). The availability of synthetic progestogens (e.g., Depostat, Provera, Primolut) which have few side effects make this form of therapy attractive. However, a clinical trial is required in which an objective assessment could be made as to the efficacy of the various progestogens.

Cancer of the Cervix Uteri

There appears to be little evidence that this form of cancer has a hormonal etiology. Such evidence that exists to implicate hormones is based on the observation that the induction of cervical cancer by chemical carcinogens is potentiated by estrogen and inhibited by progestogen. The results of epidemiological studies on women taking oral contraceptives are difficult to interpret since the sexual history of such women and their controls must be taken into account. The hormonal treatment of such cancers has not been reported to bring about objective remissions (see Kistner, 1972).

Ovarian Cancer

Because of the difficulty in early diagnosis of this cancer a large number of patients are inoperable when first seen. In a survey of the literature by Bagley *et al.* (1972) they report that about 46% of patients were in stages 1a or 1b when first seen and about 67% of these survived for more than 5 years (the range being 32% to 78%). Surgery and radiotherapy is the best treatment of the early disease. The use of stilbestrol or hydroxy-progesterone in the advanced disease has been described, but the results were disappointing since only about 15% of the patients appeared to respond (Jolles, 1962; Long and Evan, 1963; Varga and Henricksen, 1964). This response rate is not improved on that obtained by using chemotherapy (see Bagley et al., 1972). A collaborative clinical trial has been suggested by Barr et al. (1972) and others to assess the possibility of using the progestogen, gestranol hexanoate (Depostat) in the treatment of ovarian cancer. The results of this study are awaited with interest.

Prostatic Cancer

The treatment of localized prostatic cancer with stilbestrol is not the treatment of choice. The Veterans Administration Co-operative Urological Research Groups (1967) report on the use of stilbestrol at this stage of the disease concludes that any benefit derived is outweighed by the statistically significant increase in deaths from thromboembolic and cardiovascular disorders. It would, therefore, appear that surgery is the treatment of choice at the early stages of the disease.

In the more advanced stages the consensus of opinion is that stilbestrol treatment is of value because dramatic subjective and long-term objective remissions have been observed. However, the evidence in terms of sur-vival and incidence of remission do not support the view that stilbestrol treatment is beneficial in the majority of patients. In a series of 1,818 patients with prostatic cancer, those treated with stilbestrol for metastatic disease did not survive any better than a control group not treated with stilbestrol (Nesbit and Baum, 1960). Other studies have reinforced this view (Bauer et al., 1960; Emmett et al., 1960). Franks (1958) has suggested that the beneficial effects of stilbestrol is indirect and that in a majority of cases treatment is not reducing tumor growth or effecting a remission, but that the increased survival is due to relief of urinary obstruction or control of infection.

The combination of orchiectomy and stilbestrol does not seem to afford any better remission rates than one modality alone (Crowley and Duwe, 1969). Brendler and Prout (1962) observed no benefit of stilbestrol treatment in patients in relapse after orchiectomy. Testosterone has also been used in the treatment of patients with advanced prostatic cancer. The results showed no obvious exacerbation of the disease, and furthermore, one patient of the ten treated benefited for almost a year (Brendler et al., 1950; Prout and Brewer, 1967; Trunnell and Duffy, 1950).

A potent new antiandrogen, cyproterone acetate, has been used in the treatment of the advanced disease. Smith *et al.* (1973) have reported a series of 19 patients in which 18 on follow-up were found to have benefited from the treatment. These authors concluded that cyproterone acetate has a useful place in the hormonal treatment of prostatic cancer. However, Schoones (1973), in a comparative trial of cyproterone acetate and stilbestrol, reports that his preliminary results suggest that on a weight basis stilbestrol is still the antiandrogen of choice.

A small number of objective remissions may be obtained with adrenalectomy and hypophysectomy in patients with metastatic disease; hypophysectomy appears to be marginally superior to adrenalectomy (see Fergusson, 1972; Mahoney and Harrison, 1972).

Summary and Conclusions

The situation as far as prostatic and endometrial cancer is concerned appears to be more straightforward than with breast cancer. In the former, the simple concept that responsive tumors are androgen dependent and that any treatment that removes or antagonizes androgens will result in regression appears to be tenable. Similarly, the thesis that progestins act as antiestrogens in endometrial cancer is also acceptable. However, in comparison with breast cancer only a relatively small amount of research has been carried out, and these generalizations may prove to be a gross oversimplification of the true state of affairs. For example, Grattarola (1972) claims that the androgens are of key importance in endometrial cancer.

In the 80 years since Beatson described the first successful endocrine therapy an immense amount of research has been done, but the results in this chapter show how much more there is to be done before we really understand the basic biology underlying the etiology and clinical course of hormone-related cancers.

References

Albert, S., and Selye, H. (1942). The effect of various pharmacological agents on the morphogenetic actions of estradiol. *J. Pharmacol. Exp. Ther.* **75**:308.

Allen, E., and Gardner, W. U. (1941). Cancer of the cervix of the uterus in hybrid mice following long-continued administration of estrogen. *Cancer Res.* **1**:359.

Andervont, H. B., Shimkin, M. B., and Canter, H. Y. (1960). Some factors involved in the induction or growth of testicular tumors in BALB/C mice. *J. Nat. Cancer Inst.* **25**:1083.

Angrist, A., Capurro, P., and Moumgis, B. (1960). Studies on squamous metaplasia in rat bladder. II. Effects of estradiol and estradiol plus hexestrol. *Cancer Res.* **20**:568.

Armstrong, B., Stevens, N., and Doll, R. (1974). Retrospective study of the association between use of Rauwolfia derivatives and breast cancer in English women. *Lancet* **II**:672.

Athias, M. (1945). Lésions testiculaires chez des souris non cancéreuses, appartenant à une lignée très sujette au cancer de la glande mammaire. *Arquiv. Patol. (Lisbon)* **17**:397.

Athias, M., and Furtado Dias, M. J. (1941). Leseos testiculares em murganhos com adenocarcinoma espontaneo de glandula mammaria. *Arq. Patol. (Lisbon)* **13**:381.

Atkins, H. J. B., Falconer, M. A., Hayward, J. L., McLean, K. S., and Schurr, P. H. (1966). The timing of adrenalectomy and of hypophysectomy in the treatment of advanced breast cancer. *Lancet* **I**:827.

Axelrad, A., and Leblond, C. P. (1955). Induction of thyroid tumors in rats by a low iodine diet. *Cancer* **8**:339.

Bacigalupo, G., and Lingk, H. (1968). Die Urinausscheidungen von neutralen 17-Ketosteroiden. Androsteron und Aetiocholanolon bei gesunden Frauen und Frauen mit frühem und vorgeschrittenem Brustkrebs. *Arch. Geschwulstforsch.* **32**:95.

Bacigalupo, G., and Schubert, K. (1966). Some aspects of oestrogen metabolism in cases of human mammary neoplasias. *Eur. J. Cancer* **2**:75.

Bagley, C. M., Young, R. C., Canellos, G. P., and De Vita, V. T. (1972). Treatment of ovarian carcinoma: Possibilities for progress. *N. Engl. J. Med.* **287**:856.

Barlow, J. J., Emerson, K., and Saxena, B. N. (1969). Oestradiol production after ovariectomy for carcinoma of the breast. *N. Engl. J. Med.* **280**:633.

Barr, W., Edelstyn, G. A., Forster, D. M. B., Glennie, J. McD., MacRae, K. D., Menzies, D. N., O'Sullivan, J., Pitchford, A. G., Smedley, G. T., Tacchi, D., and Ward, H. W. C. (1972). Treatment of ovarian carcinoma. *Lancet* **I**:591.

Bauer, W. C., McGavran, M. H., and Carlin, M. R. (1960). Unsuspected carcinoma of the prostate in suprapubic prostatectomy specimens. *Cancer* **13**:370.

Bayliss, P. F. C., and Van't Hoff, W. (1969). Amenorrhoea and galactorrhoea associated with hypothyroidism. *Lancet* **II**:1399.

Beatson, G. W. (1896). On the treatment of inoperable cases of carcinoma of the mamma: Suggestions for a new method of treatment with illustrative cases. *Lancet* **II**:104.

Beck, J. C., Blair, A. J., Griffiths, M. M., Rosenfeld, M. W., and McGarry, E. E. (1966). In search of hormonal factors as an aid in predicting the outcome of breast carcinoma. *Proc. Can. Cancer Res. Conf.* **6**:3.

Bergsjö, P. (1965). Progesterone and progestational compounds in the treatment of advanced endometrial carcinoma. *Acta. Endocrinol. (Copenhagen)* **49**:412.

Bern, H. A., De Ome, K. B., Wellings, S. R., and Harkness, D. R. (1958). The effect of various hormonal treatments on the incidence of hyperplastic nodules and of "noduloids" in the mammary glands of C3H/HeCrgl mice. *Cancer Res.* **18**:1324.

Besser, G. M., and Edwards, C. R. W. (1972). Galactorrhoea. *Br. Med. J.* **II**:280.

Bielschowsky, F. (1953). Chronic iodine deficiency as cause of neoplasia in thyroid and pituitary of aged rats. *Br. J. Cancer* **7**:203.

Bischoff, F., Long, M. L., Rupp, J. J., and Clarke, G. J. (1942a). Carcinogenic effect of estradiol and of theelin in marsh-buffalo mice. *Cancer Res.* **2**:52.

Bischoff, F., Long, M. L., Rupp, J. J., and Clarke, G. J. (1942b). Influence of toxic amounts of estrin upon intact and castrated male marsh-buffalo mice. *Cancer Res.* **2**:198.

Biskind, M. S., and Biskind, G. R. (1944). Development of tumors in the rat ovary after transplantation into the spleen. *Proc. Soc. Exp. Biol. Med.* **55**:176.

Biskind, M. S., and Biskind, G. R. (1945). Tumor of rat testis produced by heterotransplantation of infantile testis to spleen of adult castrate. *Proc. Soc. Exp. Biol. Med.* **59**:4.

Bittner, J. J. (1958). Genetic concepts in mammary cancer in mice. *Ann. N.Y. Acad. Sci.* **71**:943.

Blair, P. B., Blair, S. M., Lyons, W. R., Bern, H. A., and Li, C. H. (1960). Effect of hormones and of parity on the occurrence of hyperplastic nodules and tumors in the mammary glands of female A/Crgl mice. *Cancer Res.* **20**:1640.

Bond, W. H. (1967). The influence of various treatments on survival rates in cancer of the breast. In *The Treatment of Carcinoma of the Breast* (A. S. Jarrett, ed.), p. 24. Excerpta Medica, Amsterdam.

Bonser, G. M., Dossett, J. A., and Jull, J. W. (1961). *Human and Experimental Breast Cancer.* Pitman Med. Publ., London.

Boot, L. M. (1970). Prolactin and mammary gland carcinogenesis. The problem of human prolactin. *Int. J. Cancer* **5**:167.

Boston Collaborative Drug Surveillance Program (1974). Reserpine and breast cancer. *Lancet* **II**:669.

Bowers, C. Y., Friesen, H. G., Hwang, P., Guyda, H. J., and Folkers, K. (1971). Prolactin and thyrotropin release in man by synthetic pyroglutamyl-histidyl-prolinamide. *Biochem. Biophys. Res. Commun.* **45**:1033.

Boyland, E. E., Godsmark, B., Greening, W. P., Rigby-Jones, P., Stevenson, J. J., and Abulfadl, M. A. M. (1958). The effect of irradiation of the pituitary on gonadotrophin excretion in women with advanced mammary cancer. In *Endocrine Aspects of Breast Cancer,* (A. R. Currie, ed.), p. 170. Livingstone, Edinburgh.

Boyns, A. R., Buchan, R., Cole, E. N., Forrest, A. P. M., and Griffiths, K. (1973a). Basal prolactin blood levels in three strains of rats with differing incidence of 7,12-dimethyl-benz(a) anthracene induced mammary tumors. *Eur. J. Cancer* **9**:169.

Boyns, A. R., Cole, E. N., Griffiths, K., Roberts, M. M., Buchan, R., Wilson, R., and Forrest, A. P. M. (1973b). Plasma prolactin in breast cancer. *Eur. J. Cancer* **9**:99.

Brendler, H. B., Chase, W. E., and Scott, W. W. (1950). Prostatic cancer: Further investigations of hormonal relationships. *Arch. Surg. (Chicago)* **61**:433.

Brendler, H. B., and Prout Jr. G. R. (1962). A co-operative group study of prostatic cancer: Stilbestrol versus placebo in advanced progressive disease. *Cancer Chemother. Rep.* **16**:323.

Briggs, M. H. (1972). Ethnic differences in urinary estrogens. *Lancet* **I**:324.

Briggs, M. H., Caldwell, A. D., and Pitchford, A. G. (1967). The treatment of cancer by progestogens. *Hosp. Med.* **2**:63.

Brown, J. B. (1958). Urinary oestrogen excretion in the study of mammary cancer. In *Endocrine Aspects of Breast Cancer,* (A. R. Currie, ed.), p. 197. Livingstone, Edinburgh.

Brownsey, B., Cameron, E. H. D., Griffiths, K., Gleave, E. N., Forrest, A. P. M., and Campbell, H. (1972). Plasma dehydroepiandrosterone sulphate levels in patients with benign and malignant breast disease. *Eur. J. Cancer* **8**:131.

Brush, M. G., Milton, P. J. D., Swain, M. C., and Moore, J. W. (1974). Endometrial cystic hyperplasia—A premalignant state or a complex endocrine disorder. In *Recent Advances in Gynaecological Cancer* (Brush and Taylor, eds.). Ballière, London.

Bryant, G. D., Siler, T. M., Greenwood, F. C., Pasteels, J. L., Robyn, C., and Hubinont, P. O. (1971). Radioimmunoassay of human pituitary prolactin in plasma. *Hormones* **2**:139.

Bulbrook, R. D. (1974). Tests of prediction. In *The Treatment of Breast Cancer* (H. J. B. Atkins, ed.), p. 177. Medical & Technical Publ., Lancaster, England.

Bulbrook, R. D., Franks, L. M., and Greenwood, F. C. (1956). The estimation of urinary 17-ketosteroids, ketogenic steroids and oestrogens in the castrated or stilboestrol-treated human male. *J. Endocrinol.* **13**:33.

Bulbrook, R. D., Hayward, J. L., and Spicer, C. C. (1971). Relation between urinary androgen and corticoid excretion and subsequent breast cancer. *Lancet* **II**:395.

Bulbrook, R. D., Hayward, J. L., Spicer, C. C., and Thomas, B. S. (1962a). A comparison between the urinary steroid excretion of normal women and women with advanced breast cancer. *Lancet* II:1235.

Bulbrook, R. D., Hayward, J. L., Spicer, C. C., and Thomas, B. S. (1962b). Abnormal excretion of urinary steroids by women with early breast cancer. *Lancet* II: 1238.

Bulbrook, R. D., Thomas, B. S., and Utsunomiya, J. (1964). Urinary 11-deoxy-17-oxosteroids in British and Japanese women with reference to the incidence of breast cancer. *Nature (London)* 201:189.

Bulbrook, R. D., Thomas, B. S., Utsunomiya, J., and Hamaguchi, E. (1967). The urinary excretion of 11-deoxy-17-oxosteroids and 17-hydroxycorticosteroids by normal Japanese and British women. *J. Endocrinol.*, 38:401.

Burrows, H. (1936). Pituitary hyperplasia in a male mouse after the administration of oestrin. *Am. J. Cancer* 28:741.

Burrows, H. (1940). Spontaneous uterine and mammary tumours in the rabbit. *J. Pathol. Bacteriol.* 51:385.

Burrows, H., and Boyland, E. (1938). Neoplasia in rabbits following the administration of 1:2:5:6-dibenzanthracene. *Am. J. Cancer* 32:367.

Burrows, H., and Hoch-Ligeti, C. (1946). Effect of progesterone on the development of mammary cancer in C3H mice. *Cancer Res.* 6:608.

Cameron, E. H. D., Griffiths, K., Gleave, N., Stewart, H. J., Forrest, A. P. M., and Campbell, H. (1970). Benign and malignant breast disease in South Wales: A study of urinary steroids. *Br. Med. J.* 4:768.

Carter, A. C., Feldman, E. B., and Schwartz, H. L. (1960). Levels of serum protein-bound iodine in patients with metastatic carcinoma of the breast. *J. Clin. Endocrinol. Metab.* 20:477.

Chou, C. Y., and Wang, C. W. (1939). Excretion of male sex hormone in health and disease. *Chin. J. Physiol.* 14:151.

Clifton, E. E., and Pan, S. E. (1948). Effect of a progesterone compound on growth of a transplanted granulosa cell tumour. *Proc. Soc. Exp. Biol. Med.* 69:516.

Clifton, K. H. (1959). Problems in experimental tumorigenesis of the pituitary gland; gonads, adrenal cortices, and mammary glands: A review. *Cancer Res.* 19:2.

Cole, M. P. (1968). Suppression of ovarian function in primary breast cancer. In *Prognostic Factors in Breast Cancer* (A. P. M. Forrest and P. B. Kunkler, eds.), p. 146. Livingstone, Edinburgh.

Cole, P., and MacMahon, B. (1969). Oestrogen fractions during early reproductive life in the aetiology of breast cancer. *Lancet* I:604.

Cramer, W., and Horning, E. S. (1936). Experimental production by oestrin of pituitary tumours with hypopituitarism and of mammary cancer. *Lancet* II:247.

Crowley, L. G., and Duwe, S. A. (1969). Current status of the management of patients with endocrine-sensitive tumors. II. Carcinoma of the prostate, endometrium, thyroid, kidney and miscellaneous tumors. *Calif. Med.* 110:139.

Cutler, B. S., Forbes, A., Ingersoll, F., and Scully, R. (1972). Endometrial carcinoma after stilboestrol therapy in gonadal dysgenesis. *N. Engl. J. Med.* 287:628.

Dao, T. L., and Nemoto, T. (1965). An evaluation of adrenalectomy and androgen in disseminated mammary carcinoma. *Surg. Gynecol. Obstet.* 121:1257.

Deshpande, N., Hayward, J. L., and Bulbrook, R. D. (1965). Plasma 17-hydroxycorticosteroids and 17-oxosteroids in patients with breast cancer and in normal women. *J. Endocrinol.* 32:167.

Deshpande, N., Jensen, V., Bulbrook, R. D., and Doouss, T. W. (1967). *In vivo* steroidogenesis by the human adrenal gland. *Steroids* 9:393.

De Waard, F., Baanders-van Halewijn, E. A. (1969). Cross-sectional data on estrogenic smears in a post-menopausal population. *Acta Cytol.* 13:675.

De Waard, F., and Baanders-van Halewijn, E. A. (1974). A prospective study in general practice on breast cancer risk in post-menopausal women. *Int. J. Cancer* **14**:153.

De Waard, F., Thyssen, J. H. H., Veeman, W., and Sander, P. C. (1968). Steroid hormone excretion pattern in women with endometrial carcinoma. *Cancer* **22**:988.

Dmochowski, L. (1953). The milk agent in the origin of mammary tumors in mice. *Adv. Cancer Res.* **1**:103.

Doisy, E. A., Veler, C. D., and Thayer, S. A. (1929). Folliculin from urine of pregnant women. *Am. J. Physiol.* **90**:329.

Dunning, W. F. (1960). Steroid-responsive neoplasms in rats and mice. In *Biological Activities of Steroids in Relation to Cancer,* (G. Pincus and Erwin P. Vollmer, eds.), p. 225. Academic Press, New York/London.

Dunning, W. F., and Curtis, M. R. (1952). The incidence of diethylstilbestrol-induced cancer in reciprocal F_1 hybrids obtained from crosses between rats of inbred lines that are susceptible and resistant to the induction of mammary cancer by this agent. *Cancer Res.* **12**:702.

Dunning, W. F., and Curtis, M. R. (1954). Further studies on the relation of dietary tryptophan in the induction of neoplasms in rat. *Cancer Res.* **14**:299.

Dunning, W. F., Curtis, M. R., and Madsen, M. E. (1951). Diethylstilbestrol-induced mammary gland and bladder cancer in reciprocal F_1 hybrids between two inbred lines of rats. *Acta. Unio Int. Contra Cancrum* **7**:238.

Dunning, W. F., Curtis, M. R., and Maun, M. E. (1949). The effect of dietary fat and carbohydrate on diethylstilbestrol-induced mammary cancer in rats. *Cancer Res.* **9**:354.

Dunning, W. F., Curtis, M. R., and Maun, M. E. (1950). The effect of added dietary tryptophane on the occurrence of diethylstilbestrol-induced mammary cancer in rats. *Cancer Res.* **10**:319.

Dunning, F. W., Curtis, M. R., Segaloff, A. (1947). Strain differences to diethylstilbestrol and the induction of mammary gland and bladder cancer in the rat. *Cancer Res.* **7**:511.

Dunning, W. F., Curtis, M. R., and Segaloff, A. (1953). Strain differences in response to estrone and the induction of mammary gland, adrenal, and bladder cancer in rat. *Cancer Res.* **13**:147.

Edelstyn, G. A., Lyons, A. R., and Welbourne, R. B. (1958). Thyroid function in patients with mammary cancer. *Lancet* **I**:670.

Ehni, G., and Eckles, N. E. (1959). Interruption of the pituitary stalk in the patient with mammary cancer. *J. Neurosurg.* **16**:628.

Eisen, M. J. (1942). Occurrence of benign and malignant mammary lesions in rats treated with crystalline estrogen. *Cancer Res.* **2**:632.

Ely, C. A. (1953). Effect of antigonadotrophic serum on testes of A-strain mice treated with estrogen. *Proc. Soc. Exp. Biol. Med.* **84**:501.

Ely, C. A. (1956). Effect of antigonadotrophic serum on recent intrasplenic ovarian implants of castrate mice. *Endocrinology* **59**:83.

Emge, L. A. (1934). The influence of pregnancy on tumour growth. *Am. J. Obstet. Gynecol.* **28**:682.

Emge, L. A., and Murphy, K. M. (1938). Effect of rapidly repeated pregnancies on transplantable mammary rat adenofibromas. *Proc. Soc. Exp. Biol. Med.* **37**:620.

Emmett, J. L., Greene, L. F., and Papantoniou, A. (1960). Endocrine therapy in carcinoma of the prostate gland. 10-year survival studies. *J. Urol.* **83**:471.

Engelsman, E., Heuson, J. C., Blonk-van der Wijst, D. and Maass, H. (1975). Controlled trial of L-Dopa in advanced breast cancer. An EORTC Breast Cancer Group Study. *Br. Med. J.* **2**:714.

EORTC Breast Cancer Group (1972). Clinical trial 2-Br-α-ergocryptine (CB154) in advanced breast cancer. *Eur. J. Cancer* **8**:155.

Ettigi, P., Lal, S., and Friesen, H. (1973). Prolactin, phenothiazine, admission to mental hospitals, and carcinoma of the breast. *Lancet* **II**:266.

Falkson, G., Van Dyke, J. J., Van Eden, E. B., van der Merve, A. M., and Falkson, H. C. (1974). Calusterone (NSC-88536): A poor substitute for fluoxymesterone (NSC-12165) in the treatment of advanced breast cancer. *Cancer Chemother. Rep.* **58**:939.

Farnsworth, W. E. (1971). Uptake of plasma androgens by human benign hypertrophic prostate. *Invest. Urol.* **8**:367.

Fels, E., and Foglia, V. G. (1960a). Ovarienimplantat in milz und hypophysektomie. *Acta Endocrinol. (Copenhagen)* **34**:1.

Fels, E., and Foglia, V. G. (1960b). E_1 factor hypofisario en la tumorigénesis experimental del ovario." *Acta Physiol. Lat. Am.* **10**:28.

Fergusson, J. D. (1972). Secondary endocrine therapy. In *Endocrine Therapy in Malignant Disease*. (B. A. Stoll, ed.), p. 263. W. B. Sanders, London.

Forsyth, I. A., Besser, G. M., Edwards, C. R. W., Francis, L., and Myres, R. P. (1971). Plasma prolactin activity in inappropriate lactation. *Br. Med. J.* **III**:225.

Fortner, J. G., George, P. A., and Sternberg, S. S. (1960). Induced and spontaneous thyroid cancer in the syrian (golden) hamster. *Endocrinology* **66**:364.

Foulds, L. (1947). Mammary tumours in hybrid mice: A sex factor in transplantation. *Br. J. Cancer* **1**:362.

Foulds, L. (1949a). Mammary tumours in hybrid mice: Hormone-responses of transplanted tumours. *Br. J. Cancer* **3**:240.

Foulds, L. (1949b). Mammary tumours in hybrid mice: Growth and progression of spontaneous tumours. *Br. J. Cancer* **3**:345.

Franks, L. M. (1958) Some comments on the long-term results of endocrine treatment of prostatic cancer. *Br. J. Urol.* **30**:383.

Franks, S., Ralphs, D. N. L., Seagroatt, V., and Jacobs, H. S. (1974). Prolactin concentrations in patients with breast cancer. *Br. Med. J.* **IV**:320.

Frantz, A. G., Habis, D. V., Hyman, G. A., Suh, H. K., Sassin, J. S., Zimmerman, E. A., Nowell, G. L., and Kleinberg, D. L. (1973). Physiological and pharmacological factors effecting prolactin secretion, including its supression by L-Dopa in the treatment of breast cancer. In *Human Prolactin,* (J. L. Pasteels and C. Robyn, ed.), p. 273. Excerpta Medica, Amsterdam.

Furth, J., and Clifton, K. H. (1958). Experimental pituitary tumours. *CIBA Found. Colloq. Endocrinol.* **12**:3.

Gala, R. R., and Loginsky, S. J. (1973). Correlation between serum prolactin levels and incidence of mammary tumors induced by 7,12-dimethylbenz(*a*)anthracene in the rat. *J. Nat. Cancer Inst.* **51**:593.

Gardner, W. U. (1937). *Some Fundamental Aspects of the Cancer Problem*, part 4. p. 67. Amer. Assoc. Adv. Sci., Washington, D.C.

Gardner, W. U. (1941). Inhibition of mammary growth by large amounts of estrogen. *Endocrinology* **28**:53.

Gardner, W. U. (1942). Persistence and growth of spontaneous mammary tumors and hyperplastic nodules in hypophysectomised mice. *Cancer Res.* **2**:476.

Gardner, W. U. (1953). Hormonal aspects of experimental tumorigenesis. *Adv. Cancer Res.* **1**:173.

Gardner, W. U. (1958). Some studies on ovarian tumorigenesis. *CIBA Found. Colloq. Endocrinol.* **12**:153.

Gardner, W. U. (1959). Carcinoma of the uterine cervix and upper vagina: Induction under experimental conditions in mice. *Ann. N.Y. Acad. Sci.* **75**:543.

Gardner, W. U. (1961). Tumorigenesis in transplanted irradiated and nonirradiated ovaries. *J. Nat. Cancer Inst.* **26**:829.

Gardner, W. U., and Allen, E. (1939). Malignant and nonmalignant uterine and vaginal lesions in mice receiving estrogens, and estrogens and androgens simultaneously. *Yale J. Biol. Med.* **12**:213.

Gardner, W. U., and Dougherty, T. F. (1944). The leukomogenic action of estrogens in hybrid mice. *Yale J. Biol. Med.* **17**:75.

Gardner, W. U., Dougherty, T. F., and Williams, W. L. (1944). Lymphoid tumors in mice receiving steroid hormones. *Cancer Res.* **4**:73.

Gardner, W. U., Kirschbaum, A., and Strong, L. C. (1940). Lymphoid tumors in mice receiving estrogens. *AMA Arch. Pathol.* **29**:1.

Gasparri, F. (1958). Pathology of the residual ovary after hysterectomy. *Riv. Ostet. Ginecol.* **13**:381.

Geschickter, C. F. (1942). Factors influencing the development and time of appearance of mammary cancer in the rat in response to estrogen. *AMA Arch. Pathol.* **33**:334.

Girard, A., and Sandulesco, G. (1936). Sur une nouvelle série de réactifs du groupe carbonyle, leur utilisation à l'extraction des substances cétonique et à la caractérisation microchimique des aldéhydes et cétones. *Helv. Chim. Acta* **19**:1095.

Glenn, E. M., Richardson, S. L., and Bowman, B. J. (1959a). A method of assay of antitumor activity using a rat mammary fibroadenoma. *Endocrinology* **64**:379.

Glenn, E. M., Richardson, S. L., Lyster, S. C., and Bowman, B. J. (1959b). Inhibition of mammary fibroadenoma of female rats by steroids of the androstane series. *Endocrinology* **64**:390.

Glenn, E. M., Richardson, S. L., Bowman, B. J., and Lyster, S. C. (1960). In *Biological Activities of Steroids in Relation to Cancer* (G. Pincus and Erwin P. Vollmer, eds.), p. 257. Academic Press, New York/London.

Gorbman, A. (1949). Tumorous growths in the pituitary and trachea following radiotoxic dosages of I^{131}. *Proc. Soc. Exp. Biol. Med.* **71**:237.

Gordon, G. S., Halden, A., and Horn, Y. (1973). Calusterone (7β, 17α-dimethyltestosterone) as primary and secondary therapy of advanced breast cancer. *Oncology* **28**:138.

Grattarola, R. (1970). The urinary androgen metabolite pattern in patients with atypical endometrial hyperplasia (adenomatous hyperplasia). *Int. J. Gynecol. Obstet.* **8**:830.

Grattarola, R. (1972). Androgenic cause of breast carcinoma and endometrial hyperplasia. *Cancer Cytol.* **12**:25.

Grauer, R. C., and Robinson, G. H. (1932). Lactation in transplantable benign mammary adenomas in rats. *Am. J. Cancer* **16**:191.

Graves, G. Y., and Harris, N. S. (1952). Carcinoma in the male breast with axillary metastases following stilbestrol therapy. *Ann. Surg.* **135**:411.

Green, J. A. (1956). The effect of hormone administration on the growth, morphology, and secretion of a transplanted mouse granulosa-cell tumor. *Cancer Res.* **16**:417.

Greene, H. S. N. (1941). Uterine adenomata in the rabbit. III. Susceptibility as a function of constitutional factors. *J. Exp. Med.* **73**:273.

Greene, H. S. N., and Newton, B. L. (1948). Evolution of cancer of the uterine fundus in the rabbit. *Cancer* **1**:82.

Greene, H. S. N., Newton, B. L., and Fisk, A. A. (1947). Carcinoma of the vaginal wall in the rabbit. *Cancer Res.* **7**:502.

Greenwald, P., Nasca, P. C., Burnett, W. S., and Polan, A. (1973). Prenatal stilbestrol experience of mothers of young cancer patients. *Cancer* **31**:568.

Griesbach, W. E., Kennedy, T. H., and Purves, H. D. (1945). Studies on experimental goitre. VI. Thyroid adenomata in rats on brassica seed diet. *Br. J. Exp. Pathol.* **26**:18.

Griesbach, W. E., and Purves, H. D. (1960). Basophil adenomata in the rat hypophysis after gonadectomy. *Br. J. Cancer* **14**:49.

Gross, J. (1973). Hormone profiles in Israelis of differing susceptibility to breast cancer. In *Proceedings of the 1st Breast Cancer Task Force Working Conference.* Williamsburg, Va.

Guérin, M. (1954). *Tumeurs Spontanees des Animaux de Laboratoire*. Le Grand & Cie, Paris.

Gutierrez, R. M., and Williams, R. J. (1968). Excretion of ketosteroids and proneness to breast cancer. *Proc. Nat. Acad. Sci. USA* **59**:938.

Guyda, H., Hwang, P., and Friesen, H. (1971). Immunologic evidence for monkey and human prolactin. *J. Clin. Endocrinol. Metab.* **32**:120.

Haddow, A., Watkinson, J. M., Paterson, E., and Koller, P. C. (1944). Influence of synthetic oestrogen upon advanced malignant disease. *Br. Med. J.* **II**:393.

Hardy, J. D., Richardson, E. M., and Dohan, F. C. (1953). The urinary excretion of corticoids and 17-ketosteroids following major operations. *Surg. Gynecol. Obstet.* **96**:448.

Harran-Ghera, N., Pullar, P., and Furth, J. (1960). Induction of thyrotropin-dependent thyroid tumors by thyrotropes. *Endocrinology* **66**:694.

Hayward, J. L. (1970). *Hormones and Human Breast Cancer. Recent Results in Cancer Research*, Vol. 24. Springer-Verlag, Berlin.

Hayward, J. L., Atkins, H. J. B., Falconer, M. A., MacLean, K. S., Salmon, L. F. W., Schurr, P. H., and Shaheen, C. H. (1970). Clinical trials comparing transfrontal-hypo-physectomy with adrenalectomy and with transethmoidal hypophysectomy. In *The Clinical Management of Advanced Breast Cancer* (J. Joslin and N. Gleave, eds.), p. 50. Tenovus, Cardiff.

Hayward, J. L., Bulbrook, R. D., and Greenwood, F. C. (1961). Hormone assays and prognosis in breast cancer. *Mem. Soc. Endocrinol.* **10**:144.

Heilman, F. R., and Kendall, E. C. (1944). Influence of 11-dehydro 17-hydroxycorticosterone (compound E) on growth of malignant tumour in mouse. *Endocrinology* **34**:416.

Heiman, J. (1944). Effect of testosterone propionate on the adrenals and on the incidence of mammary cancer in the R111 strain of mice. *Cancer Res.* **4**:31.

Heiman, J. (1945). The effect of progesterone and testosterone propionate on the incidence of mammary cancer in mice. *Cancer Res.* **5**:426.

Heiman, J., and Krehbiel, O. F. (1936). The influence of hormones on breast hyperplasia and tumour growths in white rats. *Am. J. Cancer* **27**:450.

Heinomen, O. P., Shapiro, S., Tuominen, L., and Tururen, M. I. (1974). Reserpine use in relation to breast cancer. *Lancet* **II**:675.

Hellman, L., Fishman, J., Zumoff, B., Cassouto, J., and Gallagher, T. F. (1967). Studies of estradiol transformation in women with breast cancer. *J. Clin. Endocrinol. Metab.* **27**:1087.

Herbst, A. L., Ulfelder, H., and Poskanzer, D. C. (1971). Adenocarcinoma of the vagina. Association of maternal stilbestrol therapy with tumor appearance in young women. *N. Engl. J. Med.* **284**:878.

Hertz, R. (1968). Experimental and clinical aspects of the carcinogenic potential of steroid contraceptives. *Int. J. Fertil.* **13**:273.

Heston, W. E., and Deringer, M. K. (1954). Occurrence of tumors in agent-free strain C3H$_f$ male mice implanted with estrogen-cholesterol pellets. *Proc. Soc. Exp. Biol. Med.* **82**:731.

Heuson, J. -C. (1974). Hormones by administration. In *The Treatment of Breast Cancer* (H. J. B. Atkins, ed.), p. 113. Medical & Technical Publ., Lancaster, England.

Hilf, R., Bell, C., Goldenberg, H., and Michel, I. (1971). Effect of Fluphenazine HCl on R3230AC mammary carcinoma and mammary glands of the rat. *Cancer Res.* **31**:1111.

Homburger, F., Borges, P., and Tregier, A. (1957). The production of uterine sarcomas in hydro-uteri of mice receiving testosterone. *Proc. Am. Soc. Cancer Res.* **2**:215.

Horning, E. S. (1954). The influence of unilateral nephrectomy on the development of stilboestrol-induced renal tumours on the male hamster. *Br. J. Cancer* **8**:627.

Horning, E. S. (1956a). Observations on hormone-dependent renal tumours in the golden hamster. *Br. J. Cancer* **10**:678.

Horning, E. S. (1956b). Endocrine factors involved in the induction, prevention and transplantation of kidney tumours in the male golden hamster. *Z. Krebsforsch.* **61**:1.

Horning, E. S., and Whittick, J. W. (1954). The histogenesis of stilboestrol-induced renal tumours in the male golden hamster. *Br. J. Cancer* **8**:451.

Huggins, C., and Bergenstal, D. M. (1952). Inhibition of human mammary and prostate cancers by adrenalectomy. *Cancer Res.* **12**:134.

Huggins, C., and Hodges, C. V. (1941). Studies on prostatic cancer. I. The effect of castration, of estrogen and of androgen injection on serum phosphatases in metastatic carcinoma of the prostate. *Cancer Res.* **1**:292.

Huggins, C., and Mainzer, K. (1957). Hormonal influences on mammary tumors of the rat. *J. Exp. Med.* **105**:485.

Huggins, C., Mainzer, K., and Briziarelli, G. (1958). Molecular structure of steroids and phenanthrene derivatives related to growth of transplanted mammary tumors. *Recent Progr. Horm. Res.* **14**:77.

Huggins, C., Stevens, R. E., and Hodges, C. V. (1941). Studies on prostatic cancer. II. The effects of castration on advanced carcinoma of the prostate gland. *Arch. Surg.* **43**:209.

Isler, H., Leblond, C. P., and Axelrad, A. A. (1958). Influence of age and of iodine intake on the production of thyroid tumors in the rat. *J. Nat. Cancer Inst.* **21**:1065.

Jabara, A. G. (1959). Canine ovarian tumours following stilboestrol administration. *Aust. J. Exp. Biol. Med. Sci.* **37**:549.

Jabara, A. G. (1962). Induction of canine ovarian tumours by diethylstilboestrol and progesterone. *Aust. J. Exp. Biol. Med. Sci.* **40**:139.

Jacobs, L. S., Snyder, P. J., Wilber, J. F., Utiger, R. D., and Daughday, W. H. (1971). Increased serum prolactin after administration of synthetic thyrotropin releasing hormone (TRH) in man. *J. Clin. Endocrinol. Metab.* **33**:996.

Joint Commitee on Endocrine Ablative Procedures in Disseminated Mammary Carcinoma (1961). Adrenalectomy and hypophysectomy in disseminated mammary carcinoma. *J. Am. Med. Assoc.* **175**:787.

Jolles, B. (1962). Progesterone in the treatment of advanced malignant tumours of breast, ovary and uterus. *Br. J. Cancer* **16**:209.

Jones, E. E. (1941). The effect of testosterone propionate on mammary tumors in mice of the C3H strain. *Cancer Res.* **1**:787.

Jull, J. W., Shucksmith, H. S., and Bonser, G. M. (1963). A study of urinary oestrogen excretion in relation to breast cancer. *J. Clin. Endocrinol. Metab.* **23**:433.

Juret, P. (1968). Urinary androgen excretion as prognostic factors before hypophysectomy. In *Prognostic Factors in Breast Cancer* (A. P. M. Forrest and P. B. Kunkler, eds.), p. 393. Livingstone, Edinburgh.

Kaplan, H. S., Brown, M. B., and Marden, S. N. (1951). Adrenocortical function and radiation-induced lymphoid tumor of mice. *Cancer Res.* **11**:629.

Katz, J. L., Ackman, P., Rothwax, Y., Sachar, E., Weiner, H., Hellman, L., and Gallagher, T. F. (1970). Psycho-endocrine aspects of cancer of the breast. *Psychosomatics* **22**:1.

Katz, J., Kunofsky, S., Patton, R. E., and Allaway, N. C. (1967). Cancer mortality among patients in New York mental hospitals. *Cancer* **20**:2194.

Kelley, R. M., and Baker, W. H. (1961). Progestational agents in the treatment of carcinoma of the endometrium. *N. Engl. J. Med.* **264**:216.

Kennedy, B. J. (1968). Progestogens in the treatment of carcinoma of the endometrium. *Surg. Gynecol. Obstet.* **127**:103.

Kent, J. R., and Young, H. H. (1964). Plasma testosterone levels in patients with prostatic carcinoma. *Surg. Forum* **15**:485.

Kirkman, H. (1957). Steroid tumorigenesis. *Cancer* **10**:757.

Kirkman, H. (1959). Estrogen-induced tumors of the kidney in the Syrian hamster. *Nat. Cancer Inst. Monogr.* **1**:1.

Kirkman, H., and Bacon, R. L. (1950). Malignant renal tumors in male hamsters *(Cricetus auratus)* treated with estrogens. *Cancer Res.* **10**:122.

Kirkman, H., and Bacon, R. L. (1952a). Estrogen-induced tumors of the kidney. I. Incidence of renal tumors in intact and gonadectomized male golden hamsters treated with diethylstilboestrol. *J. Nat. Cancer Inst.* **13**:745.

Kirkman, H., and Bacon, R. L. (1952b). Estrogen-induced tumors of the kidney. II. Effect of dose, administration, type of estrogen, and age on the induction of renal tumors in intact male golden hamsters. *J. Nat. Cancer Inst.* **13**:757.

Kistner, R. W. (1972). Endometrial hyperplasia and carcinoma *in situ*. In *Endocrine Therapy in Malignant Disease*. (B. A. Stoll, ed.), p. 305. W. B. Saunders, London.

Konoplev, V. P. (1959). Hepatomas in male rats induced with synestrol (Hexestrol) and testosterone propionate. *Vopr. Onkol.* **5**:138.

Kortweg, R., and Thomas, F. (1939). Tumor induction and tumor growth in hypophysectomised mice. *Am. J. Cancer* **37**:36.

Kullander, S. (1956). Studies in spayed rats with ovarian tissue autotransplanted to the spleen. *Acta. Endocrinol. (Copenhagen) Suppl.* **22**:27.

Kumaoka, S., Sakauchi, N., Abe, O., Kusama, M., and Takatani, O. (1968). Urinary 17-ketosteroid excretion of women with advanced breast cancer. *J. Clin. Endocrinol. Metab.* **28**:667.

Lacassagne, A. (1932). Apparition de cancer de la mamelle chez la souris mâle, soumis à des injections de folliculine. *C R Acad. Sci. Paris* **195**:630.

Lacassagne, A. (1937). Sarcomes lymphoides apparus chez des souris longuement traitées par des hormones oestrogènes. *C R Seances Soc. Biol. Paris* **126**:193.

Lacassagne, A., and Raynard, A. (1939). Sur le mécanisme d'une action préventive de la testostérone sur le cancer mammaire de la souris. *C R Seances Soc. Biol. Paris* **131**:586.

Lathrop, A. E. C., and Loeb, L. (1916). Further investigations on the origin of tumours in mice. III. On the part played by internal secretion in the spontaneous development of tumours. *J. Cancer Res.* **1**:1.

Law, L. W. (1954). Genetic studies in experimental cancer. *Adv. Cancer Res.* **2**:281.

Leikin, S., Rice, E. C., Bell, D. F., Jr., and Waters, R. J. (1952). Treatment of acute leukemia in children. *J. Pediatr.* **41**:40.

Lemon, H. M. (1969). Endocrine influences upon human breast cancer formation: A critique. *Cancer* **23**:781.

Lemon, H. M., Wotiz, H. H., Parsons, L., and Mozden, P. J. (1966). Reduced estriol excretion in patients with breast cancer prior to endocrine therapy. *J. Am. Med. Assoc.* **196**:112.

Lipschutz, A. (1950). *Steroid Hormones and Tumors*. Williams & Wilkins, Baltimore.

Lipschutz, A. (1957). *Steroid Homeostasis: Hypophysis and Tumorigenesis*. Heffer, Cambridge.

Lipschutz, A., and Vargas, L. Jr. (1941). Structure and origin of uterine and extragenital fibroids induced experimentally in the guinea-pig by prolonged administration of the oestrogens. *Cancer Res.* **1**:236.

Lipschutz, A., Vargas, L., Jr., and Ruz, O. (1939). Antitumorigenic action of testosterone. *Lancet* **II**:867.

Loeb, L. (1948). Aging processes in the ovaries of mice belonging to strains differing in the incidence of mammary carcinoma. *AMA Arch. Pathol.* **46**:401.

Loeser, A. A. (1939). Male hormone in the treatment of cancer of the breast. *Acta Unio. Int. Contra Cancrum.* **4**:375.

Loeser, A. A. (1941). Mammary carcinoma: Response to implantation of male hormone and progesterone. *Lancet* **II**:698.

Loeser, A. A. (1954). A new therapy for prevention of post-operative recurrences in genital and breast cancer. A six year study of the prophylactic thyroid treatment. *Br. Med. J.* II:1380.

Long, R. T., and Evans, A. M. (1963). Diethylstilbestrol as a chemotherapeutic agent for ovarian carcinoma. *Mod. Med.* 60:1125.

Loraine, J. A., Stong, J. A., and Douglas, M. (1957). The value of pituitary gonadotrophin assays in patients with mammary carcinoma. *Lancet* II:575.

Luft, R., and Olivecrona, H. (1953). Experiences with hypophysectomy in man. *J. Neurosurg.* 10:301.

Mackenzie, I. (1955). The production of mammary cancer in rats using oestrogens. *Br. J. Cancer* 9:284.

MacMahon, B. (1974). Risk factors for endometrial cancer. *Gynecol. Oncol.* 2:122.

MacMahon, B., Cole, P., and Brown, J. B. (1973). Etiology of human breast cancer. *J. Nat. Cancer Inst.* 50:21.

MacMahon, B., Cole, P., Brown, J. B., Aoki, K., Lin, T. M., Morgan, R. W., and Woo, N. C. (1974). Urine oestrogen profiles of Asian and North American women. *Int. J. Cancer* 14:161.

MacMahon, B., Cole, P., Lin, M., Lowe, C. R., Mirra, A. P., Ravnihar, B., Salber, E. J., Valoras, V. G., and Yuasa, S. (1970a). Age at first birth and breast cancer risk. *Bull. W.H.O.* 43:209.

MacMahon, B., Lin, T. M., Lowe, C. R., Mirra, A. P., Ravnihar, B., Salber, E. J., Trichopoulos, D., Valoras, V. G., and Yuasa, S. (1970b). Lactation and cancer of the breast: A summary of an international study. *Bull. W.H.O.* 42:185.

Mahoney, E. M., and Harrison, J. H. (1972). Bilateral adrenalectomy for palliative treatment of prostatic cancer. *J. Urol.* 108:936.

Mardones, E., Iglesias, R., and Lipschutz, A. (1954). Physiological action of 19-norprogesterone in the guinea-pig. *Proc. Soc. Exp. Biol. Med.* 86:451.

Mark, J., and Biskind, G. R. (1941). The effect of long term stimulation of male and female rats with estrone, estradiol benzoate, and testosterone propionate administered in pellet form. *Endocrinology* 28:465.

Marmorston, J. (1966). Urinary hormone metabolite levels in patients with cancer of the breast, prostate and lung. *Ann. N.Y. Acad. Sci.* 125:959.

Marmorston, J., Lombard, L. J., Myers, S. M., Gierson, H., Stern, E., and Hopkins, C. E. (1965). Urinary excretion of neutral 17-ketosteroids and pregnanediol by patients with prostatic cancer and benign prostatic hypertrophy. *J. Urol.* 93:276.

Marrian, G. F. (1930). LII. The chemistry of Oestrin. 111. An improved method of preparation and the isolation of active crystalline material. *Biochem. J.* 24:435.

Martin, F. I. R. (1964). Urinary gonadotrophins in postmenopausal women with breast cancer. *Br. Med. J.* II:351.

Matthews, V. S., Kirkman, H., and Bacon, R. L. (1947). Kidney damage in the golden hamster following chronic administration of diethylstilbestrol and sesame oil. *Proc. Soc. Exp. Biol. Med.* 66:195.

McEndy, D. P., Boon, M. C., and Furth, J. (1944). On the role of thymus, spleen and gonads in the development of leukemia in a high leukemia stock of mice. *Cancer Res.* 4:377.

McEuen, C. S. (1938). Occurrence of cancer in rats treated with oestrone. *Am. J. Cancer* 34:184.

McKerns, K. W. (1974). *Hormones and Cancer.* Academic Press, New York.

Meakin, J. W., Allt, W. E. C., Beale, F. A., Brown, T. C., Bush, R. S., Clark, R. M., Fitzpatrick, P. J., Hawkins, N. V., Jenkins, R. D. T., Pringle, J. F., Rider, W. D., Bulbrook, R. D., and Hayward, J. L. (1974). Ovarian irradiation and prednisone following surgery and radiotherapy for carcinoma of the breast. *Proc. 11th Int. Cancer Congress (Florence) Abst.* 3:533.

Meissner, W. A., Sommers, S. C., and Sherman, G. (1957). Endometrial hyperplasia, endometrial carcinoma, and endometriosis produced experimentally by estrogen. *Cancer* **10**:500.

Millar, M. J., and Noble, R. L. (1954a). The morphology and growth characteristics of a transplantable mammary fibroadenoma in the rat. *Br. J. Cancer* **8**:485.

Millar, M. J., and Noble, R. L. (1954b). Effects of exogenous hormones on growth characteristics and morphology of transplanted mammary fibroadenoma of the rat. *Br. J. Cancer* **8**:495.

Mittra, I., and Hayward, J. L. (1974). Hypothalamic–pituitary–thyroid axis in breast cancer. *Lancet* **I**:885.

Mittra, I., Hayward, J. L., and McNeilly, A. S. (1974). Hypothalamic–pituitary–prolactin axis in breast cancer. *Lancet* **I**:889.

Moon, H. D., Simpson, M. E., Li, C. H., and Evan, H. M. (1950). Neoplasms in rats treated with pituitary growth hormone. II. Adrenal glands. *Cancer Res.* **10**:364.

Mühlbock, O. (1956). The hormonal genesis of mammary cancer. *Adv. Cancer Res.* **4**:371.

Mühlbock, O., and Boot, L. M. (1959). The mechanism of hormonal carcinogenesis. In *CIBA Foundation Carcinogenesis* (G. E. W. Wolstenholme and M. O'Connors, eds.), p. 83. Churchill, London.

Mühlbock, O., Van Nie, R., and Bosch, L. (1958). The production of oestrogenic hormones by granulosa cell tumours in mice. *Ciba Found. Colloq. Endocrinol.* **12**:78.

Murphy, J. B., and Sturm, E. (1944). The effect of adrenal corticol and pituitary adrenotropic hormones on transplanted leukemia in rats. *Science* **99**:303.

Murphy, J. B., and Sturm, E. (1949). The effect of diethylstilbestrol on the incidence of leukemia in male mice of the Rockefeller Institute leukemia strain (RIL). *Cancer Res.* **9**:88.

Murray, W. S. (1928). Ovarian secretion and tumour incidence. *J. Cancer Res.* **12**:18.

Murray, R. M. L., Mozaffarian, G., and Pearson, O. H. (1972). Prolactin levels with L-Dopa treatment in metastatic breast carcinoma. In *Prolactin and Carcinogenesis* (A. R. Boyns and K. Griffiths, eds.), p. 158. Alpha Omega Alpha Publ., Cardiff.

Murray, R. M. L., and Sarfaty, G. (1974). Prolactin in early and advanced breast carcinoma. *Proc. 11th Int. Cancer Congr. Abstr.* **2**:122.

Mustacchi, P., and Gordan, G. S. (1958). *Frequency of Cancer in Estrogen-Treated Osteoporotic Women*, p. 163. C. V. Mosby, St. Louis.

Napalkov, N. P. (1959). Experimental thyroid tumours induced by a combined action of 6-methylthiouracil and 2-acetylaminofluorene. *Vopr. Onkol.* **5**:578.

Nathanson, I. T., and Andervont, H. B. (1939). Effect of testosterone propionate on development and growth of mammary carcinoma in female mice. *Proc. Soc. Exp. Biol. Med.* **40**:421.

Nesbit, R. M., and Baum, W. C. (1960). Endocrine control of prostatic carcinoma: Clinical and statistical survey of 1818 cases. *J. Am. Med. Assoc.* **143**:1317.

Nilsen, P. A., and Kolstad, P. (1973). Hormonal treatment of pre-invasive and invasive carcinoma of the corpus uteri. In *Symposium on Endometrial Cancer* (M. G. Brush, R. W. Taylor, and D. C. Williams, eds.), p. 115. Heineman, London.

Nissen-Meyer, R. (1965). Castration as part of the primary treatment for operable female breast cancer. *Acta Radiol. Suppl. (Stockholm)* 249.

Nissen-Meyer, R. (1967). The role of prophylactic castration in the therapy of human mammary cancer. *Eur. J. Cancer* **3**:395.

Nissen-Meyer, R., and Sanner, T. (1963). The excretion of oestrone, prenanediol and pregnanetriol in breast cancer patients. *Acta Endocrinol. (Copenhagen)* **44**:334.

Nissen-Meyer, R., and Vogt, J. H. (1961). Five years' experience of the treatment of metastatic breast cancer. *Mem. Soc. Endocrinol.* **10**:124.

Noble, R. L. (1964). Tumors and hormones. In *The Hormones* (G. Pincus, K. V. Thimann, and E. B. Astwood, eds.), p. 559. Academic Press, New York.

Noller, K. L., Decker, G. D., Lanier, A. P., and Kurland, L. T. (1972). Clear-cell adenocarcinoma of the cervix after maternal treatment with synthetic estrogens. *Mayo Clin. Proc.* 47:629.

O'Bryan, R. M., Gordan, G. S., Kelley, R. M., Ravdin, R. G., Segaloff, A., and Taylor, S. G., III (1974). Does thyroid substance improve response of breast cancer to surgical castration? *Cancer* 33:1082.

Pan, S. C., and Gardner, W. U. (1948). Carcinomas of the uterine cervix and vagina in estrogen- and androgen-treated hybrid mice. *Cancer Res.* 8:337.

Pearson, O. H., Llerena, O., Llerena, L., Molina, A., and Butler, T. (1969). Prolactin-dependent rat mammary cancer: A model for man? *Trans. Assoc. Am. Physicians (Phila.)* 82:225.

Peters, M. V. (1968). The effect of pregnancy in breast cancer. In *Prognostic Factors in Breast Cancer* (A. P. M. Forrest and P. B. Kunkler, eds.), p. 65. Livingstone, Edinburgh.

Pierson, H. (1937). Weitere Follikulinversuche. Perforierende Plattenepithelwucherungen im Uterus des Kaninchens mit Knorpel- und Knochenbefunden. *Krebsforsch.* 47:1.

Podilcak, M. D. (1961). The significance of oestrogen hormones in the development of experimental tumours of the lactic gland. *Neoplasma* 8:237.

Prout, G. R., Jr., and Brewer, W. R. (1967). Response of men with advanced prostatic carcinoma to exogenous administration of testosterone. *Cancer* 20:1871.

Purves, H. D., and Greisbach, W. E. (1946). Studies on experimental goitre. VII. Thyroid carcinomata in rats threatened with thiourea. *Br. J. Exp. Pathol.* 27:294.

Purves, H. D., and Greisbach, W. E. (1947). Studies on experimental goitre. VIII. Thyroid tumours in rats treated with thiourea. *Br. J. Exp. Pathol.* 28:46.

Ravdin, R. G., Lewison, E. F., Slack, N. H., Gardner, B., State, D., and Fisher, B. (1970). Results of a clinical trial concerning the worth of prophylactic oophorectomy for breast carcinoma. *Surg. Gynecol. Obstet.* 131:1055.

Repert, R. W. (1952). Breast carcinoma study: Relation to thyroid disease and diabetes. *J. Mich. State Med. Soc.* 51:1315.

Rivière, M. R., Chouroulinkov, I., and Guérin, M. (1960). Actions hormonales expérimentales de longue durée chez le hamster du point de vue de leur effet cancérigère. *Bull. Assoc. Fr. Etude Cancer* 47:558.

Röpcke, G., and Boot, L. M. (1972). Prolactin and the ovarian hormones in carcinoma of the mammary gland in mice. Proceedings of the IVth International Congress on Endocrinology, Washington. In *International Congress Series*, No. 273. *Endocrinology*, p. 1232.

Roth, L. (1939). Carcinoma of the prostate in a Scottish terrier. *J. Am. Vet. Med. Assoc.* 95:232.

Rudali, G., Jullien, P., and Juliard, L. (1959). Action des hormones sur la leucomogenèse des souris. *Rev. Fr. Etud. Clin. Biol.* 4:607.

Saez, S. (1971). Adrenal function in cancer: Relation to evolution. *Eur. J. Cancer* 7:381.

Saluja, P. G., Hamilton, J. M., Gronow, M., and Misdorp, W. (1974). Pituitary prolactin levels in canine mammary cancer. *Eur. J. Cancer* 10:63.

Sarfaty, G., Tallis, M., and Pitt, P. (1973). Basic results of a study of bilateral adrenalectomy for advanced breast cancer. Urinary steroids and related data in 148 patients. *Med. J. Aust.* 2:877.

Schenken, J. R., and Burns, E. L. (1943). Spontaneous primary hepatomas in mice of strain C3H. III. The effect of estrogens and testosterone propionate on their incidence. *Cancer Res.* 3:693.

Schinzinger, A. (1889). Über Carcinoma mammae. *Zentr.-Org. Ges. Chir.* 29:55.

Schlotthauer, C. F., and Millar, J. A. S. (1941). Carcinoma of the prostate gland in dogs: A report of three cases. *J. Am. Vet. Med. Assoc.* **99**:239.

Schoonees, R. (1973). Antiandrogen therapy in carcinoma of the prostate. *S. Afr. Med. J.* **47**:722.

Schweppe, J. S., Jungman, R. A., and Lewin, I. (1967). Urine steroid excretion in post-menopausal cancer of the breast. *Cancer* **20**:155.

Segaloff, A., and Dunning, W. F. (1945). The effect of strain, estrogen, and dosage on the reaction of the rat's pituitary and adrenal to estrogenic stimulation. *Endocrinology* **36**:238.

Segaloff, A., Gordon, D., Carabasi, R. A., Horwitt, B. N., Schlosser, J. V., and Murison, P. J. (1954). Hormonal therapy in cancer of the breast. VII. Effect of conjugated estrogens (Equine) on clinical course and hormonal excretion. *Cancer* **7**:758.

Selye, H. (1940). Interactions between various steroid hormones. *Can. Med. Assoc. J.* **42**:113.

Selye, H. (1944). Experimental investigations concerning the role of the pituitary in tumorigenesis. *Surgery* **16**:33.

Shimkin, M. B. (1945). Hormones and mammary cancer in mice. In *A Symposium on Mammary Tumors in Mice*, p. 85. Am. Assoc. Adv. Sci., Washington, D.C.

Shimkin, M. B. (1957). In *Cancer* (R. W. Raven, ed.), Vol. 1, p. 161. Butterworth, London/Washington.

Shimkin, M. B., and Wyman, R. S. (1946). Mammary tumours in male mice implanted with oestrogen-cholesterol pellets. *J. Nat. Cancer Inst.* **7**:71.

Shutt, D. A., Smith, I. D., and Shearman, R. P. (1974). Oestrone, oestradiol-17β and oestriol levels in human foetal plasma during gestation and at term. *J. Endocrinol.* **60**:333.

Silberberg, M., and Silberberg, R. (1945). Significance of the age factor and sex glands in experimental leukemia in mice. *Proc. Soc. Exp. Biol. Med.* **58**:347.

Silberberg, M., and Silberberg, R. (1949). Role of age in estrogen-induced lymphoid tumors of mice. *AMA Arch. Pathol.* **47**:340.

Skinner, L. G., England, P. C., Cottrell, K. M., and Selwood, R. A. (1974). Serum oestradiol-17β in normal pre-menopausal women and in patients with benign and malignant breast diseases. *Proc. Br. Assoc. Cancer Res.* Univ. of Leeds, Abst. No. 13.

Smith, F. W., Gardner, W. U., Li, M. H., and Kaplan, H. (1949). Adrenal medullary tumours (pheochromocytomas) in mice. *Cancer Res.* **9**:193.

Smith, R. B., Walsh, P. C., and Goodwin, W. E. (1973). Cyproterone acetate in the treatment of advanced carcinoma of the prostate. *J. Urol.* **110**:106.

Sommers, S. C. (1955). Endocrine abnormalities in women with breast cancer. *Lab. Invest.* **4**:160.

Stoll, B. A. (1972). *Endocrine Therapy in Malignant Diseases.* W. B. Saunders, London.

Suntzeff, V., Burns, E. L., Moskop, M., and Loeb, L. (1938). On the proliferative changes taking place in the epithelium of vagina and cervix of mice with advancing age and under the influence of experimentally administered estrogenic hormones. *Am. J. Cancer* **32**:256.

Symeonidis, A. (1948). Mammakrebserzeugung bei Mäusen durch Progesteron verabreicht während der Gravidität. *Acta Unio. Int. Contra Cancrum* **6**:163.

Symmers, W. St. C. (1968). Carcinoma of breast in transsexual individuals after surgical and hormone interference with the primary and secondary sex characteristics. *Br. Med. J.* **2**:83.

Tanaka, H., Manabe, H., Koshiyama, K., Hamanaka, Y., Matsumoto, K., and Uozumi, T. (1970). Excretion patterns of 17-ketosteroids and 17-hydroxycorticosteroids in surgical stress. *Acta Endocrinol.* **65**:1.

Terenius, L. (1971). Effect of anti-oestrogens on initiation of mammary cancer in female rats. *Eur. J. Cancer* **7**:65.

Thorn, G. W., Jenkins, D., and Laidlaw, J. C. (1953). The adrenal response to stress in man. *Recent Progr. Horm. Res.* **8**:171.

Trunnell, J. B., and Duffy, Jr., B. J. (1950). The influence of certain steroids on the behaviour of human prostatic cancer. *Trans. N.Y. Acad. Sci.* **12**:238.

Truscott, J. D., (1964). Treatment of endometrial cancer by the instillation of a progestational agent. In *Recent Advances in Ovarian and Synthetic Steroids* (R. P. Shearman, ed.), p. 140. G. D. Searle, High Wycombe.

Tullos, H. S., Kirschbaum, A., and Trentin, J. J. (1961). Role of gonadotrophic hormone in the initiation and progression of adrenal tumors in ovariectomized mice. *Cancer Res.* **21**:730.

Turkington, R. W. (1972). Prolactin secretion in patients treated with various drugs: Phenothiazines, tricyclic antidepressants, reserpine and methyldopa. *Arch. Int. Med.* **130**:349.

Ulrich, P. (1939). Testostérone (hormone mâle) et son role possible dans le traitement de certains cancers du sein. *Acta Unio. Int. Contra Cancrum* **4**:377.

Van Nie, R., Bendetti, E. L., Mühlbock, O. (1961). A carcinogenic action of testosterone, provoking uterine tumours in mice. *Nature (London)* **192**:1303.

Varga, A., and Henrikson, E. (1964). Effect of 17-alpha-hydroxyprogesterone 17-*N*-caproate on various pelvic malignancies. *Obstet. Gynecol.* **23**:51.

Vessey, M. P., Doll, R., and Sutton, P. M. (1971). Investigation of the possible relationship between oral contraceptives and benign and malignant breast disease. *Cancer* **28**:1395.

Vessey, M. P., Doll, R., and Sutton, P. M. (1972). Oral contraceptives and breast neoplasia: A retrospective study. *Br. Med. J.* **3**:719.

Vessey, M. P., Mears, E., Andolesk, L., and Ogrinic-Oven, M. (1972b). Randomised double-blind trial of four oral progestagen-only contraceptives. *Lancet* **I**:915.

Veterans Administration Co-operative Urological Research Group (1967). Carcinoma of the prostate: Treatment comparisons. *J. Urol.* **98**:516.

Wallach, S., and Henneman, P. H. (1959). Prolonged estrogen therapy in post-menopausal women. *J. Am. Med. Assoc.* **171**:1637.

Wang, D. Y. (1969). Plasma androgens in breast cancer. In *The Human Adrenal Gland and Its Relation to Breast Cancer* (K. Griffiths and E. H. D. Cameron, eds.), p. 71. Alpha Omega Alpha Publ., Cardiff.

Wang, D. Y., Bulbrook, R. D., Herian, M., and Hayward, J. L. (1974). Studies on the sulphate esters of dehydroepiandrosterone and androsterone in the blood of women with breast cancer. *Eur. J. Cancer* **10**:477.

Wang, D. Y., and Swain, M. C. (1974). Hormones and breast cancer. In *Biochemistry of Women: Methods for Clinical Investigation* (A. S. Currey and J. V. Hewitt, eds.), p. 191. Cleveland Rubber Co. Press, Cleveland.

Wilson, R. A., Brevetti, R. E., and Wilson, T. A. (1963). Specific procedures for the elimination of the menopause. *West. J. Surg.* **71**:110.

Woolley, G. W. (1951). Cortisone, related steroids and transplanted tumors of the mouse. *Cancer Res.* **11**:291.

Woolley, G. W., and Little, C. C. (1946). Prevention of adrenal cortical carcinoma by diethylstilboestrol. *Proc. Nat. Acad. Sci. U.S.A.* **32**:239.

Wynder, E. L., Bross, I. J., and Hirayama, T. (1960). A study of the epidemiology of cancer of the breast. *Cancer* **13**:559.

Young, H. H., and Kent, J. R. (1968). Plasma testosterone levels in patients with prostatic carcinoma before and after treatment. *J. Urol.* **99**:788.

Zondek, B. (1936). Tumour of the pituitary induced with follicular hormone. *Lancet* **I**:776.

Zumoff, B., Bradlow, L. H., Gallagher, T. F., and Hellman, L. (1971). Decreased conversion of androgens to normal 17-ketosteroid metabolites: A non-specific consequence of illness. *J. Clin. Endocrinol. Metab.* **32**:824.

Chapter 11

VIROLOGY

DAVID P. HOUCHENS AND
ENZO BONMASSAR

Introduction

Virology has played and continues to play an important role in the field of oncology. Although the first indication that a cell-free filtrate could transmit leukemia in chickens was seen early in this century (Ellerman and Bang, 1908), it was not until 3 years later that a virus was definitely found to be the etiologic agent of an animal tumor (Rous, 1911). Since that time animal tumors of viral origin have been found in many species of animals, but to date there has been no definite proof that viruses serve as etiologic agents in human malignancies. Although virus particles have been isolated from several types of human tumors, the establishment of proof that viruses induce human tumors has been limited only to association.

In this chapter some of the basic oncogenic virus studies in animals will be presented. Then studies of attempts to demonstrate human oncogenic viruses will be shown, and finally the concept of antiviral therapy for the control of these viruses will be discussed.

Properties of Viruses

A virus has been defined by Luria and Darnell (1967) as: "An entity whose genome is an element of nucleic acid, either DNA or RNA, which

David P. Houchens and Enzo Bonmassar • Immunochemotherapy Section, Laboratory of Experimental Chemotherapy. Drug Research and Development Division of Cancer Treatment. National Cancer Institute, Bethesda, Maryland 20014, U.S.A. The authors wish to thank Miss Cynthia Fair for typing this chapter.

reproduces inside living cells and uses their synthetic machinery to direct synthesis of specialized particles, the virions, which contain the viral genome and transfer it to other cells."

DNA viruses which produce neoplasia (Table 1) are polyoma, SV 40, papilloma, adenoviruses, herpesviruses, and poxviruses, while RNA-containing oncogenic viruses (oncornoviruses) (Table 2) are the leukemia and sarcoma viruses in birds, rodents, and cats. These oncogenic viruses change the growth properties of cells they infect, thus causing transformation. Eckhart (1972) states that three kinds of information are important for understanding how transformation occurs: (1) The function of the viral genes involved; (2) how viral information is maintained in the transformed cell; and (3) how viral gene products interact with cellular gene products to change cell growth regulation.

DNA viruses can either cause lytic-type infection, which causes destruction of the infected cell and the production of more viral particles, or temperate infection in which infectious progeny are not produced and only a portion of the host cells are transformed. On the other hand, RNA viruses do not produce lytic-type infections and are continually released by the infected host cells.

The polyoma, SV 40, and papilloma viruses make up the group called papova virus (Melnick, 1962). They contain protein and DNA in a circular form and range in size fron 40–55 nm. Adenoviruses, which cause respiratory diseases in humans and are oncogenic in rats, mice, and hamsters (Huebner *et al.*, 1963; Rabson *et al.*, 1964; Trentin *et al.*, 1962), are larger than papova viruses and contain linear double-stranded DNA (Pereira *et al.*, 1963). Herpesviruses have DNA that is linear and double stranded (Kieff *et al.*, 1971). They have been found in most species of animals and generally persist for the life of the infected animals (Roizman, 1969).

RNA tumor viruses generally are about 100 nm in diameter (Bernhard *et al.*, 1958), with 1% RNA (Beard, 1963) and sometimes a small amount of DNA which is possibly of cellular origin (Varmus *et al.*, 1971). RNA tumor viruses are classified into A-, B-, and C-type particles based on structure (Sarkar *et al.*, 1972). The sarcoma and leukemia virus particles are C-type, having a central spherical nucleoid with a unit membrane envelope around it, while the murine mammary tumor viruses are B-type particles. These have a spherical nucleoid that is eccentrically located and enclosed in an inner membrane, which in turn is enclosed in an outer unit membrane. A-type particles are the precursors of either B- or C-type particles.

Avian RNA viruses have been classified into subgroups based on their host range in chickens (Vogt and Ishizaki, 1965). Similarly, murine viruses have been classified into subgroups based on their host range in mice by Hartley *et al.* (1970). Other characterizations of RNA tumor viruses have been based on studies of group-specific antigens (Gilden *et al.*, 1971),

RNA-dependent DNA polymerase (Baltimore, 1970; Temin and Mizutani, 1970), and viral envelope antigens (Aoki and Todaro, 1973). More recently, Aoki (1974) has proposed a reclassification of murine C-type viruses based on viral envelope antigens as demonstrated by immunoelectron microscopy.

For more detailed information on morphology, composition, and classification of tumor viruses, the reader is directed to reviews by Benyesh-Melnick (1974), Gross (1970), and Tooze (1973).

Animal and Human Studies

DNA-Virus-Induced Tumors

Several reviews on the role of viruses in human neoplasia have been written recently (Allen and Cole, 1972; Epstein, 1971; Gross 1970; McAllister, 1973; Rauscher, 1970). The present discussion is limited, and more lengthy presentations of specific studies may be found in these reviews.

According to McAllister (1973), adenoviruses, herpesviruses, and B- and C-type RNA viruses could be candidates for human cancer viruses. Some of the evidence for each of these types as well as other tumor viruses is discussed below.

Fibromas, Papillomas, and Warts

Advances in the isolation of oncogenic viruses were made rapidly, beginning with the isolation of the Shope rabbit fibroma virus (1932). This agent was found to be transmitted by mosquitoes and was related to the myxoma virus which was isolated by Sanarelli (1898).

Papillomas caused by virus were reported in rabbits (Shope, 1933), dogs (DeMonbreun and Goodpasture, 1932), horses (Cook and Olson, 1951), and cows (Magalhães, 1920). Warts in humans should be mentioned at this point because of the similar morphology of the human wart virus to the Shope papilloma virus in rabbits (Strauss et al., 1949). While most human warts regress, warts in rabbits are often transformed into carcinomas.

Adenoviruses

There have been at least 31 serological types of human adenoviruses which have been isolated. The fact that certain human adenoviruses are oncogenic in animals was mentioned in the previous section. There are also

TABLE 1. Properties of DNA Oncogenic Viruses

Nomenclature	Host of origin	Tumor induction in vivo	Tumor transformation in vitro	Morphology	Viral antigens	Virus-dependent antigens of tumor cells[a]
Papova viruses						
Papilloma						
Rabbit	Rabbit	Rabbit	—	Icosahedral symmetry (40–55 nm)	—	—
Canine	Dog	Dog	—			
Bovine	Cow	Cow	Cow			
Human	Man	Man	—			
Polyoma	Mouse	Mouse	Mouse		Major capsid polypeptide, Minor capsid polypeptide, Internal histone-like proteins	T, U. TSTA, S
		Hamster, rat	Hamster, rat			
SV 40	Monkey	Hamster	Hamster, mouse monkey, human			
Adenoviruses						
Human	Man	Hamster	Hamster, rat	Icosahedral symmetry (70–80 nm)	A (group and type specific, capsid) B (subgroup specific, capsid)	T (not cross-reacting with papovaviruses)
Simian	Monkey		Human			
Bovine	Cow	Rat, mouse				

Virus	Host	Tumor host	Tumor bearing host	Symmetry (size)	Virus antigens	Tumor antigens
Avian	Chicken				C (type specific, fiber) P (group specific, major core protein)	TSTA
Herpes viruses						
Human	Man			Icosahedral symmetry (100 nm)	Various	TSTA
Type 2	Man	Hamster	Hamster			
EB	Man	Monkey	Man, monkey			
Monkey	Monkey	Monkey	—			
Avian (Marek's)	Chicken	Chicken	—			
Frog (Lucké)	Frog	Frog	—			
Rabbit	Rabbit	Rabbit	—			
Poxviruses						
Molluscum contagiosum	Man	Man	Man	Complex symmetry (230 × 300 nm)	Various	TSTA
Yaba	Monkey	Monkey	—			
Fibromamyxoma	Rabbit, Deer	Rabbit, Deer	—			

[a] All antigens are distinct from virus antigens. (T) virus-specific tumor antigen, in the nucleus of tumor cells; (U) in the nuclear membrane, induced by SV 40 only; (TSTA) tumor-specific transplantation antigens, virus specific, found in human cell membrane; (S) surface antigen, virus specific, distinct from TSTA.

TABLE 2. Properties of Oncornoviruses (RNA Tumor Viruses)

Nomenclature	Host of origin	Tumor induction *in vivo*	Cell transformation *in vitro*	Morphology (particle type)	Antigenic structure of viruses and tumor cells[a]
Avian					
Leukemia (ALV)	Chicken	Chicken	Chicken		
Sarcoma (Rous)	Chicken	Avian, rodent Monkey	Avian, rodent monkey, human	C	ts, gs-1, TSTA
Murine					
Leukemia (MuLV)					
Moloney (MLV)					
Friend (FLV)	Mouse	Mouse, rat, Hamster	Mouse, rat, Hamster	C	ts, gs-1, gs-3 TSTA
Rauscher (RLV)					
Gross (GLV)					
Radiation (RadLV)					
Graffi					
Sarcoma (MSV)	Mouse	Mouse, rat, Hamster	Mouse, rat, Hamster	C	ts, gs-1, gs-3 TSTA
Mammary (MTV) (Bittner)	Mouse	Mouse	—	B	ts, gs-1

Feline				
Leukemia (FeLV)	Cat	Cat	—	C	ts, gs-1, gs-3
Sarcoma (FeSV)	Cat	Cat, rabbit, dog, monkey	Cat, rabbit, dog, monkey, human	C	ts, gs-1, gs-3
Bovine	Cow	—	—	C	—
Primates				
Sarcoma (wooley monkey)	Monkey	Monkey	Monkey	C	ts, gs-1, gs-3
Lymphosarcoma	Ape			
Mammary				
Carcinoma, monkey (Mason-P fizer)	Monkey	—	Monkey	B (?)	ts, gs-1

"(ts) Type-specific or subgroup-specific antigens (glycoproteins), associated with the virion envelope, cross-reacting within each subgroup: five avian, two murine, and three feline. Found in the virion envelope and virus-infected cells; (gs) group-specific antigens (basic polypeptides) associated with the virion core. (gs-1) Species-specific (cross-reacting within the same species), (gs-3) interspecies-specific (cross-reacting with different mammalian species). They are located in the virion core, virus-infected cells, virus-free tumor cells, some normal cells; (TSTA) tumor-specific transplantation antigens associated with tumor cell membrane. They are cross-reacting among FLV, MLV, and RLV (FMR group) and are distinct from GLV, MTV, and RSV. They are responsible for tumor rejection in presensitized hosts.

some adenoviruses of animals (Hull *et al.*, 1965; Darbyshire, 1966) which are oncogenic in newborn mice (Table 1). Infective virus has not been recovered from tumors induced by human adenovirus, although virus particles have been isolated from tissue-cultured cell lines of hamster tumors which were initiated by human adenovirus (Connor and Marti, 1966). Human cell cultures were transformed when exposed to adenovirus 12 (Todaro and Aaronson, 1968). This transformed cell line could not be maintained by passage. Although no complement-fixing antibody to adeno-virus antigens is seen in cancer patients (Gilden *et al.*, 1970), it has been reported that there is antibody to these antigens as measured by the fluorescent antibody technique (Lewis *et al.*, 1967). On the other hand, Gilden and his colleagues (1970) reported that there was no difference in the patients showing positive fluorescent antibody compared to the normal control group.

Polyoma Virus

Gross (1953) inoculated newborn C3H mice with extracts from leu-kemic Ak mice. Instead of developing leukemia, these mice developed parotid adenocarcinomas. Gross showed that the extracts from the leu-kemic mice actually contained two virus types, one for leukemia and one for the adenocarcinoma. The name polyoma virus was given to this parotid tumor agent because it was later found to induce other tumors such as renal carcinomas, mammary carcinomas, and liver hemangiomas (Stewart *et al.*, 1958). The polyoma virus has been found in many strains of normal mice (Rowe, 1961) but does not produce tumors when it multiplies in adult animals. In trying to determine just how polyoma virus is able to cause malignant transformation, Benjamin (1966) was able to show that messen-ger RNA transcribed from the polyoma virus was produced by each transformed cell.

SV 40 Virus

Simian virus 40 (SV 40) was first isolated by Sweet and Hilleman (1960) when it was tested on kidney cells of monkeys other than the host type. This virus is similar to polyoma in structure and like the polyoma virus it does not seem to cause disease in its natural host. On the other hand, it does produce tumors in newborn hamsters (Girardi *et al.*, 1962). Because human vaccines such as polio and adenovirus are produced in monkey kidney cell cultures, it is important to determine if these vaccines are infected with SV 40. In fact, the SV 40 was found in some vaccine preparations and methods were devised to inactivate the SV 40 in further vaccines (Hayashi and LoGrippo, 1962). Of course, the ideal way to prevent SV 40 contamination of human vaccines is to use cell cultures that are free of the virus.

Herpesviruses

In order to determine oncogenic potential, Rapp (1973) pointed out the need to study carefully viruses such as the herpesviruses which infect both man and animals, persist for long periods in the body, and cause a number of clinical illnesses. Herpesviruses have been shown to produce tumors in a wide variety of animals: Luckè frog carcinoma (Luckè, 1938) and Marek's disease in chickens (Churchill and Biggs, 1967), rabbits (Hinze, 1971), guinea pigs (Hsiung and Kaplow, 1969), and monkeys (Melendez et al., 1969). Attenuated vaccine to Marek's disease has been produced and is effective in the prevention of the naturally occurring disease in chickens (Churchill et al., 1969).

One virus that "meets the criteria" of a human tumor virus, according to Rapp (1973), is the Epstein–Barr virus (Epstein et al., 1964), a herpesvirus isolated from lymphoblasts of patients with Burkitt's lymphoma (Burkitt, 1962). Virus-specific DNA has been found to be incorporated into cells of Burkitt lymphoma patients (zur Hausen and Schulte-Holthausen, 1970). Furthermore, it has been found that a large portion of adults have antibody titers to this virus. This led to the finding that the Epstein–Barr virus is the etiologic agent of infectious mononucleosis (Henle et al., 1968).

Herpes simplex II virus has been isolated from the male genito-urinary tract (Centifanto et al., 1972), and antibodies to this virus have been shown in a greater number of women with cervical carcinoma than in control groups (Rawls et al., 1969). This has led to speculation concerning sexual transmission of the virus.

RNA-Virus-Induced Tumors

Mice have been used more extensively for the study of virus-induced tumors than any other species. This has been due, in part, to the development of inbred strains of mice which respond uniformly in individual studies or have a high incidence of spontaneous tumors. Gross (1951) was able to transmit leukemia from the high-incidence leukemic Ak strain mice to the low-incidence C3H strain. He found it necessary to use newborn mice for induction of the leukemia. After the work of Gross, numerous murine leukemia viruses were isolated, each being named for the discoverer. Among these were the Graffi (Graffi *et al.*, 1955), Friend (1957), Moloney (1960), and Rauscher (1962) viruses. Gross (1970) questioned whether most murine leukemia viruses are actually the same virus isolated from different sources. The evidence shown in the various types of classification of RNA viruses mentioned above seems to refute that point.

Later studies demonstrated that sarcomas could be produced in mice by induction with viruses from leukemia-virus-infected mice (Moloney, 1966; Kirsten and Mayer, 1967). The sarcoma viruses were found to be defective in that the leukemia virus was needed as a "helper" (Hartley and Rowe, 1966).

Two avenues of study of the RNA tumor viruses in animals give promise for determining the role of viral etiology of human tumors. Mention of the RNA-dependent DNA polymerase (reverse transcriptase) has already been made (Baltimore, 1970; Temin and Mizutani, 1970). This enzyme has been found in all RNA-tumor viruses and is necessary for the production of DNA from an RNA template. Gallo *et al.* (1970) found that the leukemic cells of three patients had reverse transcriptase while the normal lymphoblasts had none. Thus, if this enzyme is necessary for malignant transformation, its inhibition would prevent transformation. The other study which is of interest is the induction of *in vitro* viruus expression by deoxyuridine analogues. One study of this phenomenon has been in the virus-free Balb/3T3 cells (Aaronson *et al.*, 1971). It is possible that nondetectable virus is present in human tumor cells and can be expressed under the proper stimulation in *in vitro* culture. This, in fact, has been reported (Stewart *et al.*, 1972) in human tumor cells in culture. Virus particles resembling animal C-type RNA tumor viruses have been isolated from human tumors (Dmochowski and Bowen, 1973). In one study (Newell *et al.*, 1968), an attempt was made to correlate the number and distribution of virus-like particles in leukemic patients with histological diagnosis, clinical status, white blood cells, and platelet counts. No such correlation could be made.

The discovery that mammary tumors in mice were induced by virus through transmission in milk to nursing animals (Bittner, 1936) has led to a great deal of speculation and study in the human breast cancer problem. It was not until later that it was realized that there was more than one type of mouse mammary tumor virus and that unlike the Bittner virus, some were passed to the offspring through the sperm and eggs (Mühlbock and Bentuelzen, 1969). The mammary tumors in mice seem to be genetically and hormonally controlled and do not develop in male mice unless they are given estrogens (Boot *et al.*, 1972). A recent review of the etiology of human breast cancer (MacMahon *et al.*, 1973) presents evidence for the-possible role of viruses in this disease. Moore *et al.* (1971) found a high incidence (60%) of B-type virus particles in milk from women with a family history of breast cancer. However, later evidence by Sarkar and Moore (1972) showed no differences in women with or without a family history of the disease.

Hypotheses of Viral Oncogenesis

There have been several hypotheses proposed to explain the mechanism of viral carcinogenesis. The two major theories are the protovirus hypothesis (Temin, 1964, 1971) and the viral oncogene hypothesis (Huebner and Todaro, 1969). These two hypotheses emphasize the relationship of RNA tumor viruses with their host cells. Final proof of either of these hypotheses would answer many of the questions involving the interaction of viral genetic information with host nucleic acid as well as the process of transformation of normal to neoplastic cells. Briefly, the theories are the following.

Protovirus Hypothesis

Temin postulated that the oncogenic virus acts through a provirus mechanism in which the viral genome is incorporated into the host-cell nucleic acid by virion-RNA-directed DNA polymerase. The neoplastic state may then be induced by any mechanism which disrupts the unstable protovirus. The malignant transformation of the cells may not be accompanied by viral production, thus the difficulty in recovering oncogenic viruses from human tumors.

Viral Oncogene Hypothesis

This theory states, unlike the protovirus hypothesis, that the oncogenes or genetic information for cell transformation are incorporated in germ cells as well as somatic cells of most vertebrates. These oncogenes have been transmitted since early in the evolutionary process and are normally suppressed, but on the proper stimulation from various carcinogenic agents, they could be expressed.

Antiviral Therapy

Therapeutic approaches to neoplasia have taken several directions including radiation, chemotherapy, and, more recently, immunotherapy. The use of drugs has had some serious drawbacks because most of these agents are toxic, not only to tumor cells, but also to normal cells. At the same time, moderate to severe immunosuppression of the patient is often an undesired side effect. If, in fact, certain human tumors have a viral etiology, then agents that have antiviral capabilities may be of considerable importance. Two recent reviews have discussed such studies and have listed agents in some detail (Chirigos and Papas, 1974; Goldberg and Goldin, 1973). One of these reviews (Chirigos and Papas, 1974) states that the treatment of mammalian oncogenic viral diseases is directed toward drugs that block some virus-specific process, interferon and interferon inducers, drugs that inhibit the reverse transcriptase, and finally stimulation of the host defense mechanisms.

The development of interferon has been summarized by Hilleman (1970). Interferon is a protein whose production is stimulated by nucleic acid or numerous synthetic inducers such as polyinosinic–polycytidylic acid (poly I:C), tilorone, statolon, and pyran copolymer (Field *et al.*, 1967; Wheelock, 1970). Interferon is species specific and seems to act at the level of inhibition of the translation process of viral replication by preventing attachment of viral messenger RNA to the host-cell ribosomes (Hirschman, 1971).

Chirigos and Papas (1974) have listed numerous compounds that have been reported to have activity against reverse transcriptase. Among these are: antibiotics such as rifamycin, streptovarycin, actinomycin D, and adriamycin; polymers such as polynucleotides; and substrate analogues like cytosine arabinoside. These various enzyme inhibitors react at different inhibition sites, any of which result in the reduction or prevention of enzyme activity.

In recent years, the use of nonspecific stimulators of the immune system has been studied extensively. One such stimulator, *Mycobacterium bovis* (BCG) has also been reported to have an effect against murine leukemia and sarcoma viruses (Larson *et al.*, 1972; Schwartz *et al.*, 1971). The mechanism may not be directly antiviral but may be due instead to the immune stimulation of the host.

References

Aaronson, S. A., Todaro, G. J., and Scolnick, E. M. (1971). Induction of murine C-type viruses from clonal lines of virus-free Balb/3T3 cells. *Science* **174**:157.
Allen, D. W., and Cole, P. (1972). Viruses and human cancer. *N. Engl. J. Med.* **286**:70.
Aoki, T. (1974). Murine type-C RNA viruses: A proposed reclassification, other possible pathogenicities, and new immunological function. *J. Nat. Cancer Inst.* **52**:1029.
Aoki, T., and Todaro, G. J. (1973). Antigenic properties of endogenous type-C viruses from spontaneously transformed clones of Balb/3T3. *Proc. Nat. Acad. Sci. U.S.A.* **70**:1598.
Baltimore, D. (1970). Viral RNA-dependent DNA polymerase. *Nature (London)* **226**:1209.

Beard, J. W. (1963). Avian virus growths and their etiologic agents. *Adv. Cancer Res.* **7**:1.

Benjamin, T. L. (1966). Virus-specific RNA in cell productively infected or transformed by polyoma virus. *J. Mol. Biol.* **16**:259.

Benyesh-Melnick, M. (1974). Oncogenic Viruses. In *Review of Medical Microbiology*. Lange, Los Altos, Calif.

Bernhard, W., Bonar, R. A., Beard, D., and Beard, J. W. (1958). Ultrastructure of viruses of myeloblastosis and erythroblastosis isolated from plasma of leukemic chickens. *Proc. Soc. Exp. Biol. Med.* **97**:48.

Bittner, J. J. (1936). Some possible effects of nursing on the mammary gland tumor incidence in mice. *Science* **84**:162.

Boot, L. M., Röpcke, G. and Kwa, H. G. (1972). Hormonal factors in the origin of mammary tumors. In *RNA Viruses and Host Genome in Oncogenesis* (P. Emmelot and P. Bentvelzen, eds.). North Holland, Amsterdam.

Burkitt, D. (1962). Determining the climatic limitations of a children's cancer common in Africa. *Br. Med. J.* **II**:1019.

Centifanto, Y. M., Drylie, D. M., and Deardourff, S. C. (1972). Herpesvirus type 2 in the male genitourinary tract. *Science* **178**:318.

Chirigos, M., and Papas, T. (1974). Immunological and chemotherapeutic prevention and control of oncogenic viruses. In *Advances in Pharmacology and Chemotherapy*. (S. Garattini, A. Goldin, F. Hawking, and I. Kopin, eds.). Academic Press, New York.

Churchill, A. E., and Biggs, P. M. (1967). Agent of Marek's disease in tissue culture. *Nature (London)* **215**:528.

Churchill, A. E., Payne, L. N., and Chubb, R. C. (1969). Immunization against Marek's disease using a live attenuated virus. *Nature (London)* **221**:744.

Connor, J. D., and Marti, A. (1966). Isolation of adenoviruses from tissue cultures of adenovirus type 12 induced hamster tumors. *Proc. Am. Assoc. Cancer Res.* **7**:14.

Cook, R. H., and Olson, C., Jr. (1951). Experimental transmission of cutaneous papilloma of the horse. *Am. J. Pathol.* **27**:1087.

Darbyshire, J. H. (1966). Oncogenicity of bovine adenovirus type 3 in hamsters. *Nature (London)* **211**:102.

DeMonbreun, W. A., and Goodpasture, E. W. (1932). Infectius oral papillomatosis of dogs. *Am. J. Pathol.* **8**:43.

Dmochowski, L., and Bowen, J. (1973). The search for a virus in human cancer. *Proc. Nat. Cancer Conf.* **7**:697.

Eckhart, W. (1972). Oncogenic viruses. *Annu. Rev. Biochem.* **41**:503.

Ellerman, V., and Bang, O. (1908). Experimentelle Leukämie bei Hühnern. *Zentralbl. Bakt. Abt. I (Orig.)* **46**:595.

Epstein, M. A. (1971). The possible role of viruses in human cancer. *Lancet* **I**:1344.

Epstein, M. A., Achong, B. G., and Barr, Y. M. (1964). Virus particles in cultured lymphoblasts from Burkitt's lymphoma. *Lancet* **1**:702.

Field, A. K., Tytell, A. A., Lampson, G. P., and Hilleman, M. R. (1967). Inducers of interferon and host resistance. II. Multistranded synthetic polynucleotide complexes. *Proc. Nat. Acad. Sci. U.S.A.* **58**:1004.

Friend, C. (1957). Cell-free transmission in adult Swiss mice of a disease having the character of a leukemia. *J. Exp. Med.* **105**:307.

Gallo, R. C., Yang, S. S., and Ting, R. C. (1970). RNA dependent DNA polymerase of human actue leukaemic cells. *Nature (London)* **228**:927.

Gilden, R. V., Kern, J., Lee, Y. K., Rapp, F., Melnick, J. L., Riggs, J. L., Lennette, E. H., Zbar, B., Rapp, H. J., Turner, H. C., and Huebner, R. J. (1970). Serologic surveys of human cancer patients for antibody to adenovirus T antigens. *Am. J. Epidemiol.* **91**:500.

Gilden, R. V., Oroszlan, S., and Huebner, R. J. (1971). Coexistence of intraspecies and interspecies specific antigenic determinants of the major structural polypeptide of mammalian C-type viruses. *Nature (London)* **231**:107.

Girardi, A. J. Slotnick, V. B. and Hilleman, M. R. (1962). Search for virus in human malignancies. I. *In vitro* studies. *Proc. Soc. Exptl. Biol. Med.* **110**:776.

Goldberg, A. I., and Goldin, A. (1973). Antiviral agents in the treatment of acute leukemia. In *Modern Trends in Oncology* (R. Raven, Raven, ed.). Butterworth, London.

Graffi, A., Bielka, H., Fey, F., Scharsach, F., and Weiss, R. (1955). Gehaüftes Auftreten von Leukämien nach Injektion von Sarkom-Filtraten. *Wien. Klin. Wochenschr.* **105**:61.

Gross, L. (1951). Spontaneous leukemia developing in C3H mice following inoculation, in infancy, with AK-leukemic extracts, or AK-embryos. *Proc. Soc. Exp. Biol. Med.* **76**:27.

Gross, L. (1953). A filterable agent, recovered from AK leukemic extracts, causing salivary gland carcinomas in C3H mice. *Proc. Soc. Exp. Biol. Med.* **83**:414.

Gross, L. (1970). *Oncogenic Viruses.* Purnell, London.

Hartley, J . W., and Rowe, W. P. (1966). Production of altered cell foci in tissue culture by defective Moloney sarcoma virus particles. *Proc. Nat. Acad. Sci. U.S.A.* **55**:780.

Hartley, J. W., Rowe, W. P., and Huebner, R. J. (1970). Host range restrictions of murine leukemia viruses in mouse embryo cell cultures. *J. Virol.* **5**:221.

zur Hausen, H., Schulte-Holthausen, H. (1970). Presence of EB virus nucleic acid homology in a virus-free line of Burkitt tumor cells. *Nature (London)* **227**:245.

Hayashi, H., and LoGrippo, G. A. (1962). Inactivation of vacuolating virus (Sv-40) by beta-propiolactone. I. Evaluation in tissue culture. *Henry Ford Hosp. Med. Bull.* **10**:463.

Henle, G., Henle, W., and Diehl, V. (1968). Relation of Burkitt's tumor-associated herpes-type virus to infectious mononucleosis. *Proc. Nat. Acad. Sci. U.S.A.* **59**:94.

Hilleman, M. R. (1970). Double-stranded RNAs (Poly I:C) in the prevention of viral infections. *Arch. Int. Med.* **126**:109.

Hinze, H. C. (1971). Induction of lymphoid hypoplasia and lymphomalike disease in rabbits by herpes virus sylvilagus. *Int. J. Cancer* **8**:514.

Hirschman, S. Z. (1971). Approaches to antiviral chemotherapy. *Am. J. Med.* **51**:669.

Hsiung, G. D., and Kaplow, L. S. (1969). Herpeslike virus isolated from spontaneously degenerated tissue culture derived from leukemia susceptible guinea pigs. *J. Virol.* **3**:355.

Huebner, R. J., Rowe, W. P., Turner, H. C., and Lane, W. T. (1963). Specific adenovirus complement-fixing antigens in virus-free hamster and rat tumors. *Proc. Nat. Acad. Sci. U.S.A.* **50**:379.

Huebner, R. J., and Todaro, G. J. (1969). Oncogenes of RNA tumor viruses as determinants of cancer. *Proc. Nat. Acad. Sci., U.S.A.* **64**:1087.

Hull, R. N., Johnson, I. S., Culbertson, C. G., Reimer, C. B., and Wright, H. F. (1965). Oncogenicity of the simian adenovirus. *Science* **150**:1044.

Kieff, E. D., Bachenheimer, S. L., and Roizman, B. (1971). Size, composition and structure of the DNA of subtypes 1 and 2 herpes simplex virus. *J. Virol.* **8**:125.

Kirsten, W. H., and Mayer, L. A. (1967). Morphologic responses to a murine erythroblastosis virus. *J. Nat. Cancer Inst.* **39**:311.

Larson, C. L., Baker, R. G., Ushijima, R. N., Baker, M. B., and Gillespie, C. (1972). Immunotherapy of Friend disease in mice employing viable BCG vaccine. *Proc. Soc. Exp. Biol. Med.* **140**:700.

Lewis, A. M., Jr., Wiese, W. H., and Rowe, W. P. (1967). The presence of antibodies in human serum to early (T) adenovirus antigens. *Proc. Nat. Acad. Sci. (Washington)* **57**:622.

Lucké, B. (1938). Carcinoma in the leopard frog: Its probable causation by a virus. *J. Exp. Med.* **68**:457.

Luria, S. E., and Darnell, J. E., Jr. (1967). *General Virology.* Wiley, New York.

MacMahon, B., Cole, P., and Brown, J. (1973). Etiology of human breast cancer: A review. *J. Nat. Cancer Inst.* **50**:21.

Magalhães, O. (1920). Verruga dos bovideos. *Brasil-Medico* **34**:430.

McAllister, R. M. (1973). Viruses n human carcinogenesis. In *Progress in Medical Virology*. (J. L. Melnick, ed.). Karger, Basel.

Melendez, L. V., Hunt, R. D., Daniel, M. D., Garcia, F. G., and Fraser, C. E. O. (1969). *Herpes saimiri*. II. Experimentally induced malignant lymphoma in primates. *Lab. Animal Care* **19**:378.

Melnick, J. L. (1962). Papova virus group. *Science* **135**:1128.

Moloney, J. B. (1960). Biological studies on a lymphoid leukemia virus extracted from S.37. I. Origin and introductory investigations. *J. Nat. Cancer Inst.* **24**:933.

Moloney, J. B. (1966). A virus-induced rhabodomyosarcoma of mice. *Nat. Cancer Inst. Monogr.* **22**:139.

Moore, D. H., Charney, J., Kramarsky, B., Lasfargues, E. Y., Sarkar, N. H., Brennan, M. J., Burrows, J. H., Sirsat, S. M., Paymaster, J. C., and Vaidya, A. B. (1971). Search for a human breast cancer virus. *Nature (London)* **229**:611.

Mühlbock, O., and Bentuelzen, P. (1969). The transmission of the mammary tumor viruses. *Perspect. Virol.* **6**:75.

Newell, G. R., Harris, W. W., Bowman, K. O., Boone, C. W., and Anderson, N. G. (1968). Evaluation of 'virus-like' particles in the plasmas of 225 patients with leukemia and related disease. *N. Engl. J. Med.* **278**:1185.

Pereira, H. G., Huebner, R. J., Ginsberg, H. S., and Van der Veer, J. (1963). A short description of the adenovirus group. *Virology* **20**:613.

Rabson, A. S., Kirchstein, R. L., and Paul, F. J. (1964). Tumors produced by adenovirus 12 in mastomys and mice. *J. Nat. Cancer Inst.* **32**:87.

Rapp, F. (1973). Question: Do herpesviruses cause cancer? Answer: Of course they do! *J. Nat. Cancer Inst.* **50**:825.

Rauscher, F. J., Jr. (1962). A virus-induced disease of mice characterized by erythrocytopiesis and lymphoid leukemia. *J. Nat. Cancer Inst.* **29**:515.

Rauscher, F. J., Jr. (1970). Present status of studies on the virus etiology of cancer. *Proc. Nat. Cancer Conf.* **6**:93.

Rawls, W. E., Tompkins, W. A., and Melnick, J. L. (1969). The association of herpesvirus type 2 and carcinoma of the uterine cervix. *Am. J. Epidemiol.* **89**:547.

Roizman, B. (1969). The herpesviruses: A biochemical definition of the group. *Curr. Top. Microbiol. Immunol.* **49**:1.

Rous, P. (1911). Transmission of a malignant new growth by means of a cell-free filtrate. *J. Am. Med. Assoc.* **56**:198.

Rowe, W. P. (1961). The epidemiology of mouse polyoma virus infection. *Bacteriol. Rev.* **25**:18.

Sanarelli, G. (1898). Das Myxomatosum Virus. Beitrag zum Studium ker Krankheitserreger ausserhalb des Sichtbaren. *Zentralbl. Bakt. Abt. I.* **23**:865.

Sarkar, N. H., and Moore, D. H. (1972). On the possibility of a human breast cancer virus. *Nature (London)* **236**:103.

Sarkar, N. H., Moore, D. H., and Nowinski, R. C. (1972). Symmetry of the nucleocapsid of the oncornaviruses. In *RNA Viruses and Host Genome in Oncogenesis*. (P. Emmelot and P. Bentvelzen, eds.). North Holland, Amsterdam.

Schwartz, D. B., Zbar, B., Gibson, W. T., and Chirigos, M. A. (1971). Inhibition of murine sarcoma virus oncogenesis with living BCG. *Int. J. Cancer* **8**:320.

Shope, R. E. (1932). A filtrable virus causing tumor-like condition in rabbits and its relationship to virus myxomatosum. *J. Exp. Med.* **56**:803.

Shope, R. E. (1933). Infectious papillomatosis of rabbits. *J. Exp. Med.* **58**:607.

Stewart, S. E., Eddy, B. E., and Borgese, N. (1958). Neoplasms in mice inoculated with a tumor agent carried in tissue culture. *J. Nat. Cancer Inst.* **20**:1223.

Stewart, S. E., Kasnic, G., Draycott, C., and Ben, T. (1972). Activation of viruses in human tumors by 5-iododeoxyuridine and dimethyl sulfoxide. *Science* **175**:198.

Strauss, M. J., Shaw, E. W., Bunting, H., and Melnick, J. L. (1949). Crystalline virus-like particles from skin papillomas characterized by intranuclear inclusion bodies. *Proc. Soc. Exp. Biol. Med.* **72**:46.

Sweet, B. H., and Hilleman, M. R. (1960). The vacuolating virus, SV 40. *Proc. Soc. Exp. Biol. Med.* **105**:420.

Temin, H. M. (1964). Nature of the provirus of Rous sarcoma. *Nat. Cancer Inst. Monogr.* **17**:557.

Temin, H. M. (1971). The protovirus hypothesis: Speculations on the significance of RNA-directed DNA synthesis for normal development and for carcinogenesis. *J. Nat. Cancer Inst.* **46**:3.

Temin, H. M., and Mizutani, S. (1970). RNA-dependent DNA polymerase in virions of Rous sarcoma virus. *Nature (London)* **226**:1121.

Todaro, G. J., and Aaronson, S. A. (1968). Human cell strains susceptible to focus formation by human adenovirus type 12. *Proc. Nat. Acad. Sci. (Washington)* **61**:1272.

Tooze, J., ed. (1973). *The Molecular Biology of Tumor Viruses.* Cold Spring Harbor Monograph Series. Cold Spring Harbor, New York.

Trentin, J. J., Yabe, Y., and Taylor, G. (1962). The quest for human cancer viruses. *Science* **137**:835.

Varmus, H. E., Levinson, W. E., and Bishop, J. M. (1971). Extent of transcription by the RNA-dependent DNA polymerase of Rous sarcoma virus. *Nature New Biol.* **233**:19.

Vogt, P. K., and Ishizaki, R. (1965). Reciprocal patterns of genetic resistance to avian tumor viruses in two lines of chickens. *Virology* **26**:664.

Wheelock, E. F. (1970). Applied and induced interferon in the prophylaxis and induced treatment of leukemia. *Arch. Int. Med.* **126**:64.

Chapter 12

IMMUNOLOGY OF MALIGNANT DISEASE

R. W. BALDWIN

Introduction

The view that immunological reactions play a role in modifying or even controlling malignant disease has gained wide acceptance within recent years. This has come about first from the results of well-substantiated investigations showing that many experimental animal tumors induced by chemical carcinogens and oncogenic viruses as well as those of unknown (spontaneous) etiology elicit immune rejection reactions comparable in kind, if not in degree, with those causing tissue graft rejections (Baldwin, 1973; Hellström and Hellström, 1974b; Cerottini and Brunner, 1974). Secondly, clinical studies have reached the stage where laboratory tests for tumor-immune reactions, initially developed in well-defined animal systems, have positively identified specific responses against a number of human tumors. Thirdly, these laboratory findings are consistent with the small but impressive examples from clinical studies suggesting, but not proving, that immunological reactions may in some circumstances have been responsible for host control of malignant disease. This includes reports of spontaneous remission with a variety of cancers such as melanomata, neuroblastomata, and renal cell carcinomata (Everson and Cole,

R. W. Baldwin • Professor of Tumor Biology, Cancer Research Campaign Laboratories, The University of Nottingham, Nottingham, NG7 2RD, England.

1966). One can also cite cases of patients having had surgical removal of breast carcinoma who remain clinically free of disease for many years but eventually develop recurrent growths and the regression of Burkitt's lymphoma in patients receiving minimal chemotherapy (Burkitt, 1967); these phenomena suggest the involvement of host immune responses. Finally, there are the reports of increased incidences of malignant tumors in patients who have received continuous immunosuppressive therapy following organ transplantation (Penn, 1974). For example, of 432 patients receiving renal homografts in one center, 24 developed malignant disease. This incidence (5.6%) is approximately 100 times greater than that observed in the general population in the same age group, and in many instances malignancy developed within a relatively short time (1 to 92 months) after the commencement of immunosuppressive therapy (Penn, 1974).

Within this framework of knowledge, therefore, it is pertinent to consider whether the detection of host immune reactions to *tumor-associated antigens* can be employed for immunodiagnosis. Also, are the immune responses in the cancer-bearing patient of sufficient magnitude to provide a basis for immunotherapy and if so, how can they be augmented?

Immunological Rejection of Tumors

The concept that tumor-specific immune responses may be effective in modifying tumor growth is principally based upon studies showing that immunity can be induced against many, although by no means all, experimentally-induced animal tumors (Hellström and Hellström, 1969; Baldwin, 1973). This was originally established with tumors induced in animals by a variety of methods including treatment with chemical carcinogens and oncogenic viruses and transplanted into inbred (syngeneic) recipients, these being genetically compatible in order to exclude any possible contribution by immune responses directed against normal tissue transplantation antigens. Employing these model systems, it has been established that hosts *preimmunized* in a variety of ways against tumor cells were protected against a subsequent challenge with the immunizing tumor. For example, surgical resection of a developing tumor graft (Figure 1) often provides complete protection against subsequent challenge with cells of the resected tumor. Tumor immunity can also be induced by implanting tumor cells in a manner that prevents their continuous growth. This may be achieved, for example, by administering tumor cells attenuated by X- or γ-irradiation (10 to 15,000 rads) or by treatment with drugs such as mitomycin C (Rios and Simmons, 1974). In some instances it is also possible to induce immunity by implanting tumor cells at sites, e.g., intradermally, which do not adequately support tumor growth (Zbar *et al.*, 1969) or by injecting tumor cells in

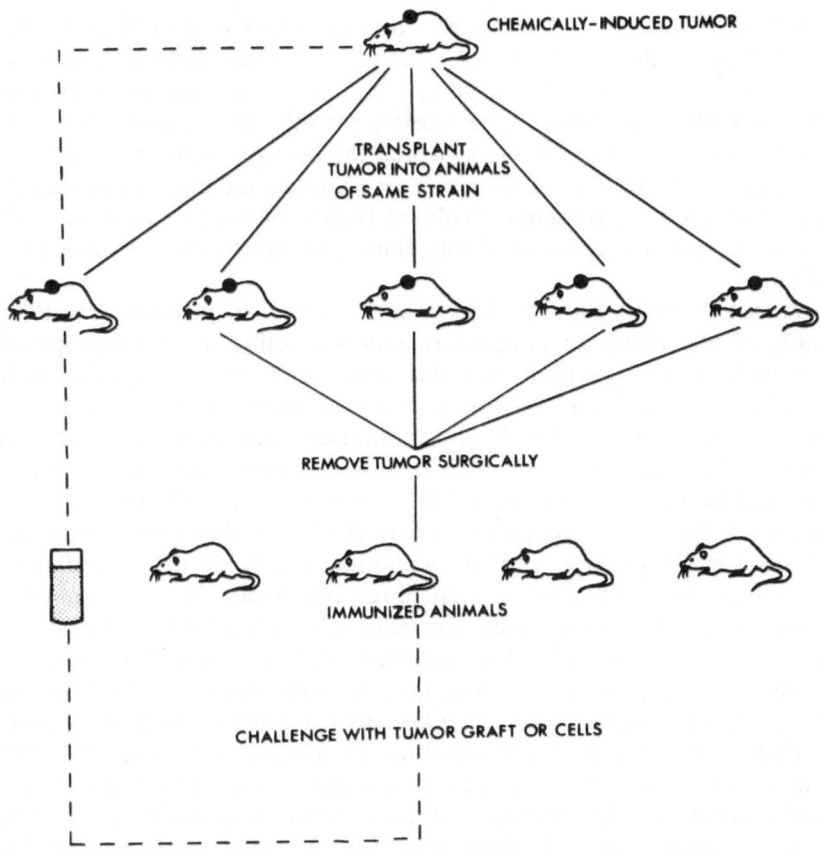

Figure 1. Induction of immunity to chemically induced tumors. Tumors induced in syngeneic (inbred) animals are transplanted to other members of the strain. Tumor implants are completely resected and this leads to the development of a specific immunity against a further challenge with the same tumor.

admixture with bacterial adjuvants such as bacillus Calmette Guérin (BCG). With the latter treatment, the adjuvant mediates an as yet ill-defined response, but probably involving macrophages, which results in the rejection of the implanted tumor cells and so frequently produces immunity in the host against further challenges with the same tumor.

The tumor-associated antigens involved in the induction of tumor immunity are known to be expressed within the cell surface membrane of tumor cells and with a number of examples it has been possible to isolate these substances employing extraction procedures similar to those developed in studies on human transplantation (HL-A) antigens (Baldwin, 1973;

Baldwin and Price, 1975). However, immunization with subcellular fractions of tumor cells or even with "purified" tumor antigens often does not
produce an immune response which protects the host against a subsequent
challenge with viable tumor. The reasons for this are not clear, but probably reflect alternative pathways in which the host processes tumor antigen
when presented in different forms. These studies indicate, however, that
immunotherapeutic protocols involving treatment with dead tumor cells,
tumor homogenates, or isolated subcellular fractions must be viewed with
caution.

Although many experimental animal tumors *do* possess neoantigens
capable of producing an immune rejection reaction against transplanted
tumor cells, this is not uniformly the case. For instance, experimentally-
induced and spontaneous mammary carcinomata as well as spontaneously
arising fibrosarcomata in rats often lack immunogenicity as defined by their
capacity to induce immunity against tumors transplanted into syngeneic
hosts (Baldwin and Embleton, 1974). It is not correct, therefore, to conclude from the many experimental animal studies that human malignant
cells necessarily express similar neoantigens capable of functioning as
rejection antigens. For obvious ethical reasons, evaluation of immunity in
patients against transplanted cancer cells is unacceptable, although some
years ago it was observed that malignant cells obtained from surgically
resected growths and reimplanted intradermally did not "take" readily,
and that large numbers were required to establish even limited growth
(Southam, 1967). Even so, these findings do not establish conclusively that
immune factors are involved, and so for the present direct evidence for
immune reactions directed against neoantigens expressed upon human
malignant cells is provided principally by *in vitro* tests of cell-mediated and
humoral immunity (see p. 285). There is a further complication in interpreting these data, however, since while the *in vitro* tests indicate that a patient
responds immunologically to antigens on malignant cells, it cannot be
concluded that this immune response functions to produce tumor rejection.
This is illustrated by studies with several tumor types including mammary
carcinomata in rats which are not able to produce an effective tumor
rejection response against tumor cells transplanted into compatible hosts.
Nevertheless, all of these tumors possess neoantigens against which the
tumor-bearing host responds, these immune reactions being detected
employing a variety of *in vitro* assays such as lymphocyte cytotoxicity
(Baldwin and Embleton, 1974).

Specificities of Tumor-Associated Antigens

The above findings indicate that tumors may express different types of
neoantigen, not all of which are able to produce immune responses capable

of causing tumor cell killing (Table 1). Tumor rejection antigens associated with chemically induced tumors almost invariably are characteristic components of individual tumors, since immunization of compatible hosts against a single tumor provides protection against a subsequent challenge with the same tumor, but not with others, even when induced by the same carcinogen and of similar histological type (Baldwin, 1973). In comparison, the tumor-associated antigens demonstrated by *in vitro* methods on tumors which are not able to elicit tumor rejection reactions differ in their specificity in being either common to several tumors irrespective of their etiology and histological type or in some cases, e.g., rat mammary or colon carcinomata, show histological-type specificites. These tumor-associated antigens have been identified as reexpressed embryonic products, since they can also be detected upon embryo cells at certain stages of embryonic development (Baldwin and Embleton, 1974; Steel and Sjögren, 1974).

Tumor rejection antigens associated with virus-induced tumors generally show virus-related specificities in that immunity elicited against one tumor will also be effective against other tumors induced with the same virus, even though they may be of a different histological type. The antigens involved in these responses may be virus-coded products or new antigens synthesized by the transformed cell (Levy, 1974; Deinhardt, 1974), and in this case some of these have also been identified as reexpressed embryonic antigens (Coggin and Anderson, 1974). In this context, it is pertinent to note that the immune responses detected by *in vitro* methods against human tumors, e.g., by cytotoxic reactions of peripheral blood lymphocytes, indicate that the antigens responsible show histological-type specificity. For example, lymphocytes from a patient with colon carcinoma react with cells of the patient's tumor and other colon carcinomata but not with those from breast carcinoma or melanoma (Hellström and Helström,

TABLE 1. Specificity of Host Responses to Tumor-Associated Antigens on Experimental Animal and Human Tumors

Tumor type	Specificity of tumor antigen detected by	
	Tumor rejection	Lymphocyte cytotoxicity *in vitro*
Chemically-induced	Individually distinct None detected	Individually distinct Cross-reacting and/or histological-type specific (embryonic antigens)
Virus-induced	Cross-reacting (virus specific)	Cross-reacting (virus specific/embryonic antigens)
Human	?	Cross-reacting (histological-type specific)

1974b). This suggests that the tumor antigens being detected may be reexpressed embryonic antigens, but formal proof of this postulate has still to be provided.

Rejection Reactions in the Tumor-Bearing Host

In experimental animal systems where tumor rejection responses can be demonstrated against transplanted tumor cells, they also develop in the tumor-bearing host. This has been defined as *concomitant immunity* and is detected in tests showing that an animal with a tumor developing at one site and which is beyond host control can, nevertheless, reject a challenge with cells of the same tumor implanted at another site. This indicates that tumor immune responses are only able to suppress growth of limited numbers of tumor cells variously estimated to be between 10^5 and 10^7 cells. It can be predicted, therefore, that immunotherapeutic procedures normally will only be able to deal with limited amounts of tumor and so will be applicable for the treatment of "minimum residual disease." Also, since tumor-bearing hosts can be shown to have developed an effective immune response to tumor implanted at a second site, this implies that either the response was too weak or developed too slowly to cause rejection of the primary tumor or, alternatively, some other factor may have modified this initial response. These observations are pertinent to the concept of circulating blocking factors which abrogate tumor rejection responses (see p. 287) and also to the view that immunotherapy may have clinical application in some circumstances.

Mechanisms of Tumor Cell Killing

In Vivo Studies

As well as permitting unequivocal demonstration of tumor-associated rejection antigens, studies with transplanted animal tumors have provided an assessment of the relative roles of sensitized lymphoid cells and serum antibody in the rejection process (Cerottini and Brunner, 1974; Hellström and Hellström, 1974b). In general, it is accepted that cell-mediated immunity is of primary importance, since it is frequently possible to transfer immunity to normal compatible hosts with lymphoid cells from tumor-immune, or in some cases tumor-bearer, donors. These cells may be obtained from a number of sources including lymph nodes, spleen, peritoneal exudates, thoracic duct lymph, and peripheral blood, but the precise nature of the effector cell is still unclear (see p. 285).

The role of tumor-specific antibody is more problematical. Early studies demonstrated a number of contradictory effects when attempts were made to transfer immunity against transplanted tumor cells with serum from tumor-immune donors: Different studies showed weak suppression of tumor growth or, quite frequently, no significant effect. In some cases, passively transferred serum even produced enhancement of tumor growth, suggesting that tumor-specific antibody plays no significant role in tumor rejection and may even act antagonistically, favoring tumor survival. This view is now thought to be too extreme in light of studies showing that antibody may produce a cytotoxic effect either through fixation of complement or probably even more effectively through cooperation with normal lymphoid cells (MacLennan, 1972). This so-called "cell-dependent antibody killing" has been proposed, for example, to account for the therapeutic effects of antibody against a transplanted rat lymphoma (Hersey, 1973).

In Vitro Studies

Characterization of effector mechanisms involved in immunological reactions against tumor cells, and also serum factors modifying cell-mediated immunity has depended largely upon the development of in vitro assays of tumor cell killing (Hellström and Hellström, 1974b; Cerottini and Brunner, 1974). The colony inhibition technique, originally introduced by I. Hellström (1967) was the first test with sufficient precision and sensitivity to allow measurement of the cytotoxic action of sensitized lymphoid cells on tumor cells in tissue culture. In this assay, tumor cells are seeded at low density in small plastic Petri dishes and after a period (generally 24 h) to allow attachment of the cells, lymphoid cells from test or control donors are added. The dishes are then cultured for 3 to 7 days, and after this time, remaining tumor colonies are stained and counted. The extent of target cell killing is shown by a reduction in the numbers of colonies surviving after exposure to sensitized lymphoid cells, e.g., taken from tumor-bearing individuals compared with those in control dishes treated with lymphoid cells from appropriate controls (normal individuals, or patients with non-malignant disease or an unrelated malignancy). This test has subsequently been modified as a *microcytotoxicity assay* in which survival of individual tumor cells is measured. In this technique (Figure 2) tumor cells, usually obtained from primary or short-term cultures, are seeded into the wells of sterile microtest plates and incubated to allow cell adhesion to the plastic surface of the wells. The tissue culture medium is then replaced with a suspension of lymphoid cells either from the sensitized host or appropriate controls, and after incubation for periods of between 36 to 72 h the numbers of surviving tumor cells is determined. This is frequently carried out by visual counting of remaining cells although variants have been introduced in the technique using tumor cells labeled with radioactive markers (e.g., [^{14}C]proline and [^{125}I]iododeoxyuridine). Release of radioactivity from ^{51}Cr-labeled tumor cells has also been used as an index of tumor cell

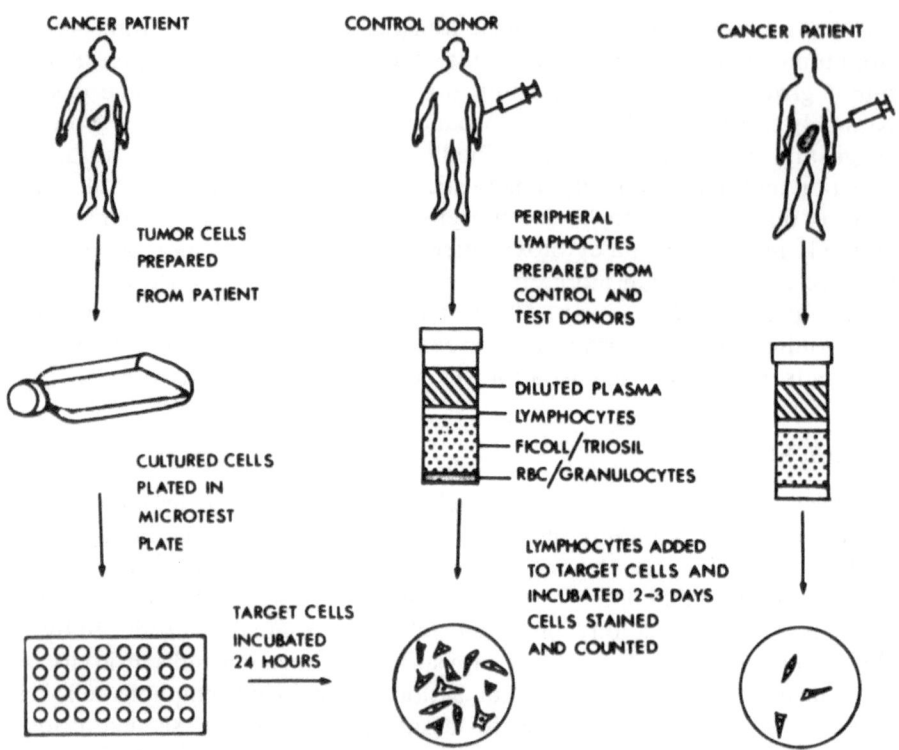

Figure 2. Microcytotoxicity test for demonstrating *in vitro* reactivity of peripheral blood lymphocytes from cancer patients against malignant cells. Malignant cells from *in vitro* cultures are plated (100 to 200 cells/well) in each of a series of wells in a microtest plate. After incubation to allow adhesion to plastic surface of the wells, the cells are exposed to peripheral blood lymphocytes and the cytotoxic effect of patients' cells is compared with that of controls. Peripheral blood lymphocytes are prepared in a number of ways, one which involves separation on a Ficoll/Triosil gradient, and cytotoxicity is assayed by visual counting of surviving tumor cells (cf. Baldwin *et al.*, 1973a; Hellström and Hellström, 1974a; Cerottini and Brunner, 1974).

destruction. This assay has the advantage of brevity, lasting only a few hours, but unfortunately few tumor types release the isotope in a satisfactory manner.

It was originally believed that cytotoxic reactions detected against tumor cells *in vitro* were mediated by thymus-derived (T) lymphocytes since this type of cytotoxic effector cell has been implicated in the immune response to allografted tissues (Cerottini and Brunner, 1974). Here, target cell killing can be produced without any contribution from Bursa-equivalent (B) lymphocytes or macrophages. The relative importance of T- and non-T-lymphocytes and macrophages in tumor cell killing is much less clear, however, and it is likely that this will vary between different tumor types (Herberman *et al.,* 1974; Cerottini and Brunner, 1974). This is emphasized by *in vitro* studies with murine sarcoma virus-induced tumors where effector cells involved in the ^{51}Cr-release assay of cell-mediated cytotoxicity have been identified as T cells (Plata *et al.,* 1974). On the other hand, both T- and "B-like" lymphocytes have been found to be involved at different stages of tumor growth when cytotoxicity was assayed by the microcytotoxicity test (Lamon *et al.,* 1973). Finally, it can be shown that macrophages are cytostatic for these tumors employing another *in vitro* assay (Senik *et al.,* 1974). An example of non-thymus-dependent lymphocyte cytotoxicity in human cancer is provided by studies on the reactivity of peripheral blood lymphoid cells from patients with transitional cell carcinoma of the urinary bladder (O'Toole *et al.,* 1974). The T- and B-lymphocyte subpopulations were separated by passing blood samples through columns of immunoglobulin-coated glass beads. With this technique, B-cells are retained through interaction with cell surface immunoglobulins and/or F^c receptors while T-cells are eluted. Analysis of the cytotoxicity of these subpopulations showed that the eluted cells were inactive, indicating involvement of a non-thymus-derived effector cell. These examples indicate that the simple concept implicating cytotoxic T-cells in tumor cell killing must be revised, and several effector cell types have now been described.

   As yet, it is not possible to specify whether all of these types play a significant role *in vivo.* For the present, therefore, attempts to monitor the effects of therapy on a patient's immune competence must include an assessment of the levels of each type of lymphoid cell.

Serum Factors Modifying Cellular Immunity to Tumors

   Lymphocyte cytotoxicity for tumor cells *in vitro* can be demonstrated in tumor-bearing patients as well as those in clinical remission, although there is evidence to suggest that the degree of reactivity may vary according to the extent of the disease (Hellström and Hellström, 1974a). The presence of lymphocytes in the tumor-bearing host which at least *in vitro* can effect cytotoxic reactions against the tumor may appear paradoxical. This led to the proposal that cellular immunity in tumor bearers may be diminished by circulating factors which specifically modify this response, so providing the tumor with an escape mechanism from host immunological control. This concept was originally proposed and developed by the Hellströms and their colleagues (Hellström and Hellström, 1974b) who employed the *in vitro* microcytotoxicity assay to show that serum from tumor-bearing individuals specifically "blocked" tumor cells from killing by lymphocytes sensitized to the tumor. In these studies, tumor cells plated *in vitro* in microtest wells (Figure 2) were first treated with tumor-bearer serum or in controls, normal serum, to allow the "blocking factor" to interact with tumor antigens expressed upon the surface of the target tumor cell (Figure 3). Sera were then removed, and the susceptibility of tumor cells to killing by sensitized lymphoid cells was determined. Blocking activity was originally demonstrated in experimental animal studies showing that serum from mice bearing Moloney virus-induced sarcomas abrogated the cytotoxicity of sensitized lymph node cells (Hellström and Hellström, 1970). This assay has subsequently been employed to detect blocking substances in serum from animals bearing many types of tumor (chemically or virally induced as well as those of spontaneous origin) and also in patients with different types of malignancy including malignant melanoma,

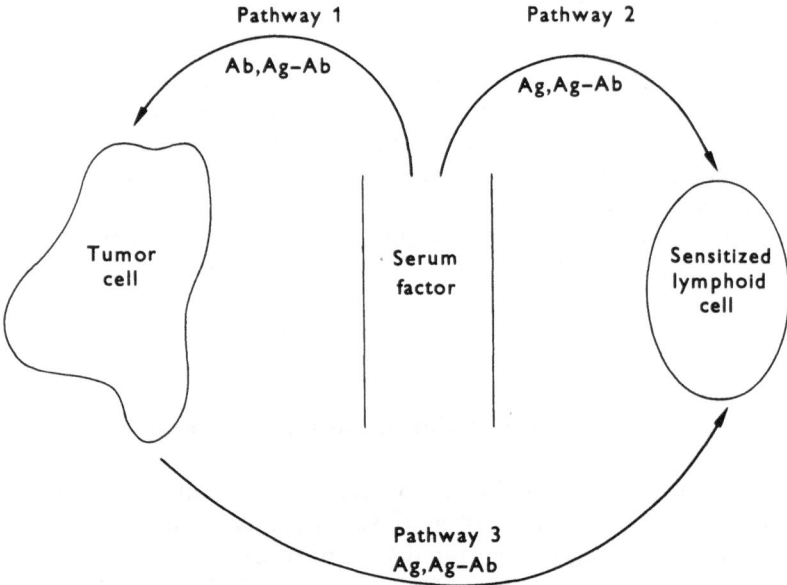

Figure 3. Diagrammatic representation of possible pathways in which host factors may abrogate cell-mediated immunity against tumor cells. *Pathway 1 (blocking):* Tumor-specific antibody or circulating immune complexes with an antibody receptor available may bind to (and mask) neoantigens on tumor cells, so preventing their recognition by sensitized lymphoid cells. *Pathway 2 (inhibition):* Circulating tumor antigen on immune complexes in tumor antigen excess may specifically interact with sensitized lymphoid cells, so inhibiting their reactivity. *Pathway 3 (inhibition):* Specific inhibition of sensitized lymphoid cells may be brought about by their interaction with tumor antigen and/or immune complexes released from tumor cells as a consequence of their interaction with tumor-specific antibody.

neuroblastoma, and carcinoma of colon, breast, bladder, lung, etc. (Baldwin, 1973; Hellström and Hellström, 1974b).

Nature of Serum Blocking Factors

Serum blocking was initially believed to be mediated by "blocking antibodies" interacting with tumor-cell surface antigens (Figure 3). This conclusion was supported by experiments showing that blocking factor could be removed from tumor-bearer serum by absorption with tumor cells and then eluted from these coated tumor cells using conditions (e.g., washing with low pH buffers) which are known to disrupt immune complexes. The concept that blocking was mediated by antibody alone became untenable, however, when it was found that this activity disappeared very soon after complete surgical resection of tumor (Baldwin et al., 1973c), or when tumors regressed spontaneously (Hellström and Hellström, 1970). In this context, it is relevant to note that loss of blocking activity only occurred following complete tumor resection, suggesting that this assay may be employed for detecting residual malignant disease.

Since it is not possible in all instances to ascribe blocking reactions to antibody alone, it was suggested that the reactivity of tumor-bearer serum may involve tumor-specific immune complexes, and this has subsequently been verified in further studies. It has been shown, for example, that the blocking factor in the serum from mice bearing Moloney virus-induced sarcomas can be absorbed onto intact tumor cells eluted with low pH buffer and separated at this pH by a membrane ultrafiltration technique into a high molecular weight (>100,000 daltons) component containing immunoglobulins and a low molecular weight (between 10,000 and 100,000 daltons) component which does not contain immunoglobulin. Neither of these fractions alone displayed blocking activity when added to cultured tumor cells, although this was restored when the two fractions were recombined (Sjögren et al., 1971). Consistent with these studies, sera taken several days following surgical resection of transplanted rat hepatomata have been shown to lack blocking activity; but instead, cytotoxic antibody was demonstrable. In this case, blocking activity could be produced by the addition of soluble tumor-specific antigen (prepared by papain solubilization of tumor membrane) to the serum, this resulting in the formation of tumor-specific immune complexes (Baldwin et al., 1972).

Further conclusive evidence for the involvement of tumor-specific immune complexes in blocking reactions is provided by studies showing that the blocking activity of tumor-bearer serum can be neutralized (unblocked) by the addition of tumor-immune serum. For example, serum obtained from mice following regression of Moloney virus-induced sarcomas and rats after surgical resection of developing hepatoma transplants specifically neutralized the blocking activity of the appropriate tumor-bearer serum (Hellström and Hellström, 1970; Robins and Baldwin, 1974).

Serum Inhibitory Factors

Interpretation of blocking reactions is complicated by the long incubation periods involved in the microcytotoxicity test (Figure 2) which has been widely used for their detection. In addition to antibody or immune complex binding to tumor cells, it is feasible that release of bound reactants may occur as a consequence of cell membrane synthesis and regeneration and these may directly interact with sensitized lymphoid cells (Figure 3). This suggests an alternative pathway in which serum factors may *inhibit* the reactivity of sensitized lymphoid cells either by direct interaction or via products released from tumor cells (Figure 3). As already discussed, more than one type of effector cell may be involved in tumor-immune rejection reactions and so at present, only a broad outline of factors modifying their reactivity can be given. Nevertheless, studies with several experimental tumor systems have revealed that the cytotoxicity of sensitized lymphoid cells can be specifically inhibited by treatment with tumor-bearer serum. The cytotoxicity of lymph node cells from hepatoma-immune rats (Baldwin *et al.*, 1973d) and spleen cells from MSV-tumor-bearing mice (Plata and Levy, 1974) can be abolished by exposure to tumor-bearer serum.

The characteristics of the inhibitory factors in tumor-bearer serum have not been unequivocally defined, but circulating tumor antigen and/or immune complexes have been implicated. This is supported, for example, by the finding that the inhibitory factor in the serum of rats bearing transplanted hepatomas can be neutralized by the addition of tumor-specific antibody (Robins and Baldwin, 1974), this being akin to the "unblocking" effects of immune serum at the level of the target tumor cell (Hellström and Hellström, 1974b). In addition. there is conclusive evidence that the cytotoxicity of sensitized lymphoid cells can be specifically inhibited by exposure to solubilized tumor-specific antigen. This was originally established in a rat hepatoma system where the cytotoxicity of lymph node cells from tumor-immune rats was abolished by exposure to papain-solubilized tumor-specific antigen (Baldwin *et al.*, 1973d, 1974). Similar studies employing virus-induced sarcomata in mice have established that solubilized tumor-specific antigen can abrogate the cytotoxicity of sensitized spleen cells as well as a T-cell subpopulation (Plata and Levy, 1974). Moreover, with a rat sarcoma model it has been shown that tumor antigen "shed" from the cell surface during *in vitro* culture inhibits the cytotoxicity of sensitized lymph node cells (Currie and Alexander, 1974).

With human tumors, in particular carcinoma of colon and melanoma, specific inhibition of blood lymphocyte cytotoxicity has been obtained following exposure to papain-solubilized tumor antigen preparations (Baldwin *et al.*, 1973b, 1974; Embleton and Price, 1974). These observations are complementary to other studies on patients with widely disseminated malignant melanoma where peripheral blood lymphocytes initially exhibited little cytotoxicity *in vitro* for melanoma cells, but reactivity appeared after repeated washing of the lymphocytes (Currie and Basham, 1972; Currie, 1973). The conclusion that lymphocyte reactivity was again inhibited by exposure to tumor-bearer serum (Currie and Basham, 1972). Subsequently it has been reported (Currie and McElwain, 1975) that monitoring of serum inhibitory activity may be a useful parameter in assessing the efficacy of immunotherapy protocols.

In Vivo Role of Serum Factors

The conclusion from the *in vitro* studies is that circulating factors including tumor-specific antigen, antibody, and immune complexes may play a biologically important role in the tumor-host relationship by inhibiting the cell-mediated arm of the tumor immune response. Blocking of tumor cells by tumor-specific immune complexes or antibody may also be important. The crucial question still unresolved is whether the effects of tumor-bearer serum observed *in vitro* play a significant role *in vivo*. The most conclusive evidence for this so far is provided by tests showing that passive administration of large quantities of tumor-immune serum into rats bearing polyoma virus-induced tumors resulted in the disappearance of blocking activity when tumor-bearer sera were tested *in vitro*, and this treatment often arrested tumor growth or even produced regressions (Bansal and Sjögren, 1972). This type of correlation does not prove, however, that tumors regressed because of the disappearance of blocking factors since other interpretations are possible; e.g., regressions may be mediated by antibody (complement or cell-dependent) responses. An alternative approach has been to demonstrate enhanced tumor growth following administration of blocking substances. This was shown in the rat polyoma system where injection of tumor-bearer serum into normal rats facilitated growth of implanted tumor (Bansal *et al.*, 1972). Similarly, injection of tumor antigen either as irradiated tumor cells or subcellular fractions of tumor homogenates into tumor-immune mice abrogated resistance against challenge with mammary carcinoma cells (Vaage, 1972, 1974).

Although these studies support the *in vitro* data for a role of circulating factors in modifying immunity in the tumor-bearing host, this hypothesis must still be viewed as unproven but providing a working basis for further studies. One approach has been to characterize the different serum factors during progressive tumor growth and although different experimental tumor systems differ in some aspects, the notable feature in most cases is an initial release into the circulation of tumor-specific antigen, either free or in immune complex (Baldwin *et al.*, 1973d) Bowen *et al.*, 1975; Thomson *et al.*, 1973a,b). These findings further support the view that tumor antigen release, either into the circulation or into the microenvironment of a tumor mass, plays a prominent role in modifying tumor-immune rejection reactions.

Immunodiagnosis

Immunodiagnosis of human malignant disease is based upon two concepts, both of which have been verified in a number of specific instances.

(1) Patients with malignant disease can recognize neoantigens on their tumor cells and this leads to the development of cellular and humoral immune responses against these neoantigens which can be detected in a variety of ways. Cellular immunity can be detected *in vitro* by the cytotoxicity of peripheral blood lymphocytes for cultured tumor cells or by the leukocyte migration test which measures the capacity of tumor cells or extracts to inhibit leukocyte migration test which measures the capacity of tumor cells or extracts to inhibit leukocyte migration in an appropriate medium (Cochran *et al.*, 1974). In addition, cell-mediated immunity can be detected in patients by their capacity to elicit delayed hypersensitivity responses against purified tumor antigen extracts injected intradermally (Herberman, 1974).

Humoral immunity has been demonstrated in a few examples, e.g., melanoma by the complement-dependent cytotoxicity of patients' serum for cultured tumor cells, although these (assay) studies require confirmation (Wood and Morton, 1970; Lewis, 1972; Baldwin *et al.*, 1973a). Antibody responses may be demonstrated more reproducibly, however, by binding assays. This is exemplified by studies in malignant melanomata (Lewis *et al.*, 1969) and Burkitt's lymphoma (Klein, 1971), employing a membrane immunofluorescence technique to show that patients' serum contains antibody reacting specifically with the tumor-associated antigens expressed either on the cell surface membrane or within the cytoplasm (cf. reviews by Lewis, 1972; Moore, 1975).

These tests provide evidence that a patient responds immunologically to new antigens associated with a developing malignancy and therefore may be aids to diagnosis. At present, however, it should be emphasized that none of these tests, except perhaps in the serological studies of Burkitt's lymphoma, and other malignant diseases associated with the Epstein–Barr virus (Klein, 1971), have developed to a stage where they can be used routinely. It should also be emphasized that immunological tests of cell-mediated immunity do not necessarily indicate that the immune response detected *in vitro* is one involved directly in tumor rejection.

(2) The second concept is that human tumors secrete into the blood and other body fluids tumor-associated substances which can be detected and measured quantitatively by immunological methods. This has been established, for example, in hepatocellular carcinoma where an "α-fetoprotein" is secreted and a so-called "carcinoembryonic antigen" is associated with colorectal carcinomata. Both of these tumor-associated substances belong to a class of antigens referred to as *oncofetal antigens*, i.e., they are present in malignant cells and also in tissue at certain stages of fetal development. Immunoassay of these substances in cancer patients indicates that the malignant lesion is secreting the antigen and therefore may have value for diagnosis. These tests do not, however, provide any information about the role of the oncofetal antigens in the tumor-host relationship, particularly with regard to their involvement in tumor immune rejection responses.

Immunodiagnosis of oncological diseases may be proposed for a number of areas of clinical management including (a) screening populations for the presence of clinically undetectable disease; (b) differential diagnosis of malignant disease; (c) differential diagnosis of benign and malignant lesions; (d) prognostic evaluation; (e) monitoring of therapy; (f) detection of residual or recurrent tumor. The tests employed for these purposes ideally should be simple to perform, inexpensive, and readily reproducible. They should also be highly specific for the malignant disease in question. At present, few if any of the proposed tests meet these criteria and so in most cases they are not yet applicable for routine clinical evaluation of malignant disease.

Carcinoembryonic Antigen

Carcinoembryonic antigen (CEA) originally identified by Gold and Freedman (1965) is associated with glandular tumors of the gastrointestinal tract, especially the colon and rectum, but also of the pancreas and stomach. This glycoprotein is not present at high levels in extracts of adult normal colon or other normal adult tissues, but it can be detected in fetal gastrointestinal tissues, hence its description as carcinoembryonic antigen. Interest in the use of CEA assays for diagnosis of gastrointestinal cancer developed from the observation that significant levels were detectable in the serum of patients with colorectal cancers, whereas in all other cases (nondigestive malignancies, nonmalignant and normal controls) serum values were negative. This has led to the development of a number of different assays for measuring serum levels of CEA, mostly involving radioimmunological methods (cf. Neville and Laurence, 1974). In principle these assays measure competitive binding of CEA in patients' serum and a known amount of added purified radiolabeled CEA to anti-CEA antibody prepared in a xenogeneic host (e.g., goat). The general conclusion now reached employing these CEA assays in a number of centers is that the test is at present impractical as a general population screen. For example, 10% of the population had elevated CEA serum concentrations (Table 2). Also, there is no statistically valid proof that the CEA test is useful as a diagnostic adjunct when malignancy is suspected, and at the present time, the assay is probably of most value for follow-up of patients (Neville and Laurence, 1974). This was originally demonstrated by Gold's group who found that CEA levels fell to normal values a few days after surgical resection of tumor, and the value of sequential CEA assay is illustrated in Figure 4. In this case, CEA levels remained elevated until after chemotherapy when a clinical response was accompanied by decreases in CEA levels.

α-Fetoprotein

Another tumor-associated fetal protein which has received considerable attention is α-fetoprotein (αFP), this being associated with hepatocellu-

TABLE 2. Occurrence of Elevated CEA Concentrations in Various Clinical States[a]

Clinical state	Percent with CEA concentration above normal
Healthy volunteers	10
Nonsmokers	3
Smokers[b]	19
Former smokers	7
Nonmalignant disease	34
Pulmonary emphysema	57
Alcoholic cirrhosis	70
Ulcerative colitis	30
Gastric ulcer	45
Breast disease	15
Endotermal carcinoma (colerectal, pulmonary, gastric, pancreatic)	73
Nonentodermal carcinoma (breast, head and neck, other)	59
Noncarcinoma (leukemias, lymphomas, sarcomas)	40
Suspected malignancy, not confirmed	17

[a]Originally compiled from CEA-Roche: *A Clinical Monograph* (1974). These data are all based on the Z-gel assay, with the upper limit of normal taken as 2.5 ng/ml (reprinted from *Transplant. Rev.* **20**, 1974.
[b]Elevations of CEA concentrations in smokers have not been carefully studied with assays other than the Z-gel assay.

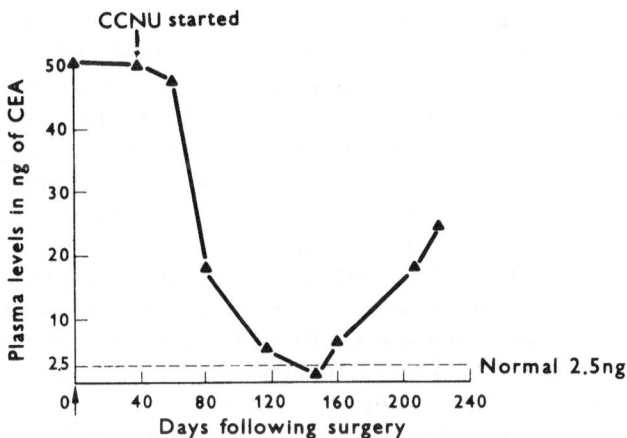

Figure 4. This illustrates the monitoring of the colonic carcinoma extent by measuring the level of CEA in plasma. In this patient the initial operation consisted of laparotomy and biopsy only. The CEA level remained elevated following the operation. Forty days later, CCNU chemotherapy was initiated. At that time, the patient's abdomen was estimated to contain between 800 and 1,000 g of tumor. The patient showed a marked clinical response accompanied by a decrease in CEA level. The CEA levels rose again between 30 and 60 days before clinical examination which indicated a relapse and increasing amounts of tumor (Holyoke *et al.*, 1972).

lar carcinoma (cf. Ruoslahti *et al.*, 1974). The early claims that increased αFP serum levels were diagnostic for hepatic tumor have not been substantiated following the introduction of sensitive radioimmunoassay procedures for its detection. For example, increased αFP levels are associated with other liver diseases including hepatitis, cirrhosis, and trauma as well as in pregnancy, although these increases are usually quantitatively much less than those observed in primary liver carcinoma. Further evaluation on the value of αFP assays are in progress, and in this connection a coordinating group for αFP (People's Republic of China, Peking) has reported a massive screening of 500,000 individuals and this should resolve its value for screening purposes.

Immunotherapy

Immunotherapy may be introduced prophylactically in order to prevent the induction of malignant disease or therapeutically for the treatment of a clinically established malignancy. The possibility of preventing human malignant disease by prior immunization with tumor-associated antigens or possibly putative human tumor viruses is at present unwarranted, although it is pertinent to note that this form of therapy, e.g., by prior immunization with oncogenic viruses (Hilleman, 1974) or even fetal cells (Coggin and Anderson, 1974), can suppress viral oncogenesis in animals. For the present, therefore, the question to be answered is whether therapeutic immunotherapy can play any role in the treatment of human malignant disease.This may be achieved by augmenting an existing tumor-specific immune response in the patient, either by active immunization with tumor antigen or by passively transferring immune factors (antibody, sensitized lymphoid cells, immunological mediators, e.g., transfer factor). Also, if the concepts developed from *in vitro* studies on the role of humoral factors modifying cell-mediated immunity prove to have *in vivo* significance, treatment may be introduced for the removal of circulating tumor antigen or immune complexes, so increasing the effectiveness of any existing host response. Finally, treatment may be introduced to nonspecifically stimulate immune responses in the patient, using a variety of adjuvants (see McKhann and Gunnarsson, 1974, for review of possible methods). Many of these manipulations have been validated employing experimental tumor systems, but in most examples, treatment is only able to deal with small numbers of tumor cells (variously estimated to be between 10^5 and 10^7 cells). Basically, therefore, immunotherapy is likely to be most effective for the treatment of small metastatic deposits of malignant cells or for so-called "minimum residual disease."

Active Immunotherapy

Nonspecific immunotherapy may be introduced by administration of immunological adjuvants, the most popular at present being BCG and *Corynebacterium parvum*. This form of treatment has produced widely varying effects when tested upon experimental tumor systems leading to regression of some tumors, whereas in other instances there has been no response or even enhanced tumor growth (Bast *et al.*, 1974). Nevertheless, many of the immunotherapy protocols now being introduced for the treatment of human malignant disease include immunostimulation with adjuvants, especially BCG. The effectiveness of this form of treatment remains unproven, although promising results have been obtained in patients with disseminated malignant melanoma (Gutterman *et al.*, 1974), when comparing the response to chemotherapy with chemotherapy and BCG administered by scarification.

Active specific immunotherapy by further stimulation of the tumor-bearing host has been demonstrated in experimental tumor systems. This may be achieved in a number of ways, e.g., injection of irradiated or mitomycin-C-treated cells, and in most instances this response can be enhanced by incorporating the tumor cells in a vaccine containing BCG or another adjuvant (McKhann and Gunnarsson, 1974; Bast *et al.,* 1974). This approach was pioneered by Mathé and colleagues (1969) in lymphoblastic leukemia and subsequently by Powles and associates (Powles *et al.,* 1973; Powles, 1974) in acute myelogenous leukemia. In these trials viable or radiation-attenuated tumor cells and BCG, injected at separate sites during the remission phase of the disease, have given clinically significant effects. For example, in the AML trial (Powles, 1974) of 19 patients in the control group who received chemotherapy only during the remission phase, 7 remained alive (median survival, 43 weeks) and 5 were in their first remission (median remission length, 27 weeks). Of the 23 patients who received immunotherapy, 16 remained alive (median, 78 weeks) and 8 were in their first remission (median, 45 weeks). These leukemia studies represent the most promising examples of immunotherapy, but at present effective treatment of solid tumors has not been achieved.

Adjuvant Contact Therapy

The immunotherapeutic response to attenuated tumor cells can be enhanced by injecting them in admixture with adjuvants such as BCG. Moreover, experimental animal tests have shown that directly contacting adjuvants with tumor *in vivo* may cause tumor rejection. This was originally established in a guinea pig hepatoma model showing that intralesional injections of BCG induced tumor regression and also prevented the development of lymph node metastases (Zbar *et al.,* 1972). This approach has subsequently been employed with other experimental transplanted tumors to induce regression of local tumor growth and has been extended to show that adjuvant contact can induce rejection of "metastatic disease"; e.g., intravenous injection of BCG can prevent the development of pulmonary metastases (Baldwin and Pimm, 1973a,b).

Clinically this approach is analogous to that originally introduced by Morton and his colleagues (1970) for the treatment of recurrent intradermal and subcutaneous malignant melanoma where intralesional injection of BCG resulted in regression of the injected nodules. Occasionally, also noninjected nodules regressed, suggesting a possible influence of a host immune response. These observations have since been confirmed and extended in a number of studies (reviewed by Bast *et al.,* 1974), but there are still reservations to the approach. First, although approximately 50% of injected nodules regressed, the response in noninjected lesions was low (14%). Second, visceral metastases have not responded to treatment, and a number of complications have been reported following repeated intralesional injections of BCG (Sparks *et al.,* 1973). Chills, fever, and malaise may occur and hepatic dysfunction has been observed. Granulomatous hepatitis was detected in 3 of 25 patients receiving intralesional BCG and 2 patients have died from apparent reactions to this form of treatment (Sparks *et al.*, 1973; Bast *et al.*, 1974).

Adoptive Immunotherapy

In principle it should be possible to transfer immune factors, e.g., from patients in remission, but the practicality of this approach remains to be proven (cf. McKhann and Gunnarsson, 1974). Animal studies employing tumors transplanted into syngeneic hosts have shown that immunity can be readily transferred with lymphoid cells, but the applicability of this approach in clinical cancer is limited because transferred lymphoid tissue will provoke an immune response in the recipient which may rapidly bring about its destruction. Alternative approaches involving administration of immunological mediators such as transfer factor (Lo Buglio and Neidhart, 1974) or tumor immune antiserum are being investigated. There is no convincing evidence at the present time, however, to show that these manipulations are therapeutically effective.

References

Baldwin, R. W. (1973). Immunological aspects of chemical carcinogenesis. *Adv. Cancer Res.* **18**:1.

Baldwin, R. W., and Embleton, M. J. (1974). Neoantigens on spontaneous and carcinogen-induced rat tumours defined by *in vitro* lymphocytotoxicity assays. *Int. J. Cancer* **13**:433.

Baldwin, R. W., Embleton, M. J., Jones, J. S. P., and Langman, M. J. S. (1973a). Cell mediated and humoral immune reactions to human tumours. *Int. J. Cancer* **12**:73.

Baldwin, R. W., Embleton, M. J., and Price, M. R. (1973b). Inhibition of lymphocyte cytotoxicity for human colon carcinoma by treatment with solubilized tumour membrane fractions. *Int. J. Cancer* **12**:84.

Baldwin, R. W., Embleton, M. J., and Robins, R. A. (1973c). Cellular and humoral immunity to rat hepatoma-specific antigens correlated with tumour status. *Int. J. Cancer* **11**:1.

Baldwin, R. W., Price, M. R., and Robins, R. A. (1973d). Inhibition of hepatoma-immune lymph node cell cytotoxicity by tumour-bearer serum and solubilized hepatoma antigen. *Int. J. Cancer* **11**:527.

Baldwin, R. W., Embleton, M. J., Price, M. R., and Robins, R. A. (1974). Immunity in the tumor-bearing host and its modification by serum factors. *Cancer* **34**:1452.

Baldwin, R. W., and Pimm, M. V. (1973a). BCG immunotherapy of pulmonary growths from intravenously transferred rat tumour cells. *Br. J. Cancer* **27**:48.

Baldwin, R. W., and Pimm, M. V. (1973b). BCG immunotherapy of local subcutaneous growths and post-surgical pulmonary metastases of a transplanted rat epithelioma of spontaneous origin. *Int. J. Cancer* **12**:420.

Baldwin, R. W., and Price, M. R. (1975). Cell membrane-associated antigens in chemical carcinogenesis. *Biomembranes* **8**:89.

Baldwin, R. W., Price, M. R., and Robins, R. A. (1972). Blocking of lymphocyte-mediated cytotoxicity for rat hepatoma cells by tumour specific antigen-antibody complexes. *Nature New Biol.* **238**:185.

Bansal, S. C., Hargreaves, R., and Sjögren, H. O. (1972). Facilitation of polyoma tumor growth in rats by unblocking sera and tumor eluate. *Int. J. Cancer* 9:97.

Bansal, S. C., and Sjögren, H. O. (1972). Counteraction of the blocking of cell mediated tumor immunity by inoculation of unblocking sera and splenectomy: Immunotherapeutic effects on primary polyoma tumors in rats. *Int. J. Cancer* 9:490.

Bast, R. C., Zbar, B., Borsos, T. and Rapp, H. J. (1974). BCG and cancer. *N. Engl. J. Med.* 290:1413,1458.

Bowen, J. G., Robins, R. A. and Baldwin, R. W. (1975). Serum factors modifying cell mediated immunity to rat hepatoma D23 correlated with tumour status. *Int. J. Cancer* 15:640.

Burkitt, D. (1967). Chemotherapy of jaw tumours. In *Treatment of Burkitt's Lymphoma* Ed. by (J. H. Burchenal, ed.), Vol. 8, p. 94. UICC Monograph Series. Springer: Heidelberg.

Cerottini, J. C., and Brunner, K. T. (1974). Cell mediated cytotoxicity, allograft rejection and tumor immunity. *Adv. Immunol.* 18:67.

Cochran, A. J., Grant, R. M., Spilg, W. G., Mackie, C. E., Ross, C. E., Hoyle, D. E., and Russell, J. M. (1974). Sensitization to tumour associated antigens in human breast carcinoma. *Int. J. Cancer* 14:19.

Coggin, J. H., and Anderson, N. G. (1974). Cancer, differentiation and embryonic antigens: Some central problems. *Adv. Cancer Res.* 19:105.

Currie, G. A. (1973). The role of circulating antigen as an inhibitor of tumour immunity in man. *Br. J. Cancer (Suppl. I)* 28:153.

Currie, G. A., and Alexander, P. (1974). Spontaneous shedding of TSTA by viable sarcoma cells: Its possible role in facilitating metastatic spread. *Br. J. Cancer* 29:72.

Currie, G. A., and Basham, C. (1972). Serum mediated inhibition of the immunological reactions of the patient to his own tumour: A possible role for circulating antigen. *Br. J. Cancer* 26:427.

Currie, G. A., and McElwain, T. J. (1975). Active immunotherapy as an adjunct to chemotherapy in the treatment of disseminated malignant melanoma: A pilot study. *Br. J. Cancer* 31:143.

Deinhardt, F. (1974). Antigens associated with DNA virus induced tumors. In *Progress in Immunology II* (L. Brent and J. Holborrow, eds.), Vol. 3, p. 271. North-Holland, Amsterdam.

Embleton. M. J., and Price, M. R. (1975). Inhibition of *in vitro* lymphocytotoxic reactions against tumour cells by melanoma membrane extracts. *Behring Inst. Mitt.* 56:157.

Everson, T. C., and Cole, W. H. (1966). *Spontaneous Regression of Cancer.* W. P. Saunders, Philadelphia.

Gold, P., and Freedman, S. O. (1965). Specific carcinoembryonic antigens of the human digestive system. *J. Exp. Med.* 122:467.

Gutterman, J. G., Mavligit, G., Gottlieb, J. A., Burgess, M. A., McBride, C. E., Einhorn, L., Freireich, E. J., and Hersh, E. M. (1974). Chemoimmunotherapy of disseminated malignant melanoma with dimethyl triazeno imidazole carboxamide and bacillus Calmette-Guérin. *N. Engl. J. Med.* 291:592.

Helström, I. (1967). A colony inhibition (CI) technique for demonstration of tumor cell destruction by lymphoid cells *in vitro*. *Int. J. Cancer* 2:65.

Hellström, I., and Hellström, K. E. (1970). Colony inhibition studies on blocking and nonblocking serum effects on cellular immunity to Moloney sarcomas. *Int. J. Cancer* 5:195.

Hellström, I., and Hellström, K. E. (1974a). Cell-mediated immune reactions to tumor antigens with particular emphasis on immunity to human neoplasms. *Cancer* 34:1461.

Hellström, K. E., and Hellström, I. (1974b). Lymphocyte-mediated cytotoxicity and blocking serum activity to tumor antigens. *Adv. Immunol.* 18:209.

Hellström, K. E., and Hellström, I. (1969). Cellular immunity against tumor antigens. *Adv. Cancer Res.* 12:167.

Herberman, R. B. (1974). Delayed hypersensitivity skin reactions to antigens on human tumors. *Cancer* **34**:1469.

Herberman, R. W., Ting, C. C., Kirchner, H., Holden, H., Glaser, G. M., Bonnard, G. D., and Lavrin, D. (1974). Effector mechanisms in tumour immunity. In *Progress in Immunology* (L. Brent and J. Holborrow, eds.), Vol. 3, p. 285. North-Holland, Amsterdam.

Hersey, P. (1973). New look at antiserum therapy of leukaemia. *Nature New Biol.* **244**:22.

Hilleman, M. R. (1974). Human cancer virus vaccines and the pursuit of the practical. *Cancer* **34**:1439.

Holyoke, D., Reynoso, G., and Chu, T. M. (1972). Carcinoembryonic antigen (CEA) in patients with carcinoma of the digestive tract. *Ann. Surg.* **176**:559.

Klein, G. (1971). Immunological studies on Burkitt's lymphoma. *Postgrad. Med. J.* **47**:141.

Lamon, E. W., Wigzell, H., Klein, E., Andersson, B., and Skurzak, H. M. (1973). The lymphocyte response to a primary Moloney sarcoma virus-induced tumor in BALB/c mice: Definition of active subpopulations at different times after infection. *J. Exp. Med.* **137**:1472.

Levy, J. P. (1974). Antigens associated with C type RNA virus-induced tumors. In *Progress in Immunology II* (L. Brent and J. Holborow, eds.), Vol. 3, p. 249. North-Holland, Amsterdam.

Lewis, M. G. (1972). Circulating humoral antibodies in cancer. *Med. Clin. North Am.* **56**:481.

Lewis, M. G., Ikonopisov, R. L., Nairn, R. C., Phillips, T. M., Fairley, G. H., Bodenham, D. C., and Alexander, P. (1969). Tumour-specific antibodies in human malignant melanoma and their relationship to the extent of the disease. *Br. Med. J.* **ii**:547.

Lo Buglio, A. F., and Neidhart, J. A. (1974). A review of transfer factor immunotherapy in cancer. *Cancer* **34**:1563.

MacLennan, I. C. M. (1972). Antibody in the induction and inhibition of lymphocyte cytotoxicity. *Transplant. Rev.* **13**:67.

Mathé, G., Amiel, J. L., Schwarzenberg, L., Schneider, M., Cattan, A., Schlumberger, J. R., Hayat, M., and De Vassal, F. (1969). Active immunotherapy for acute lymphoblastic leukaemia. *Lancet* **1**:697.

McKhann, C. F., and Gunnarsson, A. (1974). Approaches to immunotherapy. *Cancer* **34**:1521.

Moore, M. (1975). Serological approach to tumour specific antigens. In *Proceedings of the XIth International Cancer Congress*. Excerpta Medica, Amsterdam.

Morton, D. L., Eilber, F. R., Malmgren, R. A., and Wood, W. C. (1970). Immunological factors which influence response to immunotherapy in malignant melanoma. *Surgery* **68**:158.

Neville, A. M., and Laurence, D. J. R. (1974). Report on the workshop on the carcinoembryonic antigen (CEA): The present position and proposals for future investigation. *Int. J. Cancer* **14**:1.

O'Toole, C., Stejskal, V., Perlmann, P., and Karlsson, M. (1974). Lymphoid cells mediating tumor-specific cytotoxicity to carcinoma of the urinary bladder. Separation of the effector populations using a surface marker. *J. Exp. Med.* **139**:457.

Penn, I. (1974). Chemical immunosuppression and human cancer. *Cancer* **34**:1474.

Plata, F., Gomard, E., Leclerc, J. C., and Levy, J. P. (1974). Comparative *in vitro* studies of effector cell diversity in the cellular immune response to murine sarcoma virus (MSV)-induced tumors in mice. *J. Immunol.* **112**:1477.

Plata, F., and Levy, J. P. (1974). Blocking of syngeneic effector T cells by soluble tumor antigens. *Nature (London)* **249**:271.

Powles, R. (1974). Immunotherapy for acute myelogenous leukemia using irradiated and unirradiated leukemia cells. *Cancer* **34**:1558.

Powles, R. L., Crowther, D., Bateman, C. J. T., Beard, M. E. J., McElwain, T. J., Russell, J., Lister, T. A., Whitehouse, J. M. A., Wrigley, P. F. M., Pike, M., Alexander, P., and Hamilton Fairley, G. (1973). Immunotherapy for acute myelogenous leukaemia. *Br. J. Cancer* **28**:365.

Rios, A., and Simmons, R. L. (1974). Active specific immunotherapy of minimal residual tumor: Excision plus neuraminidase-treated tumor cells. *Int. J. Cancer* **13**:71.

Robins, R. A., and Baldwin, R. W. (1974). Tumour specific antibody neutralization of factors in rat hepatoma bearer serum which abrogate lymph node cell cytotoxicity. *Int. J. Cancer* **14**:589.

Ruoslahti, E., Pihko, H., and Seppälä, M. (1974). Alpha-fetoprotein: Immunochemical purification and chemical properties. Expression in normal state and in malignant and nonmalignant liver disease. *Transplant. Rev.* **20**:38.

Senik, A., De Giorgi, L., Gomard, E., and Levy, J. P. (1974). Cytostasis of lymphoma cells in suspension: Probably non-thymic origin of the cytostatic lymphoid cells in mice bearing MSV-induced tumors. *Int. J. Cancer* **14**:396.

Sjögren, H. O., Hellström, I., Bansal, S. C., and Hellström, K. E. (1971). Suggestive evidence that the blocking antibodies of tumor bearing individuals may be antigen-antibody complexes. *Proc. Nat. Acad. Sci. U.S.A.* **68**:1372.

Southam, C. M. (1967). Evidence for cancer-specific antigens in man. *Progr. Exp. Tumor Res.* **9**:1.

Sparks, F. C., Silverstein, M. J., Hunt, J. S., Haskell, C. M., Pilch, Y. H., and Morton, D. L. (1973). Complications of BCG immunotherapy in patients with cancer. *N. Engl. J. Med.* **289**:827.

Steele, G., and Sjögren, H. O. (1974). Embryonic antigens associated with chemically induced colon carcinomas in rats. *Int. J. Cancer* **14**:435.

Thomson, D. M. P., Eccles, S., and Alexander, P. (1973a). Antibodies and soluble tumour specific antigens in blood and lymph of rats with chemically-induced sarcomata. *Br. J. Cancer* **28**:6.

Thomson, D. M. P., Sellens, V., Eccles, S., and Alexander, P. (1973b). Radioimmunoassay of tumour-specific transplantation antigen of a chemically-induced rat sarcoma: Circulating soluble tumour antigen in tumour bearers. *Br. J. Cancer* **28**:377.

Vaage, J. (1972). Specific desensitization of resistance against a syngeneic methylcholanthrene-induced sarcoma in C3Hf mice. *Cancer Res.* **32**:193.

Vaage, J. (1974). Circulating tumor antigens *versus* immune serum factors in depressed concomitant immunity. *Cancer Res.* **34**:2979.

Wood, W. C., and Morton, D. L. (1970). Microcytotoxicity test—Detection in sarcoma patients of antibody cytotoxic to human sarcoma cells. *Science* **170**:1318.

Zbar, B., Bernstein, I. D., Bartlett, G. L., Hanna, M. G., and Rapp, H. J. (1972). Immunotherapy of cancer: Regression of intradermal tumors and prevention of growth of lymph node metastases after intralesional injection of living *Mycobacterium bovis*. *J. Nat. Cancer Inst.* **49**:119.

Zbar, B., Wepsic, H. T., Rapp, H. J., Borsos, T., Kronman, B. S., and Churchill, W. H. (1969). Antigenic specificity of hepatomas induced in strain-2 guinea pigs by diethylnitrosamine. *J. Nat. Cancer Inst.* **43**:833.

DIAGNOSTIC ASPECTS
ENDOSCOPY

P. R. SALMON

The diagnosis of gastrointestinal disease has been influenced profoundly by the introduction of fiber-optic endoscopy. Although endoscopic examination of the interior of the bowel was first recorded by Bozzini (1807), Kussmaul (1869) was the first to examine successfully the interior of the stomach employing a 13 mm diam hollow metal tube which was swallowed by a cooperative sword swallower. The illumination source, devised by Desormeux of Paris, was, however, insufficient for the purpose.

Mickulicz-Radecki (1881) employed the new electric incandescent lamp as a source of illumination and successfully examined the stomach through a rigid hollow tube, while Mackenzie (1881) and later Von Hacker (1904) devised efficient rigid esophagoscopes not dissimilar to modern rigid instruments. Modern gastroscopy began with the introduction by Wolf, an instrument technician, and Schindler (1936), a gastroenterologist, of a semiflexible, efficient gastroscope based on short focal-length lenses and prisms. Whereas gastroscopy has been practiced since the 1930's, it is only since the introduction of the fully flexible fiber-optic endoscope into clinical medicine (Hirschowitz *et al.*, 1958) that a complete examination of the stomach was made possible, and hitherto blind areas such as the gastric fundus, cardia, roof of the antrum, and posterior wall of the body of the stomach were regularly visible endoscopically.

P. R. Salmon • Senior Lecturer in the Department of Medicine, University of Bristol and Bristol Royal Infirmary, Bristol, England.

Progress in biomedical engineering since 1958 has resulted in considerable advances in the design and manufacture of fiber-optic endoscopes (Salmon, 1974a,b, 1977) so that now the entire gastrointestinal tract can be examined endoscopically. The most important single advance was the introduction of the operating channel and flexible biopsy forceps so that a "target biopsy" capability was available. To this facility brush cytology was added (Williams *et al.*, 1968) so that current fiber-optic endoscopes can now provide a tissue diagnosis in addition to the visual impression.

The manufacturers have ably met the demands of the medical profession and developed larger instruments capable of examining the esophagus, stomach, and duodenal bulb at the same examination: duodenoscopes capable of examining not only the second part of the duodenum but also of cannulating the papilla of Vater for choledocho-pancreatography; enteroscopes capable of examining the small intestine beyond the ligament of Treitz; and colonoscopes capable of total colonoscopy.

Design of rigid laparoscopes has also improved greatly over the past decade so that the contents of the peritoneal cavity, in particular the liver, gallbladder, spleen, mesentery, and even the pancreas can be examined, palpated, and subjected to target biopsy under direct vision. In addition color photography, using high-quality still or cine cameras, can be employed to document macroscopic pathology for records or for teaching purposes.

In this chapter the various parts of the digestive tract are considered separately, although in reality they are often examined together as part of a combined procedure (e.g., esophago-gastro-duodenoscopy). The role of endoscopy in diagnosis, especially in cancer diagnosis, is emphasized.

Esophagus

Endoscopic examinations may be performed by three main types of instrument.

Rigid Esophagoscopes (Hollow, Rigid Tubes). This type of instrument introduced by Mackenzie (1881) was fully established by the work of Chevalier Jackson in Philadelphia. Endoscopes of this type are still in use for esophagoscopy underlying the need for training in the use of rigid and semirigid endoscopes at the present time. The particular value of this type of endoscope now is for removal of relatively large foreign bodies and for aiding esophageal dilatation.

Semirigid Esophagoscopes. These instruments, introduced by Boros (1947) and developed by others (Hufford, 1949; Katz, 1966), employ lens-optic telescopes introduced via a hollow sheath with a short flexible distal obturator. This type of instrument producing a proximal image at the observer's eye encouraged the use of endoscopy in the diagnosis of esophageal lesions.

Flexible Fiber-Optic Esophagoscopes. Soon after the introduction of the fiber-optic gastroscope (Hirschowitz and colleagues 1958) the fore-oblique fully flexible fiber-optic esophagoscope was developed (Lo Presti and Hilmi, 1964). This instrument could be passed with a greater margin of safety than rigid endoscopes and without more than light sedation. This instrument and modern fiber-optic endoscopes developed from it (Salmon, 1974a) have facilities for distal tip manipulation, an operating channel of not less than 5-Fr gauge doubling as an aspiration channel, air insufflation and lens washing facilities, and an external light source with light transmission via an integral fiber-optic light guide.

Indications for Esophagoscopy

At the present time it is exceptional for esophagoscopy to be performed alone unless the rigid esophagoscope is employed, or an esophageal obstruction (e.g., stricture) is being assessed. Combined esophago-gastro-duodenoscopy with a modern fiber-optic "panendoscope" has a number of significant advantages. The cardia can be examined from both within the esophagus and from below by inversion within the stomach. Mallory-Weiss tears can also be observed where they arise in the intraabdominal esophagus. Concomitant pathology, often primary, may be assessed; for example, a fundal neoplasm invading the esophagus or duodenal ulcer disease with pyloric pathology, antral gastritis, and gastroesophageal reflux resulting in peptic esophagitis.

In spite of the important advantage of a combined examination of the upper gastrointestinal tract there are indications for focusing endoscopic examination on the esophagus.

There is a strong case for investigating all patients with dysphagia by radiology and endoscopy (Bennett 1976). A negative barium swallow cannot rule out a small neoplasm or mucosal pathology, whereas radiological demonstration of a lesion requires endoscopic confirmation, tissue diagnosis, and esophago-gastro-duodenoscopy, with inversion and examination of the fundus and cardia from within the stomach.

Strictures are easy to miss, both radiologically and endoscopically, but may often be expected if a careful history of bolus obstruction is obtained. The Schatzki ring (Schatzki 1963), a ring stricture at the squamo-columnar junction unyielding to food but allowing the tip of the endoscope (and liquid) to pass easily through it is a good example.

The single most important function of endoscopy in dysphagia is to exclude cancer. This can only be achieved if the endoscope is put to its fullest use and adequate tissue is obtained for the histopathologist. In the case of an esophageal stricture the differential diagnosis lies between a Schatzki ring (supra), a peptic stricture (Barrett syndrome), or a malignant stricture. With good radiology it is often possible to diagnose the Schatzki ring since the distending force of a barium suspension is more like that applied in eating and drinking. Barium and bread or a barium-impregnated marshmallow may be used also to locate the site of bolus obstruction in this condition. Endoscopy subsequently demonstrates either no obvious stricture for the reasons given or an easily distensible stricture sometimes associated with an obvious hiatus hernia distally. Benign esophageal strictures may be associated with heterotopic columnar epithelium and a peptic esophageal ulcer (Barrett syndrome). Esophagitis is not necessarily present (Heitmann *et al.*, 1971). These cases are often difficult to diagnose with certainty by radiological means. Endoscopic examination of strictures should concentrate on recording the level of the stricture; the appearance of the esophageal mucosa proximally; whether there is evidence of esophagitis, infiltration, or other change; and its approximate diameter. Biopsies should be taken from the proximal aspect of the stricture and from the mucosa at several sites proximal to it. Brush cytology may be performed within the stricture by rotating the brush within the narrowed area. At a later stage (at least 1 week later) if the stricture is too narrow to pass either the endoscope or a narrow endoscope (e.g., A.C.M.I. F7) through it, dilatation should be attempted. This may be performed by using the Eder–Puestow stringless guided bougié (Lilly and McCaffery 1971) and dilating the stricture in stages to 40 Fr. At this stage a narrow endoscope with adequate distal tip deflection (e.g., F7) must be employed to pass beyond the stricture and examine the lower esophagus and fundus and cardia of the stomach in order to exclude an infiltrating fundal carcinoma. A good pathologist can provide considerable assistance in interpretation of the endoscopic findings. To afford him the best opportunity, however, he should be given full clinical details of the case. Biopsies from a lower esophageal stricture showing a mixture of squamous and columnar mucosa, perhaps with minor inflammatory changes and a core of connective tissue with an overgrowth of muscularis mucosa, may be difficult to interpret by itself. With the added information of a ring, easy to negotiate with the endoscope but causing bolus obstruction, the diagnosis of a Schatzki ring may be made.

Peptic strictures are of two basic types: (a) Circumferential, where there is maximal submucosal fibrosis, but with shallow peptic ulceration, and (b) deep peptic ulceration, usually localized, well defined, and with gastric mucosa on its distal margin. Local fibrosis may be considerable, but circumferential fibrosis is much less.

Various tumor types occur within the esophagus. Squamous carcinoma is the most important. Adenocarcinoma (with varying degrees of differentiation), usually found in the lower esophagus, represents either gastric carcinoma spreading upwards or a true esophageal adenocarcinoma arising from mucous glands or areas of gastric metaplasia. Occasionally a tumor arises from both types of epithelium (adenoacanthoma). Bronchial carcinoma, malignant melanoma, metastatic carcinoma, carcinosarcoma, leiomyoma, leiomyosarcoma, or neurofibroma may also be found on occasions within the esophagus.

Stomach

Endoscopic examination of the stomach now provides a complete view of the gastric mucosa. This has been brought about by the advent and development of fiber-optic endoscopes resulting in instruments of more than 100 cm working length with effective distal-tip deflection and biopsy facilities. Both forward- and side-viewing instruments are available (Salmon 1974a), but for 95% of examinations a modern forward viewing endoscope is sufficient. In the remaining cases the roof of the antrum, or proximal lesser curve, may not be seen adequately so that a lateral-viewing endoscope is required. The decision to employ such an instrument can only be made during examination with a forward-viewing endoscope which is then withdrawn, and the second instrument is passed. Endoscopy may prove invaluable in the diagnosis and management of gastric cancer but can only do so if used intelligently.

In spite of improved methods of diagnosis and surgery mortality from gastric cancer remains very high, because most cases are diagnosed only after the onset of symptoms, at a stage at which the mortality is greater than 90%. Although the gastroscope has been employed since 1932 to diagnose gastric cancer it is only since the 1950's that endoscopes have been employed to detect cancer at a treatable stage sufficient to improve the prognosis.

In 1950, Uji *et al.* at Tokyo University Hospital developed the gastro-camera allowing intragastric photographs to be taken by a distal miniature camera mounted on a flexible tube.

Over the next 15 years various Japanese workers (Tasaka and Sakita, 1966) adapted this instrument which currently incorporates a coherent viewing bundle. Total photographic documentation of the stomach is thus possible with these instruments which take 32 photographs (4 × 5 mm; 5 × 5 mm; or 5 × 6 mm size) that can subsequently be projected or enlarged (Heinkel, 1975). This technique was developed as a screening procedure in order to detect gastric cancer at a treatable stage. Japan shares the highest gastric cancer mortality in the world (68.57/100,000 population, male) with Chile (58.43/100,000, male) and Russia (60/100,000, male), and it was this statistic that prompted the development.

As a result of a comparison of the findings of gastrophotography, radiology, surgery, and histopathology the concept of "early gastric cancer" was developed (Sakita, 1966). This form of mucosal cancer is defined as a cancer of the stomach that is limited to the mucosa or submucosa. When it extends into the muscle wall it is called advanced cancer. The macroscopic classification of "early gastric cancer" is complex. Basically three types are described, viz, protruded type (I); superficial (II); and excavated type (III). Type II is further subdivided into three groups.

The Japanese classification has taught us to biopsy the central part of flat or slightly depressed lesions and to biopsy the edge of deeply excavated or ulcerated lesions. There are difficulties encountered with the complex Japanese classification. First, 15–20% of endoscopically diagnosed early gastric carcinomas (employing published endoscopic criteria) are in reality advanced carcinomas (Ariga, 1970; Okuda, 1972) when surgical biopsy is obtained. Second, the subjectivity of endoscopic appearance is demonstrated by the variation within Japan of the various types of early gastric cancer (Ueno et al., 1970; Yamagata and Masuda, 1973), even within the same hospital reported in different years. Hermanek and Röesch (1973) suggested a simplified classification for early gastric cancer, differentiating only polypoid forms (formerly Types I, IIa, IIb, IIa, and IIb) and ulcerating forms (formerly Types IIc, III, IIc and III, III and IIc, and combined forms which include IIc and/or III lesions). This classification abolishes the discrepancies between endoscopic and pathological classification so often found with the Japanese classification. Japanese papers (e.g., Hayashida and Kidokora, 1970) state that Types I and IIa have a worse prognosis than Types IIc and III, but even this prognostic index does not stand up to statistical analysis, nor from the above is the classification sufficiently reliable to expect such data to emerge. From the simplified classification new facts may emerge, but at the present time few centers outside Japan have recorded sufficient numbers of early gastric cancer to make any such assessment, though it is clear the disease is not confined to Japan (Machado et al., 1976).

Advanced gastric cancer, comprising the great majority most often seen (including Japan) are described by the Borrmann classification (Borrmann et al., 1926) which consists of four types of lesion:

Polypoid gastric carcinoma	Type I
Ulcerating, noninfiltrating carcinoma	Type II
Ulcerating, infiltrating carcinoma	Type III
Scirrhous carcinoma (localized or diffuse)	Type IV

The importance of these two main groups of gastric cancer are reflected in the much better survival figures for "early gastric cancer" (Table 1).

**TABLE 1. Five-Year Survival Rates for
Gastric Cancer by Depth of Invasion[a]**

Gastric cancer	Percentage of survival
Mucosa	96.5
Submucosa	88.1
Muscularis propria	51.5
Subserosa	51.6
Serosa	25.0–36.7

[a] From the National Cancer Center Hospital, Tokyo,
Japan, 1962–64.

The committee on early gastric cancer of the National Hospitals of
Japan showed that of 652 registered cases of early gastric cancer sent for
surgery from 1964–1969, 17 (2.6%) died of recurrent cancer as opposed to
25–36.7% of advanced cancers at the serosa of the stomach. In general, the
prognosis worsened with the depth of invasion, independent of cancer
extent within the stomach, and this provides the principal justification for
adopting the criteria for "early gastric cancer."

In Japan, the use of the gastrocamera both for screening asymptomatic
patients and for examining patients with upper gastrointestinal symptoms
has increased the cancer detection rate (Table 2) in a country where nearly
half of the 190,000 cancer deaths each year are due to gastric cancer. The
0.6% detection rate, of which half were defined as early gastric cancer,
makes the procedure a valuable one in Japan. There are no convincing
figures from Europe demonstrating a clear value of gastrocamera screening,
although some centers have demonstrated cancer detection in selected
populations (Oshima, 1971).

The value of endoscopy in the diagnosis of gastric cancer is the ability
to detect visual criteria of malignancy and to make a tissue diagnosis where
doubt exists.

TABLE 2. Incidence of Gastric Cancer (Japan): Mass Surveys

Procedure	Number of cases	Percent Advanced cancer	Percent Early cancer
70 mm X-ray[a]	958,702	1608 (0.15)	212 (0.02)
70 mm X-ray[b]	109,392	188 (0.05)	54 (0.12)
Gastrocamera[c]	6,967	19 (0.27)	19 (0.27)
X-ray[d]	8,161	24 (0.29)	18 (0.22)

[a] Ariga, 1970.
[b] Sakita, 1966.
[c] Fujita, 1970.
[d] Sakita, 1971.

Endoscopic Criteria

With projecting or polypoid lesions it is always wise to consider the lesion malignant until proven otherwise. Biopsy and cytology should be performed in all these cases. The differential diagnosis of gastric ulceration may likewise prove difficult, and the same procedure should be followed with adequate tissue obtained for the histopathologist.

Macroscopic features suggesting ulcer cancer include an irregular ulcer margin with step formation, nodular to polypoid rigid, irregular margin wall formation, rigidity, and "clubbing" of neighboring folds. Ulcers greater than 21 mm dia as measured radiographically have about four times the chance of being malignant than smaller gastric ulcers (Wenger et al., 1971).

Tissue Diagnosis

The ability to obtain biopsy and cytology samples from gastric lesions has greatly improved the diagnosis of gastric cancer, especially ulcer cancer (Williams et al., 1968; Prolla et al., 1972; Kasugai and Kobayashi, 1974). A minimum of six biopsies is now considered essential in the diagnosis of malignant gastric ulcer. It is our practice to perform four-quadrant biopsy from the edge of the ulcer where possible and then to biopsy the base and the surrounding mucosa, especially where it is nodular, or where a fold appears to be interrupted by the ulcer.

Brush cytology likewise is providing a more accurate diagnosis of gastric cancer when combined with multiple target biopsies. The reasons for this are not hard to find. In the first place biopsies may only provide necrotic surface debris, while a brush preparation may collect cells from a wider area including cancer cells. Of particular importance is the sampling error inherent in target biopsy, while a brush preparation can collect cells from the full circumference of the ulcer.

Of 751 proven gastric cancers, 697 (92.8%) were correctly diagnosed by target biopsy. Of 238 mucosal cancers 234 (97.5%) were correctly diagnosed, and 463 of 513 advanced cancers (90.3% were likewise diagnosed correctly (Kasugai and Kobayashi, 1974).

Various studies report high diagnostic yields by various cytological methods. Thus Kasugai (1968) obtained 80.9% accuracy by routine gastric lavage and 96% by gastric lavage under direct vision. A 95.2% accuracy was obtained by target brush cytology (Kobayashi et al., 1970) and an 85.7% accuracy by the imprint smear technique (Yoshii et al., 1970).

The brush cytology technique is of particular value where a stricture prevents passage of the endoscope. Brushings from within the stricture may produce a diagnostic yield in a high percentage of cases (45 of 52 cases, 87%, Kasugai and Kobayashi, 1974). Kasugai and his colleagues at the Aichi cancer center tend to employ brush cytology in the above situation, or where biopsy is negative, but it would seem more sensible to combine this with biopsy on all occasions as presently practiced in the U.K.

Life Cycle of Malignant Gastric Ulcer

Retrospective studies of gastrocamera films have demonstrated that certain malignant ulcer cancers (often early gastric cancers) have a "malignant cycle" of healing, followed by relapse, as in a benign gastric ulcer. There are cases on record of such a cycle advancing slowly over several years (Sakita, 1971). The obvious importance of endoscopy and tissue diagnosis in all cases of gastric ulcer, whether they "heal" with medical treatment or not, is largely unheeded at the present time but has been advocated in the U.K. for the past 7 years (Gear et al., 1969).

Duodenum

Examination of the duodenal bulb is almost invariably indicated for suspected or known duodenal ulcer disease (Salmon et al., 1972). Malignant disease is rare at this site. With currently available duodenoscopes, the first and second part of the duodenum can be inspected adequately and biopsies can be obtained if necessary. A lateral-viewing duodenoscope (F5-A, JFB-2, FDS) is required for detailed inspection of the medial wall of the second part of the duodenum and periampullary region. These instruments all provide biopsy facilities.

Benign duodenal tumors are recorded in about 0.2% of postmortems (River et al., 1956), but malignant tumors are much less common (Sheehy and Floch, 1964). Many so-called primary duodenal tumors are in fact probably infiltrating pancreatic neoplasms. Ampullary cancer may rarely prove to be a carcinoma of the papilla of Vater, melanosarcoma, leiomyosarcoma, round cell sarcoma, or malignant ectopic tissue infiltrating from the adjacent pancreas, duodenum, lymph nodes, or bile duct.

Endoscopic Retrograde Choledocho-Pancreatography (ERCP)

One of the most important endoscopy developments in the past few years was the development by Machida Seisakusho in 1968 of an endoscope (FDS) capable of cannulating the papilla of Vater. This development was followed by Olympus and later American (A.C.M.I.) instruments capable of the same maneuver. By means of these endoscopes a 5-Fr gauge catheter can be manipulated by endoscopic control into the papillary orifice followed by injection of contrast medium. Although Watson (1966) had visualized the papilla of Vater with a fiber-optic endoscope and McCune *et al.* (1968) had cannulated the papilla in a few patients employing a modified Eder fiber-endoscope, it was these new endoscopes that allowed endoscopic retrograde choledocho-pancreatography on a wide scale, so that ERCP is now a clinically feasible and practicable technique. The techniques required are both endoscopic and radiological. The endoscopic techniques have been described by Cotton *et al.* (1972), Salmon *et al.* (1972), Salmon (1974a), and Salmon (1975b).

The endoscope is initially employed for upper gastrointestinal endoscopy and particularly for examining the second part of the duodenum. By these means irregularities of the mucosa and encroachment of the duodenum can be observed. The intramural bile duct can also be seen, and dilatation resulting from low bile duct obstruction can be detected readily (Salmon, 1975a).

The papilla of Vater may be examined in detail and multiple target biopsies can be obtained. Selective cannulation of the pancreatic duct and bile duct are now possible in more than 80% of patients. The clinicoradiological indications are shown in Table 3.

ERCP is proving of value in the diagnosis and management of pancreatic cancer. Although in the majority of cases the lesion is strictly speaking advanced this technique often results in an earlier diagnosis and the avoidance of further investigations and an exploratory laparotomy and may assist the surgeon in defining the local anatomy preoperatively, and help in planning the type of operation to be performed.

TABLE 3. ERCP: Clinicoradiological Indications[a]

Disease	Indications
Pancreatic disease	Undiagnosed abdominal pain (suspected to be pancreatic in origin)
	Relapsing pancreatitis (diagnosis and assessment)
	Assessment of patients after pancreatic surgery
Biliary tract problems	Undiagnosed upper abdominal pain (suspected to be biliary in origin)
Jaundice	Persistent undiagnosed jaundice
	Recurrent undiagnosed jaundice

[a]Salmon, 1977.

Pancreatic Cancer

Assessment of pancreatic main duct and side duct filling is made and parenchymography may also be employed with careful screening control to detect "parenchymal field defects" (Kasugai *et al.*, 1974). After adequate filling of the main pancreatic duct to the tail, undercouch films are taken in various projections. The use of delayed films, sequential radiographs, and a video-tape recorder may help in individual cases.

The biliary tree should also be outlined where possible to detect cancers involving the bile duct.

One of the advances offered by ERCP in pancreatic cancer is the decision as to whether a Whipples procedure or palliative procedure such as a choledocho-jejunostomy should be performed. A clear decision can be made usually by this means. In some cases selective celiac angiography may also be of value.

Endoscopic pancreatography has now virtually replaced operative pancreatography (Doubilet, 1959) due to its relative safety. Most series show 5–10% of their total ERCP cases to have pancreatic cancer. For example, Kasugai *et al.* (1974) demonstrated carcinoma in 14 of 380 cases (5%) while our series includes nearly 10% of our total examinations (Salmon 1975c).

The experience of various centers has demonstrated four basic types of pancreatic cancer (Ogoshi and Hara 1972; Stadelmann *et al.*, 1974) dependent on whether there is a main duct stricture (Type I), complete duct obstruction (Type II), tapering obstruction (Type III), or cavernous filling of the gland parenchyma (Type IV). The differential diagnosis between chronic pancreatitis may often be difficult. In this case and in the "minimal change pancreatogram" pure juice pancreatic cytology is proving of value (Shida, 1973; Hatfield *et al.*, 1974; Hatfield and Smithies, 1975). These latter workers found in 19 proven cases of pancreatic cancer that pure juice cytology alone was diagnostic in 11 cases (58%), ERCP alone in 12 cases (63%); whereas both together gave a correct diagnosis in 17 cases (90%).

As with most other procedures the results of several investigations provide a total picture of greater diagnostic value than any one procedure. With ERCP the results of clinical examination, barium radiology, pancreatic exocrine function studies, pancreatic scintigraphy, etc., must all be taken into account before making the final diagnosis.

Jaundice

The second major problem that may be helped by means of ERCP is persistent or obstructive jaundice. When the serum bilirubin is greater than

3 mg%, or in the presence of impaired hepatic function (with or without jaundice), oral or intravenous contrast media invariably fail to visualize the biliary system. The diagnosis of obstructive jaundice can be made usually from the history, presence of pruritus, lack of urinary urobilinogen, and results of liver function tests. The addition of lipoprotein-X (low-density lipoprotein), a mitochondrial antibody test, liver biopsy, and organ imaging techniques may give additional information, but all lack the precision of determining the anatomical site of obstruction.

Transhepatic cholangiography is potentially hazardous and should only be employed using the Chiba technique (Okunda *et al.*, 1974), preferably where previous ultrasonography has demonstrated dilated bile ducts. Direct laparoscopic puncture of the gallbladder is possible but rarely performed, while transjugular cholangiography (Weiner and Hanafee, 1970) is likewise seldom practiced.

Endoscopic cholangio-pancreatography (ERCP) may be performed early in the course of jaundice and results in high-quality radiographs allowing an accurate diagnosis of extrahepatic cholestasis and a decision as to whether laparotomy should be performed. When viral hepatitis and drugs (including alcohol) can be reasonably excluded, the diagnostic yield is about 70% (Salmon *et al.*, 1973a; Blumgart *et al.*, 1974). Details are shown in Tables 4 and 5.

An important group (see Table 5) consists of those patients with a normal biliary tree who can be spared a laparotomy. Other series demonstrate a similar success rate in jaundice (Oi, 1973; Liguory *et al.*, 1973). Our

TABLE 4. Jaundice: Diagnostic Value of Endoscopy and ERCP [a]

	Number of cases
Total	146
Examined by endoscopy/ERCP	145
Duodenum entered	144
Papilla seen	140
Papilla cannulated	116 (80%)
Diagnostic information	
ERCP	102 ⎫
	⎬ (75%)
Endoscopy (biopsy positive)	7 ⎭
Useful information	
Endoscopy	11
No diagnostic information	24 ⎫
Misleading information	⎬ (17%)
Endoscopy	1 ⎭

[a] Blumgart *et al.*, 1974.

TABLE 5. Jaundice: Diagnoses by Endoscopy and ERCP[a]

	Number of cases
By means of ERCP	
Gallstones	31
Pancreatic or bile duct cancer	25
Sclerosing cholangitis	5
Postoperative stricture	8
Abnormalities of gallbladder	7
Miscellaneous	
Dilated duct (postcholecystectomy)	1
Debris in dilated duct	
(postsphincterotomy)	1
Hydatid cyst	1
Tuberculous abscess	1
Normal ducts	22
Endoscopic diagnosis (biopsy positive)	
Ampullary carcinoma	3
Pancreatic carcinoma	2
Gastric carcinoma	1
Stomal ulcer	1
Total	109
Useful information on endoscopy	
Distorted duodenum (probably	
pancreatic cancer)	11

[a]Blumgart *et al.*, 1974.

results suggest that percutaneous transhepatic cholangiography may still be necessary to delineate the proximal limits of an obstruction demonstrated by retrograde cholangiography. In these cases the intrahepatic bile ducts will almost certainly be dilated allowing a high success rate with this technique.

Laparoscopy

Laparoscopy has been largely ignored in the U.K. as a means of diagnosing upper abdominal pathology. On the Continent considerable expertise and experience has accumulated over a number of years. In the diagnosis of gastrointestinal disease laparoscopy is useful in defining the cause of unexplained hepatomegaly by inspection and biopsy, establishing the presence of surface metastases, in the diagnosis of hepatic cirrhosis, in the differential diagnosis of ascites and in the diagnosis of peritoneal pathology (inflammatory and neoplastic). Of particular interest at the present time are the possibilities of pancreatic laparoscopy.

Supragastric Pancreoscopy. By means of a 130° laparoscope it is now possible to inspect the pancreas through the omentum in about two-thirds of patients (Meyer-Burg, 1972). A probe may be positioned through a separate opening to palpate the pancreas, and a directed needle biopsy may be performed at sites considered to be abnormal. Meyer-Burg obtained a 56.6% success rate in 640 cases (Meyer-Burg, 1975), diagnosing 20 cases of pancreatic cancer. It seems likely that this technique will be refined and employed more often.

Infragastric Pancreoscopy. In some cases (about 30%) due to omental fat, supragastric pancreoscopy fails. In these cases infragastric pancreoscopy, whereby the gastrocolic ligament is divided by electrosurgery, may be feasible, allowing the passage of a laparoscope directly into the lesser sac for inspection, palpation, and biopsy of the body and tail of the pancreas (Strauch et al., 1973).

Enteroscopy

Endoscopic examination beyond the ligament of Treitz presents special problems. The relative fixation of the bowel at the duodenojejunal flexure makes it impossible to negotiate the angle by the usual distal-tip deflection mechanisms supplied with modern endoscopes. Peroral examination of the small bowel beyond the duodenojejunal flexure has not hitherto been possible.

Classen et al. (1972) employed a "monorail" procedure (Paoluzi, 1970) in which a long forward viewing endoscope was threaded over a previously swallowed small Teflon tube. With a 100 cm fiber-optic endoscope they were able to examine the terminal ileum in eight of ten patients. Jejuno-ileitis with multiple ulcers and polypoid mucosa was found in one patient. This technique has, not surprisingly, found little support elsewhere since it takes 3–7 days to intubate the entire bowel and, in addition, traction on the tube required during the threading procedure can damage the bowel. Not the least disadvantage is the fact that the operating channel is utilized by the "monorail-tube" so that biopsies are not possible. More recently Mita et al. (1973) and Salmon et al. (1973b) have employed a newly designed enteroscope for peroral duodeno-jejunoscopy without a guide wire.

The use of this type of forward-viewing endoscope with a stiffening wire passed down the operating channel allows intubation of the jejunum in a high percentage of patients. Neoplasms of the small bowel are rare, nevertheless the technique appears to be of use in cases of suspected duodeno-jejunal Crohn's disease, suspected small bowel lymphoma, and where a small bowel mucosal biopsy is required, but intubation has previously failed.

Colonoscopy

Although the clinical value of colonoscopy has been well documented (Niwa *et al.*, 1969; Dean and Shearman, 1970; Salmon *et al.*, 1971; Hansen, 1971; Overholt, 1971; Sakai, 1972; Williams and Muto, 1972; Teague *et al.*, 1973) the technical difficulties of performing the procedure, together with the time involved and the need for X-ray screening facilities, have limited its use at the present time. There is no doubt, however, that fiber-optic examination of the large bowel is a major advance both in the diagnosis and the management of colorectal cancer and in removal of polyps.

Most series report a positive diagnosis of large bowel symptoms in up to one-quarter of cases examined (Teague *et al.*, 1973), but this figure depends on the method of case selection.

The chief indications will be equivocal or negative large-bowel radiology, X-ray negative rectal bleeding, total colonoscopy, and endoscopic polypectomy in patients where radiology has demonstrated one or more polyps.

The findings in 255 consecutive examinations at Bristol (Teague *et al.*, 1973) are shown in Table 6.

The ability to obtain target biopsies provides absolute precision in the diagnosis of colorectal cancer and the clarity of modern endoscope optics allows a clear distinction to be made between feces and tumors, a distinction which cannot always be made by palpation at operation. Endoscopic polypectomy is undoubtedly an additional advance and at the present time the indications for surgical colotomy and polypectomy are very few.

Of 499 colonic polyps removed endoscopically in 350 patients (Wolff and Shinya, 1973), up to 5 polyps were removed at one examination (Table 7). Their size varied from 0.5 to > 5.0 cm. Polyps of less than 0.5 cm diam were not removed since their malignant potential was low. Table 8 shows the histopathology of these polyps demonstrating the great value of endos-

TABLE 6. Endoscopic Findings in 255 Consecutive Colonoscopes[a]

Proctocolitis	55
Crohn's disease	16
Polyps	17
Carcinoma	22
Normal bowel	99
Diverticular disease	15
Operative colonoscopy	12
Others (melanosis coli, amebiasis, etc.)	19

[a]Teague *et al.*, 1973.

TABLE 7. Polyps Removed per
Procedure[a]

Patient procedures	Polyps/procedure
300	1
47	2
17	3
6	4
6	5
Total 376	

[a]Wolff and Shinya, 1973.

TABLE 8. Histopathological Diagnosis in 499 Endoscopically
Removed Polyps[a]

Type polyp		Number removed
Adenomatous polyps		262
With atypia	14	
With focal carcinoma	5	
Villous adenoma		51
With atypia	4	
With superficial carcinoma	7	
Mixed villous and adenomatous polyps		108
With atypia	10	
With superficial carcinoma	5	
Miscellaneous (juvenile, inflammatory, etc.)		4
Unretrieved		33
Malignant ''polyps''		17
Total		499

[a]Wolff and Shinya, 1973.

copic excision biopsy. Occasionally peroperative colonoscopy (Espiner *et al.*, 1973) in which examination of the unopened bowel is made at laparotomy by manipulating the endoscope with the surgeon's help round to the cecum, aids in the planning of subsequent surgery. This technique, which is relatively simple, should be reserved for cases where preoperative total colonoscopy has failed and where inspection of the whole bowel, as when polypoid carcinoma is to be removed, would be of value.

References

Ariga, K. (1970). Statistique sur le cancer de l'estomac à la lumière de la campagne de dépistage faute au Japon. *Am. Gastroent. Hepatol.* **6**:307.

Bennett, J. (1976). Oesophagoscopy. In *Topics in Gastrointestinal Endoscopy* (Schiller, K. F. R. and Salmon P. R., eds.). Heineman Medical Press, London.

Blumgart, L. H., Salmon, P. R., and Cotton, P. B. (1974). Endoscopic retrograde cholangio-pancreatography in the jaundiced patient. *Surg., Gynaecol., Obstet.* **138**:565.

Boros, E. (1947). Esophagoscopy by means of a flexible instrument: A new esophagogastro-scope. *Gastroenterology* **8**:427.

Borrmann, R., Henke, F., and Lubarsch, O. (1926). *Handbuch der speziellen pathologischen Anatomie und Histologie*, Vol. 4. pt. Km, 865. Springer, Berlin.

Bozzini, P. (1807). *Der Lichtleiter,* Verlag des Landes-Industrie-Comptoirs, Weimar.

Classen, M., Frühmorgen, Koch, H., and Demling, L. (1972). Enteroskopie-Fiberendoskopie von Jejunum und Ileum. *Dtsch. Med. Woch.* **11**:409.

Cotton, P. B., Salmon, P. R., Blumgart, L. H., Burwood, R. J., Davies, G. J., Lawrie, B. W., Pierce, J. W., and Read, A. E. (1972). Cannulation of the papilla of Vater via fibre-duodenoscope. Assessment of retrograde cholangiopancreatography in 60 patients. *Lancet* **1**:53.

Dean, A. C. B., and Shearman, D. J. C. (1970). A clinical evaluation of the Olympus CF-SB fibre optic colonoscope. *2nd World Congress of Gastroent. Endoscopy (Rome and Copenhagen).*

Doubilet, H. (1959). Pancreatography. *Ann. N.Y. Acad. Sci.* **78**:829–851.

Espiner, H. J., Salmon, P. R., Teague, R. H., and Read, A. E. (1973). Operative colonoscopy. *Br. Med. J.* **I**:453.

Evans, J. A., Glenn, F., Thorbjarnson, J., and Mujahad, Z. (1962). Percutaneous transhepatic cholangiography. Discussion of the method and report of 25 cases. *Radiology* **78**:362.

Fujita, K. (1970). Cited by Sakita, T. and Oguro, Y. (1974). In *Gastrointestinal Pan-Endoscopy* (L. Berry, ed.). Springfield, Ill., Charles C Thomas, p. 280.

Gear, M. W. L., Truelove, S. C., Williams, D. G., Massarella, G. R., and Boddington, M. M. (1969). Gastric cancer simulating benign gastric ulcer. *Br. J. Surg.* **56**, 10:739.

Hansen, L. K. (1971). Colonoscopy: A study of 50 cases. *Scand. J. Gastroenterol.* **6**:687.

Hatfield, A. R. W., Whittaker, R., and Gibbs, D. D. (1974). The collection of pancreatic fluid for cytodiagnosis using a duodenoscope. *Gut* **15**:305.

Hatfield, A. R. W., and Smithies, A. (1975). Personal communication.

Hayashida, T., and Kidokora, T. (1970). End results of early gastric carcinoma. *4th World Congress of Gastroenterology (Copenhagen).*

Heinkel, K. (1975). Personal communication.

Heitmann, P., Csendes, A., Strauszer, T. (1971). Esophageal strictures and lower esophagus lined with columnar epithelium. *Digest. Dis.* **16**, 4:307.

Hermanek, P., and Röesch, W. (1973). Critical evaluations of the Japanese "Early gastric cancer" classification. *Endoscopy* **5**:220.

Hirschowitz, B. I., Curtiss, L. E., Peters, C. W., and Pollard, H. M. (1958). Demonstrations of a new gastroscope, the "Fiberscope". *Gastroenterology* **35**:50.

Hufford, A. R. (1949). Flexi-rigid, optical oesophagoscope. *Gastroenterology* **12**:779.

Kasugai, T., and Kobayashi, S. (1974). Evaluation of biopsy and cytology in the diagnosis of gastric cancer. *Am. J. Gastroenterol.* **62**, 3:199.

Kasugai, T. (1968). Gastric biopsy under direct vision by the fibergastroscope. *Gastrointest. Endosc.* **15**:33.

Kasugai, T., Kuno, N., and Kizu, M. (1974). Manometric endoscopic retrograde pancreatocholangiography. Technique, significance, and evaluation. *Am. J. Dig. Dis.* **19**,6:485.

Katz, D. (1966). Presentation at American Society of Gastrointestinal Endoscopy. Chicago, Ill.

Kobayashi, S., Prolla, J. C., and Kirsner, J. B. (1970). Brushing cytology of the oesophagus and stomach under direct vision by fiberscopes. *Acta Cytol.* **14**:219.

Kussmaul, A. (1869). Ueber die Behandlung der Magenerweiterung durch eine neue Methode (mittelst der Magen-pumpe). *Dtsch. Arch. Klin. Med.* **6**:456.

Liguory, C., Goffu, J., Gouerou, H., and Chavy, A. (1973). Diagnostic des ictères cholestatiques par cholangiographie endoscopique. *Acta Gastro-Enterol. Belg.* **36**:702.

Lilly, J. O., and McCaffery, D. (1971). Esophageal stricture dilatation: A new method adapted to the fiberoptic esophagoscope. *Am. J. Dig. Dis.* **16, 12**:1137.

Lo Presti, P. A. and Hilmi, A. (1974). Clinical experience with a new foroblique fiberoptic esophagoscope. *Am J. Dig. Dis.* (n.s.) **9**:10, 690.

Machado, G., Davies, J. D., Tudway, A. S. C., Salmon, P. R., and Read, A. E. (1976). Superficial carcinoma of the stomach. *Brit. Med. J.* **2**:77–79.

Mackenzie, M. (1881). Original communications on the use of the oesophagoscope in disease of the gullet. *Med. Ims. Gaz.* **2**:60.

McCune, W. S. Shorb, P. E., and Moscovitz, H. (1968). Endoscopic cannulation of the ampulla of Vater: A preliminary report. *Ann. Surg.* **167**:752.

Meyer-Burg, J. (1972). The inspection, palpation, and biopsy of the pancreas by peritoneoscopy. *Endoscopy* **4**:99.

Meyer-Burg, J. (1975). Personal communication.

Mickulicz-Radecki, J. (1881). Ueber Gastroskopie und Oesophagoskopie. *Wien. Med. Presse* **22**:1405.

Mita, M., Matsumoto, K., Tachikawa, H., Yamagishi, G., Oshiba, S., Miura, K., and Yamagata, S. (1973). An improved fiberintestinoscope type FIS-IYA. *1st Asian-Pacific Congress of Endoscopy, Kyoto, Japan.*

Niwa, H. (1969). Clinical study of colono-fiberscope. *Gastrointest. Endos.* **11**:173.

Ogoshi, K., and Hara, Y. (1972). Retrograde pancreato-choledochography. English version of *Jap. J. Clin. Radiol.* **17, 7**:455, Kanehara Shuppan Co., Tokyo.

Oi, I. (1973). In discussion during International Workshop, Erlangen. *Endoscopy of the Small Intestine with Retrograde Pancreato-cholangiography* (L. Demling, and M. Classen, Eds.), p. 101. Georg Thieme, Stuttgart.

Okuda, S. (1972). Differential diagnosis of early gastric carcinoma from advanced carcinoma. In *Early Gastric Cancer* (T. Murakami, ed.). University Park Press, Baltimore.

Okuda K., Tanikawa, K., Emura, T., Kuratomi S., Jinnsuchi, S., Urabe, K., Sumikoshi, T., Kanda, Y., Fukuyama, Y., Musha, H., Mori, H., Shimokawa, Y., Yakushija, F., and Matsuura, Y. (1974). Non surgical, percutaneous transhepatic cholangiography—diagnostic significance in medical problems of the liver. *Am. J. Dig. Dis.* **19**:21–36.

Oshima, H. (1971). The gastrocamera in the early detection of carcinoma of the stomach. *Proceedings of 2nd Congress of European Association of Radiology.* Int. Congress. Series No. 249, p. 79. Excerpta Medica, Amsterdam.

Overholt, B. F. (1971). Flexible fiberoptic sigmoidoscopy—Technique and preliminary results. *Cancer (Philadelphia)* **26**:123.

Paoluzi, P. (1970). Total colonoscopy by a "monorail" method. *2nd World Congress of Gastroint. Endoscopy (Rome and Copenhagen).*

Prolla, J. C., Xavier, R. G., and Kirsner, J. B. (1972). Exfoliative cytology in gastric ulcer. Its role in the differentiation of benign and malignant ulcers. *Gastroenterology. J.* **63**:33.

River, L. J., Silverstein, J. W., and Tape, P. (1956). Benign neoplasms of the small intestine. A critical comprehensive review with reports of 20 new cases. *Int. Abstr. Surg.* **102**:1.

Sakai, Y. (1972). The technique of colonofiberoscopy. *Dis. Colon Rectum* **15**:403.

Sakita, T. (1966). Diagnosis of early gastric cancer with gastrocamera. Recent advances in gastroenterology. *The proceedings of the 3rd World Congress of Gastroenterology, Tokyo* **1**:275.

Sakita, T. (1971). The Committee of early gastric cancer of the National Hospital of Japan (Chief of Committee Sakita, T.): Report on retrospective and follow-up studies of the early carcinoma of the stomach, after surgery (in Japanese.)

Salmon, P. R., Branch, R. A., Collins, C., Espiner, H., and Read, A. E. (1971). Clinical evaluation of fibreoptic signoidoscopy employing the Olympus CF-SB colonoscope. *Gut* **12**:729.

Salmon, P. R. Brown, P., Htut, J., and Read, A. E. (1972). Endoscopic examination of the duodenal bulb: Clinical evaluation of forward- and side-viewing fibreoptic systems in 200 cases. *Gut* **13**:170.

Salmon, P. R., Blumgart, L., Burwood, R., Davies, G., and Read, A. E. (1973a). Endoscopy in the diagnosis of obstructive jaundice. In *Endoscopy of the Small Intestine with Retrograde Pancreato-cholangiography*. L. Demling and M. Classen, eds.), p. 98.

Salmon, P. R., Brown, P., Burwood, R., and Read, A. E. (1973b). Examination of the duodenum and jejunum employing a new fibreoptic enteroscope. *Gut* **14, 10**:823.

Salmon, P. R. (1974a). *Fibre-optic Endoscopy*. Pitman Medical.

Salmon. P. R. (1974b). Recent developments in gastrointestinal endoscopy. In *Topics in Gastroenterology* (S. C. Truelove and J. Trowell, eds.). Blackwells Scientific Publ.

Salmon, P. R. (1975a). Endoscopic retrograde cholangio-pancreatography (ERCP). In *Modern Trends in Gastroenterology, No. 5* (A. E. Read, ed.). Butterworth, London.

Salmon, P. R. (1975b). Early diagnosis of pancreatic cancer. *12th Symposium on Advanced Medicine, Royal College of Physicians*. Pitman Medical, London.

Salmon, P. R. (1977). New clinical procedures in endoscopy of the digestive tract. *Proc. R. Soc.*

Schatzki, R. (1963). The lower oesophageal ring. Long term follow-up of symptomatic and asymptomatic rings. *Am. J. Roentgenol.* **90**:805.

Schindler, R. (1936). Gastroscopy with a flexible gastroscope. *Am. J. Dig. Dis.* **2**:656.

Sheehy, T. W. and Floch, M. H. (1964). Neoplasms of the small intestine. In *The Small Intestine*. New York, Harper & Row. pp. 319–435.

Shida, (1973). Personal communication.

Stadelman, O., Sáfrány, L., Loffler, A., Barna, L., Miederer, S. E., Papp, J., Kaufer, C., and Sobbe, A. (1974). Endoscopic retrograde cholangiopancreatography in pancreatic cancer. *Endoscopy* **6**:84.

Strauch, M., Lux, G., and Ottenjann, R. (1973). Infragastric pancreoscopy. *Endoscopy* **5, 1**:30.

Tasaka, S., and Sakita, T. (1966). Progress of gastrocamera examination. *Proceedings of the 1st Congress of the International Society of Endoscopy, Tokyo* 70.

Teague, R. A., Salmon, P. R., and Read, A. E. (1973). Fibreoptic examination of the colon: A review of 255 cases. *Gut* **14**:139.

Ueno, K., Yamagata, S., Masnda, H., Oshiba, S., Kano, A., Yago, H., Narita, A., Yamagata, H., Shirance, A., Mochizuki, F. (1970). Clinical evaluation of gastric biopsy under direct vision in diagnosis of gastric cancer. *4th World Congress of Gastroenterology (Copenhagen)*.

Uji, T. (1952). The gastrocamera. *Tokyo Med. J.* 135.

Von Hacker, V. (1904). *A system of practical surgery* (E. Bergmann, ed.), Vol. 4, p. 17. von Lea Bros.

Watson, W. C. (1966). Direct vision of the ampulla of Vater through the gastroduodenal fiberscope. *Lancet* **1**:902.

Wenger, J., Brandborg, L., and Spellman, F. A. (1971). Cancer: Clinical aspects (The VA Administration Cooperative Study on Gastric Ulcer). *Gastroenterology* **61**:598.

Weiner, M., and Hanafee, W. N. (1970). A review of transjugular cholangiography. *Radiol. Clin. North Am.* **8**:53.

Williams, C., and Muto, T. (1972). Examination of the whole colon with the fibreoptic colonoscope. *Br. Med. J.* **3**:278.

Williams, D. G., Truelove, S. C., Gear, M. W. L., Massarella, G. R., and Fitzgerald, N. W. (1968). Gastroscopy with biopsy and cytological sampling under direct vision. *Br. Med. J.* **I**:535.

Wolff, W. I., and Shinya, H. (1973). A new approach to colonic polyps. *Ann. Surg.* **178, 3**:367.

Yamagata, S., and Masnda, H. (1973). Magenkarzinom. In *Klinische Gastroenterologie* (L. Demling, ed.), Vol. I. Thieme, Stuttgart.

Yoshii, Y., Yamacka, Y., Kasugai, T., *et al.* (1970). Significance of imprint smear in cytologic diagnosis of malignant tumours of the stomach. *Acta Cytol.* **14**:249.

DIAGNOSTIC ASPECTS
RADIOLOGY

ERIC SAMUEL

The greatly extended range of available radiological investigations including thermography, ultrasound, and isotope scanning, etc., has created an increasing problem in planning the correct approach to the investigation of a suspect cancer case. It should be axiomatic in surgical practice that in any investigation, given the same accuracy, the simplest and least invasive methods should be used first.

This is merely an extension of a problem-orientated approach to medical diagnosis, and the newer techniques that have evolved in radiology will be considered in light of this approach to the diagnosis of malignant tumors of the various systems.

Abdominal Swelling

In the investigation of any abdominal swelling, convention has dictated that the best possible definition of the anatomical site of origin of the swelling should be the first step in diagnosis, and further investigations should be sequential and related to eliciting its nature. The development of ultrasound investigation has provided us with a different approach in that

Eric Samuel • Forbes Professor of Medical Radiology, University of Edinburgh and the Royal Infirmary, Edinburgh, Scotland EH3 9YW.

the nature of the swelling can be recognized with confidence as cystic, solid, or semicystic. Once its nature is recognized, the anatomical site of origin can usually be more easily determined.

The development of the ultrasound grayscale-B scan using wavebands between 2 and 6 mH has enabled solid tumors with their multiple diffuse echoes to be differentiated from the transonic swellings which are cysts or cystic tumors. By the use of these ultrashort sound waves suitably pulsed, echoes can be registered from most intraabdominal structures. Recognizing the fact that cystic swellings are transonic and consequently produce only echoes from their walls enables the outline of the cyst and its relation to its anatomical structure of origin to be visualized. Solid swellings, on the other hand, produce echoes from within and give a completely different pattern.

The first investigation in the diagnosis of a swelling in the upper abdomen should, therefore, utilize ultrasound to determine its nature (Figure 1).

Transverse and longitudinal ulstrasound scanning will enable the normal and abnormal outlines of the kidney, aorta, inferior vena cava, liver,

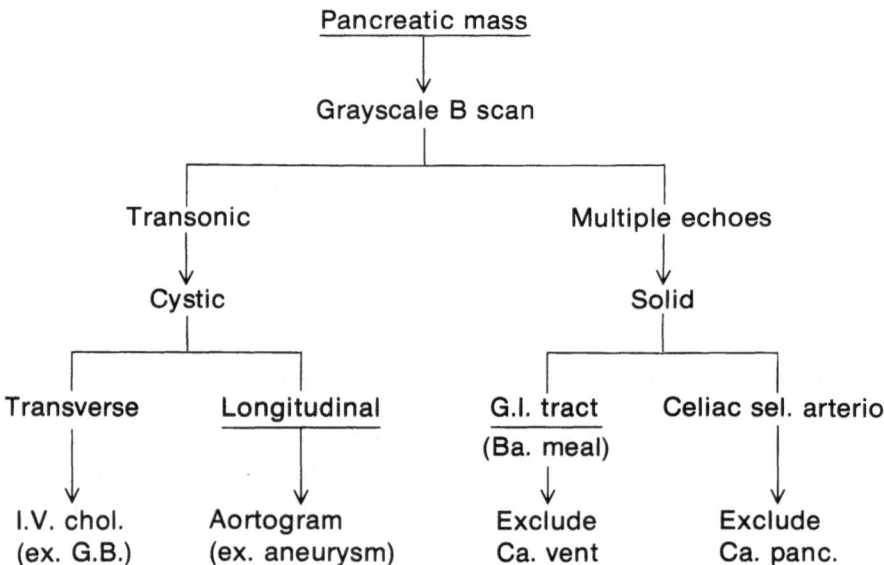

Figure 1

and spleen to be identified. Producing transverse scans at 2-cm intervals from the rib cage downwards until the pubis is reached will enable the outline of the solid visceral organs and the fluid-filled bladder to be recognized. Ultrasound has no part to play in the investigation of the small or large bowel as there is swamping of the echoes from the gas-filled bowel.

For example, in an upper abdominal swelling of suspect pancreatic origin, Figure 2, the demonstration of its cystic nature would imply the presence either of a pseudocyst or a cyst adenoma arising from that organ. The ultrasound scan will enable the size and volume of the cyst to be measured and recorded (Figures 3a and 3b). This capability of mensuration is of the utmost importance when assessing the effects of treatment.

When, however, a solid tumor is recognized by ultrasound, the problem of determining whether or not it has its origin in the pancreas may be followed by a hypotonic duodenogram which produces a double contrast view of the duodenum when the motor activity of that structure is inhibited by the injection of 1 ml of metachlorpromine. Tumors (Figure 4) arising from the pancreatic head are detected by (a) flattening of the descending loop, (b) irregularity of the mucosal folds, (c) destruction of the mucosal pattern and the presence of a filling defect, usually on the medial aspect of the curve of the duodenum. If the hypotonic duodenogram is negative, or when the tumor is thought to arise in the body or the tail of the pancreas, selective arteriography should be the next sequential step in the investigation. Selective catheterization of both the hepatic and superior mesenteric arteries may be necessary to outline the whole vascular supply of the pancreas, and until this is done no definitive decision about the presence or absence of a tumor can be made. Superselective catheterization of the pancreatico-duodenal vessels has been achieved and certainly improves the detail in the arteriogram. The arteriographic findings indicative of a tumor are (Figure 5): (1) Displacement of the pancreatic arteries and their branches; (2) the presence of abnormal vessels; (3) encasement of normal vessels by the tumor giving a characteristic local narrowing of the lumen.

This latter feature is particularly valuable in the diagnosis of malignant infiltration. Tumor staining does not usually occur with pancreatic tumors, e.g., insulinoma or a delta-celled tumor associated with the Zollinger–Ellison syndrome or the pancreatic cholera-celled tumor associated with the Weiner–Morrison syndrome Figures 6 and 7.

Isotope scanning of the pancreas with ^{99}T seleneomethione has not achieved the necessary accuracy to make it generally acceptable as a method of recognizing early pancreatic tumors. It may be that improved techniques and equipment and better radionucleotides will improve this method. Subtraction methods and computerized printouts have not really significantly improved the results of scanning to justify their expense.

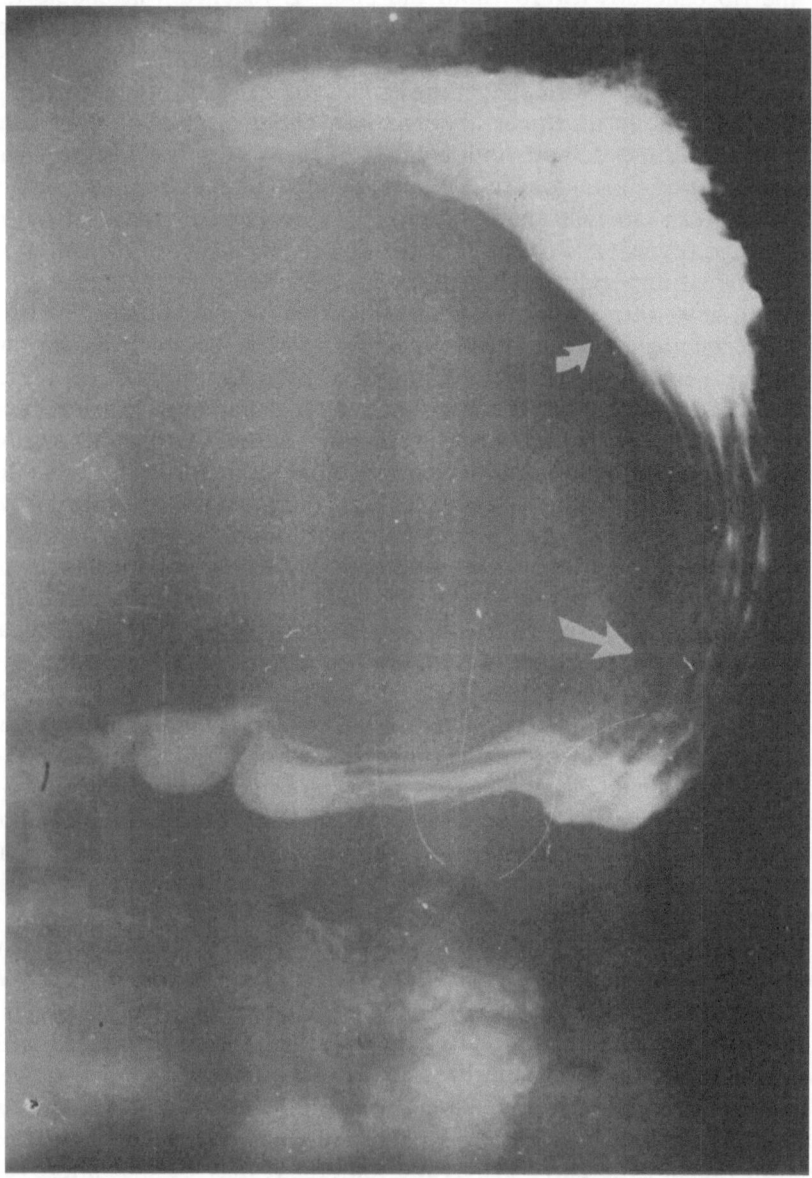

Figure 2. Barium meal examination showing stretching of the stomach by an upper abdominal mass suggesting a pancreatic origin.

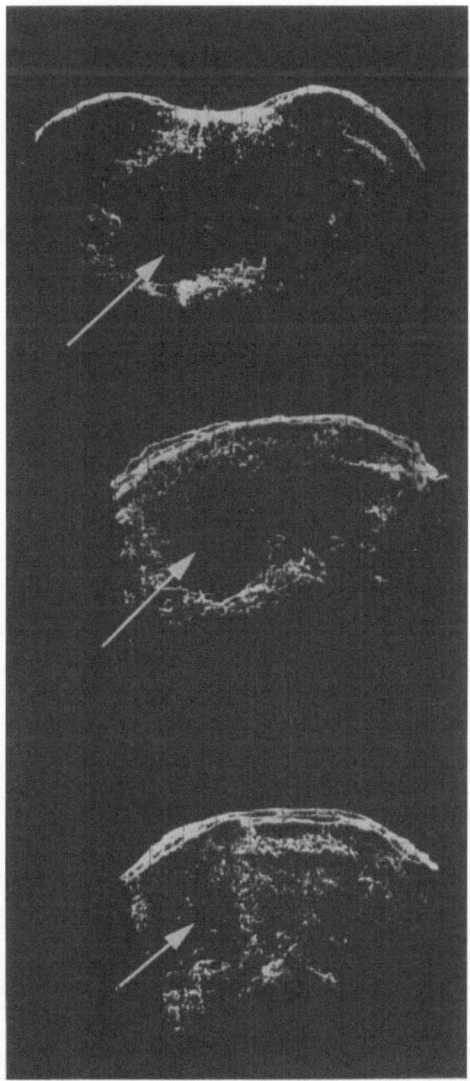

Figure 3a. Ultrasound examination showing a transonic mass with well-defined outlines indicating a pancreatic cyst.

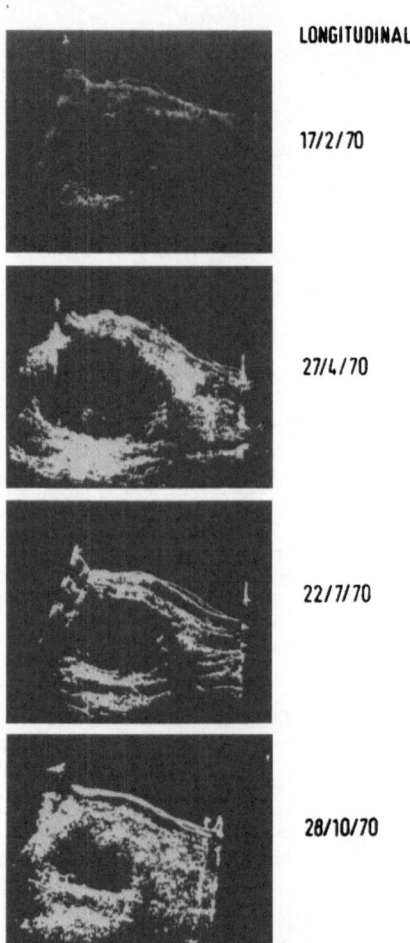

Figure 3b. Same case 1 month later showing value of echo in a follow-up examination of such cases. The area of the mass can be measured from the gradicule on the screen.

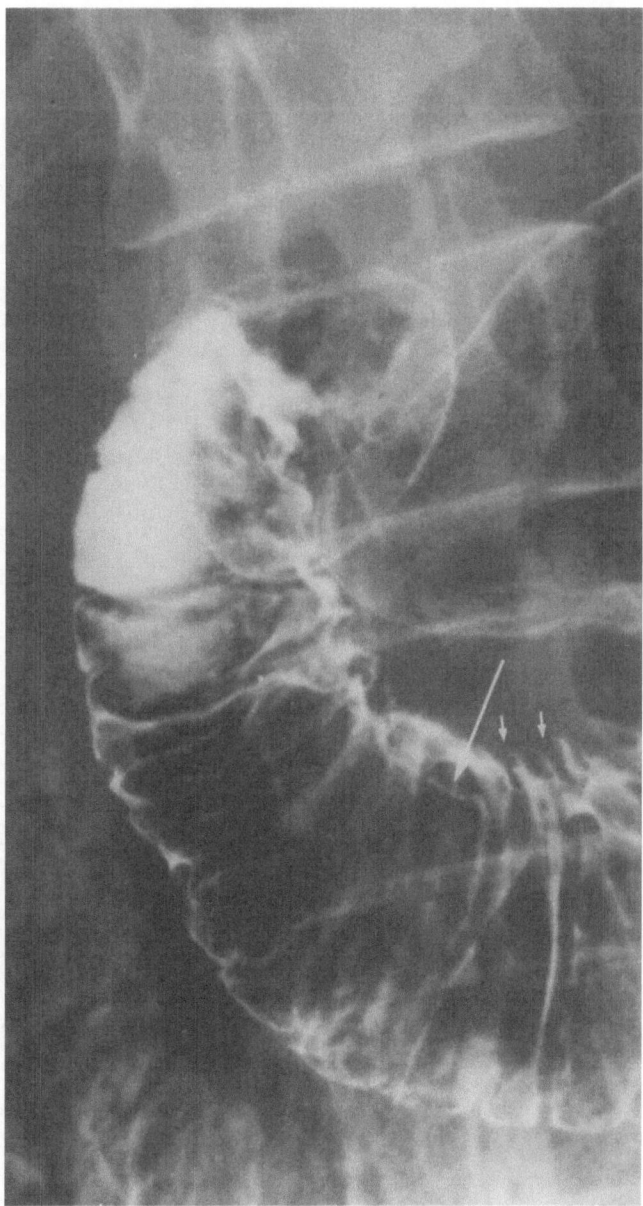

Figure 4. Hypotonic duodenogram showing the changes on the medial wall of the duodenum associated with a pancreatic tumor.

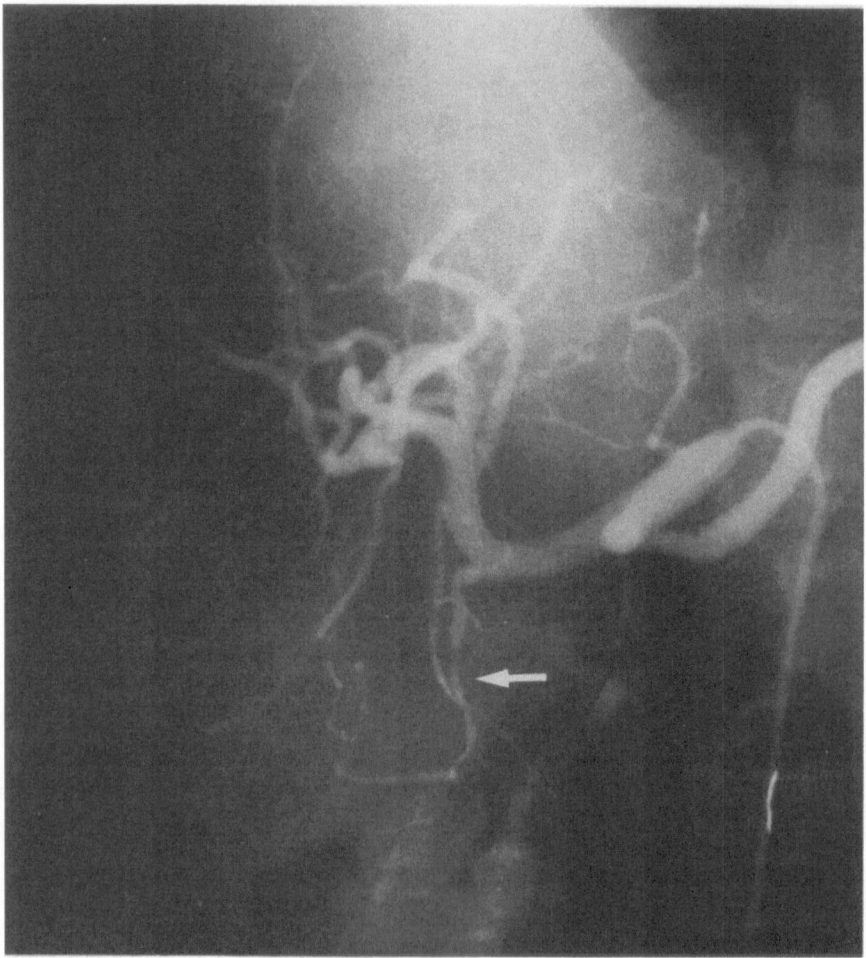

Figure 5. Pancreatic arteriogram showing displacement of vessels, cuffing of the arteries by tumor.

Renal Swelling

Ultrasound scanning of upper abdominal swelling may reveal that it is of renal origin, and this is readily achieved as the normal kidney outline and renal pelvis can be recognized by ultrasound. Transonic swelling would obviously indicate a cyst of renal origin. The sequential investigations should consist of an intravenous pyelogram valuable in confirming the finding of a normal opposite kidney and also (Figure 8) a cyst puncture which can be performed under fluoroscopic TV control; and some contrast medium introduced will exclude the presence of any tumor in the wall. Aspiration of the cyst followed by the introduction of 2–5 ml of pantopaque is claimed to prevent refilling of the cyst and certainly is of considerable assistance in following the progress of the cyst by serial X-ray examination when shrinkage of the contrast-lined cyst can be readily observed.

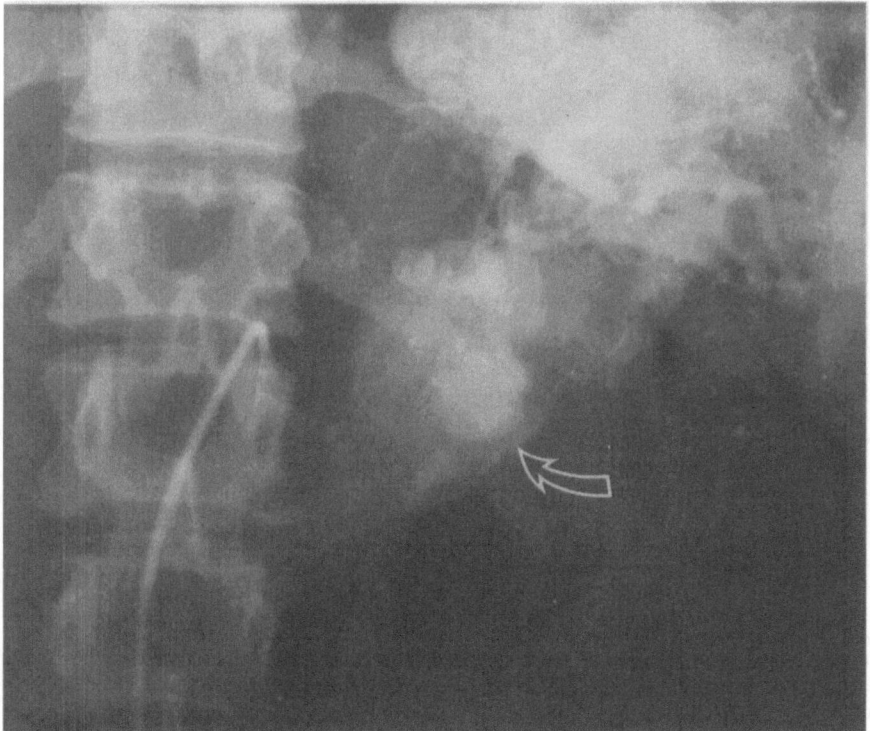

Figure 6. Pancreatic arteriogram showing tumor staining associated with an insulinoma (courtesy of Dr. Sumerling).

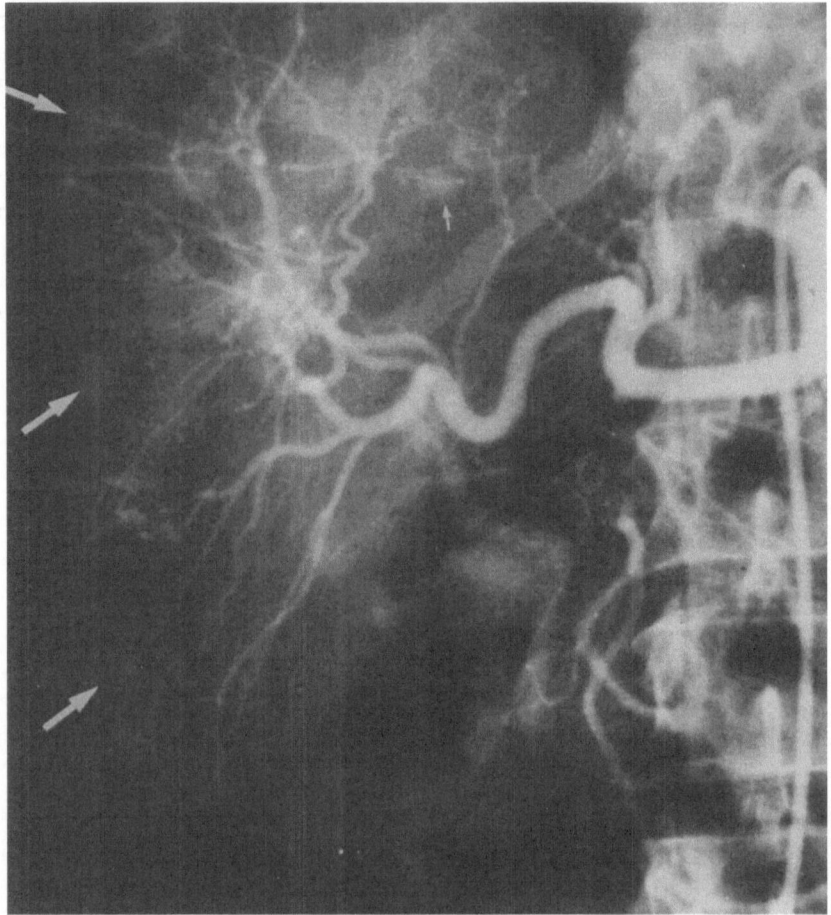

Figure 7. Hepatic angiogram showing metastatic tumor in Weiner–Morrison syndrome. The primary tumor had been removed 5 years previously and had been considered benign. Recurrence of the symptoms lead to the hepatic arteriogram which demonstrated these masses (courtesy of Dr. Buist).

PROGRAMMED INVESTIGATION

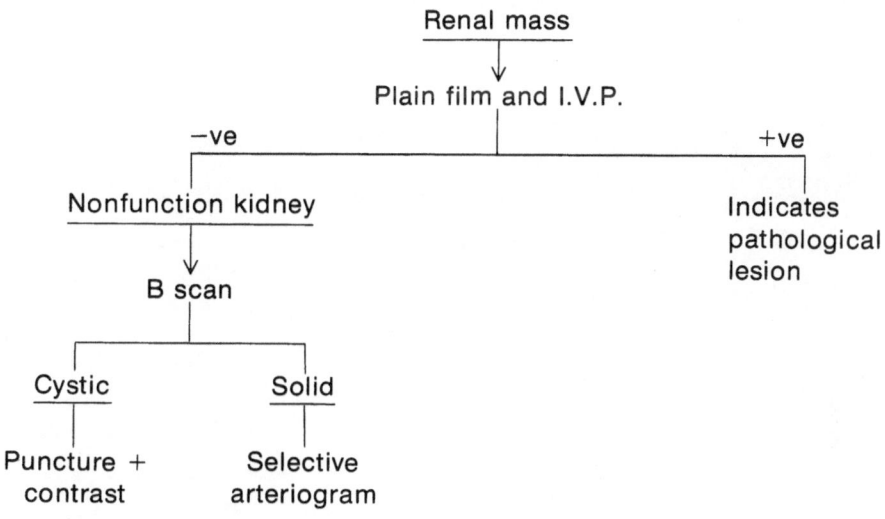

Figure 8

If, on the other hand, ultrasound shows the swelling to be solid, the relationship to the pelvis of the kidney as judged from the I.V.P. determines the next step in investigation. If the lesion is considered to be of parenchymatous origin, selective renal angiography is probably preferable to retrograde pyelography, as it enables not only a diagnosis of the nature of the swelling (Figure 9) but also its extent (Figure 10), blood supply, and spread into the renal vein and inferior vena cava. Retrograde pyelography must be the method of choice when the lesion appears to arise from the renal pelvis. Angiography is particularly disappointing in these tumors as they are usually relatively avascular.

Liver Swelling

As the liver is a frequent site of metastases from gastrointestinal cancer, any method which would allow the detection or exclusion of hepatic metastases would be of great benefit in planning the correct approach to any abdominal malignancy.

Much effort has been expended in the biochemical estimation of liver function, but it is disappointing that until there is major destruction of liver substance, biochemical changes may not be reflected.

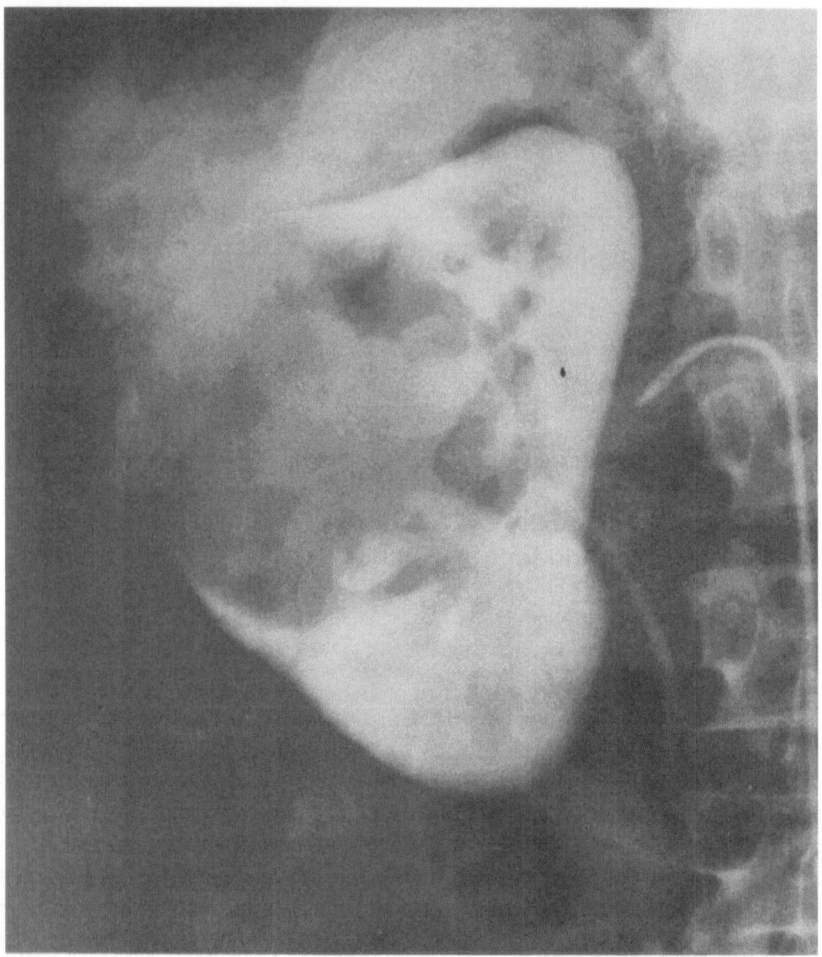

Figure 9. Nephrogram phase after a selective arteriogram. The translucent avascular smooth rounded area indicative of a cyst is clearly seen in the cortex (courtesy of Dr. Buist).

Isotope scanning using ^{99}T-labeled colloid sulfur or Rose Bengal have provided a means of detecting hepatic metastases. By scanning the liver after the injection of one of these radionuclides with a rectilinear or gamma camera, defects in the absorptive pattern of the liver caused by metastases can be seen. Scanning is carried out in the prone, supine, and lateral positions so that all lobes of the liver can be visualized. The improvement in the resolution of modern gamma cameras and scanners has

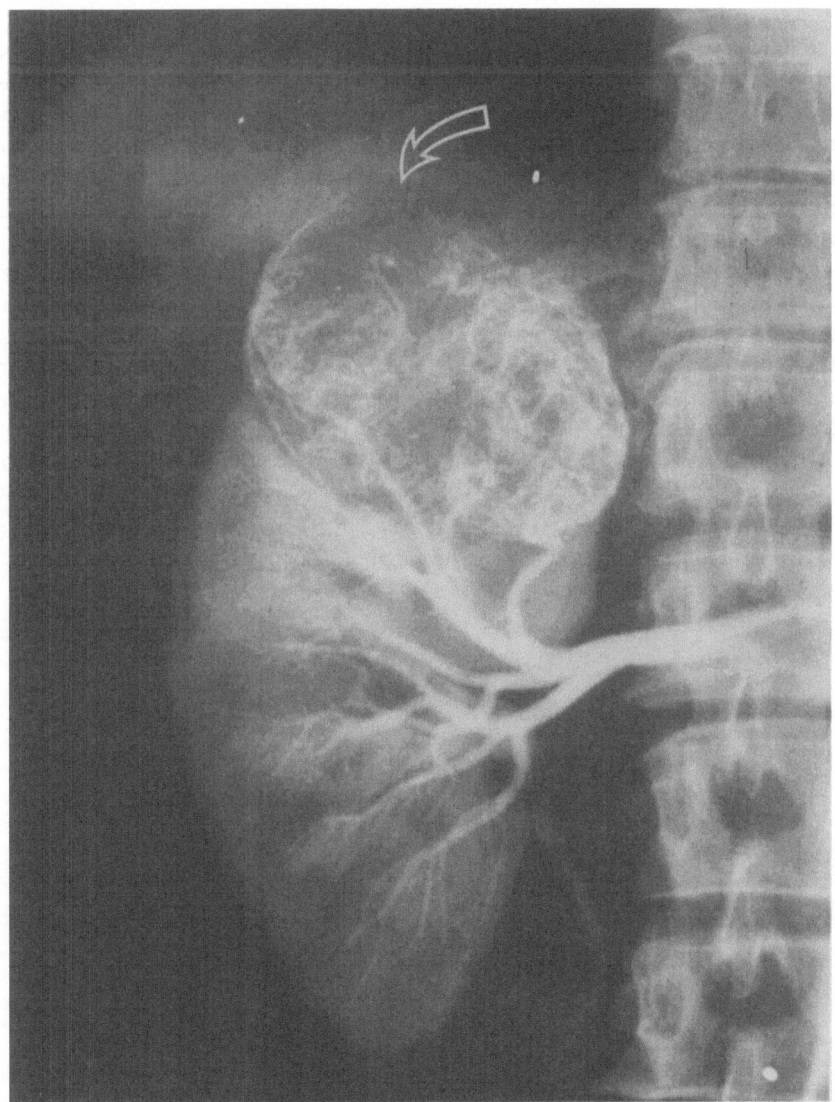

Figure 10. Selective arteriogram showing spread of tumor through capsule (courtesy of Dr. Buist).

made possible the recognition of much smaller metastases, but it is doubtful if lesions smaller than 1 cm can be seen. Even so, the degree of the resolution is such that some reservation on the overall value of this method must be made at the present time.

Dilated bile ducts and portal veins can also be recognized in good isotope scans. Isotope scanning of the liver using ^{99}T colloid sulfur in cases of obstructive jaundice has shown that it is possible to demonstrate dilated common bile ducts (Figure 11). In 17 out of 31 cases of obstructive jaundice recently studied, it was found possible to demonstrate dilatation of the bile ducts. The method, however, demands sophisticated equipment and it is possible it may be superseded by the simpler ultrasound scanning.

Grayscale ultrasound has proved to be a less complicated and less costly method of recognizing hepatic metastases and has the added advantage that large swellings can be differentiated from cystic swellings, e.g., hydatid cysts, by their transonic nature. It promises to be a ready and relatively inexpensive method of investigating the status of the liver prior to abdominal surgery.

Perhaps in the investigation of jaundice, potentially of malignant ori-

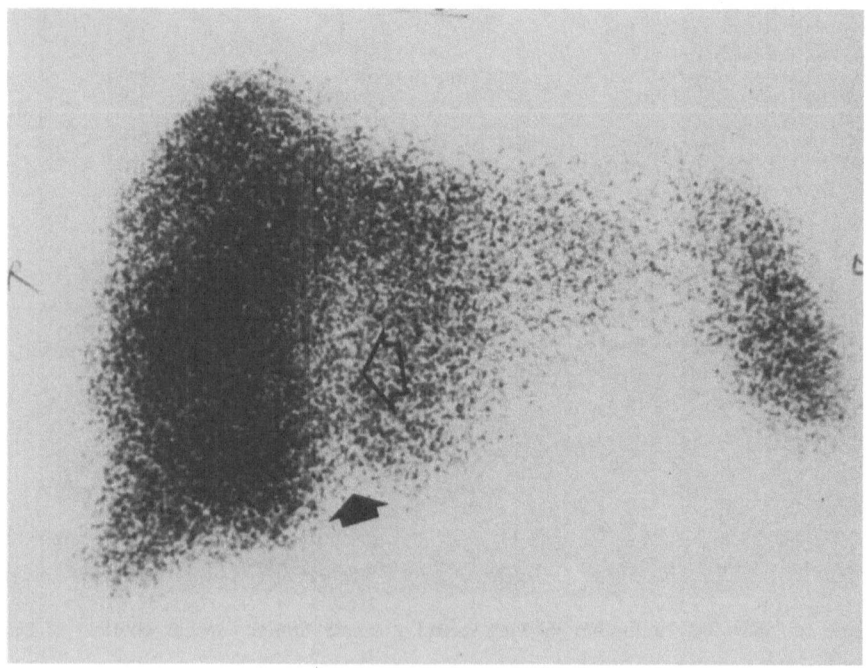

Figure 11. Isotope scan showing defects on scan caused by dilated ducts.

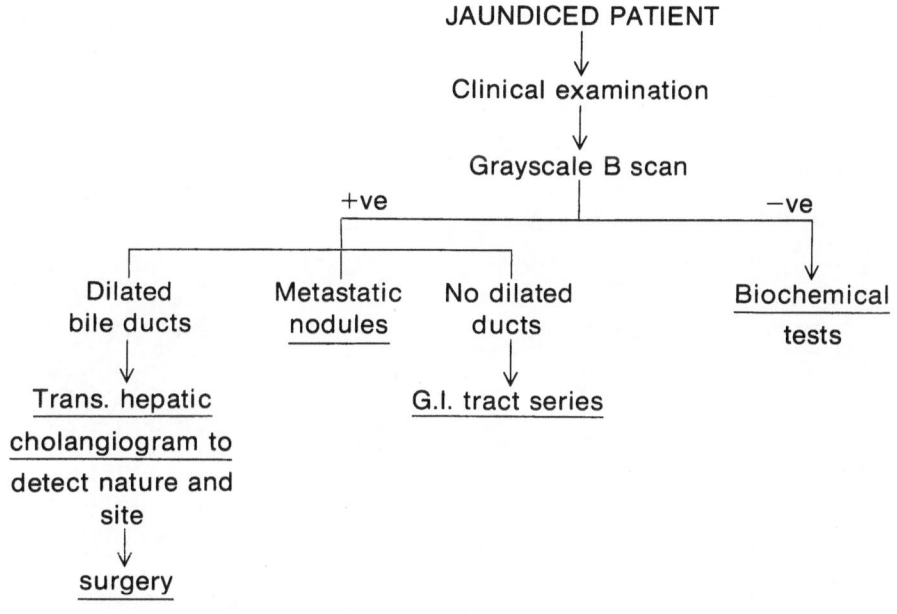

Figure 12

gin, a programmed approach will lead to the greatest saving in clinical time and indicate sooner the lines of definitive treatment. Fundamentally, the problem is the differentiation of obstructive from cholestatic jaundice (Figure 12), and as the biliary system in obstructive jaundice is generally dilated, demonstration of this feature should lead to an earlier diagnosis of its cause.

Grayscale ultrasound will enable dilated bile ducts to be seen in the liver scan, and if by the same techniques a distended gallbladder is seen, the implication is that the jaundice must be obstructive. Demonstration of the distended gallbladder is important, as dilated portal veins at the porta hepatis give ultrasound appearances almost identical with distended bile ducts (Figure 13). If distended bile ducts and a distended gallbladder are demonstrated, then the jaundice is clearly obstructive and there is need for surgical relief for its cure. The consequential investigative procedure should then be one which shows most readily the site and possibly the nature of the obstruction. This can best be achieved by a percutaneous transhepatic cholangiogram (PTC) (Figure 14), but retrograde catheterization of the bile duct by endoscopy (Figure 15), avoids the necessity of following the procedure immediately with laparotomy.

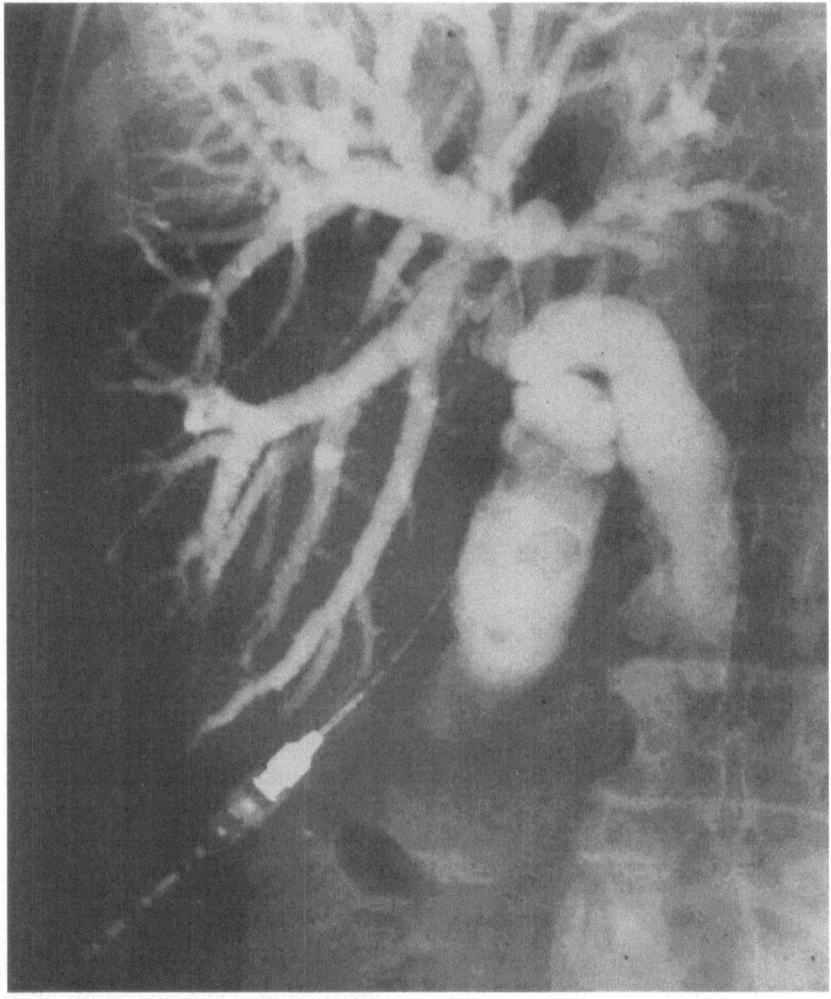

Figure 13. Transhepatic cholangiogram of the case shown in Figure 11 showing the grossly dilated duct system (courtesy of Dr. Ritchie).

With the performance of a P.T.C. under local anesthesia using the Chiba needle, with modern fluorscopic TV control, the difficulties of the method have largely vanished as the tip of the needle can be watched and the use of test injections can accurately control the site of deposition of the bolus of contrast medium in the bile ducts. The procedure should be followed within hours by surgery undertaken to relieve obstruction, other-

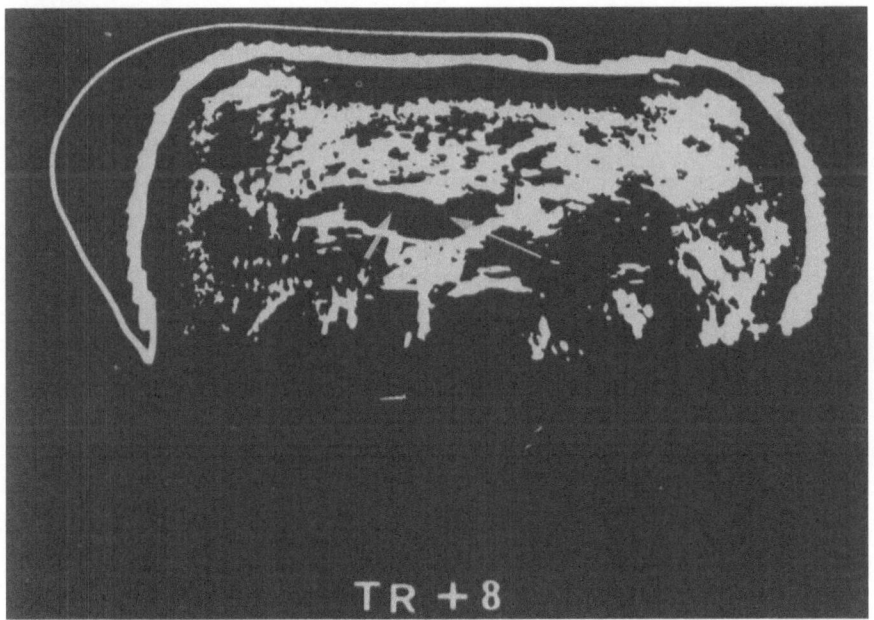

Figure 14. Transonic area in liver region indicating the major ducts (bile) dilated at the porta hepatis (courtesy of Dr. J. G. Duncan).

wise a serious leak of bile causing biliary peritonitis may occur. It is important that complete filling of the biliary tree is achieved during the examination and when this is dilated a considerable amount of contrast may be required to fill the duct system (20–30 ml); and the use of posture to fill the intrahepatic duct system may be necessary. It is our practice to perform this investigation as an immediate (1–2 h) preoperative procedure (Figure 11).

In cases where ultrasound examinations of the liver are equivocal, the investigation of the bile duct system should be undertaken by endoscopic transduodenal catheterization of the common bile duct and retrograde filling of the duct (Figure 13) in preference to transhepatic cholangiography.

This method demands a greater expertise than transhepatic cholangiography but has the advantage that it is not necessarily followed by surgical intervention. Consequently, it can be used in cases where the ultrasound examination has given equivocal results and exploratory surgery is contraindicated. If ultrasound scan fails to demonstrate distended ducts, the program of investigation must follow that shown in Figure 12. The scope of diagnostic investigation is then more widespread and difficult. Hepatic angiography may be needed to outline liver metastases and pri-

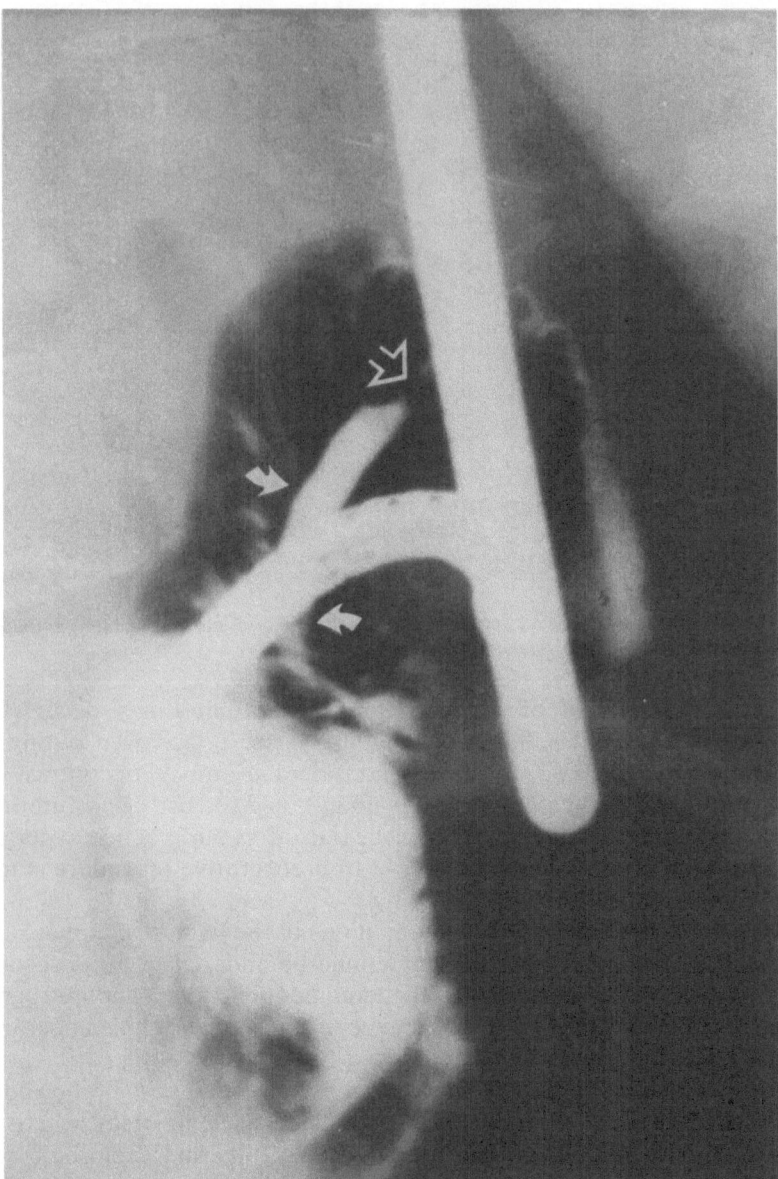

Figure 15. Transduodenal catheterization of bile duct. The filled common bile duct (solid arrows) is seen lying between the endoscopic and the carcinomatous structure of the common duct (outline arrow) is shown.

mary liver tumors, although the uptake in ^{99}T liver scans may have suggested the presence of such a tumor.

Gastrointestinal Disease

The problems we have considered so far are those where there is a clinically palpable tumor present; of greater importance is the detection of an early neoplasm of the gastrointestinal tract when no such finding is present. Carcinoma of the colon and to a lesser extent the stomach are amenable to surgical cure if the diagnosis can be made at an early stage.

Much of the impetus to the diagnosis of early gastric carcinoma has come from Japanese workers who have great experience of this special problem in Japan. Shirakabe, Ichikawa, and others have introduced the double contrast study of the stomach using a barium mixture, with air instilled through a nasogastric tube or carbon dioxide from effervescing tables being the source of the gas for the double contrast. Careful attention to gastric folds will show that many gastric ulcers are indeed early neoplasms and by careful study, infiltration of the mucosal folds with tumor around the ulcer can be recognized. When the tumor is recognized at a stage where it is localized to the mucosa and has not spread into the gastric wall (Figure 16), surgical resection has produced a 5-year survival rate which is far in excess of any figures in Western countries.

Careful techniques are needed and a good coating of the mucosa without overdistenstion of the stomach with gas (which tends to flatten the mucosal folds) will reveal flattening and destruction of these folds associated with early tumor formation.

Arteriographic studies of gastric neoplasms for delivering high doses of antimitotic drugs to tumors situated in the area supplied by the artery have not met with great success.

Bone Tumors

Arteriography has not made any real contribution to the early diagnosis of primary bone tumors. In an attempt to remedy the defects of conventional radiography, radionucleotide imaging has been used to detect the presence of early bone tumors. The use of technetium-labeled polyphosphate has had some success in the detection of metastatic tumors, but in the differentiation of primary tumors from inflammatory lesions it is of no value.

The use of isotope scanning in the detection of metastatic disease is described in chapter 13.

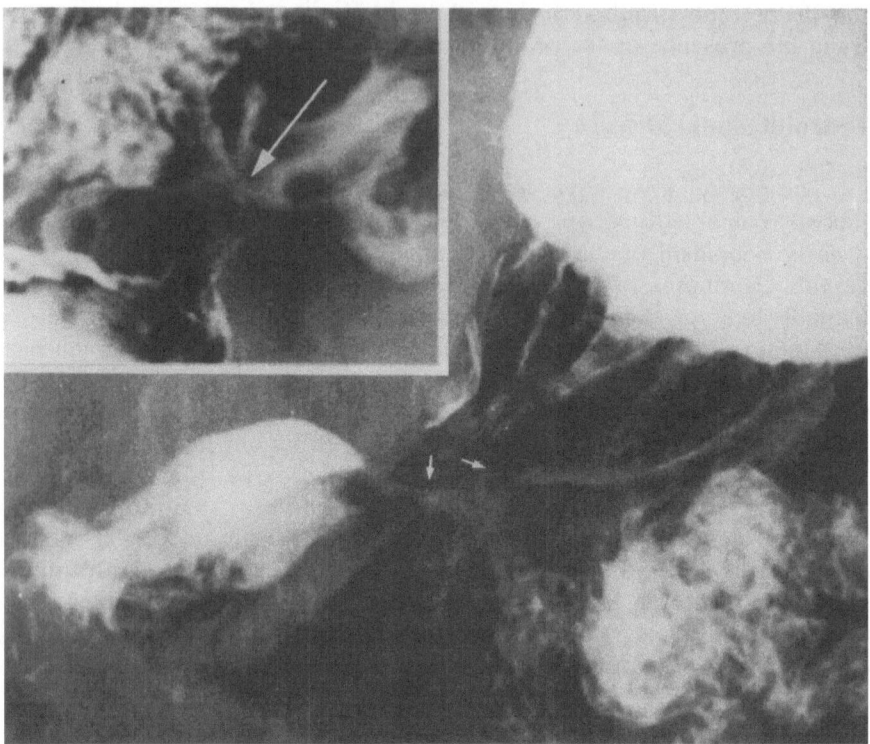

Figure 16. Double contrast views of small ulcer on lesser curvature. Note that the mucosal folds do not extend to the ulcer crater and are "cut off" leaving a clear area (infiltration) around the ulcer.

Cranial and Intracranial Tumors

The multitude of radiological examinations that have become available for the localization of intracranial lesions while achieving notable accuracy in diagnosis have, nevertheless, brought in their wake some problems in selecting the correct lines of investigation.

Figure 17 indicates the many sophisticated investigations that may be needed to reach the diagnosis of an intracranial tumor.

The development of computerized axial tomography using a new method of scanning and recording has allowed differentiation of intracranial swellings and blood clots without recourse to any invasive techniques and enables many of the complex investigations to be bypassed for a more direct approach to diagnosis (Figure 18).

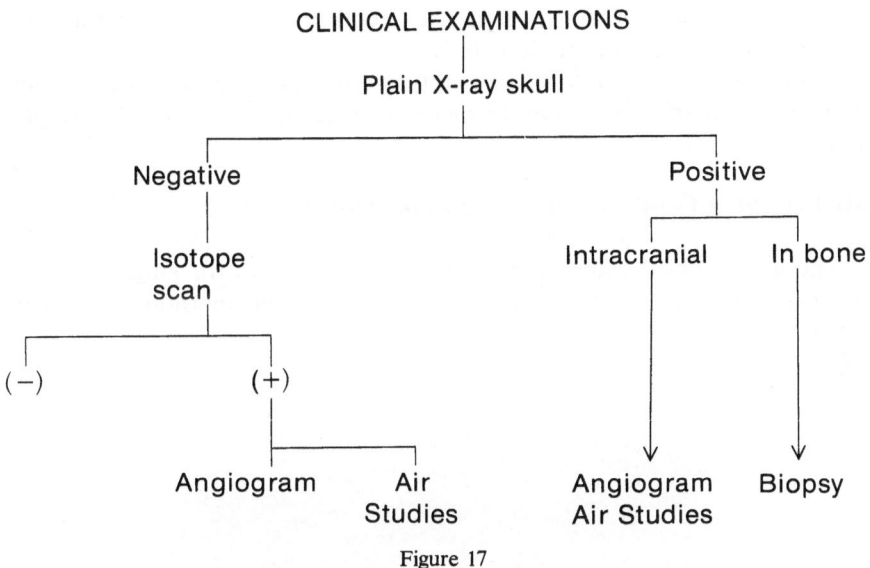

Figure 17

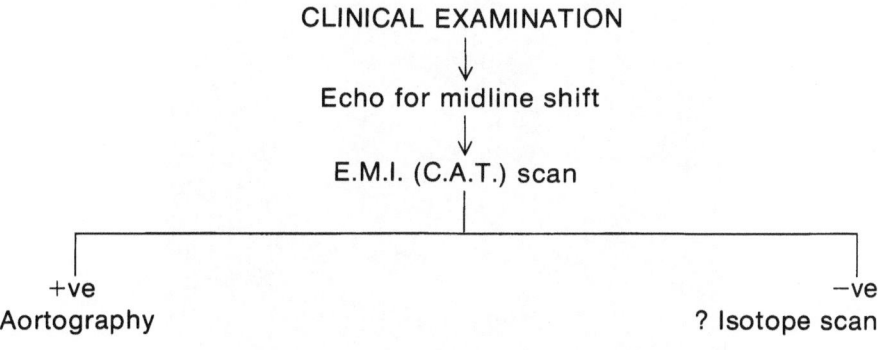

Figure 18

Although the method has not yet been fully explored, it should limit the numbers of investigations necessary for a diagnosis (Figure 19).

Radionucleotide scanning has been used extensively in the investigation of intracranial tumors, and although it has achieved considerable success, the smaller tumors (less than 1–2 cm) and the avascular tumors, e.g., metastases, may not be detected.

Angiography, although considerably more traumatic and not without hazard, is a remarkable, accurate method of detecting small intracranial tumors.

Radiology as a Guide to the Staging of Tumors

The use of chest radiographs and skeletal surveys for staging breast and other types of cancer has long been an accepted method in clinical practice.

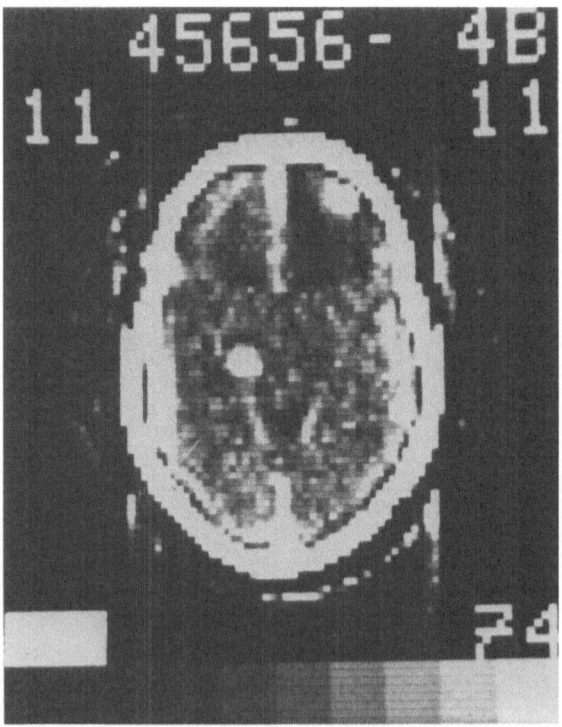

Figure 19. Transverse axial computerized scan showing area of increased densities caused by metastatic deposits (courtesy of Dr. K. Grossart).

Refinements of radiological techniques, particularly lymphangiography, have extended their usefulness in the staging of diseases of the reticulo-endothelial system.

The introduction of lymphagiograms and inferior vena cavograms have shown that many patients with Hodgkin's disease previously regarded as having localized disease (hence classified as stage 1) are shown to have disease of the retroperitoneal lymph nodes and that the disease is more advanced than it appears to be on clinical examination.

Even though both of these procedures (inferior vena cavograms and lymphangiograms) are the most sensitive available at present, it must be realized that a small but substantial proportion of cases with involvement of the abdominal lymph nodes may not be recognized by these methods.

Evaluation of possible metastatic disease in the retroperitoneal lymph nodes in seminoma of the testicle may also be made by this method. Lymphangiographic findings are thus of considerable importance in planning radiotherapeutic treatment.

Although the demonstration of distant metastases has a profound influence of the management of the case, less emphasis should be placed on the radiographic demonstration of local invasive changes in considering the best surgical procedure to be undertaken. For instance, the demonstration of renal vein or even inferior vena caval spread by a hypernephroma does not preclude the successful removal of such a tumor; it nevertheless implies that a radical nephrectomy must be planned as the primary operation. Likewise, the demonstration of infiltration of the renal capsule by arteriography has exactly the same implications for surgery. The radiological demonstration of such changes, of course, has an equally important effect in estimating prognosis in an individual case.

Combined Biochemical and Radiological Investigation

In the detection of functioning tumor, whether malignant or benign, selective catheter sampling of the venous drainage from an organ and comparison with the main venous stream, or selective drainage from the opposite vein of a paired organ, may clinch the diagnosis in such tumors.

Figure 20 shows the figures for calcitonum estimation from the venous drainage of the four parathyroid glands which allowed the diagnosis of a parathyroid adenoma to be made and the site of the parathyroid adenoma to be recognized.

Similarly, sampling of the drainage from the renal veins and inferior vena cava may be invaluable in detecting the site of an adenoma in the suprarenal gland, responsible for primary aldosterionism. Contrast studies such as shown in Figure 21 carry a possible hazard of infarction of the adrenal gland.

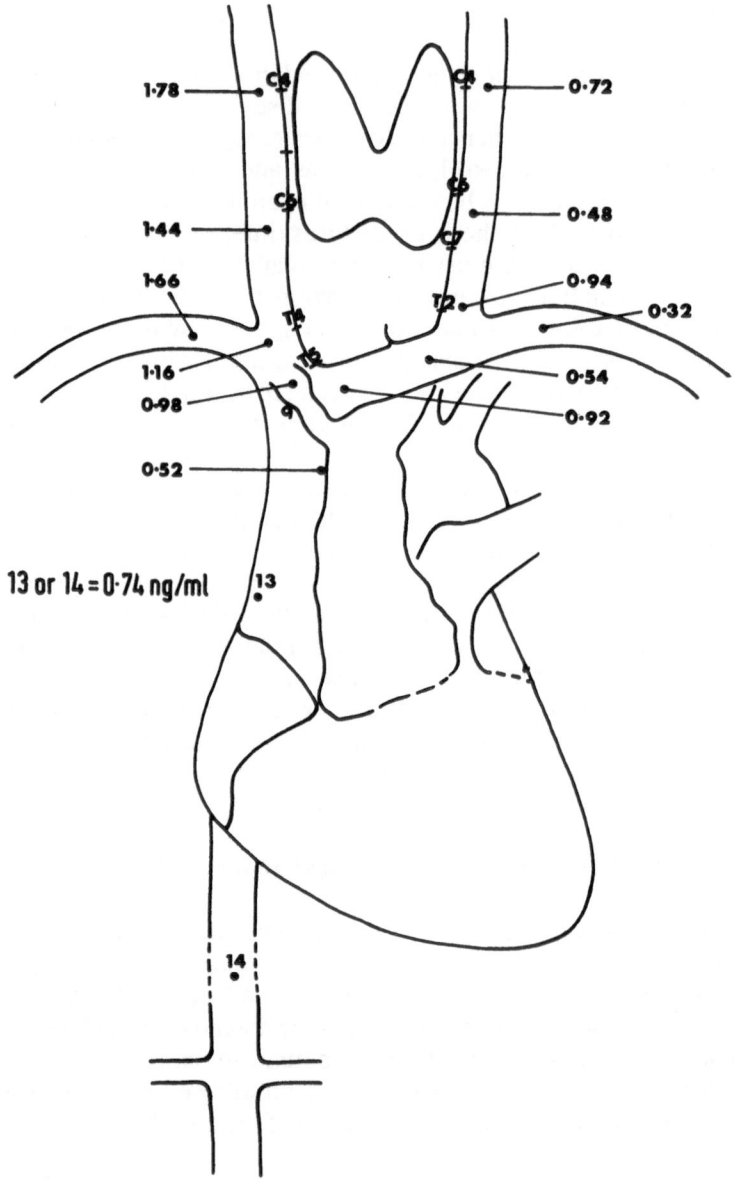

Figure 20. Calcitonum sampling from the venous drainage area of the four parathyroid sites showing a high yield (1.78 ng/ml) from the right superior parathyroid gland (courtesy of Dr. Doig and Dr. Buist).

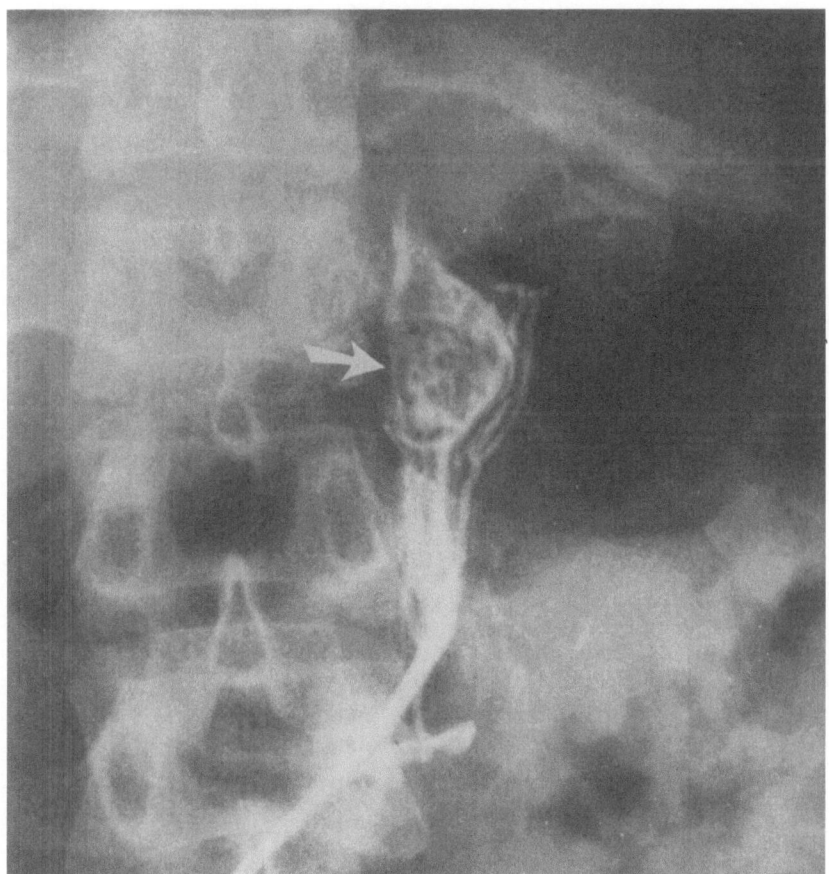

Figure 21. Adenoma of left suprarenal gland in a case of primary aldosternism showing by selective contrast injection of the suprarenal vein.

There is no doubt that with the refinement in the techniques of biochemical estimation of minute quantities of normal and abnormal hormones produced by tumors, the demand for selective venous catheterization of the draining veins under radiological control will be further increased.

DIAGNOSTIC ASPECTS
THERMOGRAPHY, MAMMOGRAPHY, AND XEROGRAPHY

ERIC SAMUEL

Radiological Diagnosis of Breast Cancer

The first radiological demonstration of a tumor in the breast was done in 1913 by Saloman who radiographed an excised breast. It was, however, soon found that with the techniques and equipment then available the demonstration of such swellings in the breast during life was not possible. Some 40 years later Lebourge (in 1951) showed that techniques and equipment had developed to such an extent that with an adequate technique tumors of the breast could be readily seen. However, he remained a relatively lone pioneer in the technique of mammography and the impetus to develop methods of detection of early disease did not come until the death rate from breast cancer was shown to have remained consistently high despite all forms of therapy. Celsus in 200 B.C. said "only in the early stages is cancer curable," and the confirmation of this undoubted fact is shown in the figures from Manchester and Edinburgh (Duncan, 1971) (Figure

Eric Samuel • Forbes Professor of Medical Radiology, University of Edinburgh and the Royal Infirmary, Edinburgh, Scotland EH3 9YW.

BREAST CANCER – LOCALIZED
AGE–CORRECTED SURVIVAL RATES

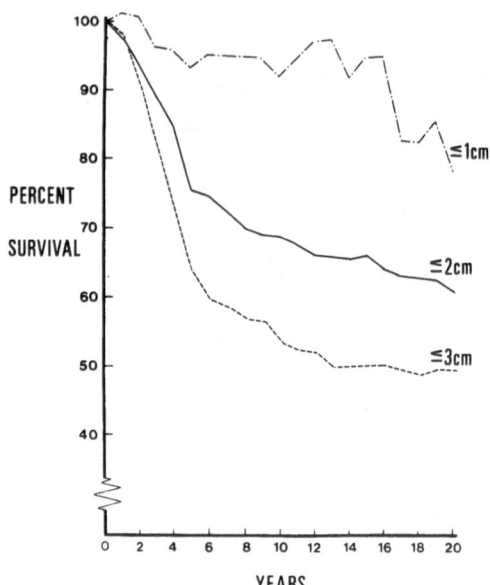

Figure 1. Corrected survival rates of breast cancer related to tumor size (courtesy of Prof. W. Duncan).

1) indicating that the length of survival of patients with breast tumors is directly related to the size of the tumor at the initial examination.

Furthermore, in the diagnosis of disease the presence of a palpable lump in itself means that the disease is already well established. Early disease in the context of the methods which will be described refers to the state when there is no swelling palpable in the breast. Many of the cancers that can be recognized by these methods are of the order of 0.5–1 mm and there is much to learn about the natural history of breast tumors and the most efficient methods of treatment when they are recognized at this stage.

The potential of recognition of breast tumors at an early stage has resulted in the advocacy of surveys of healthy women as a screening procedure. The results of the Hospital Insurance Plan in New York City (Strax *et al.*, 1970) showed that in a group of 32,000 screened women matched for age with a similar number of unscreened women the detection rate of breast cancer was 2.82/1,000 as compared with 1.7/1,000 occurring spontaneously. Perhaps of greater significance was the fact that in the screened group the percentage of axillary nodes involved was 45.8% as compared with 57.1% in the control group with a consequent 5-year crude fatality rate of 27.9% as compared with 42.1%.

Clinical examination and mammography were used as examining techniques in this survey.

Considerable interest and not inconsiderable controversy has been aroused by these surveys concerning their effectiveness, the logistics of the effort involved, and the reliability and accuracy of the methods used. The following are the methods employed in breast cancer screening.

Thermography

The normal infrared emission of the body lies in a wavelength between 4 and 15 μm, with the maximum emission at 9.2 μm. This infrared emission which is dependent on physiological factors such as skin vascularity, and convection into clothes is also influenced by processes occurring both in and deep to the skin. The thermographic appearances of the breast have been classified as (1) avascular, (2) patchy vascular, and (3) having a large venous pattern.

It has been claimed that these patterns are altered when there is local disease present in the breast. The accuracy of this has been questioned and some observers have indicated a false negative error of 40%. This would make the method unacceptable as a single screening procedure.

However, apart from the diurnal and menstrual cycle variations in the thermographic patterns of the breast, some observers have claimed that there exists a specific "thermal fingerprint" appearance for the individual (Stark and Way, 1974). If this is so then serial thermograms showing deviation from the normal pattern would indicate the development of pathological changes, albeit not necessarily malignant, in the breast.

In an attempt to exclude the subjective aspects of thermographic interpretation a new thermographic unit (AWRE) has been developed which enables a printout of 0.2°C steps of temperature 3 mm apart over an area of 13.7 × 13.7 cm of the breast. This allows a quantitative estimate of the absolute temperature change to be recorded and makes serial thermographic changes more accurate (Figures 2a and 2b).

Lloyd-Williams (1974) has suggested using this unit and following the following criteria:

(1) The demonstration of a "hot" spot.
(2) A difference in nipple temperature of 1.8°C and an absolute nipple temperature of more than 33.8°C.
(3) Using a factor A obtained by the use of the following formula:

$$A = \frac{h_1}{a_2} - \frac{h_2}{a_1} > 0.47.$$

h_1 = hot spot in affected breast
h_2 = hot spot in normal breast
a_1 = average temperature in normal breast
a_2 = average temperature in affected breast

(4) A basic temperature of > 34.5 C.

These criteria indicate a pathological change in the breast, and care

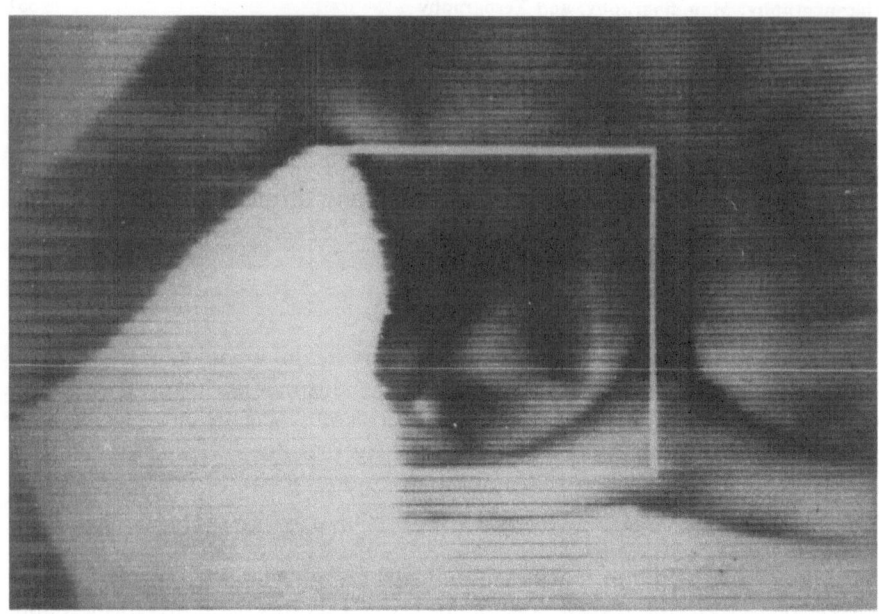

Figure 2a. Conventional thermograph taken on polaroid film.

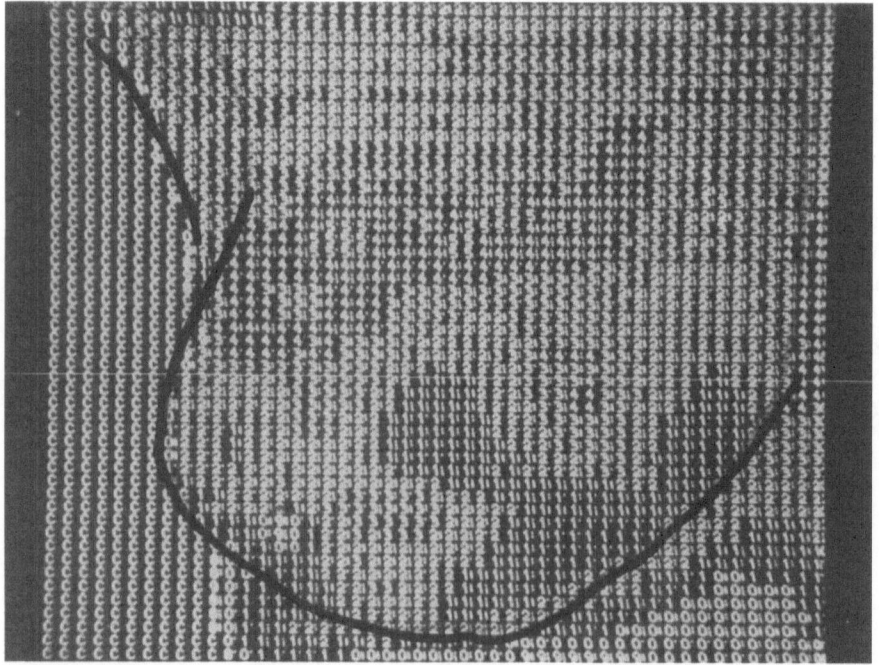

Figure 2b. Digital (quantitative) printout of same patient. (C = cold, *i.e.*, below average temperature, 0,1,2,3 = 30, 31, 32, 33°C, etc. 1· = 31.2, 1: = 31.4, 1 ⋮ = 31.6, 1| = 31.8, 2· = 32.2, 2: = 32.4°C, etc.)·

must be taken not to equate them with the development of a tumor as such changes can occur with an abscess, localized fibrocystic disease, and other conditions (Figure 3).

Possibly much of the controversy in regard to thermography has arisen from its misuse as a diagnostic tool to differentiate between neoplasms and other lumps (Nathan *et al.*, 1972).

The main function of thermography should be to identify those breasts with no palpable swelling which need further investigation (Figures 4a and 4b). Even so the accuracy of thermography as a method in fulfilling this function is still subjudice.

Mammography

The demonstration of early tumors of the breast by radiographic techniques using low-voltage X-rays (mammography) has been a major

RIGHT FRONTAL   LEFT FRONTAL

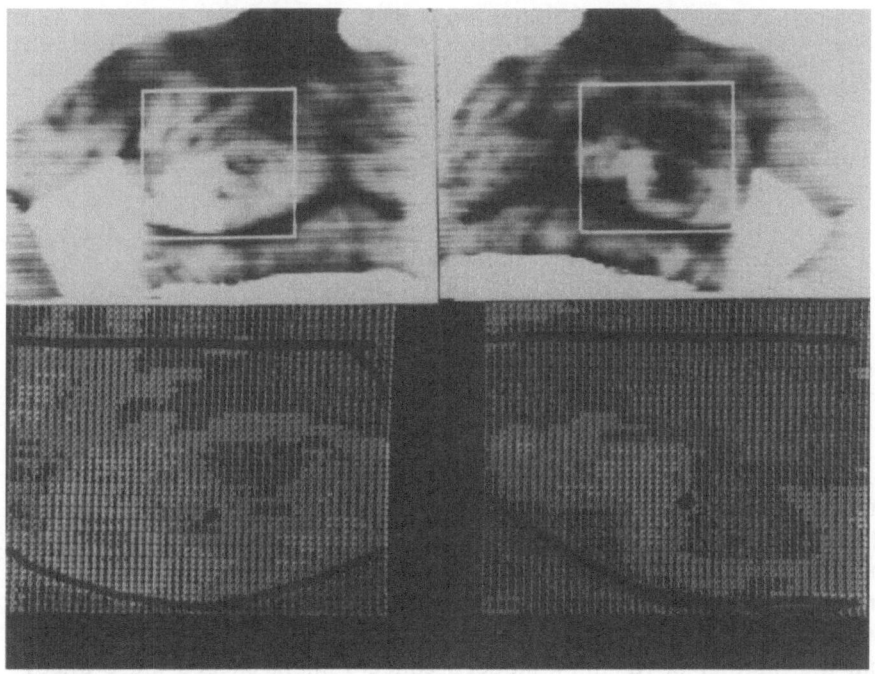

Average temp 30.2   Average temp 30.0
Maximum temp 33.2   Maximum temp 32.6
    "A" factor   0.027

Figure 3. The report of patient of Figure 2 as supplied with quantitative thermograph.

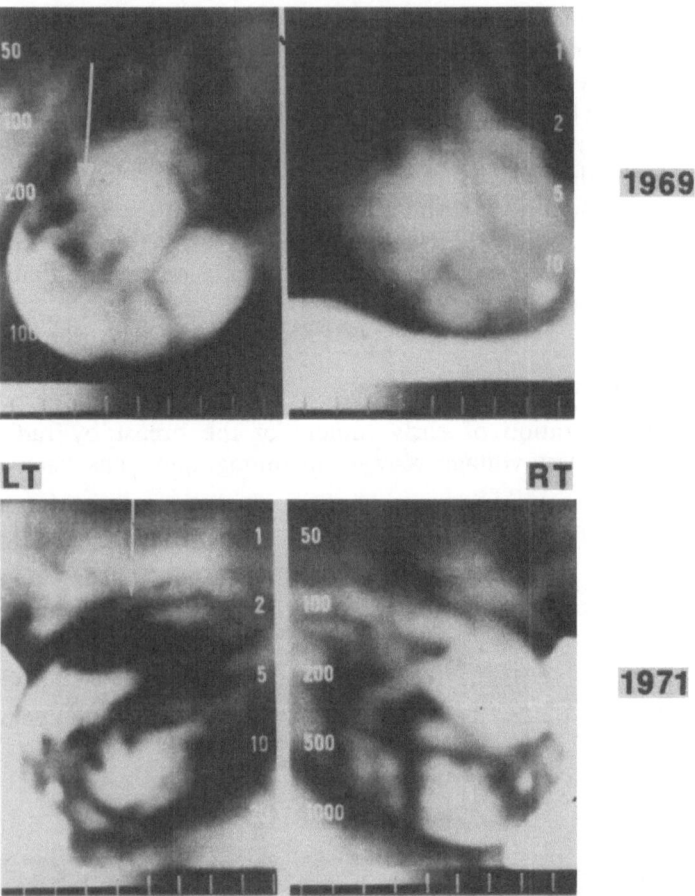

Figure 4a. Thermogram showing abnormal heat pattern in the left breast in 1969—disregarded because of the absence of a clinical sign—and in 1971.

advance in the diagnosis of early cancer of the breast. The earlier technique of mammography which involved the examination of the breast in two planes (cranio-caudal and lateral views) used industrial films to obtain maximum detail and a relatively short focal film distance. While the detail produced by these techniques was superb the radiation dose to the breast was unacceptably high. Indeed, some epidemiologists have even suggested that the number of radiation-induced cancers might exceed those uncovered by screening (Bailar, 1976). However, in relation to the radiation dose which has been known to cause carcinogenesis in the breast (Table 1) it is unlikely that the doses used in mammography would ever reach this level. However, in terms of repetitive examinations this concern in the dosage has been justified and the new low-dose techniques (Young, 1974) using a single screen in a vacuum-packed cassette and special film combinations have lowered the dose at each exposure to the order of 0.12 rad; a total of 0.3 rad to each breast. This level of radiation dosage should be well within acceptable limits.

The accuracy of mammography has also been questioned and various observers have given a percentage accuracy of between 79 and 92%. Undoubtedly, there is an inherent error in all diagnostic procedures and comparison with other X-ray procedures will give a better appreciation of

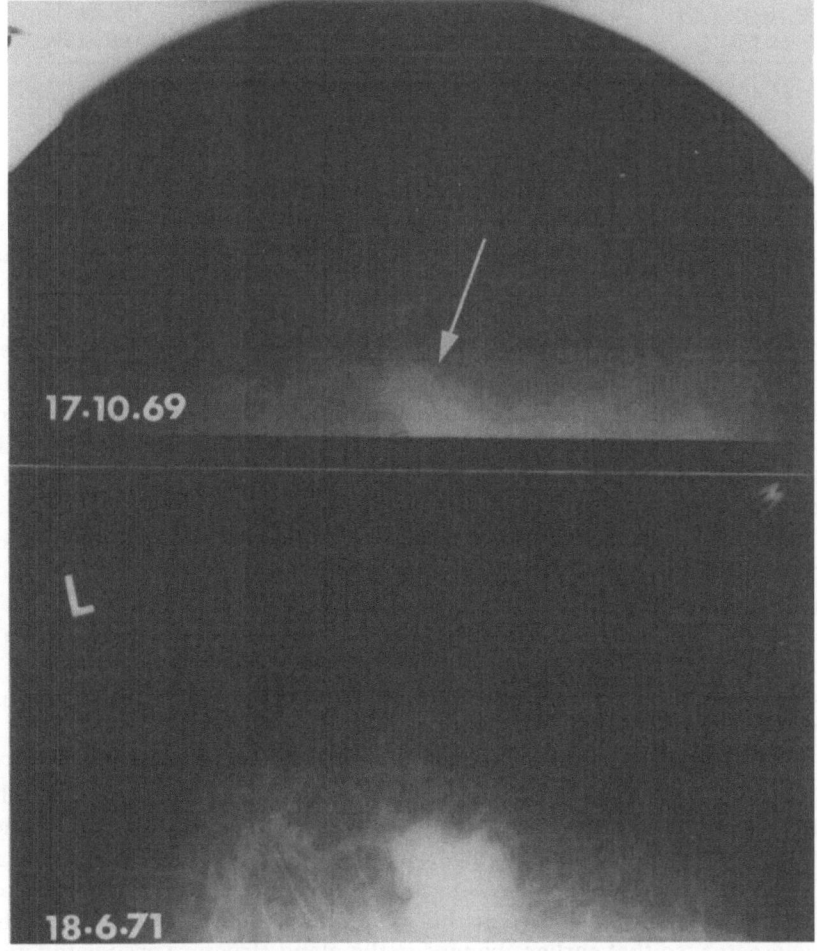

Figure 4b. Mammograms of the same case.

TABLE 1. Doses to the Breast Caused by Other Negative Radiological Procedures (Artificial Pneumothorax) and Also from Man-Made Atomic Exposure

Population of women	Cases of breast cancer per 1,000	Dose in breast (rads)
300 Recurring AP Treatment	60	1,000–4,000
600 PP Mastitis	12	40–800
Atomic Blast		
(Wanebo *et al.*, 1968)		
2119 women	2	10–89
1643 women	5	90–800
8743	1	10–49
5490	2	50–1,000

the relative accuracy of mammography in relation to other accepted radiologic procedures (Cooley *et al.*, 1960). Undoubtedly, the accuracy figures for any investigative process can be considerably influenced by the group investigated.

Mammographic diagnosis is based on: (1) The detection of a soft tissue swelling with spiculated outlines (Figure 4b). This feature becomes progressively less important in the earlier cases where swelling may not be visible. In these instances only a disturbance of normal architecture of the breast may be seen. The normal architecture of the breast as seen in the radiograph is composed of dense glandular lobulated swelling separated by thin fibrous bands with a venous pattern superimposed.

(2) The demonstration of fine pinhead calcifications. Although in themselves these are not diagnostic, their appearance in clusters is highly suggestive of an intraductal type of cancer.

Calcification may occur in other breast conditions; in vessels, when it is linear in character; in localized areas of fibrocystic disease where it is usually dense and more widespread than in carcinoma; or in fibroadenoma, when it may show areas of dense calcification.

The demonstration of early changes in the breast on mammography to some extent depends on the type of breast. In the young female the glandular structure of the breast produces a dense shadow in which it is not easy to detect swellings or calcification. Increasing years and a decrease in the glandular activity of the breast results in fatty infiltration which makes the degree of contrast between the glandular and the surrounding fatty tissue greater, so that earlier changes in the gland structure associated with malignancy can be more readily appreciated. It is perhaps fortuitous that as these breasts having large fatty infiltrates have the highest rate of error in clinical diagnosis and that it is in this group that mammography can provide its greatest assistance.

The most impressive finding in the Hospital Insurance Plan survey was that in the 49–59 age group 37% of cancers would have been overlooked if mammography had been omitted, and perhaps even more important was the fact that the group of breast cancers detected by this method showed a lower percentage of axillary node involvement and consequently a greatly improved 5-year survival (Table 2).

Xerography

The difficulties of the dense glandular breast pattern in mammographic diagnosis has led to the application of the well-known principle of xerography in the investigation of breast disease. This electrostatic method of recording X-ray images has a basic advantage, mainly that it heightens the contrast between tissues of different densities. Consequently the internal structure of the glandular portions of the breast are seen more readily. The electrostatic images produced are recorded on paper in a positive or negative mode (Figures 5 and 6). Alterations in the architecture of the breast can certainly be seen more readily than with mammography and some authorities (Wolff, 1968a,b; Gravelle, 1970) have suggested that a mammographic smear be completely superseded by xerography. The dose necessary to produce good xerograms is of the order of 1.5 rads and consequently each breast receives 2–3 rads per examination. Some authorities claim to have been able to reduce this dose, but even with the best conditions it would appear to be at least double that used in mammography. For this reason it is doubtful if xerography can be used as an unselected

TABLE 2[a]

	Number of cancers	Percentage of negative nodes	Percentage of 5 + 1 year fatalities
Detected by screening	132	70.5	16.9
Detected by mammography	44	77.3	2.3
Spontaneous in those who refused screening	73	39.7	34.5

[a]After Forrest, 1974.

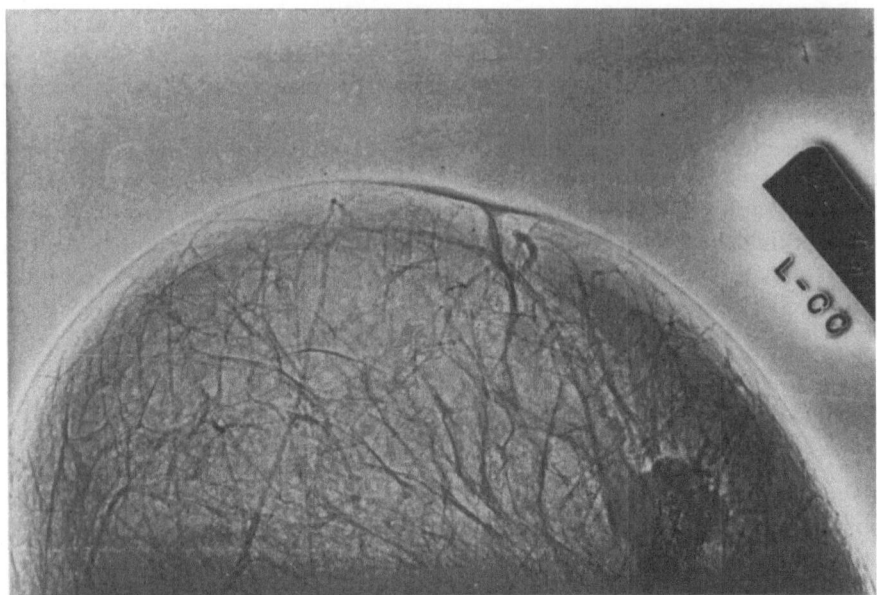

Figure 5a. Cranio-caudal view showing the tumor with characteristic outlines, spiculation, and microcalcification within the tumor.

screening procedure and furthermore, the complexities of the production of good xerograms add to its difficulties.

At the present time it would be wise to limit xerography to the examination of symptomatic women or to problem cases in which clinical examination, thermography, or mammograms have given equivocal results. It is probably not acceptable as a means of screening healthy women because of the radiation risk involved with repetitive high doses.

The results of a comparative study of 40 cases of proven breast diseases examined by mammographs and xerographs read blindly by three different radiologists at different centers are shown in Table 3.

TABLE 3. Comparative Table of Mammography and Xerography[a]

	Mammogram	Xerox
Benign lesions	92%	78.6%
Malignant lesions	64.4%	62.2%

[a]Three separate readers—score averaged 40 cases read without clinical information.

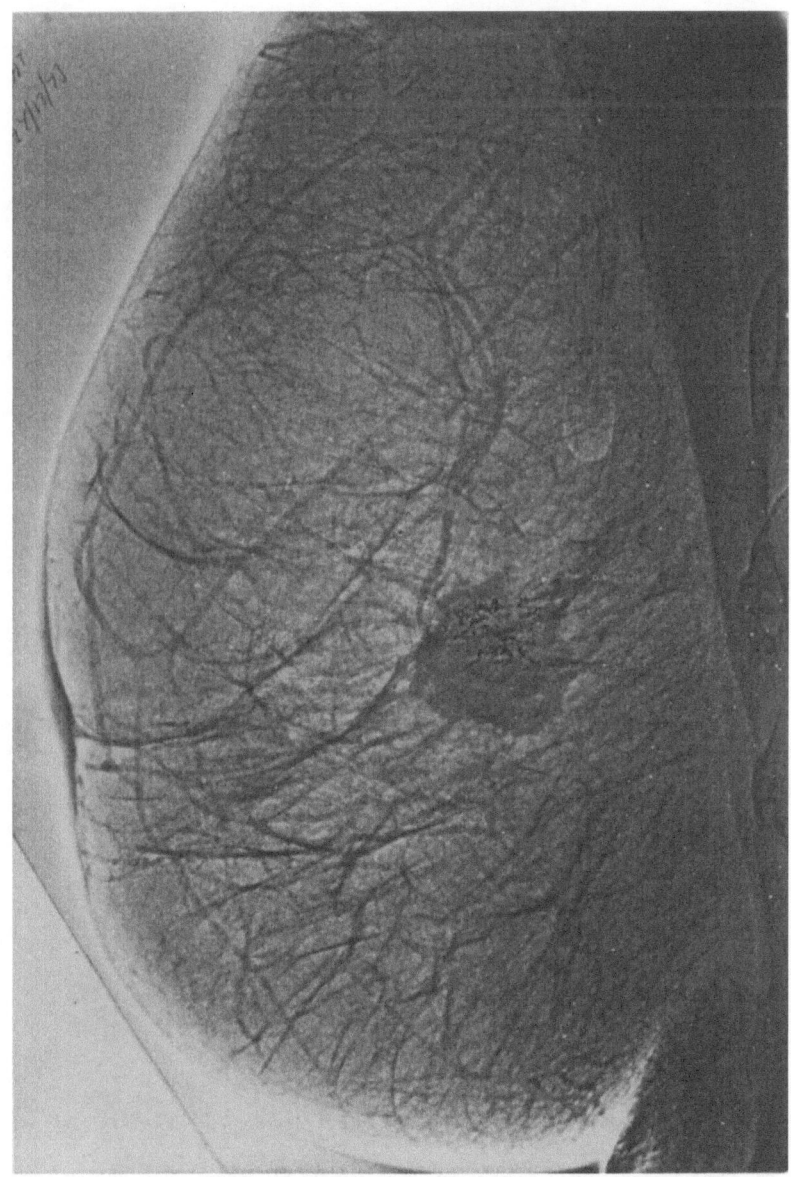

Figure 5b. Lateral view of the same case.

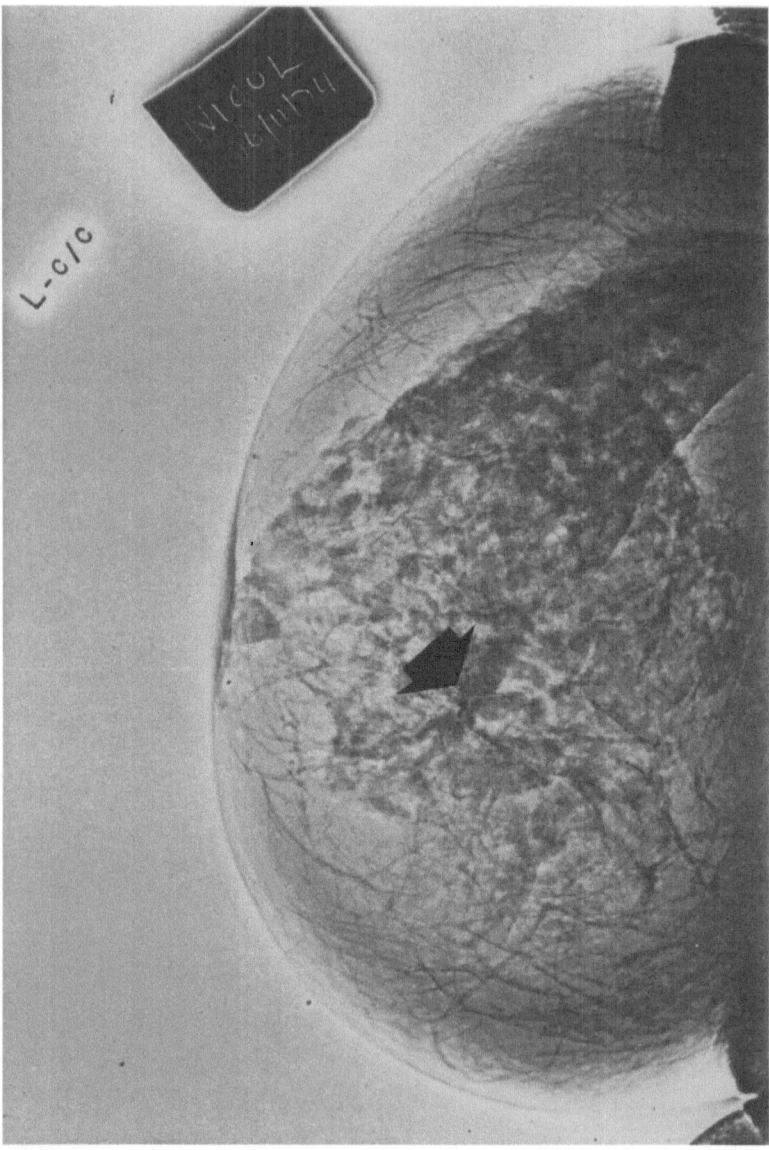

Figure 6a. Cranio-caudal view demonstrating an impalpable lesion. Note the absence of a swelling but a disturbance of breast architecture with spiculed calcification present.

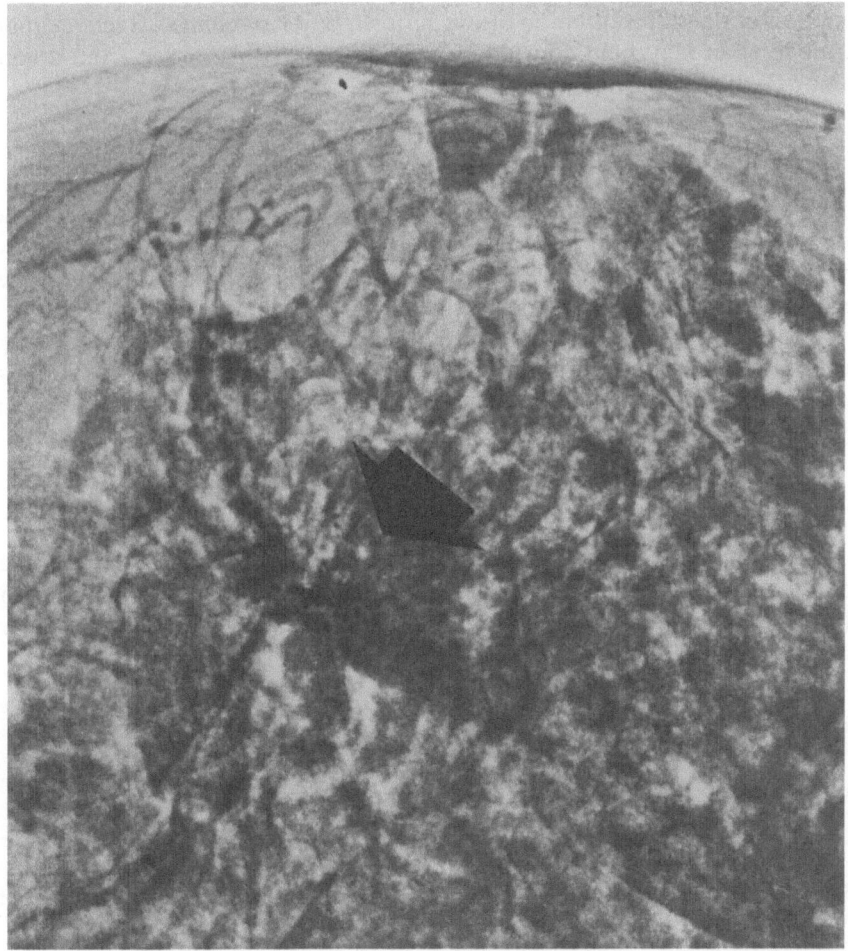

Figure 6b. Localized view of the area showing the cluster of dense calcification.

The validity of this series can be questioned as the patients were postmenopausal hospital patients who would unconsciously produce a clinical state favoring mammography as opposed to xerography.

Ultrasound

Ultrasound scanning of the breast has not achieved widespread clinical use, but with the development of the newer units it may play a useful function in the differentiation of cystic from other swellings. Even a simple A-mode scan may help considerably in differentiating a cyst from a solid tumor (Wells and Evans, 1968).

Cyst Puncture

Puncture of a palpable swelling and aspiration of cystic fluid is practiced by many surgeons. The instillation of contrast medium and air allows the outline of the cyst wall to be seen and the presence of any abnormalities or tumors in the wall to be detected.

This method, which has more widespread use in continental Europe deserves a wider application in this country. Perhaps the caution in its use is a result of the fact that associated tumors in connection with the cystic area may be overlooked (Schwartz and Siegelman, 1968).

Ductograms

Discharge from the nipple, whether serous or blood stained, is an anxiety to both patient and surgeon. Duct catheterization and the injection of contrast medium allows the outline of the affected segment to be seen.

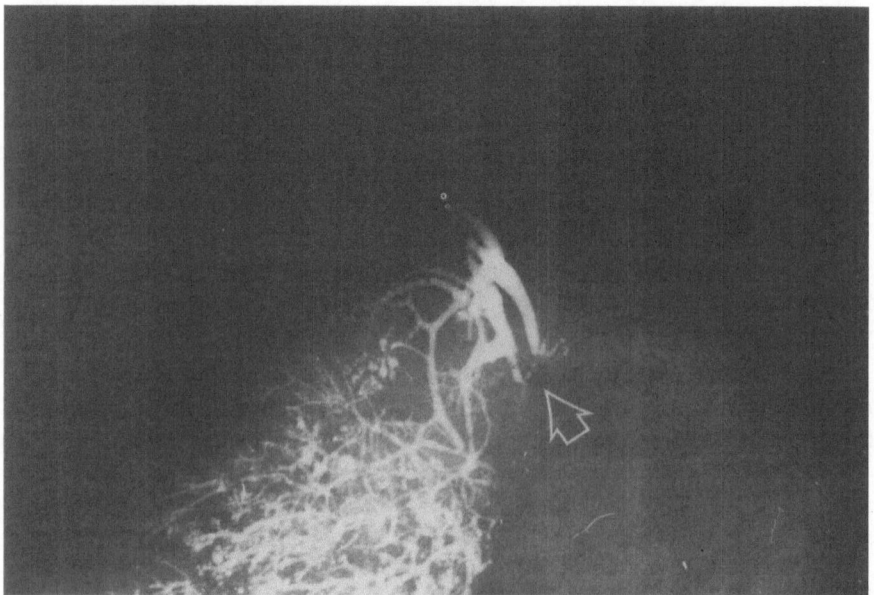

Figure 7. Ductogram showing obstruction of the ducts by an invasive malignant tumor.

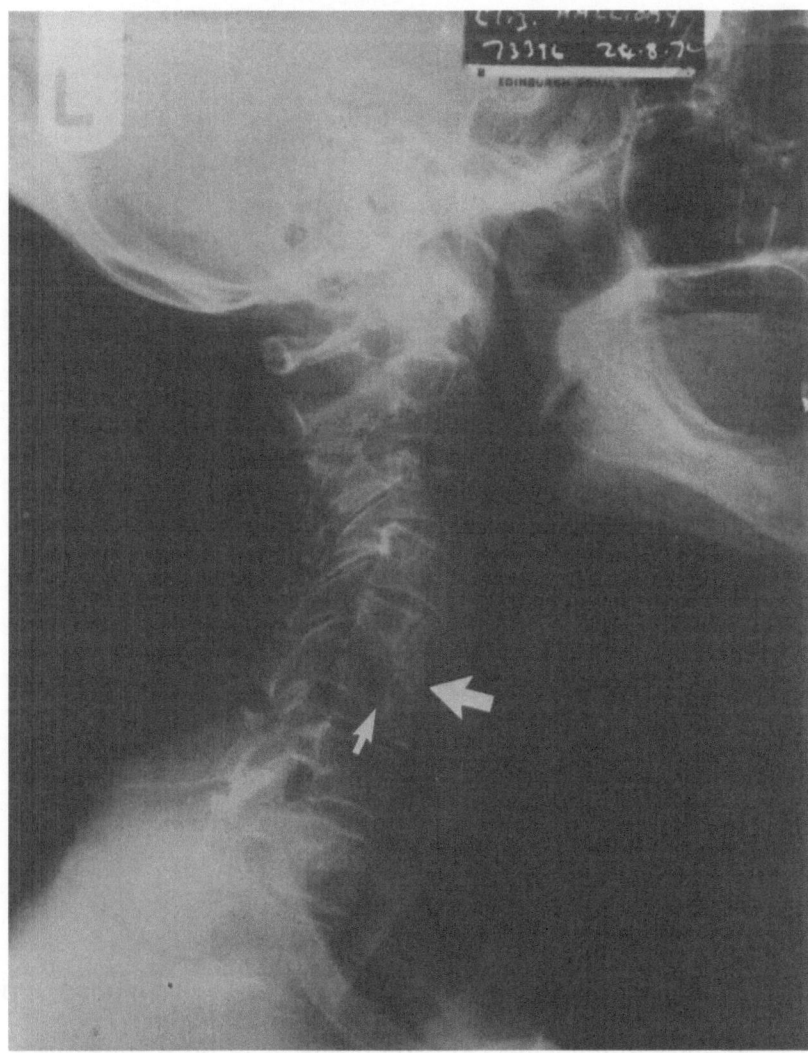

Figure 8. Lateral view of cervical region showing a pathological change in the sixth cervical vertebra.

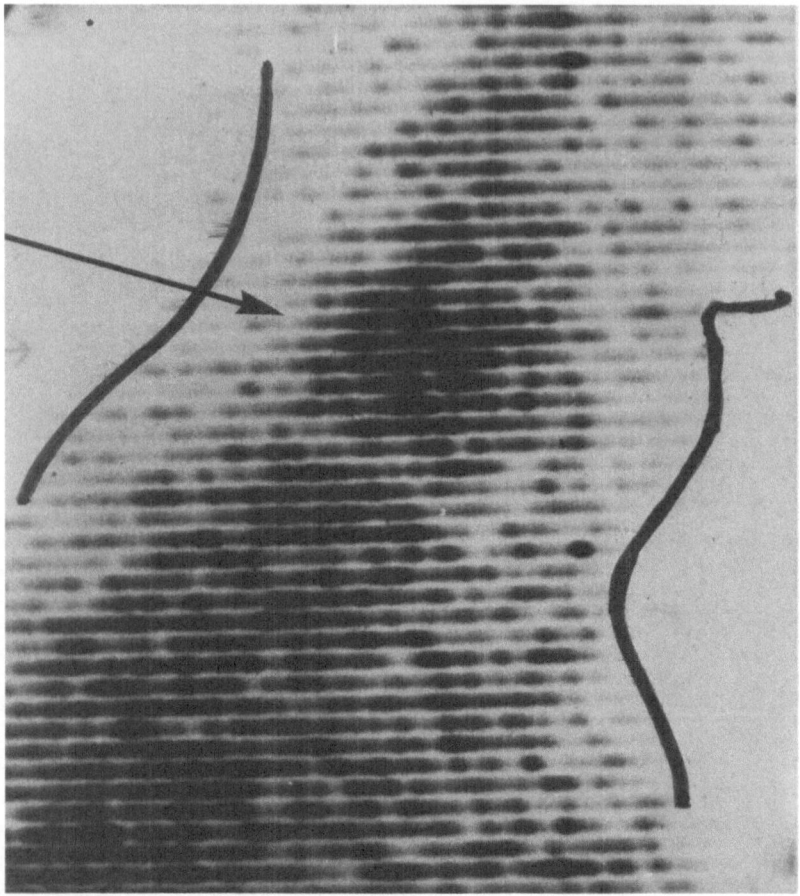

Figure 9. Isotope scan of the same case showing "hot" spot (indicating high uptake) in affected vertebra.

Papillomas and other filling defects within the breast due to more serious conditions can also be noted (Figure 7).

Associated with attempts at early diagnosis of breast diseases is the evaluation of spread of disease outside the breast (Figures 8 and 9) while the primary tumor is small or even impalpable and these features have been considered in chapter 13.

REFERENCES

Bailar, J. C. (1976). Mammography: A contrary view. *Annals Int. Med.* **84**:77–84.

Cooley, R. N., Agnew, C. H., and Rios, G. (1960). *Amer. J. Roent.* **84**:316.

Duncan, W. (1974). Personal communication.

Forrest, A. P. M. (1974). Medical Research Council Conference on Breast Cancer. MRC Reports.

Gravelle, I. H. (1970). Personal communication.

Leborgne, R. A. (1953). *The Breast in Roentgen Diagnosis*. Montevideo, Impresora Urguaya. S. A. and London, Constable.

Lloyd-Williams , K. (1974). Medical Research Council Conference on Breast Cancer. MRC Reports.

Nathan, B. E., Burn, I., and MacErlean, D. P. (1972). Value of mammography in differential diagnosis. *Br. Med. J.* **2**:316.

Saloman, A. (1913). Beiträge zur Pathologie and Klinik der Mamma Karzinoms. *Arch. Klin. Chir.* **101**:573.

Schwartz, A. M., and Siegelman, S. (1968). Nonpalpable carcinoma in fibrocystic disease of the breast. *Surg. Gynaecol. Obstet.* **126**:94.

Stark, A. M. and Way, S. (1974). The screening of well women for the early detection of breast cancer. *Cancer.* **33**:1671–1679.

Strax, P., Lenet, L., Shapiro, S., Gross, and Vinet, D. (1970). *Arch. Environ. Health.* **20**:758.

Wanebo, C. K., Johnson, K. G., and Sato, K. (1968). Breast cancer after exposure to atomic bombings of Hiroshima and Nagasaki. *N. Eng. Jour. Med.* **279**:667–671.

Wells, P. N., and Evans, K. T. (1968). An immerson scanner for two dimensional ultrasonic examination of the human breast. *Ultrasonics* **6**:220.

Wolfe, J. N. (1968, a). Xerography of the breast. *Radiology* **91**:231.

Wolfe, J. N. (1968, b). Xerography of the breast. *Oncology* **23**:113.

Young, G. B. (1974). Low dose techniques in mammography. *Brit. J. Radiol.* **47**:811–815.

Chapter 14

CYTOLOGY

O. A. N. HUSAIN

The use of cytology in the diagnosis of oncological disease dates back well over 100 years (Beale, 1878; Bamforth and Osborn, 1958).

Though the development of this scientific art was temporarily eclipsed by the advent of histology in the early part of this century, it has been returning in increasing strength ever since Dudgeon in England and Papanicolaou in the United States published their first papers on nongynecological (Dudgeon and Patrick, 1927) and gynecological (Papanicolaou, 1928) cancer detection, respectively.

Gynecological Cytology

The American practice developed predominantly along gynecological lines in the form of massive population screening program (Wilson, 1965), and the cytological effort is now running at over 30 million tests a year, much of it computer controlled.

In the U.K. a small interest developed in the use of cytology for cancer detection in sputum, urine, serous fluids, gastric washes, and tumor scrapes and imprints, and gynecological cytology was restricted to a few research or gynecological departments until 1964 when a nation-wide screening program was inaugurated (Health and Welfare Service, 1964). Five National Training Centres were created to train a cadre of pathologists and technicians and now over 2.5 million gynecological smears a year are examined by a full-time equivalent labor force of 70 pathologists and 475 technicians in over 250 laboratories in England and Wales.

O. A. N. Husain • Consultant Pathologist, Regional Cytology Centre, St. Stephen's Hospital, Chelsea, London, SW10 9TH, England.

In the wake of the cervical cytology program an interest developed in exploring the other body sites, and now a broad spectrum of cytological investigations has resulted in pathologists and technicians finding a career structure predominantly in this speciality. Because of the need to evaluate and apply quality control assessments to this field an exact and highly discriminative service is developing (Husain *et al.*, 1974).

The Cervical Smear Test

In England and Wales smears are collected from three main sources; the hospital clinics, the general practitioners, and the former Local Authority (now Community) Well Women Clinics in almost equal proportions.

The test, as originally devised by Papanicolaou (1928), was to collect some posterior fornix mucus by means of an angled glass pipet and rubber bulb and to blow out and spread the cellular secretion on to a glass slide, fix it in alcohol or a mixture of ether and alcohol, and stain it by the complex but colorful and informative Papanicolaou stain. Later, Ayre (1947) produced his special knuckle-ended spatula to scrape the cervix uteri directly at the squamo-columnar junction, the site of development of carcinoma *in situ*, producing a much more reliable sample (Wied, 1961). More recently, other techniques have been introduced, the more widely tested being the disposable plastic self-collecting irrigation pipet developed by Davis (1962) (Reagan and Lin, 1967; Anderson and Gunn, 1967). Here the technique of self-collection provides a specimen preferentially sampled at the clean, easy-to-screen, midcycle phase at about one-fifth to one-eighth of the cost of a woman's attending a traditional clinic. Of course there is no accompanying clinical examination, and the test is only 70 to 80% as reliable (Husain, 1970). Nevertheless, the pipet test appears to be more popular than the bookable clinic test (Carruthers *et al.*, 1975) and if the apparatus and technique are improved it might have a part to play in the screening for cervical and endometrial cancer, especially for the nonresponders to the clinic test.

Cervical Cancer

The practice of cervical cancer screening of the cervix uteri has now amassed an enormous literature, and numerous surveys carried out all over the world have provided much of the understanding of the natural history of the disease. It is the combination of a latent precancerous state, of something like 5 to 15 years' duration or more, an accessible organ and a simply collected and examined visual test that have provided the opportunity of eliminating this disease by periodic screening. It has also resulted in a study of this particular intraepithelial lesion in far greater detail than that of any other site of the body.

Carcinoma *in situ,* described by Schottlander and Kermauner in 1912 with numerous further reviews over the years (Friedell *et al.,* 1960), is a proliferation of an undifferentiated cell line from the basal or reserve cell layer of the endocervix. A transformation of cell type to a squamous form or metaplasia may precede this development, or it may be a separate development through a moderate to severe dysplasia directly to invasive cancer. Whichever pathway it takes, and there may well be more than one form of development of cervical cancer (Ashley, 1966), the cytology smear demonstrates the dysplastic or malignant state by the presence of cells with the characteristic irregularly enlarged and hyperchromatic nucleus and abnormal mitoses.

The nature of this lesion has been the subject of intense controversy and statistical debate. It is believed to develop primarily at the transformation zone (triggered off in some way by the sexual act), has in most temperate countries an average prevalence rate of around 5/1,000 of sexually-active women, appears to commence in the early 20's or earlier, and reaches its maximum around 35 to 40 years of age (Fidler *et al.,* 1968).

Further analysis has demonstrated a greater incidence rate in the lower socioeconomic classes in the married or divorced and the parous compared with the single or nulliparous woman and in those starting sexual activity early, or having multiple · partners, or suffering from venereal disease. Racial differences also occur, and behind it all genital hygiene and circumcision may play a significant part (Coppleston, 1969).

The conversion rate of this lesion to invasive carcinoma is still somewhat shrouded in epidemiological mystery, in spite of numerous large surveys. Green and Donovan (1970) believe that there is less than 10% progress to invasive cancer, while Boyes *et al.,* (1970) believe the figure is between 40 and 60% over periods of 5 to 15 years or more. Elaborate trials have been conducted and others have been proposed (Knox, 1966), but it has been difficult to obtain continuous follow-up of a substantial proportion of women. In British Columbia the largest and most protracted survey has now screened over 80% of its population of 690,000 women over 20 years of age, and the incidence rate has shown a significant drop from 28.4 in 1958 to 9.5 in 1973. Perhaps of greater impact is that the incidence of invasive cancer is 8 to 10 times higher in the unscreened than the screened population.

In Jefferson County, Kentucky, the female population over 20 is 210,000, and since 1956 over 90% have been screened, and the incidence of invasive cancer has decreased from 44.9 to 29.7/100,000. This is significant compared with the rest of Kentucky where the average age at death from carcinoma of the cervix is 7.6 years lower than in Jefferson County (Christopherson *et al.*, 1970). In Aberdeen, 85% of the 125,000 married women of all ages have been screened and the incidence of clinical cancer of the cervix has decreased from 26 cases in 1965 to 10 cases in 1971 (Macgregor *et al.*, 1971).

The whole success of a screening program will depend on the effective response of the population, especially of the high-risk categories, and a substantial literature has resulted from the social study of response to publicity and persuasion for self-disease (Wakefield, 1972).

There is some evidence of greater success of approaching the high-risk population by the use of health visitors in the home (Osborn and Leyshon, 1966), the use of caravans (Whitfield, 1972; Epsom, 1973) and the open-door multiple-test clinic without appointment (Donaldson and Howell, 1965).

The pattern of screening may be important. As the *in situ* state may develop in the 20's, it is sensible to start screening around 25 years, if not earlier, and repeat at two or three yearly intervals. In England and Wales the national policy is to screen women of 35 and over and repeat at 5-year intervals, and most authorities feel that with the inherent unreliability of a single test for various reasons, quoted to be from 2 to 25% (Husain *et al.*, 1974), the program would not effectively detect all cancers. As it so happens, due to the enthusiasm of the young and cytology tests being carried out at Maternity and Family Planning Clinics, 50% of the tests sent to a laboratory are from women under 35.

An important factor in planning the frequency of all screening procedures is the cost, and as the laboratory examination of the smear or cytopipet is around 50p and the clinic attendance about £2.00, then the rate per positive found will range from £38.00 for a first test in women between 35 and 45 years of age if by pipet or collected during attendance for another purpose, to something like £3,000 or £4,000 if yearly rescreening of a population of 20- to 60-year-olds occurred at a specifically established cytology (Well Women Clinic, Husain, 1973).

Endometrial Cancer

Mortality from endometrial cancer is now greater than from cervical cancer, and attempts are being made to improve the effectiveness of screening for cancer of the uterine body. The cervical scrape smear is a poor sample for endometrial cancer detection with an accuracy of about 50 to 60%, and a vaginal pool sample, though better, only reaches around 80%

(Graham and Meigs, 1949), even if the irrigation cytopipet is used (Husain, 1970).

The new techniques, the jet wash (Kanbour *et al.*, 1974) and the Barbaro lavage instrument (Wachtel *et al.*, 1973) provide almost 100% detection, but these are more complex tests, less easily applicable to routine population screening.

Nongynecological Cytology

Here cytology has more a diagnostic role than one of screening and detection, though there is an undoubted possibility in screening for certain cancers in the pulmonary and urinary tracts in high-risk categories.

Pulmonary Tract

This usually provides the second greatest demand on the cytodiagnostic department. Most commonly it is the routine examination of a deep-cough sputum specimen, usually an early morning sample that forms the basis of this examination. Around three to five specimens are examined in the average clinical case where hemoptysis, persistent cough, or X-ray shadow exists. Prior dependent drainage of the site by lying on the opposite side for 0.5 to 1 h and the use of light percussion to loosen mucus plugs are more valuable adjuncts than the use of cough stimulants or aerosols which usually contain 10 to 20% propylene glycol. Specimens can be sent fresh to the laboratory or preserved in 30% alcohol or 5% formalin if delay of more than a few hours occurs. This method, when about four smears are prepared and examined per case, has an accuracy in expert hands dependent on the number of specimens examined. Oswald *et al.* (1971) showed that the detection rate improved from 41% for the first specimen to 56% for the second, 69% for the third and 85% for four or more samples examined.

The use of bronchial washings and, more recently, the bronchial brush samples directly (Bibbo *et al.*, 1973) or by use of television localization (Hattori *et al.* 1971) has improved the diagnostic accuracy considerably, while the addition of fine needle aspiration through guide cannulae in the chest wall with its closer approach to the peripheral lesion gives an ultimate accuracy of combined approaches of up to 93% (Nasiell, 1967).

There is no conclusive published evidence of the economic value of providing a cytological screening program for lung cancer, though there appears to be reason to screen those in high-risk categories of population such as the heavy smoker and those subject to recurrent lung infections or a chronic cough as part of a comprehensive health check.

The Upper Respiratory Tract. This is also accessible to cytological sampling by swab, sponge, brush, or wash techniques for the diagnosis of early cancer of the larynx or nasal passages.

Gastrointestinal Tract

Buccal Cavity. Oral wash, or brush or swab cytology has been developed successfully in countries where these cancers have a high incidence or where large municipal or community surveys have been carried out (Stahl *et al.*, 1967; Allegra *et al.*, 1973).

Esophageal and Gastric Cytology. This is heavily practiced in Japan and other countries with high incidence rates with considerable success in the diagnosis of early or surface cancers where a much better prognosis exists (Mason, 1966; Schade, 1960).

Even the old-fashioned wash technique using up to 500 ml of normal saline through a Levin tube has produced detection rates of 93% (Schade, 1960). While the new gastro-fiberscopes, both end- and side-viewing varieties, with wash, brush, and biopsy attachments under direct viewing, have given higher figures still and much better cytological preparations from which to make the diagnosis (Fakuda *et al.* 1967; Shida *et al.* 1967).

The Japanese have an active screening program for gastric cancer combining the radioscopic and gastroscopic technique, and they claim considerable improvement in the prognosis due to detection at earlier stages of surface cancer.

Cytology of the duodenum, biliary tract, and pancreas has also developed with radioscopic guidance of ductal intubation and the use of the stimulants pancreazymin and secretin (Raskin *et al.*, 1958; Butler, 1972). Here the success rate is not high but is improving with better instrumentation and experience.

The use of the new colonoscopes with wash, brush, and biopsy attachments under direct vision is improving the detection rate and diagnosis of tumors of the large bowel (Williams and Mutot, 1972).

In the past the elaborate preparation of patients for blind irrigation washes and the detailed search for cells was a great deterrent.

All the above endoscopic techniques demand careful preparation of the patient and meticulous care of the instruments. With experience such intubations cause little distress and become acceptable by the patient.

Urinary Tract

The cytology of the urinary tract is both simple and complex: simple in its collection and presentation for microscopy, but complex in its interpretation of the cellular changes towards neoplasia, a problem very similar to that observed in histological grading of transitional cell tumors (Eposti and Zajicek, 1972).

Accuracy of cancer detection is about 80%. Freshly collected, whole output specimens of 2- to 3-h duration are necessary, preferably after exercise, as this tends to increase exfoliation from the surface of the urothelium. If not processed in the laboratory within a few hours, preservation, usually by alcohol at an ultimate strength of 20–30%, is necessary. In the laboratory specimens are centrifuged and smears are made from the deposit, or the urine is aspirated on to a Millipore filter. Some authorities issue small Millipore monitors to have about 20 ml of urine aspirated through the filter, followed by some absolute alcohol to fix the entrapped cells immediately. The filter is then sent to the laboratory at leisure (Nuovo, 1969).

Screening for cancer of those exposed to the aromatic amines in industry and chemical laboratories is now mandatory as the resulting cancers have become a proscribed disease (Case, 1966). Cytological screening of all cases of unexplained hematuria over the age of 40 also provides an economic and worthwhile service.

The use of dissolvable swabs in cytological screening of the urethra for neoplastic disease is also possible (Williams, 1968).

The Prostate. This gland has been investigated cytologically by both the massage and needle aspirate techniques. The former has a success rate of about 70% in detecting malignancy (Mason, 1967). Here massage succeeds in producing a discharge from the urethra in about one-half the cases, and a direct smear is made, the bulk of the cells for diagnosis being flushed out in the first 20 ml of urine following the massage. This is transported immediately to the laboratory where simple albuminized smears are made from the centrifuged deposit, or the cells are collected onto a Millipore or deposited from a special cytocentrifuge on to slides. As cancers of the prostate start in the subcapsular area posteriorly, such massage may be dangerous, creating a generalized spread of tumor; and this obviously presents a long way round for the cells to travel to reach the urethra.

More recently the use of the Franzen needle has overcome this problem and is now a well-established procedure. Here, the gloved index finger is sheathed to carry a long cannula so that by palpation the suspect nodule under the prostatic capsule can be located and then pierced by the fine inner needle, permitting a more direct and accurate sampling. The method is described in the next section. The results provide well over 90% accuracy (Eposti, 1966) with opportunity to sample a number of sites in the prostate. The main cause of failure is contamination by fecal material if suction is not reduced to nil before removal. Infection of the needle track is almost unknown, even in this situation.

Aspiration Cytology

The advent of the Franzen needle and syringe and stimulus from the group of workers in the Karolinska Institute in Stockholm have provided a new field of diagnostic cytology procedures which are now practiced all over the world.

No tumor site is inaccessible to the fine needle aspiration technique where the needle is inserted through the skin, without need of anesthesia, into the tumor or tissue, and suction is then applied. The needle tip is then moved to and fro within the tumor, accumulating a small quantity of cellular material inside the needle itself. On releasing the suction and withdrawal of the needle enough cellular material exists within the needle to make one or two small smears which are spread and stained by May Grünwald Giemsa as with a blood smear, or by the Papanicolaou technique.

The breast (Zajicek et al., 1967), thyroid, salivary glands (Webb, 1973), and lymph nodes are the commonest organs needled, while the lungs (through guide cannulae) and other deeply situated organs such as the pancreas, ovary, liver, and even the brain or pituitary, are sampled by this technique, using radioscopic control.

An extensive literature is developing on the subject (Eposti et al., 1968; Zajicek, 1974) and the benefits of such simple atraumatic techniques are considerable. There appears to be little danger of hemorrhage or tumor spread from such fine needle punctures so long as no suction is maintained when the needle is not in the tumor tissue itself (Zajicek, 1974; Engzell et al., 1971). In fact, in Sweden it is customary to have patients arriving at the laboratory where the pathologist on duty for that day will perform the aspiration, have the smear stained immediately, then examine and report on the case. The patient herself may even carry the report back to the clinic well within an hour of the request. In experienced hands a positive report can achieve nearly 100% reliability, though a negative result may not indicate the absence of neoplasm. It does, however, save a considerable amount of time, cost, and anxiety to obtain that sort of information so simply. A good rapport between a surgeon collecting the sample and the pathologist examining the smear provides an even more convenient service, while some surgeons become highly skilled in the interpretation of the cytological smear itself (Webb, 1973).

The diagnosis of neoplasia and other conditions in exudates from serous cavities, including the cerebrospinal fluid, has been practiced for years and provides relatively high degrees of accuracy, with practically no false positive reports, though the detection rate in fluids in the presence of cancer will vary from 40 to 85%, depending on the nature of the tumor (Spriggs and Boddington, 1968).

In cerebral surgery a quickly stained brain smear technique provides a rapid diagnosis determining the extent of tumor infiltration (Canti, 1970).

A further range of minor and incompletely investigated areas of cytological detection is developing, such as in the eye, joints, and skin (Selbach and Heisel, 1962). The use of cytology in diagnosing skin diseases dates back to the days when Tzanck (1948) produced his test for identifying the typically rounded-off acantholytic squame cells in pemphigus bullae. Now with a simple curet the differential diagnosis between small skin tumors such as sweat gland adenomas, rodent ulcers, keratoacanthomas, and squamous cell carcinomas can be made rapidly and simply (Canti, 1970).

Finally, a fairly extensive literature is developing on the cytogenetic aspects of tumor and other disease analysis. This has been confined mainly to the spontaneous preparations from serous fluids and of the cervix uteri (Spriggs *et al.*, 1962; Benedict and Porter, 1972), but the whole field of cytogenetics is expanding within and outside the cytodiagnostic departments.

References

Allegra, S. R., Broderick, P. A., and Corvese, N. (1973). Oral cytology. Seven year oral cytology screening programme in the State of Rhode Island. (Analysis of 6448 cases.) *Acta Cytol.* **17**:42.

Anderson, W. A. D., and Gunn, S. A. (1967). Premalignant and malignant conditions of the cervix uteri. Tissue validity study of the vaginal irrigation method. *Cancer* **20**:1587.

Ashley, D. J. B. (1966). Evidence for the existence of two forms of cervical carcinoma. *J. Obstet. Gynecol. Br. Commonw.* **73**:372, 382.

Ayre, J. E. (1947). Selective cytology smear for diagnosis of cancer. *Am. J. Obstet. Gynecol.* **53**:609.

Bamforth, J., and Osborn, G. R. (1958). Diagnosis from cells. *J. Clin. Pathol.* **11**:473.

Beale, L. S. (1878). *The Microscope in Medicine,* 4th Ed. Churchill, Philadelphia.

Benedict, W. F., and Porter, I. H. (1972). The cytogenetic diagnosis of malignancy in effusions. *Acta Cytol.* **16**:304.

Bibbo, M., Fennessey, J. S., Chien-Tai Lu, Straus, F. H., Variakojis, D., and Wied, G. L. (1973). Bronchial brushing technique for the cytologic diagnosis of peripheral lung lesions. *Acta Cytol.* **17**:245.

Bibbo, M., Shanklin, D. R., and Wied, G. L. (1972). Endometrial cytology on jet wash material. *J. Reprod. Med.* **8**:90.

Boyes, D. A., Worth, A. S., and Fidler, H. K. (1970). The results of treatment of 4389 cases of preclinical cervical squamous carcinoma. *J. Obstet. Gynaecol. Br. Commonw.* **77**:769.

Butler, E. B. (1972). Pancreatic cytology. In *Clinics in Gastroenterology* (H. T. Howat, ed.), Vol. 1, No. 1, p. 53. W. B. Saunders, London.

Canti, G. (1970). Lectures on the use of cytology smears in brain surgery and in the diagnosis of skin tumours. 2nd International Academy of Cytology Congress, Paris, 1965, and subsequently.

Carruthers, J., Wilson, J. M. G., Chamberlain, J., Husain, O. A. N., Patey, D. G. H., Richards, N. D., Pennicott, A., Rogers, P., Catling, R., Meade, T. W., Saunders, J., and

McEwan, P. J. M. (1975). The acceptability of the cytopipette in screening for cervical cancer. *Br. J. Prev. Soc. Med.* **29**:239–248.

Case, R. A. M. (1966). Tumours of the urinary tract as an occupational disease in several industries. *Ann. R. Coll. Surg. Engl.* **39**:213.

Christopherson, W., Parker, J. E., Mendez W. M., and Lundin F. E. (1970). Cervical cancer death rate and mass cytologic screening. *Cancer* **26**:808.

Coppleston, M. (1969). Carcinoma of the cervix. Epidemiology and Aetiology. *Br. J. Hosp. Med.* **2**:961.

Davis, H. J. (1962). The irrigation smear. A cytologic method for mass screening by mail. *Am. J. Obstet. Gynecol.* **84**:1017.

Donaldson, R. J., and Howell, J. M. (1965). A multiple screening clinic. *Br. Med. J.* **2**:1034.

Dudgeon, L. S., and Patrick, C. V. (1927). The examination of fresh tissue by the wet film method. *Br. J. Surg.* **22**:4.

Engzell, Eposti, P. L., Rubio, C., Sigurdson, A., and Zajicek, J. (1971). Investigation on tumour spread in connection with aspiration biopsy. *Acta Radiol.* **10,4**:385.

Epsom, J. E. (1973). Community cancer screening. *Modern Trends in Oncology* (R. W. Raven, ed.), Vol. I, part 2. Butterworth, London.

Eposti, P. L. (1966). Cytologic diagnosis of prostatic tumours with the aid of transrectal aspiration biopsy. A critical review of 1110 cases and a report on morphologic and cytochemical studies. *Acta Cytol.* **10**:182.

Eposti, P. L., Franzen, S., and Zajicek, J. (1968). The aspiration biopsy smear. In *Diagnostic Cytology* (L. G. Koss, ed.), 2nd Ed. p. 565. Pitman Medical, London.

Eposti, P. L., and Zajicek J. (1972). Grading of transitional cell neoplasms of the urinary bladder from smears of bladder washings. A critical review of 326 tumours. *Acta Cytol.* **16**:527.

Evans, D. M. D., ed. (1970). *Cytology Automation (Proceedings of the 2nd Tenovus Symposium, Cardiff, 1968)*. Livingstone, Edinburgh/London.

Fakuda, T., Shida, S., Takita, T., and Sawada, Y. (1967). Cytologic diagnosis of early gastric cancer by the endoscopic method with gastrofibrescope. *Acta Cytol.* **11**:456.

Fennessey, J. S. (1968). Bronchial brushing and transbronchial forceps biopsy in the diagnosis of pulmonary lesions. *Dis. Chest* **53**:377.

Fidler, H. K., Boyes, A. D., and Worth, A. J. (1968). Cervical cancer detection in British Columbia. *J. Obstet. Gynaecol. Br. Commonw.* **75**:392.

Friedell, G. H., Hertig, A. J., and Younge, P. A. (1960). *Carcinoma in Situ of the Uterine Cervix*, p. 102. Charles C Thomas, Springfield, Ill.

Graham, R. M., and Meigs, J. V. (1949). Value of vaginal smear. *Am. J. Obstet. Gynecol.* **58**:843.

Green, G. H., and Donovan, J. W. (1970). The natural history of cervical carcinoma in situ. *J. Obstet. Gynaecol. Br. Commonw.* **77**:1.

Harris, M. S., Bibbo, M. Rao, C., and Wied, G. L. (1972). Cytopreparatory technique for the endometrial jet wash specimens. *Acta Cytol.* **16**:508.

Hattori, S., Matsuda, M., Nishihara, H., and Horai, T. (1971). Early diagnosis of small peripheral lung cancer. Cytologic diagnosis of very fresh cancer cells obtained by the T. V. brushing technique. *Acta Cytol.* **15**:460.

Health and Welfare Services (1964). CMND, 2389. London, H.M.S.O.

Husain, O. A. N. (1970). The irrigation smear. *Am. J. Obstet. Gynecol.* **106**:138.

Husain, O. A. N. (1973). Cytology screening in uterine cancer. In *Modern Trends in Oncology* (R. W. Raven, ed.), Vol. 1, part 2. Butterworth, London.

Husain, O. A. N., Butler, E. B. Evans, D. M. D., Macgregor, J. E., and Yule, R. (1974). Quality control in cytology. *J. Clin. Pathol.* **27**:935–944.

Kanbour, A., Klionsky, B., and Cooper, R. (1974). Cytohistologic diagnosis of uterine jet wash preparations. *Acta Cytol.* **18**:51.

Knox, E. G. (1966). Cervical cytology: A scrutiny of the evidence. In *Problems and Progress in Medical Care* (M. McLachlan, ed.), p. 272. Nuffield Provincial Hospital Trust, OUP, London.

Macgregor, J. E., Frazer, M. E., and Mann, E. M. F. (1971). Improved prognosis of cervical cancer due to comprehensive screening. *Lancet* 1:74.

Mason, M. K. (1966). Surface carcinoma of the stomach. Pathological features and clinical significance. *Overdruk uit Tijdschrift voor Gastro-Enterolgie*, Vol. 9, No. 6, 562.

Mason, M. K. (1967). The cytological diagnosis of carcinoma of the prostate. *Acta Cytol.* 11:68.

Nasiell, M. (1967). Diagnosis of lung cancer by aspiration biopsy and a comparison between this method and exfoliative cytology. *Acta Cytol.* 11:114.

Nuovo, V. M. (1969). *Cytologic Urinaire, Encyclopédic Médico-Chirurgicale.* Editee sur Fascicules Mobiles. Paris VIe.

Osborn, G. R., and Leyshon, V. N. (1966). Domiciliary testing of cervical smears by home nurses. *Lancet* 1:256.

Oswald, N. C., Hinson, K. F. W., Canti, G., and Miller A. B. (1971). The diagnosis of primary lung cancer with special reference to sputum cytology. *Thorax* **26**:623.

Papanicolaou, G. N. (1928). *New Cancer Diagnosis: Proceedings of the Third Race Betterment Conference.*

Raskin, H. F., Wenger, J. Sklar, M., Peticka, S., and Yarema, W. (1958). The diagnosis of cancer of the pancreas, biliary tract and duodenum by combined cytological and secretory methods. I. Exfoliative cytology and a description of a rapid method of duodenal intubation. *Gast. Enterol.* **34**:996.

Reagan, J. W., and Lin, F. (1967). An evaluation of the vaginal irrigation technique in the detection of uterine cancer. *Acta Cytol.* **11**:374.

Schade, R. O. K. (1960). *Gastric Cytology.* Arnold, London.

Schottlander, J., and Kermauner, F. (1912). *Zur Kenntnis des Uteruskarzinoms; Monographische Studie über Morphologie, Entwicklung, Wachstum, nebst Beiträgen zur Klinik der Erkrankung.* Karger, Berlin.

Selbach, G., and Heisel, E. (1962). The cytological approach to skin disease. *Acta Cytol.* **6**:439.

Shida, S., Sawada, Y., and Takamura, S. (1967). Cytological diagnosis of gastric cancer by gastroendoscopical method with fibregastroscope. *Gastroenterol. Jap.* **11**: No. 2, 101.

Spriggs, A. I., Boddington, M. M., and Clarke, C. H. (1962). Chromosomes of human cancer cells. *Br. Med. J.* **II**:1431.

Spriggs, A. I., and Boddington, M. M. (1968). *The Cytology of Effusions,* 2nd Ed. Heinemann, London.

Stahl, S. S., Koss, L. G., Brown, R. C., and Murray, D. (1967). Oral cytologic screening in a large metropolitan area. *JADA* **75**:1385.

Tzanck, A. (1948). Le cytodiagnostic immédiat en dermatologie. *Ann. Dermat. Syph.* **8**:205.

Wachtel, E., Gordon, H., and Wycherley, J. (1973). The cytological diagnosis of endometrial pathology using a uterine aspiration technique. *J. Obstet. Gynaecol. Br. Commonw.* **80**:164.

Wakefield, J., ed. (1972). *Seek Wisely to Prevent.* H.M.S.O. for Department of Health and Social Security, London.

Webb, A. J. (1973). Cytologic diagnosis of salivary gland lesions in adult and paediatric surgical patients. *Acta Cytol.* **17**:51.

Whitfield, A. P. (1972). Cancer prevention: Recent encouragement in preventative measures. Cervical screening programmes and voluntary support. *Royal Soc. Health J.* **92**:282.

Wied, G. L. (1961). Techniques for collection and preparation of cytologic specimens. *Clin. Obstet. Gynaecol.* **4**:1031.

Williams, C., and Muto, T. (1972). Examination of the whole colon with the fibreoptic colonoscope. *Br. Med. J.* **III**:278.

Williams, G. (1968). Cytological screening of the urethra. *Br. J. Urol.* **XL**: No. 6, 703.

Wilson, J. M. G. (1965). Some aspects of the epidemiology of cervical cancer. *Monthly Bull. Min. Hlth.* **24**:72.

Zajicek, J., Franzen, S., Jakobsson, P., Rubio, C., and Unsgaard, B. (1967). Aspiration biopsy of mammary tumours in diagnosis and research. A critical review of 2200 cases. *Acta Cytol.* **11**:169.

Zajicek, J. (1974). Aspiration biopsy cytology. In *Monographs in Clinical Cytology, Parts I and II.* S. Karger, Basel, London, and New York.

Chapter 15

RADIOTHERAPY

THOMAS J. DEELEY

It is a reflection of current thinking that a chapter on radiotherapy should be included in a text book on surgical oncology; further that it should be written by a radiotherapist. When I trained this would have been almost inconceivable, the surgeon jealous of his technical skill often referred the patient to the radiotherapist only as a last resort for palliation when all else had failed; the radiotherapist, anxious to display knowledge and prowess of a complicated technique, somewhat forlornly tried to reproduce results equal to those of the surgeons even on patients more suitable for operation. Fortunately we have progressed considerably in recent years; the surgeon or radiotherapist no longer attempts to monopolize the treatment of the patient. Interdisciplinary cooperation has brought about a greater understanding of the part that each specialty plays in the treatment of the patient with malignant disease and patients now are referred for the method of treatment which produces the best chance of survival and the minimal incidence of complications and morbidity. There is still some confusion in many medical practitioners' minds about the role of radiotherapy in the management of the cancer patient. It is regretable that such a state should exist; in this country we are an aging population and malignant diseases are associated with the older age group, no wonder then that the incidence is on the increase and that cancer, at present the second most common cause of death, is already assuming the prime position in some parts of the country. An aging population also means that a high proportion of patients are not suitable for radical surgical procedures. Snelling in 1967 estimated that radiotherapy was used in more than one-half of patients with malignant

Thomas J. Deeley • Director. South Wales Radiotherapy and Oncology Service. Velindre Hospital, Cardiff; South Glamorgan Health Authority; Lecturer, Welsh National School of Medicine, Wales.

disease and that in the larger centers this was the method of treatment in three-quarters of the patients. We have ample evidence that the proportion of patients treated in this way is continuing to increase. Why, then, is there not more knowledge of this subject and its potentialities? The blame for this must be placed on those responsible for the teaching in the formative years of the doctor's life. Radiotherapy has been considered essentially a postgraduate study, with the result that the average newly qualified doctor during his undergraduate years obtains little or no knowledge of its therapeutic possibilities. Fortunately, this is being corrected in the curriculums of the more progressive medical schools. There are in this country only a few academic posts in radiotherapy, usually supported by no more than the minimum of academic staff. The radiotherapist cannot escape a considerable proportion of the blame; we have been too interested in the technical side of our specialty, talking about high-powered machines, measurements of radiation, radium implants, mathematics, statistics, and so on, so that we have been viewed by our medical colleagues as technicians, quasiscientists or even scientists. But a radiotherapist is a clinician directly concerned with patient care, using his scientific knowledge to advance that care by improving the results of therapy; radiotherapy is thus both an art and a science. As a clinician primarily concerned with malignant diseases the radiotherapist has been aware for many years that his work can be improved by wider knowledge of all aspects of these diseases; epidemiology, diagnosis, treatment, rehabilitation, prognosis, terminal care, and so on—a study which has in relatively recent years been designated as oncology. This is not a medical specialty, the study is too wide for any one person to be an expert in all its aspects, even though he may have a reasonably comprehensive knowledge; it is more correctly a concept. By adopting such a concept each person involved in any aspect of malignant diseases can widen his knowledge and experience of certain aspects closely related to his own specialty.

This, then, is the reason for this chapter, for by describing the nontechnical aspects of radiotherapy it is hoped that the surgeon will have a better understanding of our specialty and that even greater collaboration will result between surgeons and radiotherapists. A brief account of the development of radiotherapy will be given because there have been so many changes and advances since X-rays were first discovered. We now have available a wide selection of sophisticated apparatus used in differing ways for specific tumors or sites; it is my intention merely to introduce the names of these machines and to say little about treatment techniques. More important are the indications for radiotherapy, the types of tumor which show a sensitivity or resistance to radiation, the action of radiation on tissues, and methods of modifying these. Of particular interest is the combined use of radiotherapy and surgery and a knowledge of indications of radiotherapy as the major treatment and the contraindications of surgery. Palliation is by no means an admission of defeat; to relieve a hopeless patient of distressing symptoms even though he has a short life expectancy is, in my opinion, good medicine. Unfortunately, many patients suffer distressing symptoms and are referred for palliation only at a late stage, whereas earlier referral could have prevented both patient and family distress. We are frequently accused of producing such bad effects as fibrosis, considered to be a radiation effect on normal tissues, whereas this results more often from ablation of the tumor as much of the tissue damage has already been caused by the growing tumor and can only be replaced by scar tissue. Radiotherapy is still a young subject and our knowledge is incomplete. Radiation techniques have developed empirically over the years, the slow evaluation of the results of treatment by clinical impression, or experience, have now been supplanted by carefully controlled clinical trials with statistical analyses. Much research work is required with an increasing need for greater cooperation with other clinicians and scientists.

History

The origin of this medical specialty can be traced back to November 1895 when Wilhelm Conrad Roentgen first discovered his "new rays"; it is convenient to describe the subsequent developments during each subsequent decade.

The 1890's saw two major discoveries, X-rays by Roentgen and radium by Pierre and Marie Curie. Progress could be made very rapidly with the former if facilities for glass blowing and a suitable electrical supply were available; it is not surprising that within a few months scientists all over the world had produced similar tubes and were repeating and confirming Roentgen's experiments. These observations form the basis of modern diagnostic radiology, for different tissues were shown to absorb radiation to differing degrees and it was possible to take a photographic image of certain parts of the body. It soon became apparent that the rays could also produce changes in normal tissues and almost immediately their effects were investigated in certain incurable diseases, including cancer. Within only 2 months of their discovery they had been used in the treatment of a nasopharyngeal carcinoma, and before the close of the century the first cure was claimed. Such progress was not reported with radium because of the complicated and tedious extraction processes necessary.

The first decade of the new century was one of development; sufficient radium was available to treat a carcinoma of the cervix uteri in 1902 and X-rays were used to treat most malignant diseases and a number of nonmalignant conditions. All workers stressed the problems of reproducibility; if a good response was observed in the treatment of a particular disease there was no method of giving exactly the same treatment to another patient with the same disease. Even at this early stage workers noticed the effects of radiation on normal tissues and a few late effects were reported, but these undesirable results were out-weighed by the increasing number of cures.

The 1910's brought about a realization of the limitations of X-ray therapy, the poor penetration of the 50,000-V rays meant that only relatively superficial lesions could be given the dose necessary to ablate tumor cells. In spite of cataclysmic international hostilities this decade saw the development of machines capable of operating at about 200,000 V. New sources of radium were discovered and production increased; further laboratory work had shown that the active principle was contained in a gas radon which could be sealed in tubes and inserted directly into the tumor. Realization of the ill effects of radiation led to methods aimed at protection.

The 1920's saw new high-powered machines being used somewhat indiscriminately and giving very high doses of radiation to tissues with resulting necrosis. The greater penetration of the rays meant that more deeply situated tumors could be irradiated and also that underlying tissues, such as the lung, showed radiation effects when the breast was treated. Attempts were made to measure the dose of radiation by the biological effects produced in the skin—the erythema dose—but towards the end of this decade physical methods using ionization chambers were being developed.

The 1930's heralded the scientific era of radiotherapy with a measure of dose—the roentgen—and it was possible to reproduce treatment from patient to patient and observe the effects of varying doses both on tumors and normal tissues. Interest in biological effects was developed producing a new science called radiobiology. Radiotherapists, however, still lamented the inadequate penetration of their X-ray beams.

Progress in the next decade was again impeded by international hostilities, but ironically some technical developments used to destroy mankind eventually found application for humane purposes. The postwar years saw great advances in technology and engineering leading to the production of very high-powered machines producing rays in the range of millions of volts: linear accelerators, betatrons, and cyclotrons. Work leading to the holocaust of the atomic bomb also produced radioactive isotopes as new therapy, thus the associated science of nuclear medicine was conceived. Large quantities of radioactive cobalt became available for teletherapy machines giving beams of gamma radiation.

The 1950's saw the clinical applications of megavoltage therapy and the use of radioactive isotopes. An 8-million V linear accelerator was used clinically for the first time in August 1953, and the advantages of megavoltage therapy soon became apparent; a greater penetration of tissues, a low skin dose, less absorption in bone, and a greater accuracy in clinical set-up.

In a short time electrons and neutrons were added to the radiotherapists' armamentarium. It was now possible to give an adequate tumor dose to all sites of the body, and work began to determine the optimum treatment conditions. A new measurement of the dose within tissues—the rad (radiation absorbed dose)—was introduced. Radiobiology produced some interesting concepts and ideas for improving therapy. But radioactive isotopes, although useful diagnostically, were found to have only limited application to therapy.

In the 1960's the beginnings noted in the last decade were rationalized, and all major departments were provided with high-voltage machines. Attempts to improve the results of therapy led to a greater application of controlled clinical trials to determine the optimum treatment conditions. Advances in chemotherapy led to the introduction of many agents to be assessed, used alone or in combination with radiotherapy. The sophisticated radiation techniques which were developed demanded a more accurate knowledge of the effects of radiation both on tumors and normal tissues.

In the present decade we can expect little new in technical advances, but machine construction will inevitably be improved, leaving the radiations essentially the same. Progress in the determination of optimum treatment techniques is inevitably slow when evaluation is based on long-term survival and morbidity. Immunology and malignant diseases needs to be investigated and may have a therapeutic application. The scientific approach to malignant diseases offers new lines of research and development and demands a greater interdisciplinary cooperation between all workers in oncology.

Radiotherapy is a relatively young specialty; much of its early work was hampered by inadequate apparatus, inability to measure dose, and lack of knowledge of radiation effects, but the past two decades have seen considerable advances which will lead to a rationalization of this therapy.

Radiotherapy Equipment and Treatment Techniques

It must be presumed that the surgeon has at least some knowledge of the equipment used in the radiotherapy department. It is not the purpose of this chapter to describe this in any detail. The equipment used depends on the lesion to be treated; very superficial skin lesions may be treated with low-energy electrons from linear accelerators or radioactive strontium. Malignant skin lesions need superficial X-rays produced in the region of 60,000 to 120,000 V. Orthovoltage therapy, i.e., X-rays of 200,000 to 300,000 V, the mainstay of the department in the 1930's and 1940's, is used to treat only such relatively superficial lesions as those of lymph nodes. In many departments they have been superseded by the more penetrating rays from cobalt machines which are now the mainstay of most departments. Linear accelerators in the range of 4- to 10-million V are used to treat deep-seated tumors; betatrons with energies up to 35-million V are used to give high power beams of electrons; neutron therapy is at present limited to a few centers with cyclotrons, but smaller machines are being investigated. Hyperbaric oxygen tanks are available in some departments for use with therapy machines. Improvements have also taken place with intracavitary radiation techniques, and remote loading techniques have greatly reduced the problems of protection. The great accuracy needed with these high-powered machines has led to greater demands on mold room and workshop expertise, and diagnostic X-ray tubes are used in simulators to check the position of the radiation fields.

There is much to interest the surgeon in a modern radiotherapy department; it is suggested that visits be made to see the equipment and the patients treated. Advances have been so marked in recent years that even the experienced surgeon will benefit from a reappraisal of radiotherapy machines and the opportunity to familiarize himself with the techniques in use.

The Action of Radiation on Tissues

The physical and chemical changes produced in living tissues by irradiation are very complex and outside the scope of this chapter, indeed they are still only partially understood. Individual cells are more sensitive at the mitotic stage of the cell cycle, less sensitive at the time of DNA synthesis, and relatively insensitive in the two resting periods. Malignant cells are more likely to have a high proportion of dividing cells than the surrounding normal tissues and are thus likely to show a greater response to irradiation. More actively dividing tumors show a greater response than the more slowly growing differentiated lesions. Ideally, radiotherapy should kill off the tumor cells without causing any effect on normal cells, but this is not possible and treatment is designed to cause the maximum effect on the former with as little damage as possible to the latter. The difference in vulnerability between malignant and normal cells is referred to as the *therapeutic ratio,* and radiotherapy techniques aim at increasing this difference.

Some tumors respond to relatively low doses of radiation well within the tissue tolerance of the surrounding normal tissues. Other tumors need a dose of radiation to kill them which is almost the same as that which will kill the normal cells; and another group of tumors need doses so far in excess of that which can be tolerated by normal cells that radiotherapy is impracticable. We are thus able to define some terms used in radiotherapy.

Radiosensitivity

This is defined as the sensitivity of a particular tissue to irradiation, a *radiosensitive* tumor is killed by relatively small doses of radiation and a *radioresistant* tumor does not respond to doses of radiation which will kill normal cells.

The sensitivity of a tumor depends on various factors: the histology, anaplastic tumors on the whole being more sensitive than well-differentiated tumors; and the oxygenation of the tissues, anoxic cells being relatively radioresistant and well-oxygenated cells showing a greater response.

Radiocurability

This term is sometimes confused with radiosensitivity. While the latter term applies specifically to the effects on the individual tumor cells, the term "radiocurability" takes into account the problems of metastases. Many radiosensitive tumors also show a propensity to disseminate, and although radiation may successfully ablate the local lesion, a cure is not obtained because widespread dissemination has occurred already. Radiosensitivity can be applied also to the normal tissues. Table 1 shows the relative radiosensitivity of normal tissues and malignant tumors; it must be

TABLE 1. The Relative Radiosensitivity of Normal Tissues and Tumors

Sensitivity	Normal tissues	Sensitivity	Tumors
Radiosensitive	Lymphocytes Bone marrow Gonads Embryonic tissues	Radiosensitive	Embryonic tumors The reticuloses Anaplastic carcinoma
Moderately sensitive	Skin Small blood vessels Lens of the eye Growing tissues Lung Salivary glands	Limited sensitivity	Oat cell tumors Epithelial tumors Adenocarcinomas
Moderately resistant	Skin Thyroid gland Nerve cells		
Radioresistant	Muscle Bone Connective tissue Mature red blood corpuscles	Radioresistant	Soft tissue sarcomas Osteosarcomas Melanotic sarcomas

pointed out that these are placed in an approximate order depending to an extent on the average response for that tissue, for there is a wide spectrum of response and occasionally a much more sensitive or resistant effect may be found than is expected.

A knowledge of these relative responses helps in the planning of radiation therapy; to adjust the dose to be given to produce an effect; to select relatively sensitive tumors for treatment; to know when it is possible to treat even large tumors to a dose which is likely to be adequate in very sensitive tumors; and to avoid normal tissues which are known to be very radiosensitive.

Volume to be Irradiated

As with surgical removal, radiotherapy deals with the primary lesion and a surrounding area of apparently normal tissues where direct extension of tumor has possibly occurred. For example, in treating a visible epithelioma of the skin, the tumor and a zone of tissue extending for at least 1.0 cm around the apparent limits of the lesion are raised to a cancericidal dose, a 2.0 cm diam lesion requiring a 4.0 cm field. These requirements apply also to depth of tissue, and at least 1.0 cm must be treated below the limit of apparent extension in depth; this is not easy with the surgical removal of skin lesions and may account for recurrences where the tumor has been adequately cleared on the skin surface but not in depth. Lesions in relatively loose tissues where the tumor can infiltrate with ease into the surrounding areas may need even more clearance, and it is usual to give at least 2.0 cm clearance around a carcinoma of the bronchus.

Field Arrangement

In the treatment of any tumor, one, two, three, or more fields of irradiation may be used; usually the whole extent of the tumor is covered by each field. In deciding the arrangement of the fields it is important to avoid irradiating any normal tissue which is known to be radiosensitive. Thus, in the treatment of a carcinoma of the bronchus it would be easy to use two opposed fields, on the anterior and the posterior chest, but this would mean that the spinal cord would receive a full dose of radiation with the danger of radiation myelitis. The posterior field is therefore angled to avoid the spinal cord and passes obliquely through the paravertebral gutter.

When selecting a suitable field arrangement there are two possibilities: (a) To use as few fields as possible so arranged as to avoid areas known to be sensitive, or to irradiate only areas where it is known that any resultant fibrosis will cause the minimum of morbidity; here a small volume is raised to a high dose. (b) To use many fields angled in on the tumor so that the dose is spread over a wide volume of normal tissue, each part of which will receive a relatively small radiation dose.

Fractionation Technique

Treatment is often given daily over a number of days or weeks. The intention of fractionation of the treatment is to increase the therapeutic ratio; frequent small doses while producing effects on the tumor cells in mitosis do not have the same effect on normal tissues where there is less mitotic acitivity, and these cells therefore sustain less damage. For many years it has been customary to give daily doses for 5 days per week; the 2-day rest allowing the normal tissues to achieve some recovery; more recently investigations of fewer fractions have been made. A controlled clinical trial carried out by the author in the treatment of carcinoma of the bronchus compared daily fractionations 5 days per week for 4 weeks compared with treatments twice weekly over the same time, i.e., comparing 20 treatments with 8 treatments. The results of treatment as regards survival, morbidity, evidence of residual tumor, and metastatic dissemination were the same for each group. But instead of a daily visit to the hospital the patient came twice weekly only, so what had been dreaded by the ill patient now became almost an outing.

Before dealing more with clinical radiotherapy it is interesting to detail some of the work carried out in radiobiology and to indicate possible clinical effects.

Radiobiology

Developments in radiotherapy are limited to a certain extent by the inability to carry out direct research on patients, so that radiation techniques have evolved by a process of trial and error. Almost every department has its own techniques, each firmly supported by the radiotherapist who thinks that his technique is best. If one is so convinced it is difficult to carry out a controlled clinical trial to investigate and compare another technique; because a technique is new it does not of necessity follow that it is better. Fortunately, the growth of radiobiology has provided a means of carrying out investigations on animal tissues and human cancer cultures. Inevitably, pure scientific research of this kind has grown outside the limits imposed by patient care, and it has become a pure clinical science, unfortunately at times somewhat divorced from clinical investigation. Departments have grown up using materials disassociated from clinical problems and appearing to be unconnected with patients, but fortunately, in relatively recent years smaller departments have been developed within the radio-therapy unit and at last radiobiologists and radiotherapists are beginning to understand the problems involved in each other's work. As clinicians it is our duty to follow a line of research which is applicable to the treatment of human malignant diseases and avoid being sidetracked by some of the exciting and interesting developments in pure basic research. It is encour-aging to see that some newer radiotherapeutic techniques, such as the use of hyperbaric oxygen, have developed from basic biological research. In addition, we have been able to apply logical biological thinking to some of the clinical facts we have accumulated as a result of our empirical developments.

It is hoped that the brief explanation of radiobiology which follows will assist the surgeon in appreciating some of the problems in this specialty, in understanding, at least in part, the radiotherapy approach to these prob-lems, and in perceiving some of the trends that future developments may take.

For many years radiobiologists worked with disassociated organisms or animals, but the development of tissue-culture techniques in 1955 cre-ated the possibility of investigating radiation effects on mammalian tissues and cancer cells. After irradiation of a group of cells, some of the cells are killed, the proportion depending on the dose of radiation given. We can thus construct a typical cell survival curve (Figure 1); this curve has two parts, a shoulder which represents the period in which the dose of radiation given produced little or no effect on the surviving fraction and a straight part of the curve which is exponential. We shall use this curve to explain some of the effects seen in clinical radiotherapy and suggest ways of modifying tissue response.

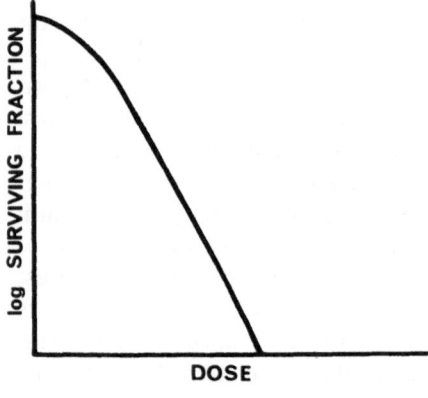

Figure 1. Typical mammalian cell survival curve after irradiation (from Deeley, 1972–3).

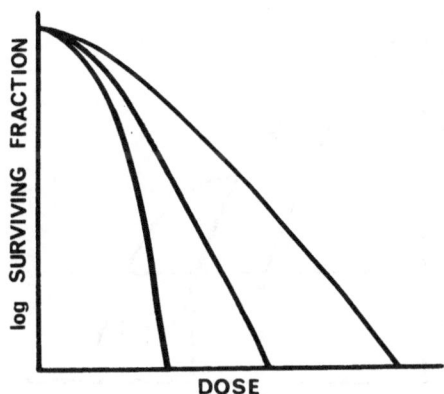

Figure 2. Cell survival curves for tumors of different histological type showing variations in both shoulder and slope of curve (from Deeley, 1972–3).

Differing Tumors

It is well known that tumors show a differing response to irradiation, which can be seen on the survival curve as different slopes or shoulders. Thus some tumors will melt away with small doses, indicating an almost negligible shoulder and steep slope, while others with a large shoulder will show little or no response to the same dose (Figure 2).

Fractionation of Dose

Radiobiological investigations have shown that the sensitivity of a particular cell depends on its position in its cell cycle at the time of the radiation, being most sensitive at the time of mitosis. Not all the cells in a tumor will be at the same stage of the cell cycle at the time of treatment; those at mitosis will be killed, a large proportion of those at the stage of DNA synthesis may be killed, while those in the intervening resting stages may show a minimal response only and may then pass into the stage of mitosis, and the tumor commences to grow again. Also, not all the cell cycles are of the same length in the same tumor, and marked differences between adjacent cells may be found in the length of the resting stage. Thus, if a single radiation treatment only is given, we have a chance of producing a response in only a limited proportion of cells. By fractionating the treatment it may be possible to increase the effect by hitting cells as they divide. But, for each fraction we have a relatively ineffective shoulder so that a greater total dose is needed to produce the same effect (Figure 3). We do not know the optimum methods of fractionation; present investigations are comparing daily fractionation with that performed two or three times weekly; or the use of split-dose techniques giving radiation for, say, 2 weeks, resting for 2 weeks, and then completing in a further 2 weeks, or

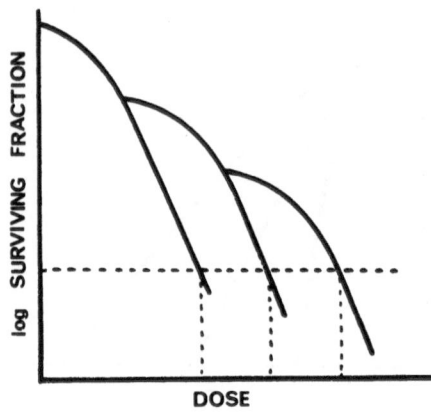

Figure 3. The effect of fractionation. To achieve the same biological effect, indicated by the horizontal dotted line, a higher dose is needed when treatment is given in two fractions and more again when given in three, and so on (from Deeley, 1972–3).

some such permutation; or of ultrasmall treatments given at about 8-h intervals rather than the usual 24 h.

An alternative method would be to induce synchronization of the cell cycles of all the cells so that they are all at the sensitive stage of mitosis at the same time and thus more sensitive; the results so far are not promising.

The Oxygen Effect

The blood supply to a tumor depends somewhat on the rate of growth of the tumor; rapidly growing cells may infiltrate around the blood vessels, whereas more slowly growing tumors will displace the vessels and possibly obstruct them. The blood supply to this kind of tumor comes from its periphery, the center receiving oxygen only by diffusion. Anaplastic tumors may have penetrating vessels and a peripheral circumferential capillary network, whereas epitheliomas have the latter only. The partial oxygen pressure across a squamous tumor is shown in Figure 4; as the tumor increases in size the partial pressure in the center decreases, and if the radius of the tumor exceeds 150 microns the center is anoxic. Further increase in size is at the expense of the tissues which necrose.

Radiobiological investigations have revealed that well-oxygenated cells respond to a lower dose of radiation than do anoxic effects, or alternatively we can say that they show a greater response to the same dose (Figure 5). The presence of even 1% of anoxic cells produces almost the same effect as if they were all anoxic. While a certain dose of radiation will kill the well-oxygenated cells at the periphery of an epithelioma, the relatively anoxic central cells will show degrees of resistance or are likely to be unaffected and grow later. We thus get the clinical picture of initial

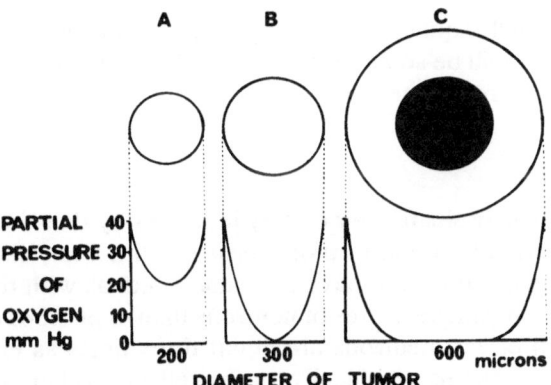

Figure 4. The partial pressure of oxygen across three tumors A, B, and C of increasing diameters. The solid black area in tumor C represents necrotic tissue (from Deeley, 1972–3).

response followed by recrudescence of the tumor. Anoxia or hypoxia may be overcome by (a) reducing all cells to the same degree of anoxia; (b) using a technique of radiation where the oxygen effect is less significant, or (c) oxygenating all the anoxic cells. The first method is applicable only where the blood supply to a tumor can be cut off for a short time, e.g., in a limb, but fails because of the nutrient arteries to bone; the second method is described later under neutron therapy. The third method can be achieved in two ways, by intraarterial injection of hydrogen peroxide, but this is limited to tumors supplied by one artery, or by the patient breathing in oxygen at high pressure while receiving treatment—hence the hyperbaric oxygen tank with oxygen at 4 atmospheres absolute. The present results suggest that hyperbaric oxygen is a useful adjuvant to radiotherapy, the best results

Figure 5. Survival curve for a population of mammalian cells containing 1% anoxic cells and 99% oxygenated cells, compared with an anoxic and an oxygenated cell population (from Deeley, 1972–3).

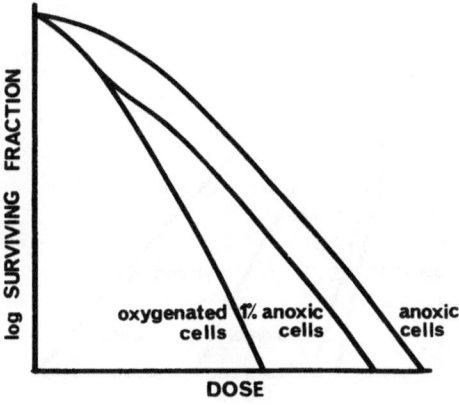

being obtained with squamous tumors; they are, however, by no means conclusive, and it will be some time before we can definitely decide that this therapy should be recommended for all radiotherapy centers.

Neutron Therapy

Fast neutrons dissipate their energy in tissues by their interaction with the elements normally found in those tissues. With neutrons, the relative anoxia of the tissues does not have the same effect as with the photons of X-rays; in addition, smaller doses of neutrons than of photons are needed to produce a given effect, neutrons are about three times as effective as X-rays. Figure 6 shows this graphically on the cell survival curve. At present there is only one cyclotron in the U.K. capable of giving a satisfactory beam of neutrons; although in use for many years we have no clear idea of its effectiveness. More recently smaller generators have been developed. Their output is relatively low, but it is hoped that in the near future the use of neutron therapy will be satisfactorily evaluated. Neutron sources ^{252}Cf and ^{242}Cm–Be are now available in a form suitable for implantation directly into tumors. Negative π mesons are a further source of radiation giving similar effects to neutrons, these accelerating machines are very expensive and only one or two are available at present.

Modification of Radiosensitivity

The radiosensitivity of a tumor may be modified in two ways: (a) by making the cell more sensitive (Figure 7); and (b) by adding to the effect of radiation by independently diminishing the cell population (Figure 8). Radiosensitizers should affect the response of radiation on the cell without

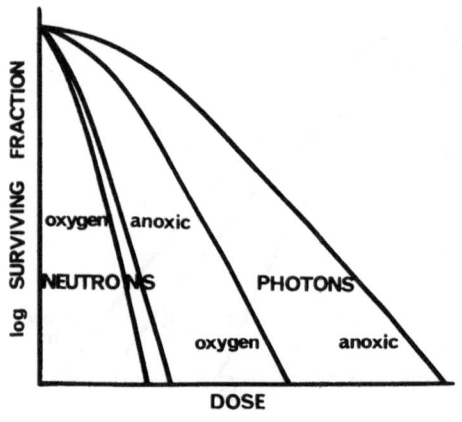

Figure 6. Survival curves showing the effects of irradiation on oxygenated and anoxic cell populations. Note the greater relative biological efficiency with neutrons and the relative effects of anoxia (from Deeley, 1972–3).

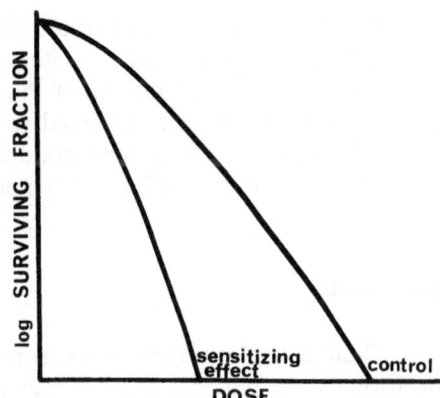

Figure 7. Survival curve showing that radio-sensitizers change the slope (from Deeley, 1972–3).

themselves having any antitumoral action. Perhaps the best-known radiosensitizer is Synkavit, 2-methyl-1-4-naphthoquinone sodium bisulfate; if given before radiation it produces slightly better survival rates than when radiation alone is used; the long-term survival rates, however, do not appear to be affected. Although the clinical results are not very encouraging, we have evidence that the sensitivity of the tumor within the patient can be modified and the search for more effective agents must continue. An interesting prospect is the use of coexistent ultrasonic radiation to cause some modification of the radiation effect, but much more animal work needs to be done before this is used clinically. A very likely line of research was to cause a reduction in the number of surviving cells with a cytotoxic agent and then reduce the fraction even further by irradiation. At present there is little evidence to suggest that the final results of such combined therapy affect the results of treatment in any way.

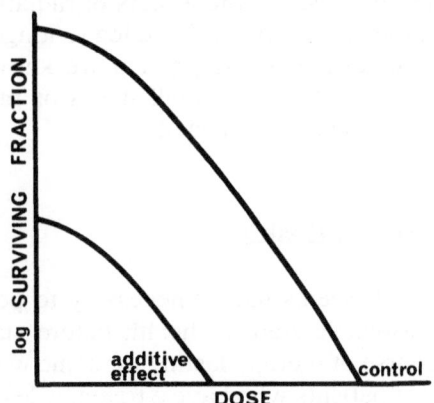

Figure 8. Survival curve to show an additive effect; the slope of the curves is the same but the initial number of malignant cells is reduced (from Deeley, 1972–3).

The foregoing has illustrated the complexity of tissue response to radiation, a response which is affected by many factors and innumerable permutations or combinations of these factors. To improve the results of therapy there is an obvious need to unravel some of the complexity, to determine optimum treatment conditions, and to obtain a greater knowledge of the biological effects of irradiation.

The Host

Clinical radiotherapy is even more complex because of the further addition of the patient; the changes already described *in vitro* are taking place in the modified surroundings of the host, so we have to consider further the normal tissues surrounding the tumor, the general condition of the patient, the possibility of dissemination of the tumor, the immunological implications of the growth, and the effect that radiation may have on these.

Normal Tissues

All growing tissues are affected to some extent by the energy released within them by irradiation; if the effect caused is minimal, recovery will occur, but if growing cells are damaged death will ensue and the dead cells will be replaced by fibrous tissue. However, the radiotherapist is frequently blamed for all radiation fibrosis, and it must be pointed out that much of the fibrosis is the result of ablation of the tumor and its replacement by fibrous tissue, in other words a successful response. The development of megavoltage therapy and other radiation techniques has called for a reappraisal of the effects of radiation on normal tissues. The improved results of treatment have led to longer survival rates with possible risk of carcinogenesis. At present we know relatively little about the possible genetic effects of small doses of radiation, and long-term studies over many years are needed.

General Health

It seems hardly necessary to point out that the patient must be in a reasonable state of health before starting treatment and able to stand a course of therapy lasting for some weeks. It is, however, only too frequent that patients who have a treatable lesion have their referral delayed to such an extent that by the time they reach the radiotherapist they are moribund.

Such practices can only occur because the clinician has an incomplete or negligible knowledge of radiotherapy.

The patient may need supportive treatment before radiotherapy begins, anemia may result in poor oxygenation of tissues and clinical results have shown poor effects when the hemoglobin is low; thus all patients presenting with hemoglobin of less than 70% are transfused. Hypertension is also associated with a poor radiation response; dehydration and malnutrition are treated, and general nursing care is given. Infection will compete with the oxygen available to the tumor tissues and adds to the patient's general toxic state, and it is treated with the appropriate antibiotic. Apprehensive or distressed patients will benefit from appropriate tranquilizers. These general requirements are in fact similar to those needed for patients undergoing operations.

Metastases

Local radiotherapy will obviously not affect a tumor which has already disseminated widely; the most common cause of failure of treatment of malignant diseases is the presence of metastases which were not clinically evident at the time that treatment started. The detection of occult metastases has been greatly improved by the use of certain radioactive isotopes capable of detecting bone metastases often before diagnostic radiological techniques, or liver and brain metastases before clinical manifestations. With technical refinements it is hoped that it will be possible to select suitable patients before embarking on a radical course of radiotherapy, and unsuitable patients will be spared a long course of hopeless treatment.

Immunology

Considerable interest has been aroused in recent years in the normal body defense mechanisms to foreign organisms such as tumor cells. Recent tests have been devised which may possibly lead to methods of immunodiagnosis. These include MEM (macrophage electrophoretic mobility), CEA (carcinoembryonic antigen), LT (lymphocyte transformation tests), and SCM (structuredness of the cytoplasmic matrix); such tests may help further in the selection of suitable patients for radiotherapy and in possible prognostic evaluation. They cannot be described further in this chapter and the interested reader is referred to the current literature. Immunological responses may play an important part locally around the tumor, or generally throughout the whole body. The artificial stimulation of such responses suggests possible therapeutic applications, but at present only relatively little work has been carried out using nonspecific immunological agents; it is possible that these may be combined with radiotherapy in the future.

The Tumor

It is, of course, necessary to know that we are dealing with a malignant tumor before starting therapy, and while every effort should be made to obtain histological confirmation it must be realized that delay increases the risk of dissemination, and in a proportion of patients the diagnosis is made on the clinical findings only. Open surgical biopsy frequently results in some delay while the wound heals, as here it is unwise to start radiation as primary healing may be delayed. The advantages of open operation are that the limits of the tumor may be explored and a suitably large piece of tissue may be obtained for a thorough histological examination. The author feels that there are considerable advantages to needle or drill biopsy, for a general anesthetic and hospital admission are not required. A small incision only is made in the skin, paraffin section can be obtained within 24 h, and radiotherapy can be started without delaying wound healing (Deeley, 1974).

Existing cytological techniques have a high degree of accuracy, not only in detecting tumor cells, but in ascertaining the particular type of tumor. Examination of sputum, gastric washings, pleural and peritoneal fluid, scrapings, or washings taken at endoscopy may all be sufficient for diagnosis.

Delineation of the tumor is essential for the radiotherapist; this implies fixing the limits of the tumor and defining the method of spread and the lymph nodes which may be involved. The extent of the tumor may be determined from clinical examination, surgical exploration possibly with metal clips or markers, endoscopic examination, diagnostic radiological techniques, and so on. More sophisticated techniques are being investigated in an attempt to define the limits of the tumor, including thermography, infrared photography, radioisotope studies, ultrasonics, tomography, and transaxial tomography.

The Treatment of Malignant Disease

Following the initial clinical examination of the patient a decision is made about the treatment to be given. This may be radical, designed to cure or to control the progress of the disease, perhaps for the patient's normal life, or otherwise to palliate distressing symptoms. It should be emphasized that malignant diseases can be cured; but some confusion may be caused by the term *cure*. This literally means that no surviving cancer cells remain in the body, but such a statement cannot be checked clinically. To assess the results of treatment we have two possible alternative ways.

(a) To assess the survival rate at a fixed time, conventionally 5 years, which is applicable to squamous lesions of the mouth and pharynx but not to other lesions. For example, it is totally inadequate for Hodgkin's disease and carcinoma of the breast and probably too long for carcinoma of the bronchus.

(b) To estimate the survival rate at a time when the probability of the patient dying from the disease is no greater than the probability of dying for the normal population of the same age group. This is the time of *normal life expectancy* and varies with the disease treated. Thus it is about 2 years for carcinoma of the corpus uteri, 3 years for carcinoma of the bronchus, 5 years for mouth and pharynx cancer, 7 years for carcinoma of the cervix uteri, and so on.

The latter is thus a better index of the efficacy of treatment and is more realistic than vaguely talking about cures; admittedly, a few patients will still die from their disease, but so will members of the normal population who will develop the disease.

Control of malignant diseases may be achieved by radiation, a palpable tumor remaining but not increasing in size. For example, an inoperable carcinoma of the rectum treated by radiation may leave a swelling palpable on rectal examination, but the surface may re-epithelialize with the relief of distressing symptoms. A technique of radiotherapy—*growth restraint technique*—aims at giving sufficient radiation usually at weekly intervals to keep a tumor under control.

Palliation implies that sufficient radiation is given to relieve distressing symptoms, including pain, ulceration, discharge, bleeding, and unsightly tumor, when there is no chance of a cure or control. Treatment is stopped when palliation is achieved and may be given again if symptoms recur. There is a belief that radiotherapy once given cannot be repeated, if radical treatment fails and symptoms cause distress, palliative treatment can then be given and the possible late effects of radiation can be ignored because the patient will not live long enough to develop them.

Methods of Treatment

The three main methods of radical treatment used in malignant diseases are surgery, radiotherapy, and chemotherapy, used alone or in various combinations. Experience has suggested that in certain diseases one method may be more successful than another, or one method may be definitely contraindicated; at yet other sites either surgery or radiotherapy may give equal results, but one treatment may be preferred because the other produces unacceptable morbidity or late effects. It is, of course, impossible to be dogmatic about any tumor at a particular site; each patient must be considered as an individual problem and the best method of treatment must be prescribed.

The following is a brief guide to the use of radiotherapy in certain malignant diseases.

Lesions where Radiotherapy Is the Treatment of Choice

Here radiotherapy is used because there is a good chance of cure because the lesion is radiosensitive; surgery is often contraindicated because of the extent of the disease involving structures which cannot be removed, and the operation would be disfiguring or would lead to severe disability. In some sites surgery and radiotherapy would give a satisfactory survival, but the morbidity resulting from operation is not acceptable. Examples are: sensitive tumors such as those of embryonal origin; neuroblastoma; medulloblastoma (here it is necessary to irradiate the whole of the CNS because of the method of spread); reticuloses (needing wide fields to cover adjacent lymphatic sites); moderately sensitive tumors of epithelial origin, such as those of the mouth and pharynx, larynx (surgery requires laryngectomy, whereas radiotherapy usually leaves the patient with a good voice), cervix uteri, anus, skin, and bladder; operable anaplastic or oat cell tumors; and inoperable squamous or adenocarcinomas of the bronchus.

Lesions where Either Surgery or Radiotherapy May Give Equally Good Survival, but where One Method May Be Preferred to the Other in Any Individual Patient

For example, carcinoma of the corpus uteri, penis, scrotum, and certain bone tumors; all these lesions are relatively radiosensitive. In skin cancer radiotherapy may be preferred to surgery if the tumor is fixed to bone or involves certain structures such as the eyelid where surgery would be difficult and may leave an unsightly scar or may obstruct the tear duct. Carcinoma of the breast is usually treated by surgery, but in patients who have a fixed lesion radiotherapy may be indicated.

Advanced Inoperable Lesions where Radiotherapy while Achieving Good Palliation May also Produce a Small Percentage of Cures or Control the Lesion for Some Considerable Time

For example, carcinoma of the esophagus, bronchus, kidney, bladder, rectum, and cecum, and advanced breast carcinoma and cerebral tumors.

Palliative Radiotherapy Given with No Chance of Cure and Aimed at Relieving Distressing Symptoms where the Tumor Is Already Widespread

These include bone metastases where often there is dramatic response to treatment; superior vena caval obstruction, but if there are no metastases the lesion is treated radically; advanced, fixed, ulcerated lesions of the skin, breast, etc., causing an offensive discharge or appearance; advanced tumors causing bleeding, for example, in the bladder, bronchus, mouth, etc; metastases in lymph nodes or skin producing symptoms; advanced tumors of the esophagus causing dysphagia.

Lesions where Radiotherapy Is Contraindicated because of the Relative Radioresistance of the Tumor

These include osteogenic sarcoma, where the definitive treatment is surgery followed by chemotherapy. Radiotherapy is indicated where the lesion develops in an inoperable site; many soft-tissue sarcomas, but radiotherapy is indicated if the lesion is inoperable because some show unexpected radiosensitivity; malignant melanoma—very occasionally an inoperable lesion may prove to be radiosensitive; and adenocarcinoma of the gastrointestinal tract; but lesions of the rectum and cecum do sometimes respond to radiotherapy.

This list may appear somewhat confusing because some lesions appear under more than one heading; usually an operable lesion is treated by surgery, but if it involves a vital organ which cannot be removed then radical radiotherapy is indicated. Even in known radioresistant, inoperable tumors radiotherapy should be tried because these tumors sometimes show an unexpected radiosensitivity and may be ablated or at least controlled for sometime, or distressing symptoms may be relieved.

In some operable lesions radical radiotherapy may in fact produce better results; for example, oat cell and anaplastic tumors of the bronchus where histological confirmation has been made on biopsy have a better survival if treated by radiotherapy, whereas squamous lesions and adenocarcinomas are best treated by surgery.

It was stated already that it is impossible to be dogmatic, for each patient needs careful appraisal, usually by both surgeon and radiotherapist, hence the great advantage of combined clinics.

Combined Therapy

Radiotherapy and Surgery

There can be no obvious advantage in employing both radical surgery and radical radiotherapy when either treatment alone can be curative. A combination of the two methods may be used in three ways: (a) preoperative radiotherapy, (b) postoperative radiotherapy, and (c) complementary irradiation.

(a) **Preoperative Radiotherapy.** There is ample evidence that malignant cells may be disseminated at the time of operation and may form metastases, but not all circulating malignant cells are viable. Preoperative radiation may improve the results of surgery because:

(i) It may reduce the number of viable cells released into the blood stream or it may reduce their reproductive capabilities so they are unable to produce metastases. The cells most likely to be disseminated are near blood vessels, well oxygenated, and particularly sensitive to irradiation.

(ii) In the same way cells spilled at the operation site may be attenuated by the irradiation and thus unable to grow.

(iii) The peripheral part of the tumor with its good blood supply may be ablated by irradiation and if the tumor is cut through or if the margin taken around it is inadequate these cells may be so attenuated they will not grow. Arising from this hypothesis it would be inevitably considered possible to convert an inoperable tumor into an operable one; this is, of course, illogical and it would be contrary to normal surgical practice. The tumor is either operable or inoperable at the beginning, and no reliance should be placed on the possible effects of what may be ineffective radiation, because the dose given when surgery is to follow is very likely to be less than that needed to ablate the tumor.

(iv) It has been suggested that irradiation renders the local tissues unsuitable for the growth of malignant cells; this is speculative, for we have no factual evidence and small doses of radiation could improve the possibilities of implantation by increasing the vascularity.

The normal tissues will be unable to withstand a high dose of irradiation if this is followed by extensive surgery; inevitably there will be complications including delayed healing, breakdown of scars, tissue necrosis, bleeding, etc. Many reports of preoperative radiation using high doses have pointed out the marked increase in the number of complications. In addition, the incomplete effects of radiation may suggest to the surgeon that the tumor is smaller than he at first thought, and he is in danger of cutting through potentially malignant tissue.

More recently much lower doses of radiation have been suggested, such as a single treatment of about 500 rads given within 24 h of operation, a dose which would be sufficient to cause an attenuation of the dividing cells in most tumors. Such radiation has been suggested in the combined treatment of carcinoma of the bronchus, rectum, esophagus, bladder, and possibly breast.

(b) **Postoperative Irradiation.** If tumor has been left behind at operation we are treating a tumor which has been incompletely removed and a radical course of radiotherapy will be required. Sometimes the term "prophylactic radiation" is used but such a concept is untenable, for radiation cannot prevent malignant diseases. The meaning is that excision has been incomplete or extends up to the edge of the excised specimen, or cells have been spilled and thus radical treatment is needed. In this way it is possible to salvage a few more patients. There is no indication for radiation if the surgeon and pathologist are satisfied that excision is complete.

(c) **Complementary Radiation.** This is given as part of the planned treatment program; surgery may deal with one part of the malignant process and radiotherapy another, the two are planned to cover the whole malignant disease. Perhaps the best examples are carcinoma of the breast, where the primary lesion may be removed by simple mastectomy and the lymph node areas are irradiated to a radical tumor dose; or carcinoma of the mouth where the primary lesion may be dealt with by X- or gamma-ray therapy, or by an implant, and the cervical nodes by a block dissection.

This treatment must be planned by surgeons and radiotherapists *before* starting any therapy in combined clinics.

Radiotherapy and Chemotherapy

The use of chemotherapeutic agents to add to the radiation effects on the primary tumor has been mentioned already but these agents may be used also to treat any metastases, clinical or occult. Again the term "prophylactic chemotherapy" must not be used for cytotoxic agents will not prevent metastases but are given on the supposition that small ones exist already. Controlled clinical trials using single chemotherapeutic agents have proved to be disappointing, but it is possible that multiple agents may be more successful, and clinical trials are in progress. This subject is dealt with in chapter 16 and is not elaborated on here.

Radiation Effects

Damage can be caused to all tissues by irradiation. Initially the treatment produces a reaction similar to an inflammatory reaction with hyperemia, edema, desquamation of cells, and increase in lymphocytes, foreign body cells, and fibroblasts. The reaction will vary according to the site irradiated; thus in the skin there is initially an erythema progressing to moist desquamation; in mucous membranes there is a thick membranous reaction, as may be found in the mouth, esophagus, vagina, and rectum; in the lung, pneumonitis filling the alveoli with desquamated cells; and in lymphocytes, a hyaline membrane reaction and thickening around the small blood vessels; each structure showing its unique response. If the damage is minimal, repair will occur, and it may be impossible to detect any noticeable permanent effect. If the damage kills cells these can only be replaced by fibrous tissue; some such damage to normal tissues will inevitably occur when radical treatment is given to cure a tumor. Fibrotic effects may be permanent, for example, lung fibrosis, fibrosis causing constriction of the smaller blood vessels in the kidney leading to radiation nephritis and hypertension, cataract of the lens, etc.

At a later stage further changes may occur in the fibrotic area. For example, in fibrotic scars of the skin any abrasion or injury may break down the equilibrium of the tissues and a necrotic ulcer may develop, possibly with infection (the treatment is excision). Years later even further changes may occur leading to the development of malignant changes.

In addition to the radiation effects on normal tissues there are radiation effects on the tumor which may be replaced by scar tissue. Thus cure of a lung cancer will cause lung fibrosis with a mediastinal shift to the affected side, elevation of the diaphragm, contraction of the overlying ribs, and even scoliosis. The circumferential spread of tumors in the bladder means that ablation may cause contraction of the bladder; ablation of an annular carcinoma of the esophagus will lead to a fibrotic stricture, and so on. All these reactions are fully described in standard textbooks of radiotherapy. The surgeon must, however, be aware of the fibrotic effects resulting from irradiation. Radiographs of a postradiation chest may show fibrotic consolidation and must be differentiated from malignant disease, either primary or secondary, and from infection. Late reactions may occur in the rectum after treatment for a carcinoma of the cervix uteri. Typically these involve the anterior and lateral walls which receive the maximum dose of radiation, the so-called "horseshoe proctitis." A rectal examination may reveal thickening somewhat similar to a primary rectal tumor and even the symptoms of pain, tenesmus, mucus, and bleeding are similar.

Information to the Patient

Much has been written about informing the patient of his illness. This is not discussed here; only a plea is made that the surgeon consider carefully what information he gives about radiotherapy before referring the patient. If possible, this is left to the radiotherapist. The surgeon has obtained already the patient's confidence and the new consultant is at a disadvantage, for he is unknown and somewhat feared. However good the surgeon's intentions the treatment given subsequently by the radiotherapist may not be that described by the surgeon. For example, if the patient expects daily treatment five times weekly for 4 weeks and is given twice weekly treatments he is immediately suspicious that all might not be right. Again, external beam therapy may be given instead of a radium implant. The discovery that a lesion is not operable may lead the surgeon to give a hopeless prognosis, even though the patient may be quite treatable and curable by radiation. A greater knowledge of radiotherapeutic techniques will convince the surgeon that there are many that are tailored to suit the individual patient.

Research

Brief details are given of some research carried out in the radiotherapy department for all radiotherapists aim at developing new techniques to improve survival rates and reduce morbidity.

Controlled Clinical Trials

Most radiotherapists anxious to determine the optimum treatment conditions are involved in controlled clinical trials; some of these may be in association with surgeons, some are multicenter trials carried out in various departments at the same time and are carefully controlled. Such trials often take many years to complete.

Computers

The complex mathematics associated with the calculation of the treatment fields has been greatly simplified by the use of computer techniques; in addition it is now possible to investigate the isodose distribution in various places which were not possible before. Computers have also made the analysis of patients' case histories easier; all departments keep careful records of patients treated and meticulously follow them up until death, such records can be recorded on computer tape and analyzed.

Selection of Patients for Treatment

For many years we have searched for methods of selecting suitable patients for radical treatment, but too often a complicated course of treatment is interrupted by the appearance of previously hidden metastases which completely change the prognosis. Recent studies of immunological techniques suggest possible ways of carrying out this selection. Radioactive isotope techniques have enabled us to detect occult metastases not detectable by other techniques. Sophisticated methods of ascertaining the limits of the growth will enable us not only to cover the tumor with adequate fields but also to avoid unecessary irradiation to adjacent normal tissues.

Radiation Techniques

It seems unlikely that there will be many developments in the production of newer radiation machines, we already have sources of radiation capable of treating all lesions in the body. Further developments will involve the determination of the optimum methods of using these machines. Thus, various techniques are being investigated, including fractionation, hyperbaric oxygen, neutron therapy, radiosensitizers, and combined treatments (surgery or chemotherapy with radiation), etc. These techniques also demand a greater knowledge of the effects of radiation which is provided by radiobiological studies. It is possible that tissue culture techniques may enable us to carry out trials on the tissue obtained by biopsy and to determine the optimum radiation techniques for that particular tumor; in the same way it may be possible to determine the best cytotoxic agent which will affect the growing culture.

Rehabilitation

Definitive treatment is only part of the rehabilitation of the patient to enable him or her to resume a life of good quality. It is regrettable that many people, medical included, imagine that malignant diseases are incurable, with the result that few facilities exist for the rehabilitation of patients. There is an obvious need for research into all aspects of this important work. This subject is further considered in chapter 17.

Conclusion

Radiotherapy has an established place in the treatment of certain malignant diseases; continuing research is producing improved results of treatment, and there is a distinct possibility that existing techniques can be improved. Too frequently the radiotherapist is not consulted until the disease has reached an advanced stage. It is hoped that a broad oncological approach to the management of malignant diseases will result in a better appreciation of the value of this mode of therapy; the result could be a swing to treatment aimed at a cure rather than palliation. Throughout this chapter the importance of combined clinics has been stressed, where surgeon and radiotherapist can agree about the best method of treatment.

References

Deeley, T. J. (1972–3). Radiotherapy. In *The British Encyclopaedia of Medical Practice* (R. Richardson, ed.). Butterworth, London.
Deeley T. J. (1974). *Needle Biopsy*. Butterworth, London.
Snelling M. D. (1967). Place of radiotherapy in treatment of malignant disease. *Ann. Royal Coll. Surg. Summer Suppl.* **41**:147–150.

Chapter 16

CHEMOTHERAPY

I. W. F. HANHAM

Today a clinician who embarks on or specializes in cancer chemotherapy must have a basic knowledge of the mechanism of action of at least a dozen or more chemical agents which are active against cancer; and he must be aware of the importance of cell kinetics, dose schedules of those drugs, toxicity and its management, and the pharmacological background of the drugs he is using, particularly their mutual interactions and individual behavior. He must always be aware of the problems which can develop with individual patients.

No single cancer agent is entirely specific for any type of tumor, although there may be a broad clinical response by individual drugs in certain types of cases. Since the successful introduction of combination regimes, the complexities of chemotherapy have increased so that critical and expert judgment is required for dosages and timing of administration.

Scientific results suggest that cell kinetics are fundamental to the basis of treatment regimes. Other factors include the interrelations of drugs in combination, their timing of administration, and the order and frequency with which drugs are given in relation to the cell cycle and its metabolism.

Experimental chemotherapy today involves the international screening of 30,000–40,000 compounds each year. Only a very few of these are acceptable for experimental clinical trial, mostly due to high toxicity. New compounds are found continually which are specific against individual tumors or active in a particular part of the cell cycle. Interest also predominates in drugs which potentiate radiotherapy and increase the sensitivity of tumors.

Most patients who succumb to cancer do so from metastases in vital organs and systemic chemotherapy forms a major attempt to eradicate or

I. W. F. Hanham • Consultant in Oncology and Radiotherapy, Westminster Hospital, London, SWIF 2AP, England.

control them. Hellmann and Burrage (1969) and Salsbury *et al.* (1970, 1974) have shown in recent experimental work with 1,2-di(3,5-dioxopiperazine-1-yl) propane (ICRF 159) that blood-borne metastases can be specifically inhibited by normalization of the development of new blood vessels at the margin of experimental malignant tumors.

Present techniques have evolved rapidly since the first basic discoveries 30 years ago, when mustard compounds were shown to affect leukocytes, lymphatic tissue, and bone marrow. This was followed by the first successful introduction of a metabolic antagonist, amethopterin, in the treatment of acute lymphoblastic leukemia. Synthesis of experimental and clinical work of over 30 years has now resulted in modern combination chemotherapy with the potential cure of certain cancers such as choriocarcinoma, Burkitt's lymphoma, acute lymphoblastic leukemia, malignant tumors of the testes, and Hodgkin's disease. At the same time, chemotherapy combined with surgery and/or radiotherapy promises cure in many patients with childhood solid tumors, such as Wilm's tumor, embryonal rhabdomyosarcoma, and Ewing's sarcoma. In other malignancies, a significant degree of cell kill is reflected in a high rate of objective tumor regression and prolonged survival, although cure cannot be shown at present. These tumors include adenocarcinomas of the breast and ovary, non-Hodgkin's lymphoma, multiple myeloma, chronic leukemias, and acute myelocytic leukemia. In other diseases, chemotherapy can achieve objective regression and palliation in one-fifth to one-third of patients.

The basis of chemotherapy is a fundamental consideration of cell function in relation to the pharmacology of cytotoxic drugs.

Cell Kinetics

Mitosis involves the replication of DNA and is the process by which mature, normal dying cells such as those of the skin, gastrointestinal tract, and bone marrow are replaced; however, this same process is also involved in the renewal of cancer cells, against which chemotherapy is directed.

The cells of the body have been described as having individual, or internal, and "social," or external, functions. Individual or internal cells maintain natural products such as hemoglobin, insulin, or steroids, or constituent elements such as osteoid, keratin, or cilia. Their activities depend on the ability of genetic material in DNA to be transformed to specific RNA and proteins involved in each individual physiological process.

External function is responsible for limiting normal, nonmalignant cell growth by contact inhibition with other cells or humoral feedback. Clonogenic cells remain in reserve, maintaining their capacity to divide, if stimulated to do so, as a result of injury to, or death of, their constituent cell.

When a cell divides, the daughter cell's cytoplasm increases in size due to the metabolic activity of ribonucleic acid formed from individual proteins and molecules related to the function of that cell; this is described at the "G_1" phase. Only a few daughter cells undergo differentiation and this occurs after a replicative stimulus. These are known as immature "G" or "stem cells." These stem cells, with the appropriate stimulus, will form new DNA. "G_1" can, therefore, vary from several hours to several years.

If a cell differentiates it passes into "S" phase where there is a restricted period of intense DNA synthesis; purine and pyrimidine bases are synthesized, forming into nucleotides, and combining into new strands of DNA that are complementary to the single components of the double helix. The action of most chemotherapeutic agents is in the "S" phase, when they are particularly involved in the demand of the cell to synthesize new purine and pyrimidine bases, in the appearance of enzymes concerned in biosynthesis, phosphorylation, and polymerization of bases, and in the opening up of the double helix, with uncovering of multiple reactive sites along the individual DNA chains.

"S" phase is followed by "G_2," which is a time of metabolic consolidation. Anticancer drugs at this stage of cell activity would affect synthesis of cytoplasmic and associated DNA proteins, as well as the maintenance of cell membranes.

Mitosis or "M" phase follows and proceeds for about 1 h, but little metabolic activity occurs. The only agents active at this stage are spindle-fiber-inhibiting poisons such as Vinca and colchium alkaloids.

The new tumor daughter cells, after "M" phase or completion of mitosis, have three possible fates:

(i) About 20–80% die because of natural defects and lack of transfer of genetic information necessary to recreate their vital metabolic processes. These appear as ghost cells and represent a large natural loss of tumor cells. Chemotherapeutic drugs can also contribute to the formation of these deficient cells, because drugs acting in "S" phase create cells with sublethally damaged DNA or interfere with DNA repair; also, protein and RNA synthesis can be affected in the "G_2" phase, giving rise to nonviable cells.

(ii) Other cells pass through a rapid "G_1" into "S" phase, providing that fraction of continuously dividing cells responsible for continuous tumor growth. This faction is most sensitive to anti-DNA metabolites and enzyme inhibitors.

(iii) A few cells have low metabolic activity and enter a prolonged, dormant "G_0" phase; these will provide a base for recurrence, are inevitably a poor target for chemotherapy, and become the most difficult to eradicate.

Pharmacology

The pharmacology of anticancer drugs relates, then, to the characteristics of tumor cells against which drug intervention is aimed, and to their host, which is the patient being treated.

Action of Cytotoxic Drugs

Molecular size is important in the pharmacology of drug action. Antitumor agents may be of small molecular size, such as hydroxycarbamide (hydroxyurea), or large and complex, such as dactinomycin (actinomycin D). Size determines whether a drug can cross a cell membrane, and such transport is usually by passive diffusion or nonconcentrative facilitative diffusion, or it is actively against a concentration gradient. Drugs reach their sites of action within the cell by one of these methods, and all three are, obviously, more difficult for large than for small molecules. If there is slow transport, larger molecular weight drugs must be in contact for a longer time, and this is achieved by higher, prolonged concentration in extracellular fluid. The mechanism of drug transport into certain areas, such as the cerebrospinal fluid or chambers of the eye, excludes molecules which are large, have net charges, or lack lipid solubility, and it is an important concept in the management of disease in these areas.

A drug's solubility is important for its therapeutic use, as highly insoluble drugs must be given orally; the size of the dose of a relatively insoluble drug may also limit parenteral use because of the volume of solvent required, and this obviously is important when using an intramuscular route. The environmental physiological pH for a drug is also critical; as in the spinal fluid, transport may be slowed down or speeded up by an increase or reduction in the *net* charge of a drug molecule. Some drugs are unstable at the acid pH of the stomach, such as triethylenemelamine (TEM) which, if given by mouth, has to be preceded by a suitable alkali.

Local tissue sensitivity always requires expert supervision and administration. Comparing two antibiotics, mitomycin C and bleomycin, perivenous extravazation of mitomycin C will cause severe tissue necrosis, whereas bleomycin can be injected subcutaneously, intramuscularly, or intravenously without reaction. The damage to local tissue by a drug can be exploited by direct injection into a malignant skin lesion or superficial node, with compounds such as podophylin, dactinomycin, or thiotepa, by necrosis of malignant cells.

The irritating effects of a drug on the central nervous system will make it unsuitable for intrathecal use. But certain drugs are routinely used in prophylaxis of acute lymphatic, meningeal leukemia. Methotrexate and cytosine arabinoside can safely be given intrathecally; but other antileukemic drugs, such as 6-mercaptopurine and vincristine, are highly toxic to the central nervous system.

The antimetabolites, such as methotrexate and 5-fluorouracil, have a primary and secondary action. The primary site, with methotrexate, is by the inhibition of dihydrofolate reductase, an effect seen primarily in dividing cells; but a very high concentration of methotrexate may also affect *non*dividing tissue and act secondarily on normal liver cells when used in an intrahepatic arterial infusion.

Mustard compounds give rise to a parasympathomimetic effect and central nervous toxicity when given intraarterially into the brain or head and neck region. Cytosine arabinoside kills cells directly, as well as acting in the "S" phase, and its secondary action depends on its rate of deamination in the liver.

Characteristics of Tumor Cells

An understanding of drug reaction in tumor cells is fundamental to chemotherapy.

The content of amino acids in a cell's membrane might influence a tumor's sensitivity to a particular drug which could be responsible for L-asparaginase's action.

The rate of synthesis of cell membrane glycoproteins and degradation of cell membranes by specific glyocisidases also determines the resistance to various drugs such as daunorubicin and dactinomycin. Resistance follows a dramatic fall in the activity of the glycosidase enzymes and an increase in the activity of glycoprotein transferase. It is also possible that specific aspects of the composition or rate of synthesis of the cell are responsible for the highly tissue-specific action of the corticosteroids.

The transport of certain antitumor agents such as free purine and pyrimidine is, apparently, by passive diffusion, their neucleosides having a highly effective, facilitated transport mechanism. Most neucleotides are, however, prevented from crossing membranes as they are charged molecules; but when these compounds are formed within the cell from free bases or neucleosides by the action of intracellular phosphorylating enzymes they are retained within the cell, inhibit specific enzymes, and act as cytotoxics.

Facilitated diffusion is involved in membrane transport of methotrexate and possibly mithramycin and bleomycin. The amount of methotrexate retained within the cell is critically dependent upon its extracellular concentration. Intermittent administration of this drug greatly increases the plasma concentration for a short time, hence the intracellular concentration. But low doses and oral administration do not achieve this effect.

The effect of drugs on tumor cells will depend on whether they are

near a blood vessel, and it is influenced by diffusion; this is not the case
with cells further away or in necrotic or fibrotic tissue. Leukemia cells, on
the other hand, circulate freely, with free access to the sinusoids of the
marrow, and are the most easily affected tumor cells.

The Basis of Interrelation of Cell Kinetics and Pharmacology

If a drug enters a cell, it interreacts with its appropriate receptor,
whose availability will depend on the phase of the cell cycle. At the same
time, it is hoped to exploit the difference in sensitivity between normal and
tumor cells to create a favorable therapeutic ratio between tumor and
normal cells. This, in many cases, is achieved and normal tissue toxicity is
avoided. In the present state of knowledge it is not possible, in solid
tumors, to measure the endpoint of eradication of cells, with potential
proliferate capacity, which might remain after treatment, or to demonstrate
the phase of the cell cycle *in vivo,* for a drug to reach its maximum
therapeutic effect. The drug concentration–time relationships which are
most likely to achieve maximum destruction of neoplastic cells with minimum effect on normal cells are also not known, and treatment can be
complicated by an individual patient's variation in tolerance to a given dose
of a drug, particularly those which rely on liver metabolism, such as
methotrexate, cyclophosphamide, and 5-(3-3-dimethyl-1-trizeno)imidazole-
4-carboxamide (DTIC). It is known clinically that intermittent high dose
concentrations of drugs are more effective.

In order to kill all the cells and so eradicate disease, it is accepted,
experimentally, that:

(1) Tumor cell kill, per cell cycle, should exceed 50% of those cells.

(2) Working with a cycle-dependent drug and assuming there is always
asynchrony of dividing cells, several optimal doses should be given over a
period longer than the mean tumor-cell generation time (otherwise cells
with a longer generation time than the mean could escape).

(3) Rest periods allow for recovery of normal tissues (notably bone
marrow, where resting stem cells will be mobilized which might otherwise
be destroyed) except for periods in which the number of tumor cells should
not increase to that initially present.

(4) Cure will only be achieved if, by repeated drug course, the number
of living tumor cells can be reduced theoretically to a number less than 1,
but without inflicting lethal damage to the host's normal cells.

It is known, experimentally, that when the appropriate drug receptors
are exposed cell kill proceeds exponentially (and is often expressed as log
kill); that is, a given drug, during a given time, kills a near-constant

percentage of cells, independent of their actual number; but that number, at the start of treatment, may make it impossible to kill a sufficient amount of sensitive tumor cells without causing lethal host damage.

Cellular resistance may develop by selection of, or mutation to, less sensitive or nonsensitive variants; this can be prevented or reduced by multidrug therapy. Drug failure can also result from tumor cells escaping to sites not reached by drugs, as in meningeal leukemia. Tumor cells can also be unaffected in sites where drug action is counteracted. Leukemic cells in the gastrointestinal tract become resistant to asparaginase because normal asparagine and amino acid levels cannot be sufficiently depleted.

Cells not in cycle, such as in prolonged "G_1" phase do not have exposed sensitive drug receptors. In solid tumors they will only enter the cell cycle to proliferate, where there is clearance of replicating cells by drug treatment. However, experiments using alternating, cycle-dependent drugs such as cytosine arabinoside, and cycle-independent drugs such as cyclophosphamide, have cured tumors containing cells out of cycle.

A normal loss of proliferating cells occurs in certain tumors. During a rest from chemotherapy, the number of proliferating cells will not increase to that present at the start of treatment. Tumors which have high, normal proliferative cell loss, such as Burkitt's lymphoma and choriocarcinoma, appear to be more easily cured. It also follows that tumors in which *all* cells continue to proliferate actively are more difficult to cure than those with a stemline compartment which is not actively proliferating and so increasing in size.

The most important principle in chemotherapy should be to treat a tumor as early as possible, as this gives the optimum result.

(1) The number of cells to be killed initially should be in the curable range (surgery and/or radiotherapy can be used to reduce the number of cells to this level).

(2) In large tumors, drug penetration is reduced by poor vascularity, so that cells with proliferative capacity, located in necrotic areas, will often survive.

(3) Immunological competence is gradually repressed over the long term by the tumor itself and is, therefore, unlikely to have an additive therapeutic effect.

(4) As tumor volume increases, the growth fraction will decrease, and so tumor cell generation time may increase, being less cell-cycle-dependent, with individual treatments.

Experimental work suggests that it may be possible to artificially synchronize asynchronous tumor cells at a chosen moment of cellular activity; drugs available at present for such clinical use would be methotrexate, 5-fluorouracil, and hydroxyurea, and this, theoretically, could ensure a maximum cytotoxic effect in the cell cycle.

Characteristics of the Tumor Host that Affect Drug Action

Children appear to be capable of tolerating larger doses of certain antitumor drugs than adults, and with increasing age the capacity to tolerate myelosuppressive drugs decreases.

Females currently producing estrogen have the disadvantage of its depressing effect on bone marrow, so exacerbating any tendency to anemia. The presence of active estrogens can affect the hepatic metabolism of numerous antitumor agents, so varying the toxicity and effectiveness of such drugs.

African children with Burkitt's lymphoma tolerate higher doses than white children, which partly explains the greater effectiveness of cyclophosphamide in this tumor in Africans. In contrast, Pinkel *et al.* (1970) has stated that American negro children with acute lymphoblastic leukemia appear to be much less responsive to an identical drug regime, in groups that are age related and socioeconomically equivalent, than their white counterparts.

Previous radiotherapy, chemotherapy, or estrogen treatment also affects a patient's capacity to tolerate myelosuppressive drugs. Binding to plasma proteins can form a basis for drug interactions, and displacement from such binding by drugs such as phenylbutazone can alter in an unpredictable way the effectiveness of a drug in an individual patient. Intracellular binding is also important as part of the pharmacological action.

Drug Excretion. Kidney excretion is critical for some drugs, such as methotrexate and cyclophosphamide. No active metabolism of methotrexate takes place in humans, and it is excreted unchanged in the kidneys by an active secretion process of the proximal, convoluted renal tubule. It is known that a large intravenous "fraction" of methotrexate is excreted quickly by this route before there is sufficient time for it to intoxicate the bone marrow. In contrast, a patient's bone marrow can only tolerate a small *daily* oral dose, as the rate of excretion is so much slower. The toxicity of methotrexate is increased by moderate renal dysfunction and, therefore, preliminary assessment of renal function is essential.

Cyclophosphamide is excreted by the kidneys, as the original compound and in its activated form, but when the patient's urine is concentrated it requires only a small fraction of the activated compound to cause hemorrhagic cystitis, which is more common when using higher intravenous fractions than in oral therapy. Concurrent treatment with barbiturates, phenothiazones, or phenylbutazone can cause alteration in hepatic metabolism of certain drugs, and so affect their activation and toxicity.

Drug Metabolism. Cyclophosphamide is activated in the patient's liver by hydrolysis of parent compound, but if there are metastases or other liver disease this will result in diminution of overall drug activation and decreased clinical effectiveness of a particular dose of cyclophosphamide.

Catabolism of drugs is also carried out by the liver. The deamination of cytosine arabinoside is critical to its therapeutic effectiveness. 5-Fluorouracil is also detoxicated by the liver and can produce increased hematological toxicity if the amount of functioning liver tissue is decreased by disease. Vinca alkaloids are also excreted by the liver.

Methotrexate affects renal tubular function and a mild diuresis is often seen, and it can also cause renal failure. Its secretion into the cerebrospinal fluid by the choroid plexus is low and combined with a poor transport across the blood brain barrier makes it impossible to achieve therapeutic concentration. The "outward reverse secretion" may prevent toxicity to the central nervous system when high levels of this drug are given intrathecally.

Host–Tumor Drug Interactions

In a response to a tumor *antigen,* the host may develop circulating antibodies. They are normally weak and may attach themselves to the surface of the cells. A patient may produce a lymphocyte cytotoxic tuberculin type of immunity, which theoretically could kill tumor cells but could be blocked by antibodies. Age can modify immune response; children and the very old are deficient in immunological competence. In contrast, nonneoplastic conditions such as a gammaglobulin anemia, protein depletion, autoimmune disease, and malaria can cause immunological hyperactivity.

The effect of drugs in host–tumor interactions are unpredictable; some appear to inhibit circulatory blocking antibodies more strongly than cytotoxic lymphocytes and so could have a beneficial effect in destroying blocking antibodies. But vincristine and cytoxine arabinoside may destroy cell-mediated immunity rather than humoral antibodies, and so promote tumor growth.

There is critical timing between the administration of drugs and antibody suppression. It is impossible at present to know if by giving antitumor therapy to a patient with a tumor of a type known to be associated with host tumor antigens that it will be detrimental. Patients who receive cytotoxic treatment respond for a longer period than those who have had no therapy, even if agents are immunosuppressive. In those who do *not* respond, then life may have been foreshortened by immunosuppression, without any beneficial cytotoxic effect on the tumor.

Cytotoxicity

Toxicity is not necessary to achieve clinical response, and this is particularly true with the antimetabolite 5-fluorouracil. Clinical response with intravenous 5-fluorouracil, 500 mg once weekly in breast and colonic carcinoma is in no way altered by varying the concentration, frequency, or route of administration of the drug which depends for its action on the presence of the enzymes iridine phosphorylase and pyrimidine phosphoribosyltransferase.

Higher antimetabolite levels may more effectively inhibit the high amount of enzymes present in the normal dividing cells of the host and increase toxicity without increasing response. A remission may be achieved earlier by increasing the initial dose, but the overall clinical result is no different than that of standard therapy, and there is an increased risk of toxicity.

With directly cytotoxic alkylating agents, a dose–response situation applies; the higher the dose, the more effective is the response. However, the optimum time intervals for repeated doses to the tumor cells with alkylating agents can be therapeutically prolonged, and cumulative toxicity can be avoided.

The patients most susceptible to leukopenia or thrombocytopenia are those who have had previous cytotoxic therapy, or tumor infiltration of the bone marrow, because their marrow reserve is accordingly reduced.

Most chemotherapists accept some diminution in the leukocyte count or other mild symptoms of organ toxicity as an indication that the dose is at the upper limit of tolerance of the patient. Levels of 3,000 leukocytes per mm^3 and 100,000 platelets are safe when using cytotoxic agents, but in some patients it is necessary to accept a leukocyte count of 1,000 or less to make an impact on a critical disease; a diminution of platelets below 100,000 is acceptable in the absence of purpura. However, this problem must be under the expert care of a physician who has facilities for fresh blood and platelet transfusion, reversed barrier nursing, or a vertical laminar bacteria-free air-flow environment. These supportive measures are particularly necessary in diseases such as leukemia, which are characterized by massive bone marrow replacement, or in patients on combination therapy which may reduce the amount of remaining bone marrow.

Chemotherapy palliation may take several weeks to become apparent and immediate, full supportive measures should be instituted to help patients with extensive metastases.

Effective chemotherapy can sometimes produce side effects which are, in themselves, temporarily life endangering. Hyperuricemia and renal failure may occur following adequate therapy of lymphoma or leukemia; allopurinol can prevent this condition, although it is synergistic with 6-mercaptopurine cytotoxicity and can induce secondary gout, and must be used with caution. Vomiting, dehydration, and confusion are often a manifestion of hypercalcemia, particularly in breast carcinoma following androgen or estrogen therapy. Treatment is either by mithramycin at the safe dose of one-fifth to one-tenth of the antitumor dose, or by triple phosphate infusion where 100 ml of solution is given per milligram of serum calcium above normal; or if these compounds are not available, large doses of systemic hydrocortisone may be used.

The effect of antitumor therapy on the suppression of immune response can create problems, particularly with opportunistic or autoinfection. Hersh *et al.* (1971) studied patients receiving 5-day courses of intensive chemotherapy for leukemia. The immune parameters used were macrophage entry into experimental inflammatory sites (the skin window), response to primary antigenic stimulation, and lymphocyte stimulation to phytohemagglutinin. There was a marked decrease in all these parameters while the patient was on treatment, but within 2–3 days there was complete, or nearly complete, recovery in immunological response, and in many patients immunological "overshoot" occurred during the recovery period. Therefore, with combination therapy given over 5 days every 2–4 weeks, the patient's immunological apparatus appears to be normal, whereas with continuous treatment a lesser initial degree of immunological depression occurs, but is sustained and tends to be progressive.

As there is evidence that cellular or T-cell immunity is the major restraining factor of immune response and since humoral antibodies may be enhancing or blocking this response, it is found that intermittent chemotherapy, as opposed to continuous treatment, impairs the blocking humoral function and allows for a greater cell-mediated response by preserving cellular immunity. This situation can be projected so that if active immunization is part of the treatment protocol, it will be most effective at the time of recovery or overshoot, and there is evidence that fungal, viral, and pneumocystic infections are less frequent in patients maintained on long-term, intermittent chemotherapy than in those on continuous chemotherapy.

Classification of Drugs

Some of the drugs in common use in surgical oncology, together with their action, are discussed below:

Conventional

Alkylating Agents
(i) They directly attack biochemical compounds of importance to cells, such as nucleic acids and enzymes. A critical portion of physiologically important molecules are made unavailable for normal metabolic reactions by connecting the drug and target molecule with a covalent bond.

(ii) They inhibit rapidly dividing cell populations. These rely on the availability, during the mitotic cycle, of highly reactive portions of the DNA molecule and of the enzymes involved in nucleic acid biosynthesis. DNA sites which are affected are: (a) phosphate sugar ester bonds, (b) the N-7 of guanine, and (c) cross-linking between adjacent hydrogen bonded bases on the double helix. These reactions are not cancer specific and will involve the marrow, gastrointestinal tract, hair follicles, and other rapidly dividing normal tissues of the body.

(iii) They act independently of DNA synthesis and cell division and attack preformed macromolecules such as nucleic acid. They are effective against slowly dividing normal lymphocytes and cells of lymphoma and chronic lymphatic leukemia; this is a nonmitotic cycle-linked effect and, as such, is similar to a radiation effect. Larger doses are more effective than smaller ones in creating a dose–response relationship.

The following drugs are in this classification:

(i) Nitrogen Mustard (Mustine). This compound is unstable and irritating to tissues. It is rapidly toxic, not only to malignant tissue, but also to the bone marrow and central nervous system, giving rise to myelosuppression, nausea, and vomiting.

Its use is in "emergencies," such as superior vena caval obstruction or extradural spinal cord compression, particularly from bonchial carcinoma or lymphoma. The dose is 4–6 mg intravenously. It is also part of combination therapy M.O.P.P. or M.V.P.P. in Hodgkin's disease (see Combination Therapy).

(ii) Cyclophosphamide. This drug has the unusual characteristic of platelet sparing. It is excreted in urine as its active or partly unchanged form and gives rise to hemorrhagic cystitis, with a concentrated urine. Alopecia is common, but hair can grow again during treatment. It is activated by hydrolysis of its ring structure in the liver; is poorly soluble, but stable, and is given orally or intravenously, in a large volume of solvent.

It is used in "emergencies" such as superior vena caval or extradural compression, with bronchial carcinomas or lymphomas. Dose is 1 g intravenously on 2 consecutive days.

It is also used intravenously in combination regimes, particularly in breast carcinoma, Wilm's tumor, neuroblastoma, testicular carcinoma, and, as a single agent, orally in carcinoma of the ovary.

(iii) Melphalan (Phenylalanine Mustard). This is a stable analogue of nitrogen mustard. Usually it does not cause alopecia, but it does cause cumulative bone marrow toxicity after prolonged dosage.

A large pulsed, single dose is given for carcinoma of the ovary. This dose is 30–50 mg given intravenously in 500 cc of 5% dextrose over 4–6 h and repeated every 8 weeks. In multiple myeloma it is given as part of an intermittent schedule of 2 mg twice a day for 4 days, with 5 mg of oral prednisone three times a day for 7 days.

(iv) Chlorambucil. This is a stable analogue of nitrogen mustard. It is given in an oral dose of 2–4 mg daily, 5 days a week, and is used mainly in carcinoma of the ovary and chronic lymphatic leukemia. Side effects are usually cumulative bone marrow toxicity, after many months.

(v) Thiotepa. This drug is mainly used in a direct local injection into a tumor, in intravesical instillation for bladder cancer in a dose of 30 mg, and for intrapleural or peritoneal infusion in a dose of 15–30 mg. Its main disadvantage is myelosuppression, particularly of platelets. However, it has the advantage of being nonirritating to normal tissue following local injection.

Antimetabolites. These interfere with metabolic pathways commonly involved in cell function, especially cell division. They interfere with DNA synthesis and are structural analogues of precursor molecules such as purines, pyrimidines, and their nucleosides or cofactors, such as folic acid. These drugs will interfere with biosynthetic enzymes or form spurious macromolecules, which leads to nonfunction and death of tumor cells.

These agents are mitotically linked but can also be incorporated, like 5-fluorouracil, into RNA and cause abnormalities of proteins necessary for cell function.

This group includes the following compounds:

(i) Folic Acid Antagonist (Methotrexate). Toxicity is myelosuppression, stomatitis, diarrhea, renal toxicity, and cirrhosis after prolonged use. Its importance is in acute lymphoblastic leukemia, as part of the present multicentric trial. This employs multiple, prolonged drug therapy for 30 months and includes prophylactic intrathecal methotrexate and cranial irradiation. It is also included in the treatment of choriocarcinoma, and Price and Goldie (1971) have used it as the main feature of their high-dose "pulsed" combination therapy, but this type of treatment requires careful supervision and monitoring.

Methotrexate interferes with dihydrofolate reductase, an important enzyme in one carbon metabolism, being required for C-2 and C-8 of purines, and also for conversion of deoxyuridylate to thymidylate by addition of a 5-methyl group. Activity is proportional to uptake into cells achieved with the high blood levels following intravenous administration, with rapid renal secretion and excretion. It is not metabolized in the body and, in the event of poor renal function, can remain for a long time in the tissues with marked toxicity.

Intravenous dosage varies from 5–30 mg weekly, depending on the individual patients; orally, 2.5–5.0 mg daily.

(ii) Antipurines (6-Mercaptopurine). This drug acts by interfering, at

multiple sites, with the conversion of purine prior to incorporation into DNA. Activity depends upon the phosphorylation of the drug within the target cell. It is also synergestic with allopurinol.

(iii) Antipyrimidines (5-Fluorouracil and Cytosine Arabinoside). 5-Flourouracil can cause myelosuppression, stomatis, gastrointestinal ulceration, nausea, vomiting, alopecia, and cerebellar ataxia. Cytosine arabinoside can cause myelosuppression, megaloblastic anemia, nausea, and vomiting.

5-Fluorouracil is particularly useful in adenocarcinoma of the breast and colon; cytosine arabinoside, in acute leukemias.

5-Fluorouracil interferes with the biosynthesis of nucleotides or thymidine, or with their subsequent incorporation into DNA. Its metabolites interfere with the synthesis of thymidylate from deoxyuridylate by the inhibition of thymidylate synthetase, an enzyme involved in the addition of the formyl group at C-5 of uracil. Breast and colon tumors might contain floxuridine macrophosphates which metabolize 5-fluorouracil.

The usual dose is 500 mg weekly iv.

Natural Products: Antibiotics

Dactinomycin (actinomycin D). Toxicity includes myelosuppression of all formed elements, with photosensitization of previously irradiated areas. Its side effects are dermatitis, alopecia, nausea, and vomiting.

It is used particularly in the treatment of female choriocarcinoma, but is less useful in chorionic carcinomas of the male testes.

It is currently used in the combination regime (D.A.V.E.) for Wilm's tumor. This regime is: actinomycin D, 0.6 mg/m² on days 1 and 8; adriamycin, 30 mg/m² on days 1 and 8; vincristine, 0.8 mg/m² on days 1 and 8; cyclophosphamide, 200 mg/m² on days 1 and 8. This course is given every 3–4 weeks for six treatments and then at increased intervals, and is completed after 2 years. Survival rates of 85% have been quoted in early disease.

Vinca Alkaloids. These are derived from the common periwinkle, and include vincristine and vinblastine:

Vincristine can cause cumulative neurotoxicity including acroparesthesias, loss of tendon reflexes, and weakness of the extremities, excluding the drug for maintenance therapy. Vinblastine has been substituted in combination regimes to avoid neurotoxicities. Other side effects include neuropathic adynamic ileus with remitting constipation and alopecia. Its particular value is in inducing remissions in acute lymphoblastic leukemia.

Vinblastine is myelosuppressive rather than neurotoxic and requires careful monitoring in combination regimes. It is particularly useful in Hodgkin's disease and is included in solid tumor regimes, using three or four drugs.

Both drugs act by having a spindle-fiber-inhibiting activity, causing metaphase arrest. Some inhibition of RNA and lipid synthesis has been described, in addition to its effect on the cytoplasm of neural tissue. It is excreted in the liver.

Experimental Drugs

Adriamycin. This drug is an anthracycline antibiotic, a hydroxylated analogue of daunorubicin. It is rapidly cleared from the plasma and slowly excreted in plasma and bile, being predominantly metabolized in the liver. Evaluation has shown it to give significant objective responses in adenocarcinoma of the breast (35%) and acute leukemias (25%).

Its side effects are alopecia, myelosuppression, stomatis, nausea, and vomiting. A more serious effect is cardiac toxicity which may cause fatal myopathy if the *total* dose exceeds 550 mg/m^2.

Bleomycin. This is a mixture of sulfur containing glycopeptide antibiotic. In the presence of sulfhydryl compounds, bleomycin binds to DNA and causes single-strand scission which is responsible for the inhibition of thymidine incorporation into DNA.

In man, the drug accumulates in the skin and tumor tissue, with 40% excreted over 24 h.

Clinical testing shows a significant response rate in squamous cell carcinoma at various anatomical sites; in malignant lymphomas and testicular carcinoma. Drug toxicity includes cutaneous reactions, stomatitis, alopecia, pyrexia, nausea, vomiting, and fatal pulmonary fibrosis, but there is little bone marrow toxicity in high doses. The most commonly used dose schedule is 15 mg/m^2 iv or im twice weekly.

ICRF 159 [1,2-di(3,5-dioxopiperazane-1-yl) Propane]. The cytotoxicity of this drug is not by inhibition of DNA synthesis but by the blocking of late "G$_2$" or early prophase.

Experimental evidence with Lewis lung tumor suggests that ICRF 159 inhibits metastasis formation at doses having little influence on the growth of the primary tumor implant; inhibition is produced by its effect on the invading margins of the primary tumor.

Leucopenia and thrombocytopenia are evident after a few days and are dose related, i.e., 5 g total dose. Hellmann *et al.* (1968) showed dramatic decreases in the number of circulating blast cells with no cross-resistance to other leukemic drugs.

DTIC [5-(3,3-Dimethyl-1-triazeno)imidazole-4-carboxamide]. The pharmacological action of this drug is by a mechanism including alkylation inhibition of DNA synthesis, *de novo* purine synthesis, and SH interaction.

Pharmokinetic studies show a short plasma half-life and rapid urinary excretion by a renal tubular secretory mechanism. About 46% of the administered drug is excreted in 6 h, 21% as DTIC and 20% as AIC (5-amino-4-umidazole carboxamide), its final metabolite.

Dosage schemes vary from 70–160 mg/m² a day for 10 days, every 28 days, or 250 mg/m² a day for 5 days every 21 days, or high intermittent doses of 1050–1250 mg/m² repeated every 4–5 weeks.

Toxicity includes bone marrow depression, nausea and vomiting, and a "flu-like" syndrome. Significant activity in man has been shown against malignant melanoma, with a 22% response rate, or in combination with other active drugs in malignant melanoma and sarcomas.

Streptozotocin. This is an antibiotic produced by *Streptomyces aeromogenes* which inhibits DNA and protein synthesis in *Escherichia coli*. It has a specificity for the beta cells of the pancreas and a beneficial effect in patients with metastatic islet-cell tumors with restoration of normal blood glucose and insulin levels. Doses are from 5–30 g, iv.

L-Asparaginase. This catalyzes the hydrolysis of L-asparagine into L-aspartic and ammonia. L-Asparaginase is extracted from *E. coli* and, after its administration, L-asparagine is depressed in the serum which is an essential amino acid for lymphomas and the lymphocytic component of bone marrow.

It causes chills, fever, nausea, and vomiting, and hypersensitivity reaction. Severe pancreatitis followed by induction of diabetes is not uncommon. Its value is in second-line or resistant strains of leukemia and in some lymphosarcomas.

The dose is 100–1,000 U/kg, lasting over 10–30 days.

Nitrosureas

BCNU [*1-3-bis(2-Chloroethyl)-1-nitrosurea*]. Its pharmacological action is by alkylation. It is rapidly metabolized, but breakdown of the product may be responsible for toxicity.

The clinical response is 50% in Hodgkin's disease; 42% in brain tumors; 39% in multiple myeloma; 16% in malignant melanoma; and 13% in colonic cancer.

The dose is 100 mg/m² a day for 7 days iv, with course repeated every 6 weeks.

CCNU [*1-(2-Chlorethyl)3-cyclohexyl-1-nitrosurea*]. Experimentally, this drug has a superior activity to BCNU in L1210 leukemia and great lipid solubility. It is rapidly metabolized with 50% urinary excretion in 24 h.

Clinical trials show a superiority to BCNU in Hodgkin's disease and activity against malignant gliomas, gastrointestinal cancer, carcinoma of the breast, adenocarcinoma of the kidney, bladder cancer, malignant melanoma, and squamous cell carcinoma.

Toxic effects of CCNU are nausea, vomiting, delayed leucopenia, and thrombocytopenia.

The dosage is 130 mg/m² orally, repeated every 6 weeks.

Methyl CCNU [*1-(2-Chloroethyl)-3(4-methyl-cyclohexyl)-1-nitrosurea*]. Experimentally, this is superior to both BCNU and CCNU in advanced Lewis lung tumor. It is rapidly absorbed orally and the dosage is 200 mg/m² p.o. every 6 weeks.

Combined Techniques

Combination Therapy

Treatment in disseminated cancer may destroy all malignant cells. Initially, clinically visible disease is eliminated either by surgery, radiotherapy, or chemotherapy, and a patient undergoes a remission. Once this is achieved, further treatment attempts to continue the response or, eventually, cure the patient.

In a relatively homogeneous population of cells, it takes the same treatment to reduce the number of neoplastic cells (using a log plot) from 1 million to 1,000 (1 mg of tissue), as from 10^{-12} to 10^{-9} (1 kg of tumor). This is an exponential fall, or as such has to be maintained by continuous treatment. There is evidence that this reduction in cells becomes more difficult as treatment progresses, because as more cells enter the cycle, the tumor becomes smaller, and the final, absolute reduction may require a completely different modality of treatment. Some cells may never enter the "cycle," some may be drug-resistant cells, and there are those behind pharmacological barriers which have already been discussed. One method of treatment is by stimulating the patient's cellular immune response, using BCG and this has been shown to be effective in eradicating local metastatic malignant melanoma.

Combination chemotherapy was first introduced in 1961 with the use of two or more agents in acute lymphoblastic leukemia of childhood. Prednisone and vincristine synergistically increased the remission rate to 90%. The concept then arose that agents with varying toxicity and mechanism of action could be therapeutically combined at a full dose with resultant enhanced antitumor effect. A combination of four drugs in acute lymphoblastic leukemia would produce an increased additive effect, each drug reducing the tumor cells by 10^{-3}, making a theoretical "death total" of 10^{-12} cells. A marked reduction in leukemia cells and a prolonged remission is achieved, and the more prolonged the course, the longer the sustained remission. Today, the survival of children with acute lymphoblastic leukemia with such modifications in combination treatment has resulted in a 50%, 5-year survival.

These studies with acute leukemia have now been applied to other malignant diseases, such as Hodgkin's disease. With single agents, a remission in recurrent or advanced disease was only 10–20%, but de Vita in 1968 combined four known effective agents, mustine, oncovin (vincristine), procarbazine, and prednisone (M.O.P.P.), which achieved a remission rate of 80%. Of those undergoing complete remission, 80–100% remained alive after 3 years, but this long remission is dependent on the patient *initially* undergoing a complete remission. With Hodgkin's disease, a 45%, 5-year remission was maintained after completing only six cycles of treatment, and this has now been improved to 60% by a spaced, phased intermittent course of maintenance M.O.P.P. (In the U.K., vinblastine is generally substituted for vincristine, i.e., M.V.P.P.)

Pharmacological, vascular access and cytokinetic problems make solid tumors more difficult to treat with combination chemotherapy than leukemias and lymphomas. Although cytogenic abnormalties occur with leukemia cells, these are usually represented as a single clone, whereas in a solid tumor, such as a melanoma, there are four different clones, each with a variable sensitivity to individual drugs. This clonogenic problem emphasizes the need for a multifaculty approach, not only with combination chemotherapy, but including surgery, radiotherapy, and immunotherapy in the overall management of any solid tumor.

It is now generally accepted there is no evidence that a single agent is more effective on its own than in different combinations with several other drugs. The number of drugs for a combination can range from two to five. No individual agent should create synergistic toxicity, and each should be active against the tumor, although no agent to date is specific for a particular cancer. The combinations could be made less empirical if each individual agent was phase-specific in the cell cycle, and experimental work increasingly emphasizes the need to develop cell-cycle synchronization and attempts to eliminate those clones of residual nonproliferative or insensitive cells.

However, the induction and length of remission in solid tumors to date has not been as dramatic as in some hematological malignancies; this disparity may be cytokinetic, due to multiplicity of cell clones in a single metastasis, inadequate dosage, or failure of the drug to reach potentially proliferating cells because of poor vascularity or surrounding necrosis. Exponential cell kill becomes more difficult as the tumor reduces in size, unless normal malignant cell loss is a feature of the tumor's behavior.

Long-established chemotherapy agents are, however, now routine in combination regimes, particularly in breast carcinoma, and these will be discussed later. But new experimental agents, such as the anthracyclines (adriamycin), triazenoimidazoles (DTIC) and nitrosureas (BCNU, CCNU, methyl CCNU) alone or in combination with cyclophosphamide have an improved antitumor activity.

The South West Cancer Chemotherapy Study Group of the M.D. Anderson Hospital (1973) compiled the results of single agents in osteo- and soft-tissue sarcoma, which showed a response rate with triazenomidazole (DTIC) alone of 15% and with adriamycin alone, 31%. These agents were found to be compatible and synergistic experimentally, and their combination has increased the clinical response rate to 41% with a median response over 5 months. It was then suggested that the above combination should be expanded to include cyclophosphamide and vincristine in the following regime: Adriamycin, 20–50 mg/m² on day 1, iv; cyclophosphamide, 300–500 mg/m² on day 1, iv; DTIC, 50–100 mg/m² on days 1–5, iv; and vincristine, 10 mg/m² on days 1 and 5, iv. This treatment gives a 60% remission rate in soft-tissue and bone sarcoma.

One of the most significant experimental agents to be used in combination regimes is adriamycin, being a small chemical modification (a hydroxyl group at position 14) of the other active anthracycline, daunorubicin. Adriamycin is active against human leukemia, lymphomas, breast carcinoma, and soft-tissue and bone sarcoma and is extensively used in many clinical trials of combination regimes in solid tumors.

Therapeutic Aspects

Regional Chemotherapy

This comprises all methods by which cytotoxic agents may be applied to or introduced directly into localized tumors, or tumor-bearing regions. These methods can reduce such limiting systemic effects of chemotherapy as toxic depression of bone marrow and gastrointestinal epithelium. A higher dose of an agent is distributed to a small tissue volume and the tumor utilizes or absorbs the drug before it reaches the systemic circulation.

Newton and Westbury in 1971 classified regional chemotherapy in the following way:

(1) **Surface Application (to Skin or Surgical Wounds).** Disease confined to its site of origin and nearby infiltrated tissue can be dealt with by surgical excision or radiotherapy. If these fail however, or lesions are too extensive, as in a skin cancer, topical application of 5-fluorouracil is indicated.

(2) **Intercavitary Installation (Bladder, Bowel, Pleura, Pericardium, or Intrathecal).** In the bladder, small papilliferous tumors of a few millimeters diameter may be controlled by the intravesical installations of thiotepa or

ethoglucid, but not in infiltrating carcinoma, unless as a palliative measure in excessive hematuria.

In carcinoma of the colon and rectum, bowel irrigation with 1:5,000 mercury perchloride solution has reduced the incidence of suture line recurrence following conservative excision.

Intraperitoneal or intrapleural installation of mustine hydrochloride, thiotepa, or triazequinone following paracentesis will reduce the rate of fluid reaccumulation in 50–60% of cases.

Cytosine arabinoside or methotrexate can be safely instilled into the spinal thecal cavity as a prophylactical or therapeutic measure in acute lymphatic leukemia.

(3) Interstitial. Direct injection of a cytotoxic agent into a tumor using thiotepa made up into 2% lignocaine with hyaluronidase is well tolerated by normal tissue and can have a marked local antitumor effect.

(4) Intraarterial. Intermittent injection or continuous infusion of drugs is relatively simple and can be applied to any area where an arterial catheter can be placed; few vessels are beyond surgical, operative exposure or closed catheterization by a skilled radiologist. Such anatomical areas are the head and neck, including the brain, limbs, and pelvis, and primary or secondary liver tumors can also be treated in this way.

In the head and neck, excellent regression can be achieved with epithelial cancers of the mucous membrane and skin, using a simple intraarterial injection of mustine or infusion of methotrexate, vinblastine, ethoglucid, or nitropodozide; however, the areas of therapeutic effect are limited by vascular anatomy, as there may be extension across the midline, requiring bilateral infusions. There is a high risk of complications and morbidity such as extravasation of infusate, septicemia, secondary hemmorhage, arterial thrombosis, embolism, and severe regional tissue reactions such as alopecia and leukopenia, and this method in no way replaces modern radiotherapy techniques, which are adaptable to a precise tumor area and have a low morbidity. Intraarterial chemotherapy for recurrent disease is disappointing, presumably due to obliterative endarteritis.

In the limbs intraarterial injection and infusion are technically more simple than isolated perfusion of limbs. Cannulation of the femoral or iliac arteries for injection or infusion may be effective by direct Seldinger puncture in the groin or retrograde cannulation from the dorsalis pedis or posterior tibial artery at the ankle, using a long, modified epidural catheter. This technique today is mainly in advanced malignant melanoma, using ethoglucid (epodyl), procarbazine or vinblastine.

Isolated perfusion is usually reserved for treatment of lesions involving the distal two-thirds of limbs where vascular cannulation is simple and tourniquet isolation effective. This is used exclusively for malignant melanoma in those cases where either the extent of the primary lesion or local recurrence and satellite formation makes control by surgery unlikely. The cytotoxic agent is phenylalanine nitrogen mustard (melphalan).

In the pelvis, patients with recurrent disease may have pain, discharge, and bleeding but otherwise are well; when disease has followed radiotherapy or surgery, a single injection into the aorta under generalized anesthesia, introduced via the femoral artery by Seldinger puncture, advanced to the aortic bifunction, with inflation of the tourniquets on both thighs above arterial pressure for 3 min will in many cases reduce distressing pain, bleeding, and discharge and make the quality of a distressed patient's life more acceptable.

Breast Cancer

Of all major solid tumors, breast carcinoma is one of the most responsive to chemotherapy, and if single agents are used they can achieve a 20–30% response. These drugs include: 5-fluorouracil, cyclophosphamide, methotrexate, vincristine, adriamycin, and prednisone.

Recognized indications for chemotherapy in breast carcinoma are local recurrence or dissemination disease after radiotherapy; an inflammatory or rapidly growing carcinoma with a short clinical history of disease in the immediate postmenopausal patient; or where there is a short time interval between the primary and secondary disease. Chemotherapy is also indicated when patients have failed to respond to, or relapse after, hormone therapy.

Greenspan (1963) reported one of the first combination regimes at Mount Sinai in New York, obtaining a 60% response rate (25 out of 40 patients), using a combination of methotrexate and thiotepa, and in 1966 he reported 81% remission (59 out of 73 patients) with thiotepa, methotrexate, cyclophosphamide, 5-fluorouracil, and testosterone.

Cooper (1969) of the Buffalo Medical Center reported a 90% remission rate (54 out of 60 patients) combining five drugs: 5-Fluorouracil, 12 mg/kg a day for 4 days, then 500 mg a week, iv; methotrexate, 25–50 mg a week, iv; vincristine, 35 mg/kg a week, iv; cyclophosphamide, 2.5 mg/kg a day, iv; and prednisone, 0.75 mg/kg daily, p.o.

Hanham *et al.* (1971) reported 91% remission with 64 out of 70 patients; 50% were in remission after 12 months, 30% after 24 months, and 10% were still in remission after 2 years. Their regime was given over a period of 5 days every 3 to 4 weeks, being a modification of that reported by Costanzi and Coltman (1969).

The details are as follows: Days 1 and 5, cyclophosphamide, 200–300 mg, iv; days 1 and 4, methotrexate, 10–15 mg, iv; days 2 and 5, vinblastine, 4–6 mg, iv; and days 1 and 5, 5-fluorouracil, 500 mg, iv.

This is now generally accepted as one of the standard quadruple regimes in this country for breast cancer. Vinblastine has been substituted for vincristine to avoid neurotoxicity.

Hanham (1974) reported particularly interesting responses in patients with jaundice due to liver involvement; cancer *en cuirasse* of the chest wall and intractable bone pain which had not improved with radiotherapy or hormones. Response occured where there was failure of hormonal control, ablation, or rapid deterioration and in cases where relapse occured after long-term remission with hormone treatment. Side effects were alopecia, stomatis, gastrointestinal dysfunction, and myelosclerosis. Hanham (1974) reported that alopecia is greatly reduced by the use of a scalp tourniquet maintained at 300 mm of systolic pressure for 30 min during and after the injection.

There are many and variable regimes; out of 323 patients so far studied, 244 or more than 75%, have undergone an objective remission. This compares with the remission rate in general of other therapeutic modalities as follows: Oophorectomy, 40–50%; hormonal ablative surgery, 30–40%; androgens, 20%; estrogens, 35%; single agent chemotherapy, 30%; and combination chemotherapy, 56–75%.

It is important to remember, however, that single agent chemotherapy can be used as a successful adjuvant to endocrine ablation and Wilson *et al.* (1969) showed that in those patients likely to respond poorly to adrenalectomy because of a short free interval (less than 12 months without disease), the addition of 5-fluorouracil postoperatively increased the remission rate from 10 to 59%.

Salih and Flax (1973) suggested that the sensitivity to hormones of breast tumors cultured *in vitro* might be of value in preselecting patients for a particular hormonal drug or pituitary ablation; and that in those patients who were considered to have a negative response, chemotherapy should be instituted immediately where there was early recurrence of disease.

Prophylactic chemotherapy could be considered, for example, in a late stage 2 breast carcinoma with "high" axillary nodes, where patients are at risk and are known to have a poor prognosis. Hormone sensitivity tests would exclude those primary tumors with a hormone responsiveness, and chemotherapy could be initiated on a long-term basis to prevent recurrence.

Cancer of the Colon

It is known that 30–68% of colonic cancers seen surgically have already metastasized to regional lymph nodes, and curability is closely related to this finding. A wide variation, 15–61% of cases, has been found to have venous involvement, and there is marked correlation with this and later death due to metastasis in the liver and lungs. Implantation also occurs in the peritoneum and in abdominal wounds. Half of the patients die from distant metastases and the other half from local recurrence. About 60% of patients with carcinoma localized to the colon and 39 % with regional node involvement will survive 5 years. After 5 years there is only 5–10% recurrence in this group of patients.

Radiotherapy is useful as palliation with locally unresectable or recurrent rectal carcinoma. Survival improvement has been claimed with preoperative radiotherapy by improving resectability as a result of reducing tumor bulk, reducing local recurrence at the site of excision and minimizing regional and distant metastases.

No improvement in the therapeutic index has been achieved over the original intravenous dose regime of Ansfield and Curreri (1963). Younger patients do better than the more elderly in terms of toxicity; and the results are better in patients with a long interval between primary and secondary disease. Pulmonary metastases appear to have the lowest objective response with chemotherapy.

Single agents which have been evaluated are mitomycin C and adriamycin; both drugs, however, have a lower therapeutic regression rate than 5-fluorouracil and are more toxic. Moertel and Mays (1973) compared the nitrosureas with 5-fluorouracil. In their clinical trials, BCNU was of less value than 5-fluorouracil in response rate and duration; but CCNU was as effective and methyl CCNU was probably better than 5-fluorouracil, although the latter two drugs are only available at present for limited clinical trial. There appears to be no cross-resistance to nitrosurea following the use of 5-fluorouracil.

Carter and Friedman (1974) have analyzed 2,000 cases treated with 5-fluorouracil with an overall response rate of 21%. As a result of clinical trials, the following single agents have provided a response, and Carter and Friedman (1974) listed them in order of remission rate, as: 5-fluorouracil; methyl CCNU; BCNU; mitomycin; CCNU; cyclophosphamide; methotrexate; melphalan; hexamethylmelamine; and DTIC. Any of these drugs can be used either in two, three, four, or five combinations. From the world literature, Carter and Friedman (1974) compiled the most promising results with three or more drugs as follows, although only one of these regimes includes three known active drugs against colonic carcinoma:

(a) **Three-Drug Combination.** Current Mayo clinic workers show a combination of BCNU, 5-FU, and mitomycin C to be no better than using 5-fluorouracil alone, but Sloane-Kettering workers have used a combination of 5-FU, cytosine arabinoside, and mitomycin C and have found it marginally more successful than a single agent.

(b) Four-Drug Combination. Falkson *et al.* (1974) reported that the BCNU, DTIC, vincristine, and 5-fluorouracil combination gave better results than any previously used chemotherapeutic regime and 15 of the 22 patients who received adequate doses of the drugs responded even though 9 had previously been treated with 5-fluorouracil. Priestman and Hanham (1972), in a much smaller series of cases, reported a 66% objective response in 9 cases with hepatic metastases with a mean survival time of 9 months. They used cyclophosphamide, methotrexate, vincristine, and 5-fluorouracil.

Chemotherapy and Surgery in Large Bowel Cancer

The rationale of employing chemotherapy as an adjuvant to surgery has evolved significantly over the past 15 years. It is used in an interoperative or immediate postoperative course in an attempt to sterilize clonogenic cells liberated by surgical trauma, based on the observation of circulating tumor cells and on experimental work on animal systems. However, clinically no statistically significant difference in survival in the last 15 years has been shown between those treated by postoperative adjuvant chemotherapy and a control group of 1,200 patients observed in seven studies of up to 19 months.

Human colonic carcinoma has a slow doubling time, low growth fraction, and long transit time, and no trial has persisted with therapy longer than 19 months or attempted postoperative combination regimes. To date the place of adjuvant chemotherapy is still uncertain, following surgical excision of the primary tumor.

Ovarian Cancer

Outside the confines of the true pelvis and of those cases with resectable disease, 60% present with advanced disease, and 20–50% will develop recurrent disease. Therefore, most patients with ovarian cancer require systemic therapy at some stage of their disease.

Alkylating agents are the most extensively tested, showing an initial response rate from 45–65%, with 5–15% of these continuing to respond 2 years after the initiation of therapy. No alkylating agent is better than any other, and these include melphalan, chlorambucil, cyclophosphamide, and thiotepa. There is no difference between daily oral doses, oral loading doses, intermittent intravenous doses, and intermittent, intensive intravenous doses. Intraperitoneal administration is less effective than intravenous use of the same drug, and intraperitoneal drugs are ineffective against intraabdominal disease. The response rate to alkylating agents appears to be about 42% when a tumor becomes refractory to radiotherapy, but it is over 46% in previously untreated patients, so there would appear to be some disadvantage in previous radiotherapy. There is no variation in response rate with serous, mucinous, or undifferentiated tumor histology.

Combination Chemotherapy in Ovarian Cancer

Smith and Ruttledge (1970) reported, in one of few randomized trials, a 38% response rate in 47 patients refractory to melphalan using a combination of cyclophosphamide, actinomycin D and 5-fluorouracil; however, in a direct comparison, the response rate was 45% in 47 cases treated with these ·drugs, compared with 42% for 50 patients treated with the single agent melphalan. There appears to be no therapeutic advantage in using combination therapy rather than single alkylating agents in the initial treatment.

Brandl (1970) reported on the use of cyclophosphamide, vinblastine, and triaziquone (Trenimon®), claiming an .80% objective response in 26 patients with no prior therapy, but in the trial there was no comparison with a single alkylating agent.

Combination chemotherapy has not been shown to have an advantage over single alkylating agents, although noncomparative trials have demonstrated a good response in primary disease with remission times similar to those obtained with alkylating agents; but in any solid tumor there are important theoretical reasons for finding new, effective combination regimes in an attempt to cure disease.

Most clinical trials with radiotherapy and chemotherapy have demonstrated no synergistic effect. Radiotherapy has not been shown to be superior to chemotherapy either for palliation or improving the 5-year survival. There is no evidence to suggest that radiotherapy and chemotherapy together are superior to chemotherapy alone. Complications from total abdominal radiotherapy are more frequent and severe than those of chemotherapy, and these might suggest that the latter is more appropriate in a disease in which only palliation in most cases can be achieved at present.

Conclusion

This chapter attempts to review the essential theoretical and clinical features of chemotherapeutic agents and emphasizes the need for full integration of chemotherapy into the surgical management of patients with malignant diseases. However, unless the clinician understands and is familiar with the drugs he is using, serious deleterious effects can arise. But no patient should be denied expert knowledge in their use in the correct context.

Combination chemotherapy is a major advance and is now curing patients with certain diseases; given time and continuing expert and painstaking research, many more patients with different diseases can expect prolonged therapeutic remissions and a reasonably normal life.

References

Ansfield, F. J., and Curreri, A. R. (1963). Further clinical comparison between 5-fluorouracil (5Fu) and 5-fluoro-2-deoxyuridine. *Cancer Chemother. Rep.* **32**:101.

Brandl, K. (1970). *Zentbl Gynak.* **92**:233.

Carter, S. K., and Friedman, M. (1974). Integration of chemotherapy into combined modality treatment of solid tumours. *Cancer Treat. Rev.* **1**:001.

Costanzi, J. J., and Coltman, C. A. (1969). Combination chemotherapy using cyclophosphamide, vincristine, methotrexate and 5-fluorouracil in solid tumours. *Cancer Chemother. Rep.* **53**:90.

Cooper, R. C. (1969). Combination chemotherapy in hormone resistant breast cancer. *Proc. Am. Assoc. Cancer Res.* **10**:15.

de Vita, V. T., Serpick, A. A., and Carbone, P. P. (1970). Combination chemotherapy in the treatment of advanced Hodgkin's disease. *Ann. Int. Med.* **73**:881.

Greenspan, E. M. (1966). Thiotepa, methotrexate, cyclophosphamide, 5-fluorouracil, and testosterone in advance breast cancer. *J. Mount Sinai Hosp.* **33**:1.

Greenspan, E. M., Fieber, M. M., Geeson, L., and Edelman, S. (1963). Thiotepa and methotrexate chemotherapy of advanced breast cancer. *J. Mount Sinai Hosp.* **30**:246.

Hanham, I. W. F. (1974). Chemotherapy in breast cancer. *Proc. Royal Soc. Med.* **67**:292.

Hanham, I. W. F., Newton, K. A., and Westbury, G. (1971). Seventy five cases of solid tumours treated by a modified quadruple chemotherapy regime. *Br. J. Cancer* **25**:462.

Hellmann, K., and Burrage, Karen (1969). Control of malignant metastases by ICRF 159. *Nature (London)* **224**:273.

Hersh, E. M., Whitecar, J. P., McCredie, K. B., Bodey, G. P., and Freireich, E. J., (1971). Chemotherapy, immunocompetence, immunosuppression and prognosis in acute leukaemia. *N. Eng. J. Med.* **285**:1211.

Moertel, C. G., and Mays (1973). Therapy of advanced gastrointestinal cancer with the nitrosureas. *Cancer Chemother. Rep.* **4**:27.

Newton, K. A., and Westbury, G. (1971). Indications for the treatment of cancer by regional chemotherapy. *Geriatrics* **26**:125.

Pinkel, D., Walters, T., and Bushore, M. (1970). Identification of black children with acute lymphocytic leukemia (All) as high risk patients. *Proc. Am. Assoc. Cancer Res.* **11**:321.

Price, L. A., and Goldie, J. H. (1971). Multiple drug therapy for disseminated malignant tumours. *Br. Med. J.* **4**:336.

Priestman, T. J., and Hanham, I. W. F. (1972). Results of 27 cases with hepatic metastases treated by combination chemotherapy. *Br. J. Cancer* **26**:466.

Salih, H., Flax, J., and Hobbs, J. R. (1972). *In vitro* oestrogen sensitivity of breast cancer tissue as a possible screening method for hormonal treatment. *Lancet* **i**:1198.

Salsbury, A. J., Burrage, Karen, and Hellman, K. (1970). Inhibition of metastatic spread by ICRF 159: Selective deletion of a malignant characteristic. *Br. Med. J.* **4**:344.

Salsbury, A. J., Burrage, Karen, and Hellman, K. (1974). Analysis of the antimetastatic effect of ICRF 159. *Cancer Res.* **34**:843.

Smith, J. P., and Rutledge, F. (1970). Chemotherapy in the treatment of cancer of the ovary. *Am. J. Obstet. Gyn.* **107**:69.

South West Cancer Chemotherapy Group (1973). Chemotherapy of metastatic sarcomas using combinations with adriamycin. Symposium on Clinical Pharmacology, Jacksonville, Florida. Gottlieb, J. A., coordinator.

Van Eden, E. B., Falkson, G., Van Der Merwe, A. M., Van Dyk, J. J., and Falkson, H. C. (1973). FIVB—A new combination of drugs in the treatment of cancer. *S. Afr. Med. J.* **47**:982.

Wilson, R. E., Piro., A. J., Aliapoulios, M. A., and Moore, F. D. (1969). Evaluation of adrenalectomy and hypophysectomy in the treatment of metastatic cancer of the breast. *Cancer* **24**:1322.

Chapter 17

REHABILITATION

RONALD W. RAVEN

The rehabilitation of patients who are affected in so many different ways by oncological diseases is a subject of increasing importance throughout the world. The problems of the enormous number of patients with crippling disabilities justify a place of high priority in the work of the caring professions. In addition to the relief of suffering, rehabilitation gives fresh hope to patients and families to dispel the fear and despondency they so often experience. The tremendous therapeutic advances of recent decades are resulting in an ever increasing number of cured patients for rehabilitation and resettlement.

Divisions of Rehabilitation

There are three divisions to discuss, namely, clinical research and education and training.

Clinical Rehabilitation

In its broadest sense this is the complete program of treatment carried out by the oncology team following the established diagnosis. The objective is to restore the patient to a life of longevity and of good quality. Consequently, an assessment is made of the patient's total requirements, immediate and longer term, which are governed by the particular prognosis. Many cured patients can resume their normal lives without any disability, while

Ronald W. Raven • Member of Council, Royal College of Surgeons of England; Consulting Surgeon, Royal Marsden Hospital and Institute of Cancer Research; Consulting Surgeon, Westminster Hospital, London, SW1, England.

others have a residual disability caused by the disease or the treatment, but
they can be restored to a life of good quality. For some patients life can
never be the same again, nevertheless substantial benefit is available for all;
even those with a short prognosis can be rendered self-supporting and
comfortable, easing their period of total disability. This means that the
rehabilitation program must be planned to meet the various individual
requirements.

The Oncology Team

This is composed of surgeon, physician, radiotherapist, chemotherap-
ist, family doctor, community physician, nurse, medical social worker,
physiotherapist, occupational therapist, speech therapist, prosthetist,
resettlement officer, and chaplain. The clinician to whom the patient is first
referred usually takes the final responsibility for the patient, unless this is
delegated to a colleague. Every member of the team may not be required
for each patient, but their help is always available. The active participation
of key members of the patient's family is often necessary, especially for
those with stomas and for amputees.

Collaboration between church and medicine in this work on a greater
scale is desirable, to build up patients spiritually and physically, for it is the
whole person we are treating.

The Rehabilitation Unit

For an oncology center, service, or department a special unit deals
with a sufficient number of patients to justify such an establishment for both
in-patient and out-patient treatment. All members of the team will not be
required full time in the unit, for they have other work to carry out. In many
general hospitals the work of such a unit forms part of the rehabilitation
services for all patients. The special unit, in addition to being a focal point
in this work, enables research and teaching to be carried out under ideal
conditions.

The Rehabilitation Program

This is designed for two clinical groups—patients with controllable
and uncontrollable diseases. Their prognosis varies from a few months to
many years, so the program must be flexible to meet the various requirements for the patient during the whole period from hospital into the
community. The time schedule varies from weeks to months until the
patient is restored to family life and employment. The broad spectrum of
rehabilitation is set out in Table 1.

TABLE 1. The Rehabilitation Program

Primary treatment	Surgery, radiotherapy, chemotherapy, combination therapy
Secondary treatment Restoration of nutrition Restoration of function	Physiotherapy, occupational therapy, speech therapy, stomal care, prostheses
Restoration of spirit	
Resettlement	Home, family, employment

Patients with Controllable Diseases. Many patients have no disability or deformity and are able to return to their families and employment. Other patients have residual defects caused by the disease or treatment; nevertheless, they can be rehabilitated for a life of good quality.

Patients with Uncontrollable Diseases. These patients have disability or deformity caused by the disease or treatment and a prognosis which is relatively short. Continuing treatment and supervision are required to keep them comfortable and self-supporting. Many patients are thereby able to live with their families and even to work. With the help of various team members the final period of total disability with complete dependence upon others is shortened to a minimum period of perhaps days. An atmosphere of hope is engendered around the patient and family, for no patient must be given the impression that hope is abandoned and treatment has ceased.

Special Aspects of Rehabilitation

Primary Treatment

The majority of patients with oncological diseases require surgical treatment which involves the removal of tumors, organs, and limbs. Manipulation of hormonal systems may necessitate endocrine surgery and replacement therapy. Many patients undergo radiotherapy, either alone or in combination with surgery and chemotherapy. There is a considerable expansion in the use of chemotherapy, alone or in combination with other primary treatment. The scope of this chapter does not include a detailed discussion of primary treatment, although this is fundamental in rehabilitation. The latter is usually, but not logically, regarded as the care of the patient following primary treatment.

Secondary Treatment

This commences during or at the end of primary treatment and is planned for each patient according to requirements.

Restoration of Nutrition. The majority of patients have various nutritional deficiencies requiring correction. These are especially severe with carcinoma of the alimentary tract and are corrected to enable the patient to undergo primary treatment. Nutritional deficiencies are measured by the amount of weight loss, degree of dehydration, wasting, and weakness of skeletal muscles. A complete hematological examination will reveal the severity of anemia and electrolyte and water imbalances, which are rectified by the appropriate treatment. Avitaminosis is frequent, especially deficient ascorbic acid; the relevant vitamins are therefore given. A high calorie, protein, and carbohydrate intake is necessary and given, preferably, orally. When this route is impossible, nutrition is built up by the nasogastric, intravenous, or gastrostomy methods. Blood and plasma transfusions are given when necessary. Gastrostomy feeding is valuable when patients with advanced esophageal carcinoma are treated with radiotherapy and chemotherapy. This enables the patient's nutrition to be maintained throughout the period of treatment until normal deglutition is restored. Nasogastric feeding is necessary for some weeks following laryngectomy, laryngo-pharyngectomy, and laryngo-esophago-pharyngectomy. Liquidized food with vitamin and iron supplements is an excellent way to administer nutrients by gastrostomy or nasogastric tubes. During the administration of concentrated foods the urine should be examined for glycosuria, which can appear suddenly with marked hyperglycemia. This requires urgent correction, for the patient may lapse into a coma.

All patients shoud be encouraged to resume oral feeding as soon as possible, but special problems are seen frequently. Following total gastrectomy or esophago-gastrectomy the "dumping syndrome" may occur, with persisting malnutrition. These patients tolerate proteins and fats better than carbohydrates; naturally occurring fats of high molecular weight are tolerated better than homogenized fats. Cytamen is also required after these operations, and meals should be taken dry. Steatorrhea may follow esophago-gastrectomy and pancreatectomy, and medium-chain triglycerides should be given.

Constant watch is necessary for iron deficiency anemia during several years after primary treatment, and this is treated by oral iron replacement with ascorbic acid. Anemia may be due to folic acid deficiency which is corrected by giving up to 20 mg daily.

Patients with malnutrition usually have anorexia, and if they are encouraged to start eating, thus gaining weight, their appetite frequently returns.

Restoration of Function. Bodily functions are affected in many different ways by oncological diseases and the treatment given. Various groups of patients are described for special management.

Patients with Amputations

Numerous varieties of amputations are carried out, including those of minor and major limbs, the breast, and external genitalia. These operations cause considerable psychological and physical suffering which is ameliorated by the care of various members of the team who adopt an optimistic attitude and give constant encouragement. Phantom limb pain can be very troublesome and difficult to control with sedatives. Hypnosis, early fitting of a prosthesis, and an elastic sock on the stump can be helpful.

Limb Amputees

Tumors of soft tissues and bone may require the amputation of a part or whole of a limb. Infrequently a more major amputation, either a forequarter or hindquarter amputation, is required, and in very rare circumstances even a hemicorporectomy has been performed. Before an amputation is done an explanation is made to the patient and key relatives about the operation and the prosthesis to be worn afterwards. The visit of an amputee, fully rehabilitated, to the patient and family greatly helps their morale. The prosthetist sees the patient before the amputation to make the necessary arrangements for a suitable prosthesis. The appearance of a prosthetic hand and forearm should simulate exactly the normal side; the color and texture of a lower limb prosthesis is less important, except in female amputees. These prostheses are continually improved, and it is hoped that powered limbs will be available eventually to improve function, especially of the hand.

Lower Extremity Amputations

These vary from an amputation of a part of a toe to disarticulation of the hip and hindquarter amputations. Following the small amputations patients' functions are restored quickly, and they walk without disability. The major amputees require much care to make them self-supporting. A below-knee amputation is very satisfactory, for the patient has a normal knee joint and walks well with a good prosthesis. A midthigh amputation is also satisfactory, and patients walk well with the prosthesis. The care of the stump and the prosthesis is explained to the patient. The prosthesis is fitted when the wound has consolidated, and walking exercises commence early. The usual postoperative care is given with muscle exercises under the supervision of the physiotherapist. Full ambulation is soon achieved, the patient dresses normally, and special exercises are taught which include climbing stairs, kneeling, and driving a car.

Upper Extremity Amputations

These vary from an amputation of part of a finger to disarticulation at the shoulder joint and forequarter amputations. Hand function recovers soon after partial or total amputation of a finger, but the loss of a thumb causes considerable disability. Part of a normal hand can be made to function better than any prosthesis, and this should be conserved whenever possible. Since the function of the upper extremity is more specialized and intricate than that of the lower extremity, it is more difficult to replace with a functional prosthesis. The conventional prosthesis is relatively simple and uses the power of the patient's musculature so that the patient soon recognizes its function and position. Patients with an artificial hand are trained for useful employment and other activities.

In general, young patients adapt to prostheses more easily than older patients, who have many difficulties to overcome. A temporary prosthesis is usually fitted as soon as the healing stump will allow while the permanent prosthesis is being made. The simple pylon prosthesis is particularly valuable, for it enables the patient to be ambulant and become adjusted until the permanent apparatus is provided. Prostheses are now being made of strong, light materials and fitted with comfortable, balanced and suction sockets. Considerable attention is given to the activation of prostheses with the use of various power systems for the different functions of the upper and lower extremities.

The loss of part, or the whole, of a limb is a traumatic experience for patients, who have many questions about their future lives which require detailed and sympathetic answers. They must not regard themselves as maimed and incapable; it is helpful when the prosthesis is accepted and used as part of themselves.

Other Amputations

Amputation of the External Genitalia

In both males and females these operations cause considerable upset, which is ameliorated by the sympathetic understanding of doctors and nurses. In the male a partial amputation of the penis is done when possible rather than a total amputation. In the latter operation, the urethra is implanted in the perineum to allow normal micturition; it is usually advisable to remove the testicles and scrotum.

Amputation of the Breast

Carcinoma of the breast is a dangerous and unpredictable disease. In stages I and II it is treated by mastectomy. It is beyond the scope of this chapter to discuss the type of mastectomy for various patients, but the loss of the breast, whether by simple or radical mastectomy, is psychologically disturbing for many patients, especially in the younger age groups, who fear possible repercussions on their marital, social, and business lives. Their rehabilitation begins when the carcinoma is diagnosed and the need for mastectomy is explained to the patient, husband, or other key member of the family. The sympathetic understanding of this ordeal by the surgeon and family considerably ameliorates the distress. The patient is assured that a good prosthesis will be provided for her and she can wear her usual day and evening clothes without disfigurement, so that no one will detect the deformity.

In the immediate postoperative period the presence of a sympathetic nurse is most helpful, especially for the wound dressings and when the patient first sees the scar, which may be a somewhat traumatic experience. During the first week the upper extremity is kept largely at rest, allowing the skin flaps to adhere to the chest wall to obliterate the dead space. The serum exudate diminishes rapidly to allow removal of the suction drains, usually after 3 or 4 days. At the end of the first week active arm exercises begin under the supervision of the physiotherapist, and full movements are soon achieved. Capsulitis in the shoulder joint can be troublesome, but it is usually avoided by resting the upper extremity for the first week. Sympathetic pain in the remaining breast may cause the patient some anxiety, which is allayed by the explanation that it is common and harmless. The patient will notice a loss of sensation in the affected side of the chest wall and tingling down the inner side of the arm, but this need not cause her any concern. It is helpful if a temporary prosthesis is worn as soon as the wound allows. The patient is warned against excessive overuse of the arm to avoid lymphoedema.

Postoperative Lymphoedema. A mild degree is frequent following mastectomy, but this usually causes no inconvenience. Excessive use of the limb, trivial injuries, and infections of the skin should be avoided. Constricting shoulder straps are not worn.

Severe lymphoedema may follow all types of mastectomy and is very disabling, even causing a useless limb, especially when it is associated with paralysis of the brachial plexus due to traction by the heavy limb, or malignant infiltration. Such a useless limb, without disease, may require disarticulation through the shoulder joint to give the patient relief.

The causes of lymphoedema include thrombosis or kinking of the axillary vein; residual or recurrent carcinoma in the axilla; fibrosis following axillary infection after the operation, or due to radiotherapy. Preventive treatment is, therefore, important.

Active treatment is somewhat disappointing and the limb should be supported adequately to prevent brachial plexus traction. All forms of trauma to the skin must be avoided to diminish the risk of infection and cellulitis. Compression techniques can help in reducing the swelling, and the limb is held in the elevated position whenever this is convenient. Limitation of fluid intake and a diuretic are sometimes useful. Active exercises are carried out under the supervision of the physiotherapist, for it is important to restore function, especially of the hand.

Mastectomy Leaflet. Patients who have undergone mastectomy may have many different problems to solve for which expert advice is necessary. The value of a leaflet dealing with these problems is stressed, and these are available upon request from the Marie Curie Memorial Foundation in English, French, and German. Experience proves how grateful patients are for the information and advice they contain.

Patients with an Artificial Stoma

The creation of a stoma, either temporary or permanent, is part of the operation for a number of malignant tumors and may cause considerable apprehension for the patient and family which can be relieved by explanation and training. Nurses are now becoming stomal therapists and an increasing number of stomal clinics are being established in hospitals. Before the stoma is made, patients are given an explanation about its function and care; and this is continued after the operation so that patients can manage their stomas before leaving the hospital. In addition, key members of the family should be familiar with them when patients return home. A periodic examination and discussion about stomal function should be arranged, so that any difficulty can be overcome.

Tracheostomy

A permanent tracheostomy is created as part of the operation of laryngectomy, laryngo-pharyngectomy, and laryngo-esophago-pharyngectomy for carcinoma of the larynx and hypopharynx.

During the immediate postoperative period, constant medical and nursing supervision are essential; the patient should never be left alone and suction is always available to remove the mucus in the trachea until the patient develops a good cough reflex. The air is kept moist with a humidifier placed near the tracheostomy. This will help to avoid mucus forming crusts and plugs in the trachea. The patient may succeed in coughing them out, but when large they will block the lower end of the tracheostomy tube, causing a bivalve action. It may be impossible to aspirate a large plug after removing the inner tube; it is then necessary to remove the outer tube so that with coughing and aspiration its removal may be successful. If these methods are unsuccessful bronchoscopy is done and the plug is extracted with forceps. After several days the cough reflex becomes stronger and mucus secretion diminishes.

The patient is instructed in how to remove, clean, and insert the tube. When the tracheostomy has healed and consolidated, patients usually wish to wear the tube at night; during the day a perforated metal shield is provided to cover the opening. Normal dress, including collar and tie, can be worn, so there is no visible deformity.

Gastrostomy

This operation is usually performed for patients with carcinoma of the esophagus undergoing radiotherapy and chemotherapy. It is also required when there is an esophago-bronchial fistula or a mediastinal abscess from a perforating carcinoma. Patients can be given a high calorie, balanced diet throughout treatment to mantain their nutritional state with gain of weight. Since this treatment is carried out in the hospital, gastrostomy management is done by the medical and nursing staffs. When deglutition is reestablished, the gastrostomy tube is removed and the wound heals quickly. If for any reason the gastrostomy is permanent, the patient and key relatives are instructed in the preparation and administration of the feeds before leaving the hospital.

Colostomy

This stoma may be temporary or permanent. The former variety is usually closed after a short period, but patients require instruction about the care of the permanent colostomy. A terminal colostomy is established when an abdomino-perineal excision of the rectum is done for a carcinoma, and a clear explanation is given to the patient beforehand. At the same time there is reassurance that a normal life will follow with but little disability. In addition to this professional advice, it is most helpful for the patient to be visited by someone who has a colostomy to share the experience.

During the postoperative period the patient is taught colostomy management. This includes the care of the stoma and surrounding skin to prevent excoriation. Stenosis is prevented by frequent digital dilatation. There are two methods of choice for regulating the colostomy function. Many patients are taught daily colonic irrigation which ensures satisfactory emptying of the bowel, and no further action that day. They are given the necessary apparatus for this and wear a soft dressing over the stoma with a light belt. Other patients rely on a spontaneous action in the evening or morning and wear a light plastic bag over the stoma in case of need. Patients are given advice about foods which may cause diarrhea, and they quickly learn what foods to avoid. Many are relatively young patients with good career prospects which are not jeopardized by this operation, which carries a good prognosis for earlier disease.

Ileal Conduit

Following total cystectomy for carcinoma, the best method of diverting the urine to the body surface is by an ileal conduit. This operation may be necessary also for advanced rectal carcinoma, involving the base of the urinary bladder. Before the operation is done a detailed explanation is given to the patient and key members of the family. The best position for the stoma in the anterior abdominal wall is chosen, preoperatively, with the patient standing and recumbent and with the appliance fitted. The chosen appliance is light and water tight; there are several suitable bags available. The Hollister bag is very satisfactory and easy to change, and it is discarded weekly. If a particular bag is found unsuitable by the patient there are others to choose from. The skin around the stoma may become sore and inflamed; Karaya gum in a powder is applied or Orabase seals are valuable. Infection of the urine with *Bacillus proteus* causes dermatitis requiring systemic antibiotics and local spraying with polybactrin.

Patients with Tumors in the Head and Neck

There are many problems to solve in this group of patients, who may have severe deformity or disability following surgery, radiotherapy, regional infusion, or combined treatment. Teamwork is essential by surgeons experienced in this branch of excisional and reconstructive surgery supported by colleagues in other disciplines. Excellent prostheses are available for all kinds of defects, and reconstructive surgery has attained a high standard of perfection. Primary reconstruction of soft tissue defects is done when possible using whole thickness skin grafts, especially the delto-pectoral flap. Where a prosthesis is required this is also fitted at the time of the excisional operation, even though it is a temporary type. There are indications for both methods. When a long period of hospitalization with multiple staged operations is required for elderly patients this is a disadvantage, especially when a good prosthesis can be provided quickly. There are obvious advantages, however, especially for younger patients, when a defect can be corrected by plastic surgery. When a prosthesis is worn the cavity can be inspected for recurrent disease, which is an advantage.

Radical Facio-Maxillary Resections

Different operations are necessary for tumors in the various sites. Some are carried out inside the mouth, which limits the external facial deformity, and various types of obturator are available for maxillary defects. External operations resulting in soft tissue and bone defects cause more serious disfigurement, especially when an orbital exenteration is required, but well-fitting prostheses of good appearance can be made, which patients find acceptable. These include an artificial eye, nose, and pinna.

Mastication Problems

These occur after operations on the mouth, tongue, and jaws and are solved in various ways. An upper denture is incorporated in the prosthesis after resection of the maxilla. Prostheses are available to replace a part, or the whole, of the mandible which can be inserted when the primary resection is done, or after an interval to allow consolidation of the soft tissues. Special jaw and tongue exercises are prescribed to restore speech and mastication. The soft tissues of the mouth and cheek are reconstructed whenever possible to enable normal mastication. Following total glossectomy there is much functional difficulty with speech and deglutition, but patients are helped considerably by appropriate exercises and training. Teeth, when healthy, should always be conserved and protected during radiotherapy for buccal carcinoma. Dryness of mouth is troublesome after radiotherapy, but this improves with time.

Following plastic procedures much help can be given by physiotherapists to improve tissue suppleness by massage and exercises. When permanent deformity results, patients are gradually reintroduced to society and confidence is thus regained. Help for the patient's family is also necessary to enable them to accept the altered appearance from facial defects and avoid self-consciousness.

Learning to Speak

Speech is affected after operations on the mouth, larynx, and pharynx. Satisfactory speech is soon regained after partial glossectomy with the help of the speech therapist, but considerable difficulty is experienced following total glossectomy, although eventually the patient learns to communicate when the muscles in the floor of the mouth have hypertrophied.

After laryngectomy, laryngo-pharyngectomy, and laryngo-esophago-pharyngectomy the patients are taught a new technique for speech. Some patients learn quickly and can be understood clearly, but considerable time and training is necessary for others. Following the first two operations the pharyngeal muscles are conserved so that pharyngeal speech is acquired, which is more natural with little hesitation. When the hypopharynx and cervical esophagus are removed the patient learns esophageal speech which is more difficult to acquire.

There are some patients, especially elderly, who fail to master the new technique of speech, so they are provided with an electrical larynx. This vibrator is held against the side of the neck and a monotonous variety of speech is produced, but there is clear communication.

The speech therapist should see these patients before operation to give preliminary instruction. In addition, it is useful if a patient can see and talk with another patient who has undergone the same operation, for this gives confidence. The time required to regain satisfactory speech varies up to several months.

Paralyses Caused by Tumors

Considerable additional suffering is experienced by a patient with malignant disease when a paralysis occurs, but rehabilitation will often bring amelioration, even with a major paralysis. Some patients can be made ambulant and self-dependent, even though the disease cannot be cured. The various paralyses are shown in Table 2.

Peripheral Nerve Paralysis

Cranial Nerves These are paralyzed singly, or in groups, by tumors usually malignant, which occur in various sites in the head and neck. The tumors are often primary, but metastatic tumors do occur, as for example

TABLE 2. Paralyses Caused by Tumors

---

(1) Lesions of peripheral nerves
   Cranial nerves
   Spinal nerves: plexus, cords, trunks
(2) Lesions of the central nervous system
   Cerebrum, motor area
   Spinal cord, pyramidal tracts, cauda equina

---

in the base of the skull from a primary breast carcinoma. Cranial nerve paralyses are usually permanent and can cause considerable disability, including partial or complete blindness, unilateral or bilateral; strabismus; double vision; and deafness with vertigo. A facial nerve paralysis is very disfiguring, but plastic surgery will minimize the deformity of the eyelids and angle of the mouth.

Trigeminal nerve involvement causes severe neuralgia requiring the routine treatment for its relief. Anosmia and hemiparalysis of the tongue do not cause serious disablement. Mild dysphagia may be experienced from involvement of the glossopharyngeal nerve; and some voice hoarseness results when the vagus nerve is affected. Unilateral paralysis of the sterno-mastoid and trapezius muscles affects movements of the head and shoulder, which are improved by corrective exercises.

Common causes of these paralyses include malignant tumors in the epipharynx involving the base of the skull; primary tumors in the neck, including thyroid carcinoma and glomus tumors; metastatic tumors in the base of the skull; and cervical lymph node metastases. These tumors are treated by routine methods.

Spinal Nerves. Primary and metastatic tumors cause paralyses of various kinds by affecting a nerve plexus or cord, or a single spinal nerve. It is not uncommon to find involvement of the brachial plexus and the axillary nerve trunks by metastatic breast carcinoma in the supraclavicular or axillary lymph nodes. The affected upper extremity may become a painful liability from total or partial paralysis. The treatment varies with the condition of each patient. Supraclavicular metastatic breast carcinoma is treated by local irradiation, endocrine therapy, and chemotherapy. When the carcinoma is controlled, partial function may be restored by the appropriate physical methods. For patients with a painful, paralyzed upper extremity, disarticulation at the shoulder joint is probably the best treatment to give relief. A sarcoma, either fibro- or liposarcoma, in the axilla may cause paralysis by infiltrating nerve cords or trunks. When the tumor can be excised, this should be done with the affected nerve or nerves, and function should be restored as much as possible by postoperative treatment. The tumor may infiltrate more widely, causing serious paralysis of the limb, when a disarticulation at the shoulder should be done, provided the tumor can be cleared. Otherwise a forequarter amputation is necessary. Satisfactory prostheses can be fitted for these patients as described under amputations.

Central Nervous System Paralysis

Cerebral Motor Paralysis. The cerebral motor cortex is affected by a variety of benign and malignant tumors, including metastatic tumors. The latter are frequently from primary malignant tumors in the bronchus, kidney, and breast; and malignant melanoma of the skin. All these tumors may cause hemiparesis or the more serious hemiplegia. The accurate localization with the EMI Scanner system is necessary, and it is stressed that emergency treatment is essential. When possible the tumor is excised; otherwise radiotherapy is given together with dexamethasone to relieve the increased intracranial tension. Rehabilitation techniques will often restore function, unless permanent damage has occurred. The patient's general nutritional state is maintained by routine methods. The tendency for muscle contractions to develop is prevented by the physiotherapist carrying out a full range of passive movements of the limb twice daily and splints, especially for night wear, may be necessary. The extensive area of sensory loss makes the patient unaware of temperature changes, so that excessive heat and cold are avoided to prevent tissue damage. The patient must be turned regularly to the normal side every 3 h to relieve pressure, and all pressure points must be padded for protection. In addition, the patient is placed on a ripple mattress or sheepskin rug. Restoration of function gives enormous relief to these patients, even though the life expectancy may be short because of the malignant disease.

Spinal Cord Paralysis. These are due to primary and secondary tumors pressing on various levels of the spinal cord, causing tetraplegia or paraplegia. Such pressure also occurs on the cauda equina, causing paralyses of these large nerves. These paralyses are serious and distressing, for which emergency treatment is essential for any recovery to be achieved. Some patients, for example with Hodgkin's disease, have a reasonably good prognosis, hence the necessity for effective treatment of the paralysis to restore function.

Tetraplegia

This is the most serious of all types of paralyses causing profound distress for the patients, who are often in middle age and accustomed to an active life. The psychological disturbance requires considerable sympathetic understanding and care. The pressure on the cervical segment of the spinal cord is caused by a primary or metastatic tumor. It may, for example, complicate a chordoma in the epipharynx which compresses the cord by direct extension. Metastases from a primary breast carcinoma or other site may cause compression from vertebral collapse. The possibility that this may occur and the premonitory symptomatology should be recognized so that preventive action is taken. If tetraplegia does occur, pressure on the spinal cord must be relieved immediately by laminectomy if this is possible, or otherwise by radiotherapy. When dyspnea accompanies the paralysis a tracheostomy is required. Immobilization in plaster with head traction is instituted; muscle contractures and pressure sores are prevented by routine treatment. Disturbances of micturition and defecation are dealt with by bladder catheterization and rectal enemas. The catheter is removed later when automatic micturition is established. Antibiotics are necessary to reduce the incidence of urinary infections. When the pressure on the spinal cord has been relieved the next objective of physical therapy is to mobilize the patient and restore function to the upper and lower extremities. During this phase of treatment a cervical collar is provided to support the head and prevent neck movements. Later a light cervical collar is worn for an indefinite period. General supportive treatment is given throughout to maintain the patient's nutritional state, restore morale, and encourage self-dependence. In all this work the minister, physiotherapist, occupational therapist, and family must collaborate with the clinicians, for this task requires teamwork.

Paraplegia

The problems created by paraplegia are similar to those of the preceding paralysis but are somewhat less serious. Paraplegia is more common and caused by primary tumors, benign and malignant. Generalized Hodgkin's disease may be complicated by paraplegia. In other patients metastatic carcinoma in the soft tissues or vertebrae can cause pressure on the spinal cord directly or through vertebral collapse. When vertebral metastases are known to be present precautions, including spinal support, are taken to prevent collapse.

The general management of these patients resembles that for tetraplegics. Emergency treatment is essential to relieve the pressure on the spinal cord by laminectomy when indicated, or otherwise by radiotherapy and chemotherapy. Passive movements of all affected joints are done daily to maintain a full range and avoid contractures, especially during the initial weeks of paralysis. The patient is turned in bed at intervals of 3 h during the day and night and a ripple mattress or sheepskin rug is provided, to prevent pressure sores. The latter are serious complications for they heal with difficulty and may require blood transfusion and skin grafting operations. Bladder catheterization is necessary, and antibiotics are given to minimize the risk of urinary infections. The catheter is removed later, when automatic bladder action has developed. For a time rectal enemas are necessary to prevent fecal impaction. Following the definitive treatment for the spinal cord compression, rehabilitation continues with special exercises for the paralyzed muscles and to increase the power of the remaining muscles which now have more work to do. The patient's range of activities are extended as mobility increases, with a wheelchair, walking between bars, elbow crutches, and a walking stick. Finally, the patient may be able to walk unaided.

An important aspect of the patient's rehabilitation is resettlement at home with the family and at work, provided the general health permits this, for much depends upon the degree of control of the malignant disease. Before final discharge from the rehabilitation unit, the patient is taken home for daily and weekend visits to become acclimatized with the family. In some cases stairs may be difficult to climb and new accommodations have to be provided on ground level. When disabled patients are able to drive, modifications may be required for their motor cars. The methods and objectives of rehabilitation described here are influenced by the degree of control of the malignant disease and its prognosis.

Cauda Equina Paralyses

Primary and metastatic pelvic tumors involve the cauda equina causing various paralyses in the pelvic organs, perineum, and lower extremities. Good examples are an advanced carcinoma of the rectum, uterus, or urinary bladder. It is important to recognize early any involvement of the nerves of the cauda equina, before bladder paralysis occurs, so the appropriate treatment can be given. An early symptom is neuralgic pain in the buttocks or thighs, which may be so severe that the patient cannot walk and requires bed rest with adequate sedation using methadone hydrochloride in 5 mg doses. Other manifestations at this stage include bilateral patellar and ankle clonus. As the paralysis progresses widespread sensory disturbances are found in the perineum, genitalia, and thighs. Later the urinary bladder and ano-rectal sphincters including the levatores ani become paralyzed, causing urinary and fecal incontinence.

The malignant tumor affecting the cauda equina may spread upwards to involve the lumbar nerve plexus, resulting in paralysis of the muscles of the lower extremity and deranged locomotion.

As in the other varieties of paralysis, pressure on the cauda equina should be removed quickly by excision of the tumor where possible, or otherwise treated with radiotherapy and chemotherapy. Bladder catheterization, rectal enemas, and antibiotics may be required until normal micturition and defecation are reestablished. The same general care and rehabilitation are necessary as for the other major paralyses.

Neuromyopathy

Neurological disturbances accompanying malignant diseases have long been recognized and are now attracting considerable interest because of their etiology and seriousness. They may be apparent even before the primary malignant tumor is diagnosed. Reference is made to the ectopic ACTH syndrome caused by an oat-cell carcinoma of the bronchus, where muscle weakness and wasting interfere considerably with the patient's mobility and even cause paralysis. This syndrome is caused by the carcinoma secreting polypeptide hormones. This activity must be diminished by radiotherapy and chemotherapy and urgent rectification of fluid imbalance and serum electrolyte abnormalities. The hypercalcemic syndrome may accompany osseous osteolytic metastases, hepatoma, and carcinoma of the bronchus and kidney. In this syndrome muscle weakness and hypotonia are severe, causing immobility, and the condition requires urgent treatment, otherwise it will be fatal.

Disseminated Breast Carcinoma

In this stage of the disease many patients benefit considerably from combined treatment including endocrine surgery, radiotherapy, and chemotherapy. Patients with osseous metastases may develop a pathological fracture which heals with adrenalectomy, and pain is relieved. The patients require endocrine replacement therapy and general supportive care, which enables them to enjoy lives of good quality for many years.

Pathological Fracture

This may complicate a primary bone tumor as an osteogenic sarcoma, or metastatic breast carcinoma. Patients in the latter group can often be rehabilitated by endocrine surgery for the metastatic carcinoma and from the insertion of an intramedullary nail to overcome the local fracture disability and thus restore function.

Research Rehabilitation

This subject requires more study and work to improve our methods of treatment and provide better appliances and prostheses. More information is necessary about the needs of patients with malignant diseases following definitive hospital treatment. Many are discharged without adequate preparations made for their reception into family and community life and employment. The work capacity of patients should be assessed, and any need for the modification or change of employment should be examined. Patients with a disability may require training facilities for a change of work.

Research is necessary concerning the subject of nutrition in malignant diseases, for we have little knowledge of metabolic abnormalities and their

correction. We are only beginning to understand the importance of vitamins, and especially ascorbic acid defects.

Increasing attention is being given to the care of stomas, but we need
more information about the welfare of patients with a tracheostomy, including its repercussions on family life, psychological effects, reactions to loss
of normal speech, and their resettlement and efficiency in employment.
Vocal rehabilitation needs special study with measurements of the effectiveness of speech therapy, efficiency of esophageal voice, and the various
pharyngeal vibrators which are used.

There is an increasing clinical and research collaboration in biomedical
engineering to solve various problems, including the provision of better
prostheses of different kinds. These include prostheses for voice production, especially an electronic artificial larynx, and powered limbs with a
good functioning hand.

Education and Training

This is necessary for the medical, nursing, and other caring professions to develop a high standard of teamwork and facilitate interdisciplinary communication. Teaching programs including congresses, lectures,
and seminars are required, in addition to facilities for practical experience
in hospitals and clinics on an interdisciplinary basis.

Patient counseling and education are essential to engender confidence
and secure cooperation in treatment techniques. The education of the
patient begins when the diagnosis is established, for it is desirable that the
patient knows the truth about the illness, which is communicated with
kindness and understanding in the presence of a key relative. There are few
exceptions to this rule, as when the family requests that this not be done
and it is felt that the patient cannot be told for some special reason. In these
circumstances rehabilitation is made more difficult, especially when there is
a poor prognosis.

The educational needs of the family are similar to those of the patient;
they have an important part in the work. Their education starts at the time
of diagnosis, and they gradually learn how they can help the patient's
recovery and resettlement. They may have to live with a patient who has a
disability or deformity and will be required to adjust to these new circumstances with understanding.

All members of the rehabilitation team require special knowledge of
oncology gained from work in hospitals and clinics where all types of
malignant diseases are dealt with. The close association of church and
medicine in the rehabilitation of these patients is desirable, so that some
special training should be incorporated in the training of ordinands.

COMPUTERS IN ONCOLOGY
THE USE OF COMPUTERS IN THE INVESTIGATION OF THE CELL

E. J. DAVISON

Introduction

The purpose of this chapter is to show that the use of mathematical system techniques may be used to obtain insight into the mechanism of cell behavior. In particular, it will be shown that the mathematical model of a cell can be used to find the possible mechanism which explains why a normal cell suddenly becomes tumorous. This will be done by obtaining a mathematical model of a growing cell living in a culture medium, and then systematically examining the behavior of the cell when various disturbances are applied to different parts of the mathematical model of the cell. The motivation for applying such an approach is that mathematical system techniques have been highly successful in explaining and predicting the behavior of technical–industrial processes (see, e.g., Himmelblau and Bischoff, 1968) and recently have given insight into the mechanism of various biological processes (see, e.g., Mesarovic, 1968; Diamant *et al.*, 1970; Palmby *et al.*, 1974). There has been to the author's knowledge no previous work done on this problem. The idea, however, of describing a

E. J. Davison • Department of Electrical Engineering, University of Toronto, Toronto, Canada. This work has been supported by the National Research Council of Canada under Grant A4396. The author wishes to thank E. Fabian, P. Wong, E. Mak, and J. Phillips for assistance in the computer modeling of the cell system.

cell using a mathematical model is not new. Pollard (1960) and Yeisley and Pollard (1964) described a cell using 5 and 7 differential equations, respectively. Heinmets (1964a,b, 1966) has modeled a cell using 19 differential equations to study various transient responses of the cell assuming no cell division takes place, and his qualitative model shall form the basis of the model to be described in this paper. Glueck (1969) used Heinmet's model to extend some of the latter's results. Weinberg and Zeigler (1969) studied the transient behavior of a nondividing cell using automata theoretic analysis. Other papers have been concerned with the modeling of tumor cells, per se; e.g., Jansson (1968) finds a model of tumor cells assuming that the cell population is tumorous, instead of finding a model of normal cells and then finding conditions under which these normal cells become tumorous. All the previous results use either analogue or analogue–digital computers to study the mathematical model of the cell; this study shall use solely digital computers.

In the synthesis of any model of a physical (or biological) system, certain assumptions as to what effects to include or exclude must always be made, and this is certainly true in the case of obtaining a mathematical model of a cell. It is also obvious that it is not necessarily clear (initially at least) what effects are more important and should be included, and what effects need not be included in such a model. In the case of finding conditions for a cell to become tumorous, however, one receives insight into its possible mechanism even if the model has not included enough effects; i.e., if the assumed model does not have the property of becoming tumorous, then one can assume the mechanism of tumor growth lies in those effects which have not been incorporated into the model. If the assumed model does have the property of becoming tumorous, then one can assume the mechanism of tumor growth lies in those effects which have been incorporated into the model. In the model to be described, any dynamics occurring outside the nucleus of the cell have been ignored, e.g., interaction effects of cells with neighboring cells have not been incorporated. It will be shown, however, that the present model is rich enough in structure to give "tumor-like" behavior when certain disturbances occur.

The chapter is organized as follows: section 2 describes the normal cell model, section 3 studies the behavior of the cell model under Mg^{2+} deficiency, section 4 deals with the case when the cell is subject to a split dose of ionizing radiation, and section 5 studies those disturbances which cause the cell to become "tumor-like."

Normal Cell Model

This section deals with the qualitative behavior assumed for the model of the cell.

Normal Cell Chemistry

The topic of cell chemistry is a vast one. The basic components (states) of the cell system are: genes, messengers, templates, enzymes, repressors, and activators. The following biochemical equations (Table 1), taken from Heinmets (1966), are assumed to describe the cell's behavior. (See end of chapter for definition of symbols used.) It is observed that all dynamic behavior outside the nucleus of the cell has been ignored in this model and that the extracellular nutrient pool P_e is assumed to be a constant (but its value can be varied). Figure 1 gives a block diagram for the interconnection of the various components of the cell.

TABLE 1. Complete Set of Reactions Occurring in the Cell

1. $E_p + P_n \xrightarrow{k_1} [E_p P_n]$

2. $B' + E \xrightarrow{k_2} B$

3. $G_B + P_n \xrightarrow{k_3} G_B + B'$

4. $G_C + P_n \xrightarrow{k_4} G_P + M_p$

5. $G_E + P_n \xrightarrow{k_5} G_P + M_P$

6. $G_E + [E_p P_n] \xrightarrow{k_6} G_E + E_p + M$

7. $B + M \xrightarrow{k_7} N$

8. $B + M_p \xrightarrow{k_8} N_p$

9. $C + P_a \xrightarrow{k_9} [CP_a]$

10. $N + [CP_a] \xrightarrow{k_{10}} B + C + M + E$

11. $N_p + [CP_a] \xrightarrow{k_{11}} B + M_p + C + E_p$

12. $M \xrightarrow{k_{12}} P_n$

13. $M_p \xrightarrow{k_{13}} P_n$

14. $B \xrightarrow{k_{14}} P_i$

15. $C \xrightarrow{k_{15}} P_i$

16. $E \xrightarrow{k_{16}} P_i$

17. $E_p \xrightarrow{k_{17}} P_i$

18. $P_e + E \xrightarrow{k_{18}} P_i + E$

19. $P_i + E \xrightarrow{k_{19}} P_n + E$

20. $P_i + E \xrightarrow{k_{20}} P_a + E$

21. $E_p + C \underset{k_{31}}{\overset{k_{21}}{\rightleftharpoons}} [E_p C]$

22. $E + P_i \underset{k_{32}}{\overset{k_{22}}{\rightleftharpoons}} [EP_i]$

23. $E_p + B \underset{k_{33}}{\overset{k_{23}}{\rightleftharpoons}} [E_p B]$

24. $N \xrightarrow{k_{28}} P_i$

25. $N_p \xrightarrow{k_{29}} P_i$

26. $P_i \xrightarrow{k_{30}} X$

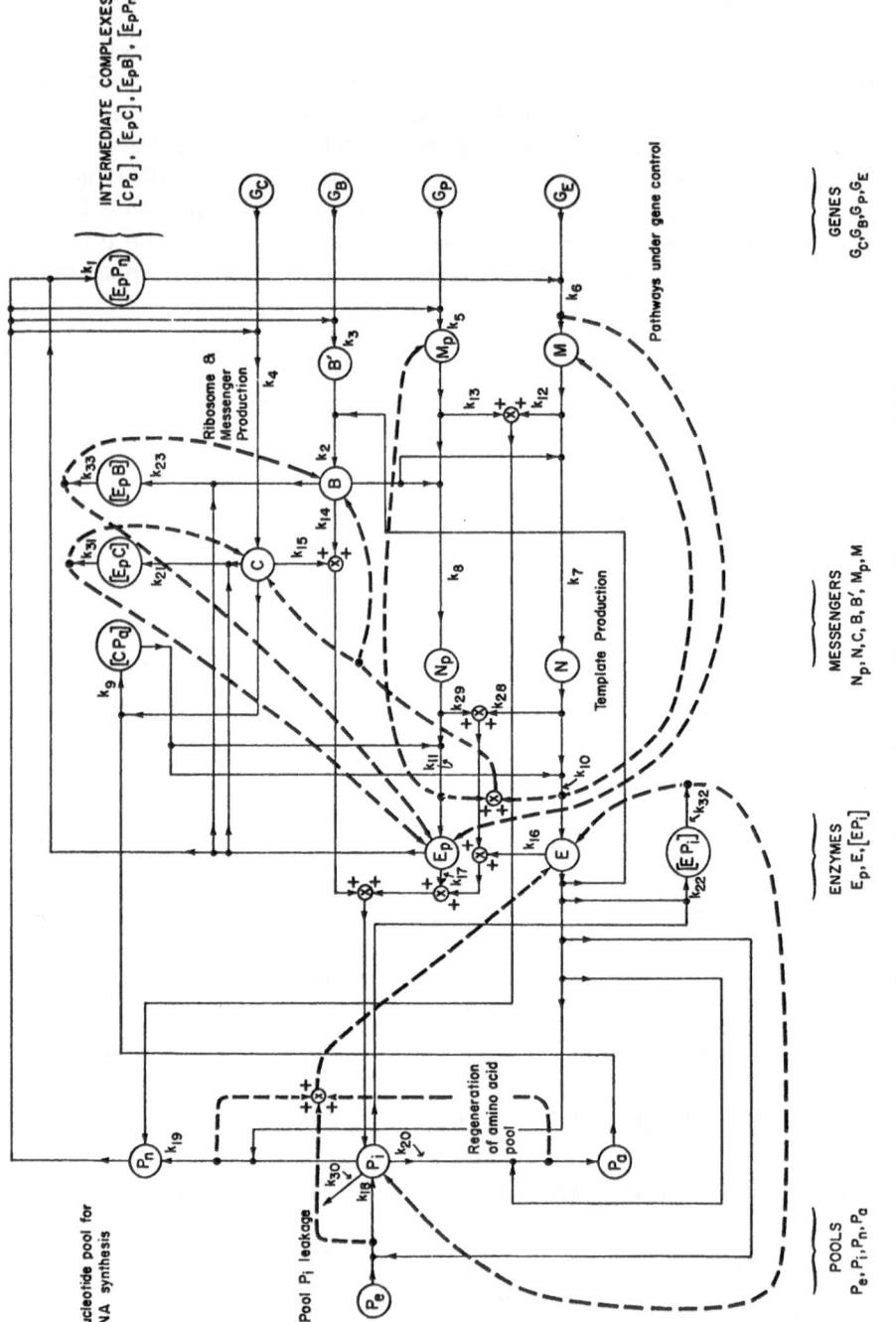

Figure 1. Flow chart showing dynamics of a cell nucleus (see Table 1).

G_E represents a group of genes required for protein synthesis, G_P is used for the synthesis of the enzyme E_p (which is the polymerase for messenger M), gene G_B produces the RNA fraction of the ribosome, while the protein fraction of ribosome is provided by the total protein E. Gene G_C produces transport RNA. The behavior of the cell system can briefly be described as follows. The complexing of messenger M with ribosome B yields template N; messenger M is produced by the interaction of the complex $[E_pP_n]$ with gene G_E. Enzyme synthesis results when templates interact with transport RNA and the amino acid pool complex $[CP_a]$. The total protein E is used to convert internal pool P_i into RNA precursors and amino acids, and to convert external pool P_e into internal pool P_i. Gene G_E is the only gene where polymerase is operating in the messenger synthesis. The formulation of polymerase E_p follows the same line represented by total protein E synthesis. The external nutrient pool P_e is converted into an internal pool P_i, where part of the pool P_i leaks out from the cell (via k_{30}), but the product is not associated with the external pool. The principal regulating element in the system is the complexing of total protein with the internal pool (Eq. 22, Table 1); this complexing is reversible, and the ratio between the two rate constants k_{22}, k_{32} determines the degree of regulation at this level. Additional regulating features are the complexing of polymerase with transport RNA (Eq. 21, Table 1) and the complexing of polymerase with ribosomes (Eq. 23, Table 1).

Mathematical Model of Cell

Using standard mass balance techniques on the chemical reaction equations of Table 1, a set of 17 simultaneous nonlinear differential equations of the type

$$\dot{x} = f(x, u, k); \quad x(0) = x°; \quad 0 \leqslant t \leqslant t^* \tag{1}$$

is obtained [see Davison (1975) for details], where $x \in R^{17}$ is the state of the cell given by

$$
\begin{array}{lll}
x_1 = E_p & x_7 = M & x_{13} = E \\
x_2 = P_n & x_8 = M_p & x_{14} = P_i \\
x_3 = [E_pP_n] & x_9 = N & x_{15} = [E_pC] \\
x_4 = B' & x_{10} = N_p & x_{16} = [E_pB] \\
x_5 = B & x_{11} = P_a & x_{17} = [EP_i] \\
x_6 = C & x_{12} = [CP_a] &
\end{array}
\tag{2}
$$

where $u \in R^5$ are the external inputs to the cell given by

$$
\begin{array}{lll}
u_1 = P_e & u_3 = G_c & u_5 = G_P \\
u_2 = G_E & u_4 = G_B &
\end{array}
\tag{3}
$$

and which must be determined, where $k \epsilon R^{29}$ is a vector of unknown rate constants for the cell which must be determined, and $x(0) \epsilon R^{17}$ are the initial conditions of the cell which must be determined; t^* is the division time of the cell, when cell division takes place, and must be determined. The above equations (1) describe the behavior of a single cell from the time of birth to the time at which cell division takes place (t^* sec later).

Mathematical Model of a Growing Cell

To describe the behavior of a growing cell, it is necessary to introduce some type of mitosis hypothesis (since the biological details as to when a cell divides are not well understood.) Considering the system (1), the following division hypothesis is made:

Division Hypothesis

Let $t^* \epsilon [0,\infty]$ be the time which globally minimizes the criterion function $J(t) \triangleq \|x(t) - 2x(0)\|$. Then if $J(t^*) < \|x(0)\|$, cell division takes place at $t = t^*$; if $J(t^*) \geq \|x(0)\|$, cell division does not take place. If cell division takes place, the initial condition of the new generated cell is equal to $(1/2)x(t^*)$.

The motivation for such a hypothesis is that a cell in steady-state behavior, i.e., with identical dynamic behavior existing from one generation of cell growth to another, will have the property that $J(t^*) = 0 < \|x(0)\|$, and $x(0) = (1/2)x(t^*)$.

Let x_i, t_i^*, $i = 1,2,3, \ldots$ denote the state and division time, respectively, of the parent cell, first daughter cell, second daughter cell etc. Then the behavior of a growing cell is thus described by the following sequence of differential equations:

$$\dot{x}_1 = f(x_1, u, k), \quad x_1(0) = x^\circ, 0 \leq t \leq t_1^*, \tag{4}$$
$$\dot{x}_{i+1} = f(x_{i+1}, u, k), \quad x_{i+1}(0) = \tfrac{1}{2} x_i(t_i^*), \ 0 \leq t \leq t_{i+1}^*, \ i = 1,2,3, \ldots$$

where t_i^*, $i = 1,2,3, \ldots$ is found so that $\min_{t_i \epsilon (0,\infty)} \|x_i(t_i) - 2x_i(0)\|$ occurs

at $t_i = t_i^*$, assuming that the constraint

$$\|x_i(t_i^*) - 2x_i(0)\| < \|x_i(0)\|, \ i = 1,2,3, \ldots \tag{5}$$

is satisfied. If (5) is not satisfied for some value of i, say I, cell division does not take place for $i \geq I$ and the cell dies.†

---

†Note that the topic of cell death is a very complex one and the fact that a cell does not participate in cell division does not, of course, necessarily imply that it is dead, e.g., the cell may differentiate. It will, however, be assumed in this study, for the sake of simplicity, that a cell which does not undergo cell division cannot survive.

Steady-state behavior in the cell is said to have taken place if there exists a scaler $t_s^* > 0$ such that

$$\lim_{i \to \infty} t_i^* = t_s^*$$

$$\lim_{i \to \infty} \| x_{i+1}(t) - x_i(t) \| = 0, \ \forall t \ \epsilon \ [0, t_s^*] \tag{6}$$

If (6) is not satisfied, the cell is abnormal and either dies or possesses some type of irregularity.

Simulation of Cell Growth

If it is assumed that the parameters k, u, x° are known, then the mathematical model of a growing cell (4) is completed specified, and it is only a matter of numerically integrating the equations (1) and carrying out a one-dimensional minimization search to obtain simulations of cell growth. In order to integrate the equations (4) an analogue or hybrid computer was *not* used because of scaling problems, and because there exist very successful algorithms for rapidly integrating large sets of differential equations (so called "stiff" methods of numerical integration) on a digital computer (e.g., see Davison, 1973). Davison (1975) gives details of the method of integration used; a typical computation time required to integrate the equations (1) on an IBM 370/165 digital computer was 0.68 sec real time.

Identification of Parameters of Cell Model

At this stage, in order to find a normal cell model it is necessary to identify parameters k, u, x° (which are not necessarily unique) so that conditions (4) to (6) are satisfied, subject to the following constraints:

$$k > 0, u > 0, x_i(t) > 0, \ \forall \ t \ \epsilon \ [0, t_i^*], \ i = 1,2,3, \ldots \tag{7}$$

where $\xi > 0$ means that all elements of the vector ξ are constrained to be positive. (The last condition of (7) is necessary since all states of the cell must be positive.) This was done by using a Monte Carlo search procedure for the parameters $k > 0$, $u > 0$, $x^\circ > 0$ and then substituting these parameters into (1), and carrying out the cell growth process described by (4),(5) until condition (6) was satisfied. For detailed properties of the normal cell obtained, see Davison (1975).

Effect of Mg²⁺ Starvation on the Cell

In order to verify the validity of the cell model obtained, the following experiment was carried out.

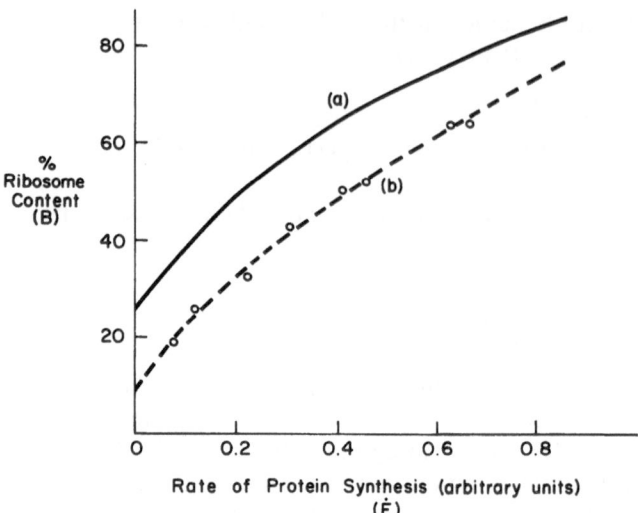

Figure 2. Comparison of experimental and theoretical recovery of cell from Mg^{2+} starvation. (a) Computed curve obtained from cell model; (b) experimental curve (McCarthy, 1962).

Let the ribosome content of the cell initially be put equal to zero (i.e., $B = 0$ at $t = 0$, or alternately $x_5(0) = 0$). Then how does the ribosome content of the cell vary with respect to rate of protein synthesis during recovery of the cell?

This experiment corresponds to an experiment McCarthy (1962) carried out in which cells of *E. coli* were starved of Mg^{2+} content so that their ribosome content almost entirely disappeared. On restoration of Mg^{2+}, the ribosome content slowly returned to its normal value.

On simulating the system (1) with all cell parameters equal to their normal values except for $x_5(0)$ which is $x_5(0) = 0$, the following results were obtained (see Figure 2).

In this case, it can be seen that the shape of the simulated cell recovery curve is almost identical to the shape of the experimental recovery curve of McCarthy (1962). The only difference between the two curves is a bias effect, which can be accounted for by the fact that the mathematical model of the cell is not intended to be a model of a specific cell, e.g., *E. coli,* but only of a representative cell.

Effect of Ionizing Radiation on a Cell

It is well known that if a cell is subject to a sufficiently large dose of ionizing radiation, the cell may eventually die. It is the purpose of this section to compare the simulated cell's response to ionizing radiation with experimental results for the case of a split-dose ionizing radiation disturbance. In order to do so, it is necessary to relate the effect of ionizing radiation on a cell to the states of the cell itself. Since the phenomenon is biologically not completely understood, this will be done by introducing a radiation effect hypothesis.

Radiation Effect Hypothesis

A dose D of ionizing radiation at time t affects a cell by destroying a certain fraction of all of the components (states) of the cell at time t; the larger the dose D is, the larger is the fraction of the cell's components (states) destroyed at time t.

The motivation for the hypothesis is that experimental evidence has indicated that ionizing radiation actually destroys part of the various components of the cell being radiated (Little, 1968).

It will be assumed then that the effect of ionizing radiation on a cell at time $t = 0$ is to cause the initial conditions of all states of the cell to be multiplied by a number r, $0 < r \leq 1$ called the *radiation factor;* the more severe the dose of radiation, the smaller is the radiation factor.

Split-Dose Experiment*

Consider now the effect of applying only one-half of the radiation dose at $t = 0$ and the other half of the dose Δ seconds later. Experimentally it has been found that the cell in this case is much less affected by the radiation now as compared to a single dose of radiation. [See, for example, Elkind *et al.* (1964) and Sinclair and Morton (1964), who studied the effect of X-ray radiation on Chinese hamster cells.]

It is of interest to see if the cell model considered also behaves in this way. The following results were obtained on simulating the cell model (4), (5), assuming that all cell parameters were normal except for the initial conditions which were all multiplied by the radiation factor $r_1 = 0.75$, and then, Δ seconds later, multiplying all resultant states of the cell by the radiation factor $r_2 = 0.75$ (see Figure 3).

This can be compared with the experimental results obtained by Sinclair and Morton (1964) given in Figure 4. As can be seen, the computed response curve is very similar to the experimental curve; in particular, it has a minimum occurring at a time slightly larger than the generation time, which agrees very well with the experimental results. (Note that the recovery curve of Figure 3 is only for one cell; for a large number of cells,

*For detailed properties of these results, see Davison (1975).

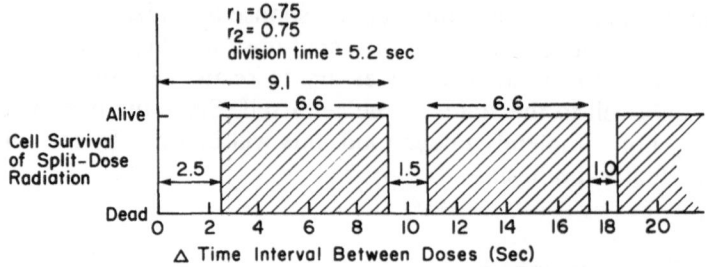

Figure 3. Computed split-dose recovery function for a single cell subject to ionizing radiation obtained from cell model. Survival is plotted as a function of the time interval between the two doses r_1, r_2.

taking into account the statistical variation of the cells, the qualitative predicted curve of Figure 4 will occur.)

Effect of Disturbances on the Cell: "Tumor-Cell" Behavior of the Cell

This section deals with the systematic study of applying various disturbances to the cell and then observing the effect of these disturbances on the cell's behavior. The results were obtained by simulating the system (4), (5) on using the normal parameters of the cell, except for a single parameter only, which was varied by a factor varying from 0.1 to 10. The single parameter was systematically chosen from the list of rate constants, external inputs, and initial conditions of the cell. In this case it was

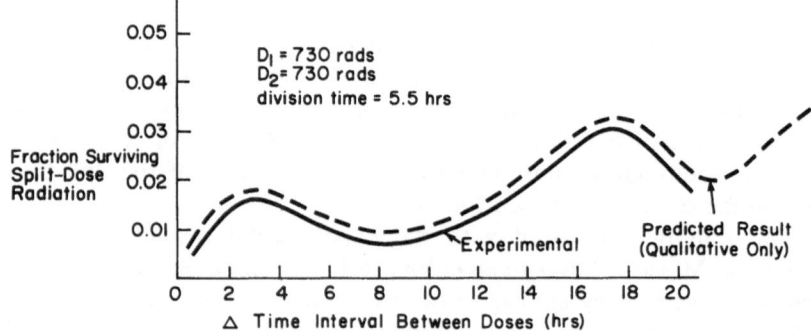

Figure 4. Experimental split-dose recovery function in cells subject to ionizing radiation (Sinclair and Morton, 1964). Survival is plotted as a function of the time interval between the two doses D_1, D_2.

observed that for some disturbances the cell dies, for other disturbances the cell basically remains normal, and for still other disturbances, the cell's division rate suddenly increases (by as much as a factor of 7!).

Perturbations which Cause Cell to Become Tumorous*

The following is a summary of all parameter perturbations which cause the cell to suddenly change into a fast-growing "tumor-like" cell with the following properties: (i) the disturbed cell is physically larger than the normal cell (typically by a factor of 10); (ii) the division time of the disturbed cell is greatly speeded up (typically by a factor of 5); (iii) the energy requirements of the disturbed cell are much greater than of the normal cell, and (iv) the disturbed cell generally behaves in an irreversible way, i.e., it is not possible to apply an opposite parameter change to the disturbed cell so that it returns to its normal behavior.

The cell becomes "tumor-like" when any one of the following changes in the normal parameters of the cell occurs:

[1] $P_e \rightarrow P_e \times 10$

[2] $G_E \rightarrow G_E \times 10$

[3] $G_P \rightarrow G_P \times \dfrac{1}{10}$

[4] $P_n(0) \rightarrow P_n(0) \times 10$

[5] $[E_pP_n](0) \rightarrow [E_pP_n](0) \times 10$

[6] $C(0) \rightarrow C(0) \times 10$

[7] $M(0) \rightarrow M(0) \times 10$

[8] $M_p(0) \rightarrow M_p(0) \times 10$

[9] $N(0) \rightarrow N(0) \times 10$

[10] $N_p(0) \rightarrow N_p(0) \times 10$

[11] $E(0) \rightarrow E(0) \times 10$

[12] $[E_pC](0) \rightarrow [E_pC](0) \times 10$

[13] $[E_pB](0) \rightarrow [E_pB](0) \times 10$

[14] $[EP_i](0) \rightarrow [EP_i](0) \times 10$

[15] $E_p + P_n \xrightarrow{k_1} [E_pP_n]$; $k_1 \rightarrow k_1 \times 10$

[16] $B' + E \xrightarrow{k_2} B$; $k_2 \rightarrow k_2 \times 10$

[17] $G_p + P_n \xrightarrow{k_5} G_p + M_\nu$; $k_5 \rightarrow k_5 \times \dfrac{1}{10}$

[18] $G_E + [E_pP_n] \xrightarrow{k_6} G_E + E_p + M$; $k_6 \rightarrow k_6 \times 10$

[19] $B + M \xrightarrow{k_7} N$; $k_7 \rightarrow k_7 \times 10$

*For details of the results obtained, see Davison (1975).

[20] $C + P_a \xrightarrow{k_9} [CP_a]$; $k_9 \rightarrow k_9 \times 10$

[21] $N + [CP_a] \xrightarrow{k_{10}} B + C + M + E$; $k_{10} \rightarrow k_{10} \times 10$

[22] $N_p + [CP_a] \xrightarrow{k_{11}} B + M_p + C + E_p$; $k_{11} \rightarrow k_{11} \times 10$

[23] $P_e + E \xrightarrow{k_{18}} P_i + E$; $k_{18} \rightarrow k_{18} \times 10$

[24] $E_p + C \underset{k_{31}}{\overset{k_{21}}{\rightleftharpoons}} [E_pC]$; $k_{21} \rightarrow k_{21} \times \dfrac{1}{10}$

[25] $E + P_i \underset{k_{32}}{\overset{k_{22}}{\rightleftharpoons}} [EP_i]$; $k_{22} \rightarrow k_{22} \times \dfrac{1}{10}$

[26] $E_p + B_i \underset{k_{33}}{\overset{k_{23}}{\rightleftharpoons}} [E_pB]$; $k_{23} \rightarrow k_{23} \times \dfrac{1}{10}$

It would be interesting to determine those external disturbances in the cell which cause the above perturbations in the cell's parameters to occur. This then would give insight into what type of external disturbances in a cell cause it to behave in a tumorous way. This is an obvious future research area.

Conclusions

This chapter provides a mathematical model of a dividing cell and studies various behavioral patterns of the resulting cell growth when the cell is subject to different disturbances. The main results of this study are the following:

(a) The cell model's behavior has agreed with experimental behavior for the case of a cell subject to Mg^{2+} starvation and then allowed to recover to nominal values.

(b) The cell model has agreed with experimental behavior for the case of a cell subject to a split dose of ionizing radiation. In this case the cell model has explained a mechanism for the rather complicated survival versus time-interval plot of cells subject to a split dose of ionizing radiation. In explaining this mechanism, there is no need to introduce extra assumptions such as "healing effects" occurring in the cell.

(c) The cell model has predicted that fast growing "tumor-like" behavior can occur in the cell when certain types of disturbances affect it; in such cases the physical size of the cell is much larger than its nominal value (typically by a factor of 10), the division time of the cell is greatly speeded up (typically by a factor of 5), and the energy requirements for the disturbed cell are much larger than for the nominal cell. Moreover, the behavior of these "tumor-like" cells is, in general, irreversible; i.e., when a disturbance of the opposite type is applied to the resultant "tumor-like" cell, the cell does not revert back to its original nominal values but continues in its "tumor-like" state. Since the mathematical model did not include any effects of extranucleus behavior in a cell (e.g., the cytoplasm) or interaction of cells with neighboring cells, this implies that tumor behavior (or malignant behavior) can be brought about by disturbances occurring solely in the chemistry of the nucleus of the cell, and hence is a very fundamental property of a cell. It would obviously be of interest to verify experimentally these predictions. This is an area of future research.

The above study has indicated that the mathematical modeling of cell processes is a method which can be used to obtain insight into the behavior of biological processes. It has the significant advantage that simulations of complex biological behavior can rapidly be carried out on a digital computer with all interior states of the process being monitored. For example, the total time required to simulate a cell dividing once was only 0.7 sec of real time on an IBM 370/165 digital computer; this includes the time to plot all 17 states of the cell as a function of time and perform data collection.

Terminology and Symbols

Pools

P_e = Extracellular nutrient pool
P_i = General intracellular metabolic pool
P_a = Amino acid pool for protein synthesis
P_n = Nucleotide pool for RNA synthesis

Enzymes

E = Total protein
E_p = RNA polymerase for messenger RNA (M) synthesis

Genes

G_E = Genes for messenger RNA (M) synthesis
G_P = Gene for messenger RNA (M_p) synthesis
G_B = Genes for the synthesis of RNA fraction of ribosome
G_C = Genes for transport RNA (C) synthesis

Messengers

M = Messenger (RNA) for protein (E) synthesis
M_p = Messenger (RNA) for E_p synthesis
B' = RNA fraction of ribosome
B = Ribosome

C = Transport RNA
N = Ribosome and messenger complex for protein (E) synthesis (template)
N_p = Ribosome and messenger complex for E_p synthesis (template)

Intermediate Complexes

$$[CP_a] \; [E_pP_n] \; [E_pC] \; [E_pB] \; [EP_i] \; X$$

References

Davison E. J. (1973). An algorithm for the computer simulation of very large dynamic systems. *Automatica* **9**:665–675.

Davison E. J. (1975). The simulation of cell behaviour: normal and abnormal growth. *Bull. Math. Biology*, **37**(5):427–458.

Diamant N. E., Rose P. K., Davison E. J. (1970). Computer simulation of intestinal slow-wave frequency gradient. *Am. J. Physiol.* **219**, (6):1681–1690.

Elkind M. M., Alescic T., Swain R. W., Moses W. B., Sutton H. (1964). Recovery of hypoxic mammalian cells from sub-lethal X-ray damage. *Nature (London)* **202**:1190–1193.

Glueck A. R. (1969) Simulation of cell behavior. Private communication, Princeton Computation Center, Electronic Associates Inc., P. O. Box 582, Princeton, N.J., Oct. 1969 (presented at Washington University, Nov. 1969).

Heinmets F. (1964a) Analog computer analysis of a model-system for the induced enzyme synthesis. *J. Theoret. Biol.* **6**:60–75.

Heinmets F. (1964b) Elucidation of induction and repression mechanisms in enzyme synthesis by analysis of model system with the analog computer. In *Electronic Aspects of Biochemistry*, pp. 415–479. Academic Press, New York.

Heinmets F. (1966) *Analysis of Normal and Abnormal Cell Growth.* Plenum Publishing Corp., New York.

Himmelblau D. M., and Bischoff K. B. (1968) *Process Analysis and Simulation* Wiley, New York.

Jansson B. (1968). Mathematical description of the growth of tumor cell populations with different ploidi-compositions. *6th Annual Symposium in Math & Computer Science in the Life Sciences*, March, Houston.

Little J. B. (1968). Cellular effects of ionizing radiation. *N. Engl. J. Med.* **278**(7):369–376.

McCarthy B. J. (1962). The effect of magnesium starvation in the ribosome content of Escherichia coli. *Biochim. Biophys. Acta* **55**:880–888.

Mesarovic M. D., ed. (1968) *Systems Theory and Biology*, Springer-Verlag, New York.

Palmby F. V., Davison E. J., and Duffin J. (1974). The simulation of multi-neurone networks: modelling of the lateral inhibition of the eye and the generation of respiratory rhythm. *Bull. Math. Biol.*, **36**:77–89.

Pollard E. (1960) Theoretical aspects of the effect of ionizing radiation on the bacterial cell. *Am. Nat.* **XCIV**: No. 874, 71–84.

Sinclair W. K., Morton B. A. (1964). Survival and recovery in X-irradiated synchronised Chinese hamster cells. *Cellular Radiation Biology Proc., 18th Ann. Symp. Fund. Cancer Res..* Univ. Houston, Texas.

Weinberg R., and Zeigler B. P. (1969) Computer simulation of a living cell: Multilevel control systems. University of Michigan Tech. Report 08228-17-T, Dec. 1969, Ann Arbor, Michigan.

Yeisley W. G., and Pollard E. C. (1964) An analog computer study of differential equations concerned with baterial cell synthesis. *J. Theoret. Biol.* **7**:485–503.

COMPUTERS IN ONCOLOGY
COMPUTERS IN ONCOLOGICAL CASE RECORDS

BARRY BARBER

Introduction to Computers

There is hardly a field of activity which has been unaffected by the development of digital computers during the last three decades. Such devices can carry out a sequence of logical instructions at high speed and can store vast quantities of information in a readily accessible form. Since the sequence of instructions, or program, can be held in store with the data it is possible to manipulate the data logically at the speed of electronic circuitry without the loss of time involved in human intervention and decision making. In general, the computer's internal instructions relate to some action to be taken in relation to one or more items of data at specified positions in the computer store. The computer's central processing unit is informed of the position of the first instruction in the program and it then follows the instructions sequentially until told to stop. Since the computer's internal instruction code can be difficult to learn to use efficiently, it is usual to simplify the programming by giving the computer instructions in a stylized language which can later be translated into machine code for internal use. Computer systems are described in terms of the size of their

Barry Barber • Chief Management Scientist, North East Thames Regional Health Authority, 40 Eastbourne Terrace, London, W2 3QR, Thames, England.

immediate access store, the speed with which information may be read from store, the variety of special instructions available to manipulate the information in store, the variety of equipment attached to the computer, and the languages that can be used for giving instructions to it. The cost of providing specified computing facilities is one of the few things that has consistently decreased.

The fundamental unit of information is a single binary element or bit; it is capable of distinguishing between two possibilities or therefore of assuming the values 0 or 1 only. In the computer store the data are stored in groups of bits, together representing an item of data to which the computer may readily obtain access. The arrangement of the store is part of the fundamental architecture of the computer. Some of the more commonly encountered groupings are of 8, 12, 16, 24, or 36 bits. An 8-bit group is called a byte, while the larger groupings are called words. A byte-orientated computer usually has instructions to handle groups of bytes to simplify the efficient use of the store. The bit groupings can be referenced directly by their position in the store, and this reference number gives the location or address of one particular group.

In general, a group of B bits can distinguish between 2^B possibilities. Thus, four bits are required to distinguish the numbers 0 to 9, six bits to distinguish between all the letters of the alphabet, and any positive integer from 0 to 1023 may be held in ten bits. The size of a computer store is usually expressed in terms of the "binary thousand" or K; this is 2^{10}, i.e., 1024. Thus, in principle, a $32K$ word store has 32×1024 places to store information that can be held in one word. Store sizes range from $4K$ words on a minicomputer to about 8 Mbytes on a large machine. Speed of access of information from the store is of considerable importance; this currently varies from 100 nsec for special high-speed storage locations to about 2 μsec for a rather slow store. The basic two-number addition time is likely to be within the range of 500 to 1000 nsec.* The user is not normally concerned with the details of the computer's instruction code, but obviously special requirements may need special facilities in the computer, and the speed with which certain types of work can be done may well be governed by the versatility of the computer's set of instructions. For instance, where a computer is required to handle a lot of numerical computation it may be desirable for it to have special floating point arithmetic instructions. Since a single computer word will only contain a finite number of numbers it is usually necessary to express numbers in a binary format corresponding to the scientific notation 0.1674×10^{-6}. A number is then stored in standard form as an integer exponent ($^{-6}$) together with a standardized number within a specified range (0.1674). A special hardware floating-point arithmetic unit is sometimes provided to handle the arithmetic on numbers stored in this floating-point format. In general, similar

*See section on Notation on p. 482.

results can be obtained by using a sequence of standard instructions, but the extra logical circuitry enables such calculations to be carried out more rapidly.

Much more equipment is required than the basic computer store and the associated processing unit. Some means of entering information and instructions is required. This may be done by electric typewriters, punched-card or tape readers, television type visual display units, or electrical signals from items of equipment. The results of the computation can be printed out on typewriter, special fast line printers, or visual display units. In addition, extra storage is often required for programs or information. This may be achieved using magnetic tape units, magnetic drums, or exchangeable disc units. The correct tapes and exchangeable discs have to be loaded when required, and the computer searches for the appropriate material. The drums and discs can provide direct access to several hundred Mbytes of information within less than 50 msec, while it may take 5 min to find the correct information on a magnetic tape. Finally, the computer's programs or instruction lists are normally written in a formalized semi-English language such as FORTRAN, ALGOL, COBOL, PL/1, or BASIC. Some of these languages provide very powerful logical facilities far removed from the machine's own instruction code that considerably reduce the programming effort required to solve problems. They are called high-level languages. Special master programs are provided by the manufacturer to enable the computer to translate these languages into its own internal code.

For certain specific tasks it is possible to obtain programs already written from particular computers, but usually it is necessary to have professional systems analysts and a programming staff to devise suitable systems for handling work with a computer. In some cases it is necessary for the computer instructions to be written in a language very close to the machine's own instruction code (low-level language). This can be particularly necessary in handling systems on small computers, or in providing an immediate response from the computer at remote terminals. The manufacturers also provide special operating programs to facilitate the handling of the computer. Such programs can simplify the provision of a really effective service from the computer by helping to run several programs, at the same time efficiently sharing the use of the various peripheral devices required by the programs.

Computers vary from rugged process-control computers capable of functioning on the factory floor and in any office or laboratory environment to systems requiring special air-conditioning and filtration equipment. The costs vary from about £1,000 for a microcomputer to well over £5 million for a major data-processing system. The physical equipment is collectively called "hardware," while the programs or lists of computer instructions are called "software." Both hardware and software may be bought or hired, or small quantities of time may be purchased or obtained free. Some computers can be linked remotely to terminals such as typewriters or visual displays so that calculations may be carried out or inquiries answered at situations remote from the location of the computer system. Computers can handle certain types of calculation or inquiry immediately on request provided the necessary programs are available on direct-access storage. The necessary data or inquiry can be entered directly through a terminal and the results can be provided immediately via the same terminal (real-time system). In other cases, the data are transformed into a suitable medium, such as punched cards, and, at a convenient time, the computer program and data are processed and the results are forwarded in due course to the user (batch processing).

The process of creating a list of instructions for a computer is called programming, while the task of loading them into the computer and supervising its functioning is called operating. Before the programming can be started, it is necessary to decide what functions can usefully be performed by the computer and how these functions will be linked to other activities; this study is known as systems analysis. After the program has been written, it must be prepared on some medium that the computer can read together with other associated information or data. This work is called data preparation. In a large computer system all these activities form the basis of different computer professions, but they may be carried out by a single person on a minicomputer.

Predictions in the computer field are exceedingly difficult to make. On the one hand, the computer manufacturers have provided immense improvements in hardware performance and have devoted much effort to the provision of special software to enable the hardware to be used more readily and efficiently. In addition, there appears to be no conceptual limit to what more and more sophisticated computer systems can do. Yet, on the other hand, the application of such systems to practical problems has been fraught with difficulties. The computer world is full of splendid schemes that may work in a few years' time, and others that have collapsed for the lack of proper attention to users' needs and to the organization they were designed to help. Successful computing systems require attention to much else besides technical detail. Computer systems can be rejected by organizations quite as effectively as the rejection of organ transplants by the human body. Considerable care has to be devoted to ensuring that the computer system is effectively grafted into the organization's psychosocial systems as well as its physical systems. Successful organizations are continually changing and developing in response to changing circumstances. Thus an inflexible computer system can easily prove to be an expensive inconvenience. Also, the gap between aspirations and attainment can be painful and acutely felt. However, there is no doubt about the usefulness and effectiveness of properly designed systems. Such systems are now in widespread use for handling financial and credit systems, airline reservations, process control systems, and much else. In the Health Service, in addition to the finance systems, there are systems for handling out-patient appointments; outline in-patient information; laboratory requesting and reporting; the analysis of information from laboratory equipment such as Auto Analyzers, Coulter Counters, and gamma cameras; the analysis of stylized specialist patient records; cancer registration; and radiation treatment planning. Taylor (1967), Whitby and Lutz (1971) and Coles (1973) all provide an introduction to computers and to some Health Service applications of computing technology. The major systems take much time to build, to implement, and to prove effective in practice. The broad concept is easy, but the practical detail can be difficult and time consuming.

Scientific Computing and Systems Development

One of the more important developments in the scientific community of the health service over the past decade has been the way in which scientists have managed to gain access to computing facilities to pursue their scientific work more effectively. Although not unique to the health service and not widely recognized, this certainly constitutes one of the major success stories of computing within that service. Medical physicists have taken a full share in developing the use of computers for ad hoc scientific calculations as distinct from the implementation of major data-processing systems. Currently, many physics departments have either a mathematician, or a physicist with particular interests in computing who endeavors to make sure that the department is adequately provided with computing facilities and programming support. There is no doubt that the programming manual has, in many respects, replaced the slide rule as the standard calculating equipment of the scientist. A medical physics department without access to computing facilities must be regarded as inadequately equipped. This is even more clear cut with regard to multidisciplinary oncology centers where data-processing systems are required as well as research facilities. The reason why scientific computing has spread so rapidly is that the computing power can be brought to bear very quickly on the problems encountered daily by scientists. This contrasts with the situation of the medical and nursing staffs where real computing power is only slowly being brought to bear on the central problems of patient care.

It is worth emphasizing the enormous difference between ad hoc scientific computing and the development of computer-based systems. The more important features of the situation are summarized in Table 1. This can be regarded only as a general guide to an obviously complex situation.

TABLE 1. Comparison of Ad Hoc Scientific Computing and Systems Development

	Scientific computing	Systems development
Staff involved	One, or at most, a few	Many
Flow charting	Often ignored	Vital
Documentation	Often nonexistent	Vital
Time to produce	Short	Long
Usage	Few times, or routine use by a few people	Routine running
Program maintenance	Often not required	Vital
Maintenance by	Single individual	Successive programmers
Education	Few staff members	Many staff members
Benefits obtained	Rapidly	Over a period of time
Dependence on individuals	Highly dependent	Independent

A great deal of scientific work can be undertaken by a single person who knows precisely what the technical problem is and proceeds to solve it, writing his programs directly in a high-level language. Such programs can be produced fairly quickly and may be used only a few times before being discarded with the experimental notebooks after the results have been obtained. Alternatively, they may be used routinely by a few people. The benefits are obtained rapidly, and only a few individuals need be involved.

The whole situation is radically different when one considers systems development. In this case, many staff personnel are likely to be involved in the systems specification, analysis, programming, data preparation, punching and computer operating, quite apart from the users of the results. Adequate flow charting and documentation are vital to the success of such a project. Much time is required before the final system can be rendered operational, and when this happens the system is expected to be routinely used thereafter. Proper arrangements have to be made for system maintenance which is likely to be carried out by a succession of different programmers. Many staff personnel have to be educated in various ways, particularly the users of the system, as any lack of communication at the time the system is designed, or during system implementation, can render the whole system ineffective. The benefits of the system can be substantial, but they are likely to accrue only over a long period of time.

The scientist's training makes it easy for him to launch into a scientific computing environment making good use of facilities very quickly. The danger arises if he unwittingly strays into the field of systems development without appreciating the great amount of effort required to ensure that such systems are developed in a highly engineered form.

Research Uses of Computers

Computing systems both large and small are now essential tools for the handling of a great deal of routine statistical analysis, model building, and scientific problem solving. It is difficult to specify in advance what problems will be solved. The scope is, in practice, limited only by the initiative, ingenuity, and inventiveness of those concerned. It is vital that the person using the computer should have a sound appreciation of the problem to be solved, otherwise the attempt to use a computer may merely put off the discovery of ignorance about the problem itself while wrestling with computer technology. Computers can be programmed only to solve problems where it is known, in principle, how to solve them. The computer utilizes its speed to carry out calculations which would be prohibitively time consuming if handled manually. However, the programmer must know, or be told, how to set about the task. The first clear need is an adequate understanding of the basic methods of conducting research. No amount of computer analysis can rectify faults in the design of controlled clinical trials or a lack of understanding of the statistical aspects of data analysis. It is now very easy to get the standard statistical calculations carried out on computers or even programmable desk calculators, but this facility makes it vital that the user should understand the statistical methods built into the programs. He must be able to assess when the techniques he is using are valid, what checks need to be carried out, and what conclusions may validly be drawn from the results presented by the computer output. All this should be the outcome of a carefully planned research program with specified objectives, and it is at this stage that good statistical advice should be sought; this is much more important than getting advice regarding computing. In general, the statistical analysis can indicate relationships between particular variables, and tests can be carried out to ascertain whether the observed data are likely to have arisen by chance, or are consistent with some specified underlying pattern. Until these various hypotheses have been properly formulated they cannot be tested against the experimental data. Some of the simpler calculations are worked through in various statistical texts (e.g., Moore, et al., 1972), and these may be used to test the accuracy and data output of unfamiliar computer programs. In some cases it is obvious immediately that the system is producing nonsensical results, but in other cases the results may appear quite reasonable but yet, in some circumstances, may be incorrect. The amount and detail of the checking required depends on the importance of the results and the consequences of error.

In addition to the use of standard statistical programs, it is often possible to use statistical systems for accumulating particular research records or surveys and generating reports from these records (e.g.,

S.P.S.S.). The scope and utility of such systems depend very much on the detail of the particular problem in hand. Finally, the research worker may be involved with such detailed and specific types of data analysis that the programs have to be specially written for his purposes.

In this case, and in the absence of trained staff to whom he may pass the problem, it may be convenient for him to learn a relatively simple programming language (e.g., FORTRAN or BASIC) which enables him to give instructions to the computer and thus direct the data analysis himself. The elements of handling such simple programming languages can readily be learned within a few days, and the ability to make rapid changes in data collection and analysis can be a vital element in the successful prosecution of research projects. Often such research analyses can be programmed by the user in less time than it takes to sit down with a professional programmer and explain the nature of the task to be carried out. Alternatively he may be able to modify programs used elsewhere to deal with his own requirements. Few organizations maintain sufficient programming staff to enable them to provide a programmer to write the frequent changes needed in the daily drive of a research project. The achievement of program changes not undertaken by the research worker in person may therefore take weeks or even months; hence the advantage of using a comprehensive statistical system such as S.P.S.S. In this discussion research is understood in its wider context, rather than as the simple listing of patients with particular characteristics to be written up as a small-scale study.

The level of access to computing facilities for research purposes depends on the amount and type of research being undertaken in an institution or by the individual research worker. However, if it is being done on other than a very occasional basis, local computing facilities of a small machine size with remote access links to larger machines are desirable. A courier service to a computer center coupled with rapid processing jobs can also be attractive. The balance of activity varies, and it is often useful to have a variety of options that can be utilized according to the nature of the work to be carried out. In general the fewer people involved directly between the research worker and the arrival of his results, the faster his work is likely to proceed. The computing facilities are merely tools to speed up the examination of evidence rather than an end in themselves.

Oncological Implications of Computer Systems

In a fast developing field it is invidious to be dogmatic about the scope and extent of future work. However, it is possible to discern the pace of past development by reading published conference proceedings (Laudet et al., 1976; Abrams, 1970, 1972; Anderson and Forsythe, 1975) or the four volumes of Stacey and Waxman (1965–1974). There are few areas of current development which were not discussed a decade ago or which do not form a logical extension of that work. Furthermore, the rate of implementation of systems is still relatively slow. Major hospital systems may take between 5 and 10 years to implement fully. This appears to be due to the complex, multidisciplinary, psychosocial systems of the hospital as well as to the intrinsic difficulty and high technical performance required by the health care situation. The major problems relate to the management of organizational change (Fairey, 1976) and to the accurate and efficient gathering of data from the environment. The easiest approach simply involves the completion of the forms. However, this activity is an additional administrative responsibility which tends to be relegated to transient clerks with no real interest in or knowledge of the matters described. This work is usually accorded a low priority and it is not surprising that the data are frequently quite inaccurate and incomplete. However, this approach has the signal advantage of leaving the organization's systems untouched. However, it was hoped that the problem of accuracy and completeness could be overcome by providing a terminal simple enough to be used by the professional staff themselves and a system designed to interact with the hospital's other systems, thus saving the need for extra data manipulation. However, it is noticeable that even in a real-time environment there is a tendency for professional staff to delegate the data entry (say, to nurses) or to batch groups of transactions. In addition, the design of such systems to be closely linked with other hospital systems is at present very time consuming and difficult. The use of visual displays with light pens for the selection of items from lists appears to have some advantages, but these devices are still relatively expensive in relation to the number of terminals required in a major hospital system. In many ways it is easier to construct a national computer system dealing with specific records than to devise detailed hospital systems. The main problem is then that of agreement about the data to be collected and a clear professional and administrative effort to ensure that accurate material is fed into the system. In principle, it should be possible to extract more information from a national cancer registry than seems possible at present. Even though specific controlled clinical trials are likely to be required to settle the details of the relative merits of particular treatments, it should be possible to extract appropriate information regarding prognosis, and the broad therapeutic effectiveness of various treatments and centers from suitably designed national systems.

Collen (1974) and Stacey and Waxman (1974) both provide extensive reviews of the current state of systems development and implementation, and Shuman et al. (1975) gives a related review of operational research in health care. The broad picture is summarized in Figure 1. The development represents a gradual climb from the lower level financial and adminis-

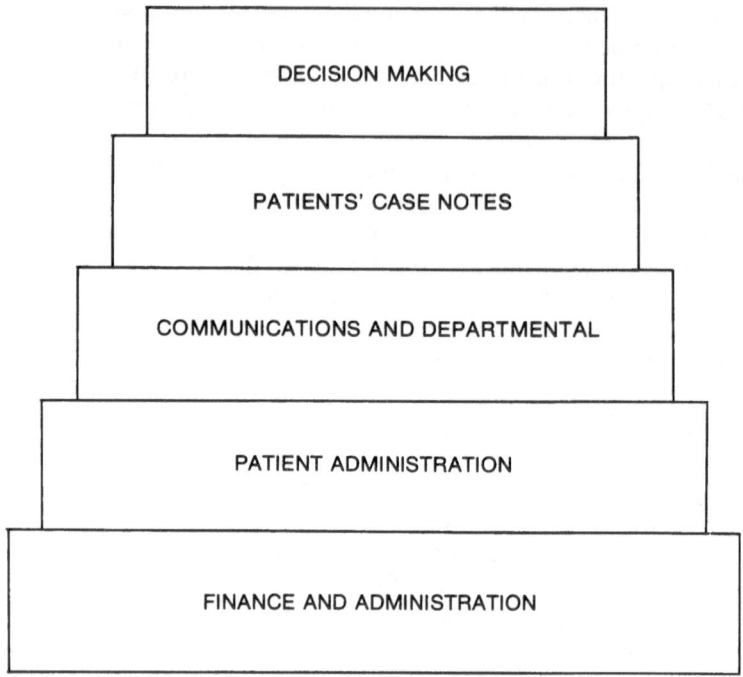

Figure 1. Development of health service computing systems.

trative systems toward the development of systems to assist with clinical decision making. Radiation treatment planning systems have been described in more detail because of their importance in oncology, while financial and general administrative systems have been ignored as part of the organizational framework rather than of special oncological interest.

Patient Administration Systems

Following the use of the computer in specialist areas, the logical starting point for the development of general Health Service computer systems was the patient administration systems. All sections of the service are concerned with patient-orientated administrative activities such as identifying patients; sending letters to them and to their family doctors; and carrying information about appointments, waiting lists, and the use of beds and clinics. These are the normal and essential preliminaries to medical care and they provide a useful area of activity for testing out computer systems before the latter can reasonably be utilized in the more critical areas of medical care. A large variety of systems of differing complexity and scope have been built during the last decade to handle these types of activity using batch processing and real-time computing facilities. This work always enables the organization to improve their associated manual systems and procedures and the process of computerization throws a great deal of light on the functioning of the organization. Also such systems provide the basis for the extension into the area of communications systems and patients' case records.

Figure 2 shows the computers supporting the patient administration system at The London Hospital. It has currently 61 visual display terminals in the various wards and departments carrying waiting lists, admission and discharge information, and an inpatient index. Also, a drug interaction notes system is available together with a clinical laboratory system with requesting and reporting facilities. Figure 3 shows a typical ward terminal. Further details are given by Barber and Abbott (1972), Abbott *et al.* (1974), and Barber *et al.* (1976). The ideas for this system were developed out of earlier work using batch processing techniques on a small second generation computer.

Communications and Departmental Systems

These systems form an interface between the activities of patient administration and the patients' case records. They often cover a small

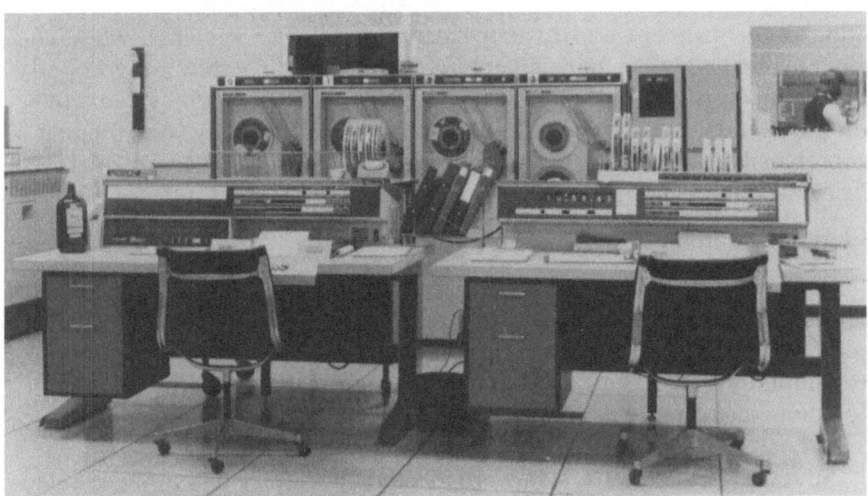

Figure 2. The London Hospital computer system.

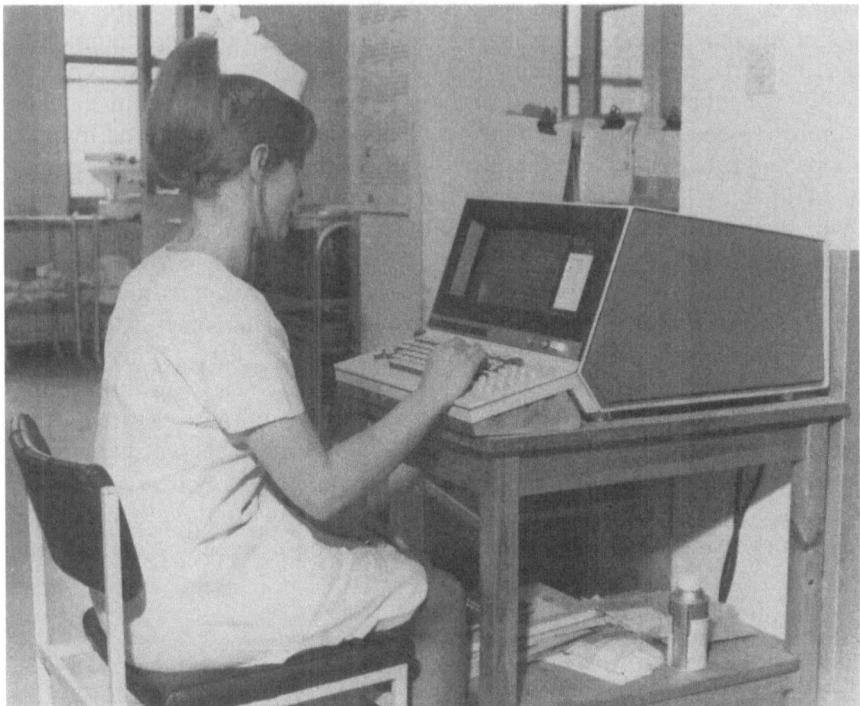

Figure 3. Computer terminal being used in a ward at The London Hospital.

section or department and include sections of other systems. They can often be handled on a departmental basis, providing they are properly linked into the rest of the organization. In many areas such systems have been particularly successful where systems aimed directly at providing a comprehensive system for handling the case records have proved to be difficult to implement.

Radiation Treatment Planning Subsystems

For over a decade efforts have been made to use computer systems to facilitate the process of radiation treatment planning. The first work involved the use of batch processing techniques, but since then small on-line computers have been used as well as terminals and small local computers linked to remote computers. Sternick (1976) is a good introduction to the field.

Several commercial systems are available for carrying out these calculations and many radiotherapy centers have written their own special programs for this purpose. In general, the limitation of batch processing systems lies in the delay between the specification of the field arrangements and the availability of the resultant field. This means that it is important that the first guesses at an appropriate field configuration should be very good if undue delay in starting treatment is to be avoided. However, where there is a direct on-line link with a computer it is possible for a large number of field configurations to be explored rapidly before selecting a most suitable arrangement. Thus half an hour's work directly on the computer may provide a good arrangement, while setting up the first run on a batch system may take almost as long and still lead to modifications, and repeated work a few hours, or even a day, later, if the first guesses are unsuitable. Arguments continue about the best computer approach to this problem, but these are much less important than the key features required by the users of the system. The ease of entering and changing data about the radiation fields, the patient's body contours, the speed of response of the system, and the ease of interpreting the results are all of far more practical importance than the technical details of the computer system used to achieve the desired result. A great deal of time can be wasted if the radiotherapists or physicists are concerned unduly with the computer technicalities instead of with clarifying their user requirements. Computer technicalities should be left to the computer professionals.

The British Institute of Radiology and the Department of Health and Social Security commissioned a study of the relative merits of the radiation treatment planning systems currently used in the United Kingdom. This report (Barber, 1973) outlined the main systems then available and illustrated the kind of information obtained from the various systems. Figure 4 illustrates the sort of graphical output provided by the system developed at The Royal Marsden Hospital for use on a D.E.C. PDP8 computer shown in Fig. 5. At present, the systems take a significant amount of effort to commission because the computer has to be provided with detailed data about the radiation beams from the installations being used. As might be expected this effort is comparable with the effort normally devoted to the commissioning of a major item of radiation equipment itself. When the information has been entered correctly into the computer, the routine operation of the system to produce treatment plans can be learned within a few days.

However, the planning process is not automatic. It requires a thorough understanding of the principles and practice of radiation treatment planning. The computer merely carries out the calculations much faster than they can be done by hand. Some attempts have been made to produce computer programs that seek the "best" plan in some defined sense from a range of plans. However, at present it is only possible in relatively

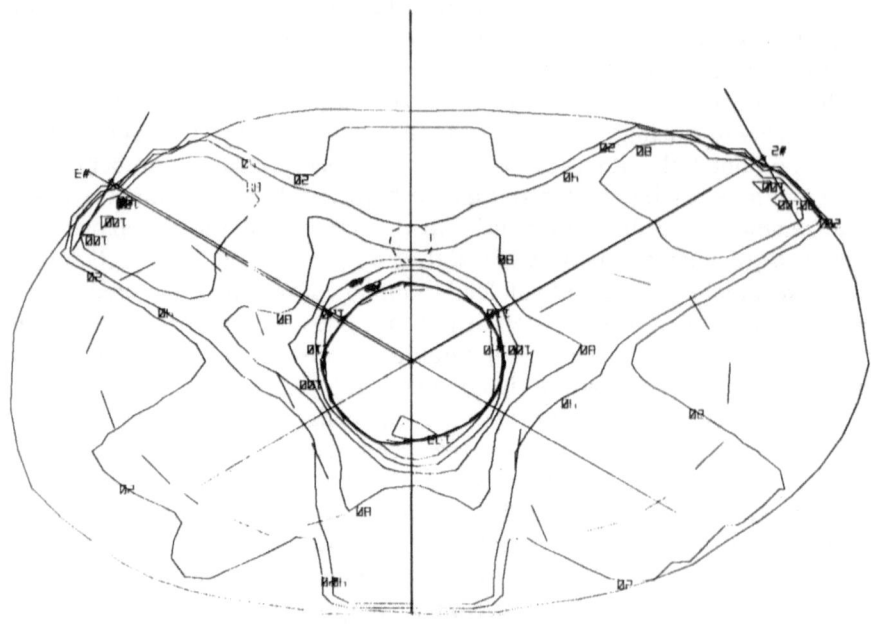

Figure 4. Treatment plan from Royal Marsden system.

restricted situations and the interactive dialogue using a direct link to a computer provides the fastest method of finding a good plan. Eventually, one may hope to devise optimal planning systems.

Barber (1973) enumerates the major activities related to treatment planning and to indicate the scope for using computers to assist in their execution. Other matters that could be handled readily by a local treatment planning computer include the storage of the finally selected plan, independent plan checking, the production of the treatment prescription, the checking of the patient set-up, and the measurement of patient contours. Such systems could be linked to a simulator to provide a "dose-computing simulator" or to the administrative and record systems of the department. Such steps are a reasonable extension of present practice and would comprise the first "automated radiotherapy systems."

Other Service Department Subsystems

In general, the service department subsystems are concerned with internal departmental functions and with requesting and reporting functions which link with the rest of the hospital organization. The balance between these various activities depends on the department concerned as well as on the particular emphasis adopted within a particular computer system. Some of the more common departments are the biochemistry, hematology, and pathology laboratories and the diagnostic X-ray department. Laboratory systems are now relatively common and much of the original drive came from a desire to handle a large volume of testing on automated equipment such as Coulter Counter and Auto analyzers. Service department subsystems can print results or make them available on a network of terminals located in the wards and clinics. One of the major hurdles is that of making sure that a sufficiently high proportion of investigation requests are made either on the computer terminals or on some computer readable medium. If this is not possible, all the relevant material has to be entered into the system as part of the departments' administrative routine. Such systems can be used to assist with the preparation of the work schedules and with technical quality control in the system. The requesting and reporting are the key activities which interface with the Patient Administration and the Patient Case Records in Figure 1. At present it appears that such systems cannot make individual urgent results available more rapidly than the previous manual system, but that they can and do routinely make a much greater volume of material available more rapidly. Requesting and reporting systems for diagnostic X-ray departments follow a similar pattern.

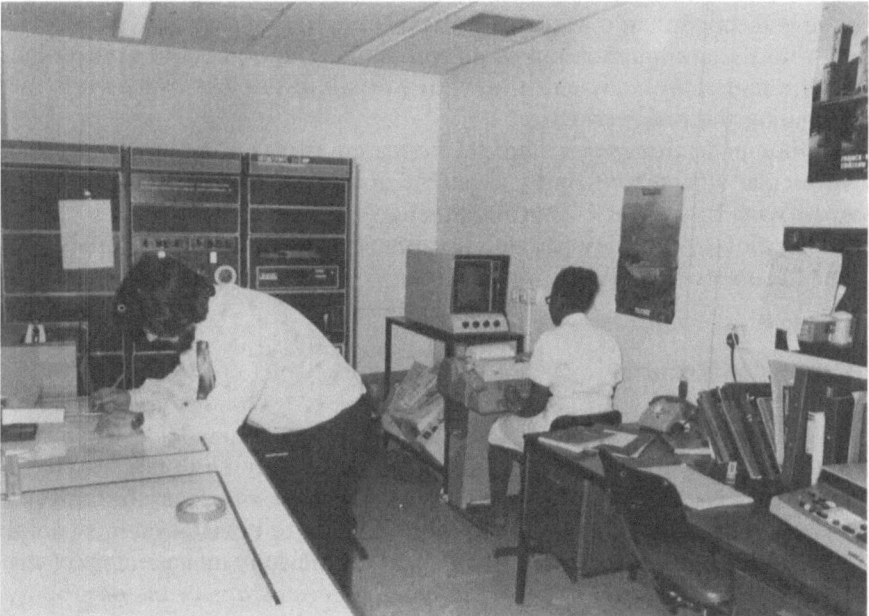

Figure 5. Royal Marsden/Rad 8 treatment planning computer system.

In addition to specific departmental systems a number of virtually self-contained health screening systems have been developed. These cater to the routine production of a battery of tests for individual patients or citizens. These systems can be readily integrated into the health care delivery system of a community or of a major hospital. The use of such systems has been relatively restricted so far in the United Kingdom, but perhaps the emphasis on community health care and preventive medicine within the reorganized National Health Service may lead to a fresh examination of the value of such systems when used in conjunction with an appropriate health care strategy.

A number of self-contained patient monitoring systems have been developed, mainly in conjunction with intensive care units to assist with the management of small numbers of acutely ill patients. The data are obtained directly from transducers attached to the patient, from conventional monitoring equipment attached to the patient, or by direct entry of data by a nurse or technician. Such systems can alert the clinician to developing problems at an early stage, and they provide a detailed description of the patient's condition and his response to treatment. They can also be geared to the administration of limited and specific forms of treatment.

The final communications subsystem of note is the development of nursing systems to assist with the ward management nursing care plans and records. The recording required in such systems is very much less in volume and scope than that of the patient's case records. Such systems can assist with the communication of information about a patient between the various nurses involved, and they can provide a flexible framework for coordinating the patient's care.

Although this only gives a brief indication of the communication and departmental systems currently available or being designed, such systems have proved to be easier to implement than the higher level systems outlined below. Also they provide a valuable guidance for developing full patient case-record and decision-making systems.

Patient Case Records

For over a decade various attempts have been made to construct computer-based patient case records. This can readily be done in stylized abstracts of relevant clinical data for the purposes of research analysis. However, it has proved to be much more difficult to devise systems useful for the routine recording of patient data and for the daily management of the patient. For the purposes of research, such records are very similar to any other survey in that key data are recorded for subsequent computer input and analysis using standard methods of form design. Such techniques are also suitable and used for collecting data for various cancer registries, so that routine statistics may be produced and cancer follow-up cards issued.

This work has been extended into the area of patient management in particular specialties and the major hospital computer systems have varying quantities of clinical information associated with the routine patient administration material, but as far as is known there is no system which completely takes over the function of the manual case records for a major general acute hospital. However, this is only a matter of time and enterprise. The main obstacle is that of finding a really fast and convenient method of entering the information into the computer and retrieving it subsequently.

Much of the material contained in the case records can be entered by clerks during the ordinary administrative process or by secretaries typing reports directly into the computer system. In addition, information from the communication and departmental systems described above can be entered automatically. Doctors' orders and requests can readily be entered into a television display type computer terminal on the ward, selecting the appropriate options from lists presented on the computer screen. However, the major problem is the entry of the results of the clinical consultation; the history, symptoms, signs, conclusions, and items to be followed up. There is some evidence to suggest that the adoption of a problem-orientated case-record approach (Weed, 1971), or some other logical structure based on an operations analysis of the use of the records, could transform the whole record gathering and storage system. The attempt to store records as they are currently organized merely perpetuates an inefficient manual system without exploiting the potential of the computer system. It is likely that development of appropriate case-record systems can be handled more easily in particular specialist areas initially. Thus an approach to case records within oncology could be a reasonable starting point for a system ultimately designed to spread throughout the whole of medicine.

Decision Making in Patient Care

Much has been said about diagnosis by computer. This has given rise to excessive hope on the one hand and excessive fear on the other. At present, it has been shown that computers can perform about as well as a good specialist in very limited specific areas. However, no general diagnostic facilities have yet been produced, though it is reasonable to expect that, when satisfactory case-record systems have been produced, the next step of utilizing computers will be in giving assistance for decision making. Anderson and Forsyth (1975, pp. 553–623) give a good indication of the current developments in this field. The key question is normally not what is the diagnosis, but rather what is the necessary action in given circumstances.

Furthermore, it is likely that computer-assisted decision making will be available as a background checklist for the highly trained specialist as well as an educational support for more junior staff. Only when this stage has been reached will it be possible to say that computers are contributing really significantly to the process of providing medical care. The present problem of medical computing is that of providing convenient systems for medical personnel who have relatively little to gain from the system and whose expected usage is at most occasional. Once effective systems have been produced to assist with decision making there will be no problem of user acceptance because of the intrinsic medical value of the suggestions and commentary provided by the systems. In addition, it can be expected that simpler and more convenient techniques will have been devised for communicating with computer systems by that time.

Conclusion

The general literature on computing science and technology is enormous, and there is no difficulty in pursuing certain specialist areas of interest with courses or in journals. Regarding medical computing, no new "principles" of computing have so far emerged, but a great deal of effort has been necessary to render systems convenient and acceptable to the users. Many of the problems are highly interesting from a technical viewpoint but often practical performance in system design and construction has been left far behind the sometimes overoptimistic objectives and hopes of the system design team. Medical, or more strictly health service, computing is now a wide-ranging activity involving many computer and health service staff members. The references quoted in this chapter are sufficient for anyone wishing to pursue specialist health service computing interests in order to assess the current state of development of various types of system. Sternick (1976) is particularly helpful in the applications of computers to radiation oncology and Shuman et al. (1975) is helpful in the general area of operational research. In addition, a much greater emphasis is being given on specific systems objectives and an evaluation of the system against these objectives. Furthermore, the attempt to evaluate such systems is slowly beginning to lead to the concept of attempting to evaluate other aspects of health care systems.

Notation

1 Mbyte $= 10^6$ bytes
1 μsec $= 10^{-6}$ seconds
1 nsec $= 10^{-9}$ seconds

References

Abbott, W., Barber, B., Cohen, R. D., Fairey, M. J., Kenny, D., and Scholes, M. (1974). *A Case Study in the Installation of a Real-Time Computer System*. The London Hospital, London.

Abrams, M. E. (1970). *Medical Computing Conference Proceedings*. Chatto & Windus, London.

Abrams, M. E. (1972). *Spectrum 71: Conference on Medical Computing*. Butterworth, London.

Anderson, J., and Forsythe, J. M. (1975). *Medinfo 74: First World Conference on Medical Informatics*. North Holland, Amsterdam.

Barber, B. (1973). Computerised dose computation. (A report prepared for the British Institute of Radiology and the Department of Health and Social Security.) The London Hospital, London.

Barber, B., and Abbott, W. (1972). *Computing and Operational Research at The London Hospital*. Butterworth, London.

Barber, B., Cohen, R. D., and Scholes, M. (1976). A review of the London Hospital computer project. *Medical Informatics*, 1:61–72.

Coles, E. C. (1973). *A Guide to Medical Computing*. Butterworth, London

Collen, M. F. (1974). *Hospital Computer Systems*. Wiley, New York.

Fairey, M. J. (1976). The management of organisational change. In *Case Studies in Operational Research in the Health Services* (B. Barber, ed.), Operational Research Society, United Kingdom.

Laudet. M., Anderson, J., and Begon, F. (1976). *Medical Data Processing*. Taylor & Francis, London.

Moore, P. G., Shirley, E. A., and Edwards, D. E. (1972). *Standard Statistics Calculations*. Pitman, London.

Shuman, L. J., Dixon Speas. R., and Young, J. P. (1975). *Operations Research in Health Care*. Johns Hopkins University Press, Baltimore.

Stacey, R. W., and Waxman, B. D. (1974). *Computers in Biomedical Research*, Vols. I–IV. Academic Press, New York.

Sternick, E. S. (1976). *Computer Applications in Radiation Oncology; Proceedings of the Fifth International Conference on the Use of Computers in Radiation Therapy*. University Press of New England. Hanover. N.H.

Taylor, T. R. (1967). *The Principles of Medical Computing*. Blackwells, Oxford Edinburgh.

Weed, L. L. (1971). *Medical Records, Medical Education and Patient Care*. Press of Case Western Reserve Univ., Chicago.

Whitby, L. G., and Lutz, W. (1971). *Principle and Practice of Medical Computing*. Churchill Livingstone, Edinburgh, London.

Chapter 19

EDUCATION IN ONCOLOGY: PROFESSIONAL AND PUBLIC

CRAWFORD JAMIESON

Oncology cannot be the sole province of a few highly specialized units. Neurosurgery can be a tight specialty because only a small percentage of the population will ever need the skills of the neurosurgeon. Even in this example the more common conditions of concussion, epilepsy, etc., are managed by the general physician, pediatrician, and surgeon who must be sufficiently familiar with the subject to make the correct decisions in the referral of patients to neurosurgical units and must be able to care for them after their discharge. A large minority of the population of this county will at some time in their lives contract an oncological disease (Registrar General, 1975) and it would be wrong to expect this vast amount of clinical material to be handled in this way.

Specialist oncological units should exist, though the need for them has not been appreciated fully to date, and the staffing and training of the doctors and scientists who work in them is not a great problem. Although Great Britain has been somewhat dilatory in this field, other nations have not, and it is possible for a dedicated individual to tailor himself a good

CRAWFORD JAMIESON • Consultant Surgeon, St. Thomas and Hammersmith Hospitals; Senior Lecturer in Surgery, Royal Postgraduate Medical School, London, England.

training here and abroad which equips him well for such a post. We are fortunate in having ample resources of scientists with whom such trainees can work. Biochemistry, cellular biology, pharmacology, histopathology, immunology, and physics are as advanced and expanding here as in any other country, and owing to the relatively small distances between our seats of learning they are accessible to anyone who is sufficiently interested. Our main lack is the large clinical unit with sufficient scope of practice to attract these workers toward becoming part of its organization and to offer the breadth of clinical material so essential to good training. An attempt to give an interpretation of the ideal role of these units is made later, but it is important first to define the objectives of professional training in oncology.

There are four convenient groups of doctors requiring education: (1) The senior specialist who trained before the management of these diseases had reached its present complexity; (2) the family doctor who is increasingly involved in the management of oncological problems; (3) the general surgeon, physician, or radiotherapist who treats those patients who present in his broad spectrum of practice; and finally (4) the young specialist who is planning a career with a major interest in the field.

Their individual requirements are considered below.

The Senior Specialist

Further education should be unnecessary for the senior specialist will probably have made every effort to learn the advances in diagnosis and treatment as they have been made and will have been stimulated by a succession of junior staff. He may, however, find it difficult to find the time to consider a claimed advance in sufficient detail or to obtain enough reliable information to allow him to make major changes in an aspect of management of his patients which has proved in his hands to be fairly reliable over a number of years. He may also, though it takes courage to admit it, not know exactly what has happened to his patients during those years. A truly balanced view of one's own practice is difficult to obtain unless one can stand back from time to time to study it. It is surprisingly difficult also to obtain the necessary information from our present design of hospital records. Gross data are included such as how many patients were treated, 5-year mortality rates, and obvious complications; but the exact stage of the disease present at the time of treatment and objective evidence of the efficacy of therapy are seldom stated with sufficient clarity to enable concrete conclusions to be made.

The senior and established specialist may, therefore, need education in methods of data collection and data analysis. He should also be able then to review his practice, not in a vacuum, but with his peers, and between them they should be able to reach conclusions of such definition that management can be modified with confidence. It would also save time if the necessary advances and new hypotheses in his fields of interest could be presented to him in a concise but undistorted form in journals, seminars, and discussion groups. Postgraduate societies should fill this role. Existing postgraduate societies are fractionated into systems, but societies are now forming with a common ground in oncology and these should offer programs of wide and common interest to a variety of specialists.

The Family Doctor

The family doctor has too much to learn already and must struggle to keep abreast with new developments in the whole of medicine. It is beyond the scope of this chapter to attempt to define the ideal undergraduate and postgraduate training of a family doctor. This is changing rapidly as medical school curricula are modernized, and it is now well recognized that the family doctor is a specialist and as such needs his own postgraduate training program. Fortunately, few work alone and a partnership of three or four allows each member to specialize to a greater or lesser degree. It is hoped, therefore, that most practices could in the future support one partner with a greater than average knowledge and interest in oncology who would be able to advise and assist in the continued education of his colleagues.

What does the family doctor need to know about oncology? He must know a considerable amount: His role as a referring physician necessitates the early recognition of symptoms and signs of oncological diseases in a busy consulting room. He must be continually on guard. It is easy for us to teach students that sudden onset of dyspepsia, weight loss, or change in bowel habit should ring alarm bells in the mind of the clinician, but these bells ring so often for less sinister reasons in the consulting room of a family doctor that his vigilance may well relax. He sees the whole unfiltered spectrum of serious and trivial, rare and common diseases, and it is a great credit to the training and dedication of these doctors that the standard of referral of patients with oncological diseases is so high.

His duty to such a patient can terminate with referral, but usually it does not. The patient, after investigation and treatment, is referred back to his care with occasional visits to the hospital for reassessment. This shared care of the patient may tax the interest, tact, and patience of a family doctor to a great extent. His needs in these circumstances are the following.

(a) He must know what happened to the patient in the hospital. He needs a prompt report from the specialist team containing diagnosis, treatment, prognosis, and a full analysis of the information given by the staff of the hospital to the patient and his relatives.

(b) He must know what may happen to the patient in the future. He is in a much better position to support his patient if he knows the natural history of the disease and the plan of management favored by the specialist to whom the patient was referred. These two points may be considered together. He may already have considerable knowledge of the behavior of the disease, but he can be assisted in his education and revision by better systems of communication with the hospital. We must continue our efforts to improve the traditional and often inadequate contact between the hospital and the family doctor.

An approximate prognosis may easily be included in a conventional discharge summary, but an outline of possible future management may be more complex but valuable in its capacity to educate and aid cohesion of efforts on the patient's behalf. The most simple examples arise from those clinical situations in which there is considered to be one ideal plan of management and the only doubt lies in its timing, or frustration by complications of therapy. A patient may be admitted with large bowel obstruction, found to have a colonic carcinoma, and treated initially by an emergency colostomy. His future management can be predicted in some detail and the patient's doctor can be sent a simple plan in addition to a full summary and account of the information supplied to the patient, e.g.,

24/8/76   Transverse colostomy for obstruction due to sigmoid colonic carcinoma.
9/9/76   Discharged.
14/9/76   To be seen in outpatient clinic.
28/9/76   Due for readmission for probable colectomy on 2/10/76.
16/10/76 Approximate date of discharge. Convalescence arranged for 2 weeks.
12/11/76 Readmission for closure of colostomy.

This simple plan may be frustrated by death or complications, but it does allow the doctor and the patient to know where they are and the future to be discussed with some confidence.

A much more complicated clinical situation may be mapped out in a similar way using a systems analysis flow chart. This may sound like an intimidating prospect but it need not be too complex, or incomprehensible, after a minimal amount of experience. A flow chart is a plan of the possible future eventualities and the treatment which each would require. Figure 1 illustrates such a chart; in this case the management in one clinic of a woman presenting with a lump in the breast (Jamieson and Dudley, 1973). These charts are composed after detailed analysis of the existing lines of management of a complex but recurring clinical problem and are then modified as necessary in use. The flow chart must fit all patients, not vice versa. Thus if a patient presents whose ideal management does not fit the chart the whole chart must be changed.

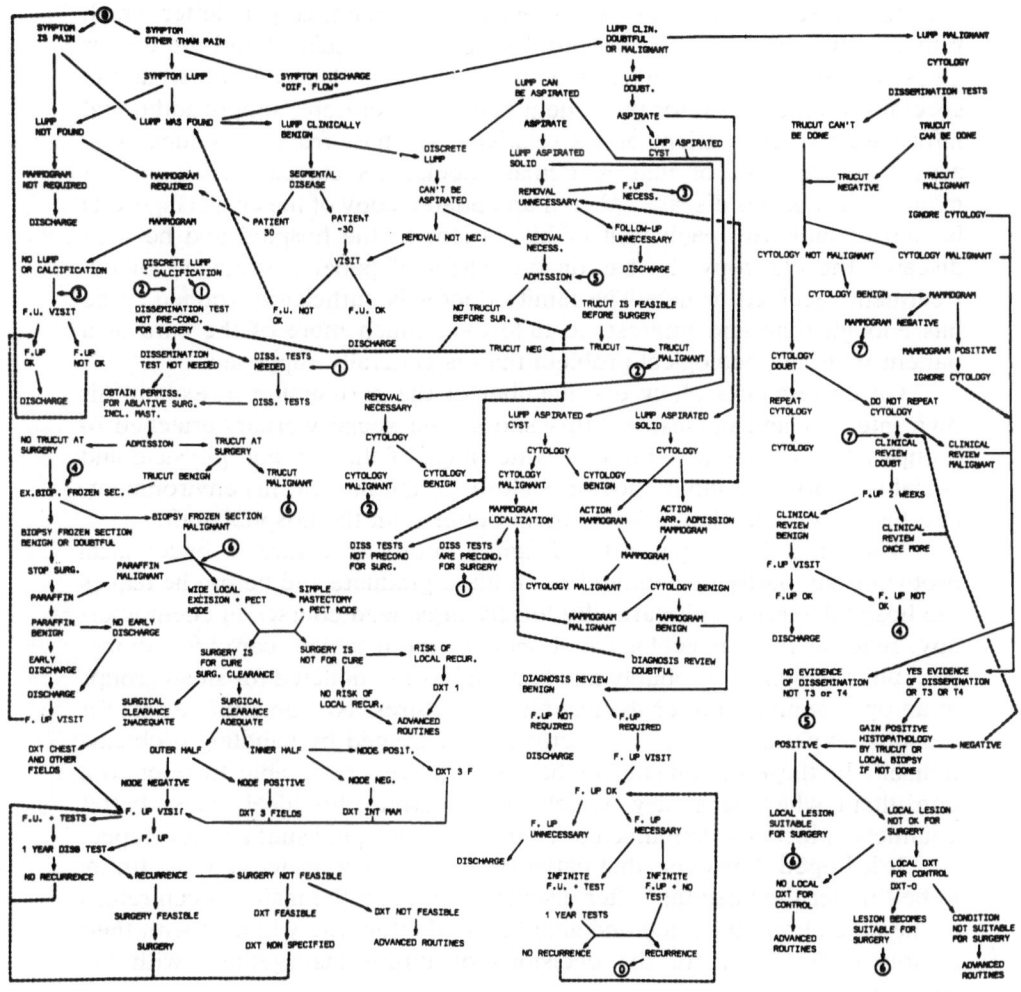

Figure 1. Systems analysis flow chart of treatment for a patient

Each chart is revised several times in the first few months of use, but alterations become progressively less necessary as defects are made apparent by varied clinical situations. The chart is also, of course, revised immediately if an advance in management is made. A major alteration of this nature brings with it a second chain of minor alterations so these flow charts are not static and rigid, but are fluid. It is quite simple to become educated in their use, and they have considerable value. Their use in an oncological unit is discussed later, but as far as the patient's family doctor is concerned, a copy of the appropriate chart which is sent to him marked with the present position of the patient and an accompanying letter which remains an important personal link between the specialist and the doctor gives him several advantages over a letter alone. He can see what the specialist intends to do for the patient and can, therefore, supply additional information to the patient or his relatives. He has, from the educational aspect, a summary of that particular specialist's current views on the management of this disease. Also, if an updated copy of the chart (Figure 1) is sent to him with each visit of his patient to the hospital and he then discards the old copy, he has on one sheet of paper a summary of the treatment received to date. The family doctor is sufficiently trained, if he has enough time and interest, to take over much more of the care of a patient with an oncological problem than is generally supposed.

Group practices allow one member of the partnership to expand his own interests and nurses, health visitors, and social workers attached to groups allow the supervision of a wide range of therapy and physical and social support. The family doctor is closer to the patient, his environment, and his family and should know them better than the hospital staff.

The education required for a family doctor in regard to oncological problems can partly be acquired as an undergraduate and before he leaves the hospital service and partly by locally organized courses in chemotherapy, relief of pain, psycological support of the disabled, care after dying, etc., all of which are probably most profitable if conducted for small groups in an open seminar rather than as formal lectures. No substitute exists for personal experience, and the doctor is best trained by handling problems himself. In these circumstances he must, however, be able to refer to a consultant when necessary, which may frustrate this ideal unless better channels of instant communication with senior hospital staff are developed.

It is hoped, however, that patients will not be considered in the future to be "under the hospital" after discharge, but that the majority can return to the care of an interested and able family doctor who will deal with their routine care and share the decisions of future management with the specialist.

The family doctor has a much wider role in oncology than this, for he is also in the front line of public education about many aspects of cancer. He can measure the value of some screening tests and persuade the public that many tumors can be cured if the patient presents soon after noticing symptoms or a lump. He is the first barrier to false hope raised by sensational but erroneous claims for advances and thus protects his patients. He must, therefore, be well informed.

The good family doctor has a difficult task to remain informed of advances in all the specialties which swamp his undergraduate and postgraduate training. This task must be made as simple as possible, but it is difficult to keep things simple without allowing them to become boring. It is clear, however, that it is the duty of the medical services of this country to supervise the interests of the family doctor and his patients. He must be given by courses, seminars, and personal contact with specialists, the information he requires to diagnose and manage oncological diseases and to advise his patients on the true nature of these diseases and the role which they, the public, should play in minimizing their ravages.

The General Specialist

This adjective and noun are basically contradictory; if you are a specialist you are not general. The radiotherapist is not a general specialist for his practice involves a great majority of patients whose diseases lie in oncology. The surgeon, physician, gynecologist, and pediatrician are necessarily, however, very general specialists. Widespread superspecialization is almost bound to be a total failure and it seems that there is sufficient agreement in the profession about this, so there is no need to list all the probable reasons. For geographical, economical, and social reasons hospitals in this country will continue to be staffed by more or less general specialists for the foreseeable future. All these doctors have to treat oncological diseases. There is no reason for attempting to condense *all* oncology into specialized hospitals because: (a) the weight of the clinical load is too great; (b) patients usually need more of the expertise of the specialist in the systems in which tumors originate than of the specialist of neoplasia as a whole; (c) patients who need considerable social support are better managed in a local environment; and (d) neither the general specialists, the family doctors, nor their patients would accept such a system of superspecialization.

We must, therefore, continue to train specialists to have a special interest in oncology in all these fields. Setting the standards for education at this level is the responsibility of the Royal Colleges of Physicians, Surgeons and Gynecologists who establish their curricula and examine for their diplomas; the actual training takes place at present in a wide variety of institutions. The postgraduate training of surgeons and physicians is at present under close review. The Royal Colleges of Surgeons has laid down desirable standards of postgraduate specialist training both before and after the examination for fellowship. There are increasing demands from developing specialties for space in these training programs and the balance of ideal training against superspecialization is most critical. What is a general surgeon? He is certainly no longer truly general. He has relinquished gynecology, orthopedics, thoracic surgery (with the possible exception of the intrathoracic esophagus), and most of urology. He never laid claim to neurosurgery, otorhinolaryngology, or ophthalmic surgery. An interested general surgeon may make occasional forays into all these fields and is expected to have a minimal standard of knowledge of their disciplines for his qualifications, but most general surgeons in this country now confine their practice to the alimentary tract and its associated viscera; the endocrine apparatus and some other soft tissue pathology which remains in common ground surrounded by the fenced off specialties. He undertakes pediatric surgery but major pediatric surgery is often referred to the few pediatric units or, more commonly, to the appropriate system specialist. Peripheral vascular surgery has not yet acquired the status of a separate speciality, but this may come in time.

Analyzed in this light, the practice of the general surgeon seems rather confined, but it does contain the bulk of the common oncological diseases, i.e., tumors of the gut and its exocrine glands, the breast, the endocrine glands, and the skin. Oncology comprises such a large part of the work of a general surgeon that it would not be feasible or popular for some surgeons to confine themselves to oncology, while the remainder relinquish their share.

Clearly all general and specialist surgeons must be trained in oncology. Are they sufficiently well trained at present? There would seem to be some deficits which need to be improved.

We still do not possess adequate records and data retrieval methods which would enable us to analyze the results of treatment easily and accurately. We are not trained to improve communications between hospitals, family doctors, and patients. A serious difficulty is that no real appraisal is made during the process of certification of postgraduate clinical diplomas of the candidate's ability to assess data. He is expected, when applying for a senior appointment, to possess the appropriate diploma and to have published articles, but neither of these qualifications gives any guarantee that he is capable of deciding for himself the true scientific value of a publication on the strength of which he may be persuaded to alter the management of his patients. We must ensure that we know the potential fallacies of mathematical analyses of case series and clinical trials, the limits beyond which the truth cannot be discerned, and whether differences between groups are important or "significant." The two words are by no means synonymous in clinical research. The doctor cannot acquire this mature and responsible attitude towards the publications which must dictate the course of future training unless he knows the elements of statistics and is taught which methods are appropriate and inappropriate to given situations. Without this he cannot assess the work of others or, indeed, his own. "Clinical impression" has little or no place in modern medicine.

This neglect of mathematical education must be one of the greatest deficits in present training and examination, but most curricula in basic sciences understress other basic subjects of considerable value to the clinician planning a career with interests in oncology. There is probably still too much emphasis on anatomy and esoteric physiology and too little cell biology, histopathology, and modern immunology in which the complement fixation test and bacterial antigens play only small parts.

Most specialists in training never leave the closed community of the hospital and are not, therefore, sufficiently conversant with the support facilities available for their patient when the patient is discharged. These facilities are, of course, local and personal and are undoubtedly the province of the family doctor. Thus there is all the more reason for him to retain control of the patient rather than the hospital, but knowledge of the possibilities and limitations of support on the part of the specialist go a long way to cementing relations with the family doctor and improving the overall efficiency of care.

Lastly, there is the continuous problem of remaining up-to-date for which there is no easy solution. It is important that the undergraduate customs of seminar and discussion continue during a career, for the habit is easier to retain than to regain. Thus it is essential that specialists in training are not allowed to become submerged completely in the clinical work of a busy appointment; postgraduate teaching and discussion must be continuous if the habit is not to be lost.

The Young Specialist Planning a Career in Oncology

Oncological physicians have now earned an accepted place in the hospital service and new chairs in the specialty are being established. These superspecialists have an important role to play in clinical practice, research, and education. Their clinical work leans toward the management of the diffuse oncological diseases such as leukemia and the reticuloses and is based mainly upon chemotherapy. Their expertise in the control of chemotherapeutic agents has also enabled them to contribute in a most valuable way to the management of some solid tumors, particularly those of children (Malpas *et al.*, 1976) and female choriocarcinoma (Goldstein, 1974). The dramatic improvement in the outlook of these tumors by combined chemotherapy and surgery represents one of the most encouraging aspects of modern therapy and a true advance. Medical oncologists have also instigated continually expanding programs of animal and clinical research into new treatments and, as a result of this research and their clinical practice, can make valuable contributions to teaching at all levels.

The surgical oncologist is less well established or defined. The primary management of solid tumors seems likely to remain surgical for the foreseeable future, but the role of the surgeon will not, it is hoped, end after the extirpation of a primary tumor. Most surgeons remain intimately involved in the care of their patients with advanced or recurrent diseases and, for the future, it seems to be increasingly likely that a combination of local treatment with systemic treatment of earlier lesions may improve results. The surgeon will have to be acquainted with the disciplines of the physician/oncologist to manage this therapy.

Thus the need clearly exists for surgeons who are prepared to specialize in oncology to the same extent as the medical oncologist if these advances are to continue. It is unnecessarily cumbersome and inefficient for combined therapy to be conducted by a committee, although intense collaboration between all specialties involved in clinical and experimental oncology is essential. Medical oncologists would not have evolved if physicians had remained content to ask their radiotherapeutic colleagues to manage chemotherapeutic regimens, and the wider disciplinary approach that this branching of the specialty brought with it probably has had tangible benefits. The surgical oncologist should add even more dimensions to the specialty. He should be able to advance the management of solid tumors, to improve clinical research into the results of surgical treatment of oncological diseases, and to help educate his junior surgical colleagues. He should also be in a position to act in an advisory capacity in cases of unusual complexity and to fulfil a valuable role in the management of rare tumors such as melanoma. He need not necessarily be trained as a general surgeon. The orthopedic surgeon, urologist, gynecologist, etc., with a special interest in oncology could make valuable contributions to his specialty. Each of these physicians must have been fully trained in his specialty in addition to his training in oncology, in the same way that a medical oncologist must first equip himself as a physician.

How can these superspecialists be trained? Appropriate programs are under construction. Basically, the establishment of a few specialist centers integrated with other disciplines of importance to oncology, in which the trainee surgical oncologist can work and study, is required. The field crosses the boundaries of surgical subspecialties, and there is no reason why a place in such a program should not be available to a member of one of the other specialties in surgery who desires to frame his main practice in the oncology of his chosen specialty.

These centers would also offer places to surgeons who do not wish to devote their careers solely to oncology, but who have a particular interest in the subject. Rotation for a shorter period of probably 1 year following completion of certification in his specialty would expose such a man to the whole work of the center and greatly aid his training. This latter group would naturally be a much larger one of superspecialists, as these are only needed in very small numbers.

The general remarks on the inadequacy of some aspects of our postgraduate education, particularly in data retrieval and in basic statistical methods, are even more important to the curriculum proposed for the surgical oncologist. Analysis of logical management by using flow charts and the efficiency of care in the form of audit are important to the full education of a specialist whose main duty will be to provide hard data on the benefits and disadvantages of new lines of therapy.

Lastly, consideration must be given, as far as the hospital service is concerned, to the education of other members of the service and particularly to surgeons and radiotherapists in understanding and accepting the role of the surgical oncologist. It is hoped that he will be accepted in this position as an advisor and tutor and not considered as a competitor for the routine cancer surgery. The expertise of the surgeon is more important than the esoteric knowledge of the oncologist in the management of most early solid tumors, and the advances that his specialty will inevitably bring to the management of late and recurrent disease will surely be welcomed.

Public Education

Cancer is rightly a dreaded disease. Atheroma is more lethal in our civilization but does not have the same sinister quality in the public image. It may be that the quicker death of a coronary thrombosis or a stroke is preferred to the possible lingering decline of some cancers.

The medical profession in this country, however, must take some blame for the terror that the word cancer breeds in patients. It is possible that we have tried too hard to shield individuals from the prognosis of their illness and the true nature of the disease from which they suffer. Patients cured by surgery may never know they had cancer and so do not spread the word that cure is possible. The difference in the general frankness and approach of the doctor to his patient in the United States and the United Kingdom have, until very recently, been most dramatic. It appears that the patient from a good center in the United States feels a bond of truth and shared adversity between himself and his clinician which is seldom found here. It can, of course, be overdone, but a tissue of half truth and evasion may be more damaging and throw an intolerable burden upon the relatives of the patient who must dissemble at a time of increasing stress when truth and a shared view of the future, even though it be bleak, can be a great support.

The increased awareness of the American citizen of the true nature of cancer makes him more ready to seek advice early, to participate in screening programs, and to act as his own early warning system in being alert for symptoms and signs of an oncological disease. We cannot change the feelings of our patients in a single stroke, but we can analyze the information we give them and strive to make it as factual as possible, within the confines of palatability. We must also continually consider the burden which any distortion of the truth places upon relatives.

The potential value of public education in reducing deaths from cancer remains to be evaluated. Logically, it would be expected that increased awareness of the danger would encourage a patient to present earlier for treatment and therefore improve the chances of cure. Knowledge of this kind is only of value, however, if it is supported by a hope of cure and not outweighted by fear of a mutilating operation. A 20-year-old study suggested that women who knew that a breast lump might be malignant procrastinated longer before seeking medical advice than women who did not know (Paterson and Aitken-Swan, 1954). A little knowledge may be dangerous, but full awareness of the facts must surely be beneficial. More must be done by all members of the medical profession and government to educate the media and the public about the true nature of cancer. The truth can only be less terrifying than its specter.

There is evidence that even when the outlook is bleak patients would prefer a frank discussion of their problems. In a recently published survey of dying patients, the majority felt that there had been too little frank discussion by their doctors and not one resented being told unpalatable facts.

References

Goldstein, D. P. (1974). Prevention of gestational trophoblastic disease by use of actinomycin D in molar pregnancies. *Obstet. Gynaecol.* **49**:475.

Jamieson, C. W., and Dudley, H. A. F. (1973). Another hospital discharge system. *Lancet* **2**:314.

Malpas, J. S., Freeman, J. E., Paxton, A., Walker Smith, J. Stansfield, A. G., and Wood, C. B. S. (1976). Radiotherapy and adjuvant chemotherapy for childhood rhabdomyosarcoma. *Brit. Med. J.* **1**:247.

Paterson, R., and Aitken-Swan, J. (1954). Public opinion on cancer. A survey among women in the Manchester area. *Lancet* **2**:857.

(1975) Registrar General's statistical review of England and Wales for the three years 1968–1970: *Suppl. Cancer.* H.M.S.O.

INDEX